Pain Management: Integrated Research

Pain Management: Integrated Research

Edited by Emerson Haynes

hayle medical

New York

Hayle Medical,
750 Third Avenue, 9th Floor,
New York, NY 10017, USA

Visit us on the World Wide Web at:
www.haylemedical.com

ISBN: 978-1-63241-788-6

The publisher's policy is to use permanent paper from mills that operate a sustainable forestry policy. Furthermore, the publisher ensures that the text paper and cover boards used have met acceptable environmental accreditation standards.

Printed in China.

Cataloging-in-Publication Data

Pain management : integrated research / edited by Emerson Haynes.
p. cm.
Includes bibliographical references and index.
ISBN 978-1-63241-788-6
1. Pain--Treatment. 2. Pain medicine. 3. Medicine--Research. I. Haynes, Emerson.
RB127 .P35 2019
617.9--dc23

Table of Contents

Preface

The main aim of this book is to educate learners and enhance their research focus by presenting diverse topics covering this vast field. This is an advanced book which compiles significant studies by distinguished experts in the area of analysis. This book addresses successive solutions to the challenges arising in the area of application, along with it; the book provides scope for future developments.

The field of medicine concerned with the approaches to ease the suffering and to improve the quality of life of those struggling with chronic pain is known as pain management or algiatry. Medical practitioners, physiotherapists, clinical psychologists, pharmacists, nurses, occupational therapists, massage therapists and mental health specialists are some of the members of a pain management team. Medications, including analgesics and anxiolytics are often used to relieve pain. Certain interventional procedures, such as epidural steroid injections, neurolytic blocks, facet joint infections, spinal cord stimulators and intrathecal drug delivery system implants can prove to be effective in pain management. This book unfolds the innovative aspects of pain management which will be crucial for the progress of this field in the future. It is a compilation of chapters that discuss the most vital concepts and emerging trends in the field of pain management. This book is a complete source of knowledge in the present status of this important field.

It was a great honour to edit this book, though there were challenges, as it involved a lot of communication and networking between me and the editorial team. However, the end result was this all-inclusive book covering diverse themes in the field.

Finally, it is important to acknowledge the efforts of the contributors for their excellent chapters, through which a wide variety of issues have been addressed. I would also like to thank my colleagues for their valuable feedback during the making of this book.

Editor

1

Effect of Pregabalin on Cardiovascular Responses to Exercise and Postexercise Pain and Fatigue in Fibromyalgia

Andrea T. White,[1,2] Kathleen C. Light,[1] Lucinda Bateman,[1,3] Ronald W. Hughen,[1] Timothy A. Vanhaitsma,[2,4] and Alan R. Light[1]

[1] *Department of Anesthesiology, University of Utah, Salt Lake City, UT 84112, USA*
[2] *Department of Exercise and Sport Science, University of Utah, Salt Lake City, UT 84112, USA*
[3] *Bateman Horne Center of Excellence, Salt Lake City, UT 84102, USA*
[4] *Department of Kinesiology, Westmont College, Santa Barbara, CA 93108, USA*

Correspondence should be addressed to Andrea T. White; andrea.white@hsc.utah.edu

Academic Editor: Marina De Tommaso

Pregabalin, an approved treatment for fibromyalgia (FM), has been shown to decrease sympathetic nervous system (SNS) activity and inhibit sympathetically maintained pain, but its effects on exercise responses have not been reported. *Methods*. Using a randomized double-blind crossover design, we assessed the effect of 5 weeks of pregabalin (versus placebo) on acute cardiovascular and subjective responses to moderate exercise in 19 FM patients. Blood pressure (BP), heart rate (HR), and ratings of perceived exertion (RPE) during exercise and ratings of pain, physical fatigue, and mental fatigue before, during, and for 48 hours after exercise were compared in patients on pregabalin versus placebo and also versus 18 healthy controls. *Results*. On placebo, exercise RPE and BP were significantly higher in FM patients than controls ($p < 0.04$). Pregabalin responders ($n = 12$, defined by patient satisfaction and symptom changes) had significantly lower exercise BP, HR, and RPE on pregabalin versus placebo ($p < 0.03$) and no longer differed from controls ($p > 0.26$). Cardiovascular responses of nonresponders ($n = 7$) were not altered by pregabalin. In responders, pregabalin improved ratings of fatigue and pain ($p < 0.04$), but negative effects on pain and fatigue were seen in nonresponders. *Conclusions*. These preliminary findings suggest that pregabalin may normalize cardiovascular and subjective responses to exercise in many FM patients.

1. Introduction

Fibromyalgia syndrome (FM) is characterized by widespread pain in muscles, joints, and deep connective tissues for at least three months. Additionally, using the American College of Rheumatology (ACR) classification criteria, FM patients report painful hypersensitivity to pressure in at least 11 of 18 tender points during clinical examination [1]. FM patients represent a heterogeneous population of chronic pain patients, making them challenging to diagnose and to treat successfully [2]. One example of this heterogeneity is that many FM patients have comorbid pain and fatigue disorders, such as myalgic encephalomyelitis/chronic fatigue syndrome (ME/CFS, hereafter referred to as CFS), migraine headaches, irritable bowel syndrome, and temporomandibular disorder, while other FM patients do not [3–5].

Heterogeneity among FM patients is also reflected in their differing response to medications, including pregabalin, the first drug licensed by the U.S. Food and Drug Administration (FDA) specifically for treatment of FM [6]. Pregabalin is a potent inhibitory ligand for $\alpha 2$-delta subunit of calcium channels in the central nervous system (CNS) that has analgesic and anxiolytic as well as anticonvulsant activity. Clinical trials of pregabalin have shown significant reduction of pain, improved sleep quality, and improved health-related quality of life in the majority of FM patients studied [6–8].

However, a common side effect of pregabalin is an increase in lethargy and sedation, which is especially problematic for FM patients with comorbid CFS who already have profound physical and mental fatigue (mental fog). Other common side effects that deter patients from continuing pregabalin use include weight gain, swelling and tingling in extremities, and dizziness. Thus, Smith and Moore [9] conclude that pregabalin has a therapeutic benefit above placebo with tolerable side effects in only approximately 50% of FM patients (pregabalin responders) while the other 50% of FM patients are nonresponders to this treatment.

It is also notable that exercise therapy (both aerobic and strength training) has been shown to reduce pain ratings and increase function in FM patients [10–12]. However, because many FM patients (especially those with comorbid CFS) experience postexertional worsening of pain, physical fatigue, and mental fog, the dropout rate of FM patients from exercise programs is high [13, 14]. This postexertional symptom worsening is thus important not just because of its impact on the person's symptoms during the next several days following each bout of exercise but also because it serves as a strong and immediate disincentive to exercise [15] and contributes to long term physical deconditioning [14]. Thus, it is clinically important to determine whether medications for FM such as pregabalin may moderate these postexercise symptoms.

To our knowledge, no previous studies have used standardized exercise tasks with extended postexercise symptom monitoring to assess effects of pregabalin versus placebo on cardiovascular responses or symptom severity in patients with FM. The most similar investigation that we could find was a study of postexercise changes in pain ratings in CFS + FM patients, rheumatoid arthritis patients, and healthy controls on placebo versus paracetamol. That study found mixed responses in CFS + FM patients, with paracetamol associated with decreased pain immediately after exercise in some but not all of these patients [16]. In our previous studies on patients with comorbid CFS + FM [17, 18], we had determined *post hoc* that patients tested while on their normal medications that included pregabalin had lower pain and mental fatigue scores both at preexercise baseline and for at least 48 hours after acute exercise than patients on other treatments (unpublished data). In these studies, the acute exercise task consisted of 25 minutes of combined arm and leg cycling at 70% of age-predicted maximal heart rate. Using this information, we hypothesized that pregabalin treatment would decrease pain and fatigue symptoms in at least some patients both at preexercise baseline and following an acute exercise challenge. We further hypothesized that pregabalin treatment would partially normalize cardiovascular differences in response to exercise seen between FM patients and healthy controls, with the caveat that this beneficial effect might be seen only in those patients who are treatment responders and/or those patients without comorbid CFS.

2. Methods

2.1. Participants. Written informed consent approved by the University of Utah Institutional Review Board was obtained from all study volunteers before participation. Our objective was to recruit 20 patients aged 18–65 from a private fatigue clinic who met the 1990 ACR criteria for FM [1] and who were not currently using pregabalin or a related anticonvulsant drug, gabapentin, or opioids to treat their pain. Current use of serotonin- and norepinephrine-reuptake inhibitors was not exclusionary [1]. Of these 20 FM patients, we intended to recruit 10 who also met both Fukuda et al.'s 1994 case definition [19] and the Canadian criteria for myalgic encephalomyelitis/chronic fatigue syndrome (CFS + FM). Sample size was estimated based on prior data showing gene expression differences between CFS/FM patients while taking pregabalin or gabapentin versus patients on neither drug [17]. Healthy age- and gender-matched controls ($n = 18$) were also recruited for participation in the exercise protocol as a comparison group. Data were collected between June 2011 and June 2013.

2.2. Study Protocol. This pilot study utilized a double-blind, placebo-controlled crossover design to examine pre- and postexercise leukocyte gene expression changes induced by pregabalin (Lyrica) in patients with FM, patients with both CFS + FM, and healthy controls. Evaluation of symptom changes, subjective ratings of pain and fatigue, and responses to an acute exercise challenge were obtained in conjunction with treatment and placebo conditions. Here, we report on cardiovascular and self-reported symptom responses to exercise with respect to treatment effects, while the gene expression results will be reported in a separate paper (Light et al., in preparation). Pregabalin and identical appearing placebo were provided by Pfizer.

2.3. Drug Treatment and Effects. Upon study entry, patients were examined (by Lucinda Bateman) at the Fatigue Consultation Clinic (FCC), where the diagnosis of CFS + FM or FM was confirmed. Patients were randomized to receive either pregabalin or placebo for 5 weeks, including a 2-week upward titration phase up to 450 mg/day. FM and CFS + FM groups were randomized in blocks in order to achieve similar numbers in each group who received pregabalin or placebo treatment first. FCC staff were not blinded to the treatment the patients received for safety reasons. At the end of 5 weeks, patients reported for exercise testing in the Department of Anesthesia at the University of Utah, as described below. All University of Utah research staff, including the PI, were blind to the diagnosis and treatment of the patients. Following a 2-week washout period supervised by FCC staff, patients then received the opposite treatment for another 5 weeks. At this time, patients again reported to the blinded staff at University of Utah and repeated the exercise task.

2.4. Exercise Task. The acute exercise challenges were conducted during the fifth week of both treatment and placebo phases. The exercise task consisted of sustained (25 min) submaximal exercise using the Schwinn Air-Dyne bicycle ergometer. For the first exercise task in week 5, work-rate was gradually increased during the first 5 minutes until each subject attained a heart rate corresponding to 65–75% of age-predicted maximum heart rate. Thereafter, work-rate was adjusted as necessary to maintain the target heart rate. For the second exercise task (after 5 weeks on the second treatment, in week 12), we replicated the first exercise session so that work-rate was equivalent for both placebo and pregabalin conditions. Healthy controls completed one exercise session using the same protocol used for patients. During each exercise task, heart rate (HR) was recorded each minute, systolic blood pressure (SBP) and diastolic blood pressure (DBP) were recorded at minutes 10 and 20, and rating of perceived exertion (RPE) was recorded every 5 minutes using a modified Borg Scale [20]. Ratings of mental fatigue, physical fatigue, and pain using a 0–100 scale were provided by the patients and controls at baseline, in the middle of the exercise, after exercise, and at 0.5, 8, 24, and 48 hours after exercise.

2.5. Classification of Patients as Responders versus Nonresponders. Patients were classified as pregabalin responders or nonresponders prior to data analysis. Classification used the "Effects of Study Medication" questionnaire that patients completed after each treatment. The first question, "How satisfied are you with the study medication you have used most recently?," was scored as 0 (not at all), 1 (somewhat), 2 (moderately), 3 (quite a bit), or 4 (very much). Then, patients circled symptoms that "got better" and symptoms that "got worse" from a list of 16 symptoms. We also recorded and tallied symptoms that were reported but not on the list.

2.6. Analysis. Initially, unpaired t-tests were utilized to determine whether FM and CFM + FM patients differed significantly for any exercise variable. Analyses of variance (ANOVAs) were used to compare controls to all patients while taking pregabalin and placebo. Repeated measures analyses with planned contrasts were used to examine treatment differences in exercise variables and subjective ratings of pain, fatigue, and exertion. Follow-up analyses examining responses in pregabalin responders and nonresponders were also performed. To ensure that differences in cardiovascular responses were not influenced by differences in physical work, these measures were adjusted for individual differences in work-rates. Significance was set at alpha <0.05.

3. Results

3.1. FM Compared to CFS + FM. The only variable that was significantly different between FM patients and CFS + FM patients was exercise work-rate ($p = 0.03$). FM patients achieved higher work-rates than CFS + FM patients on both placebo and pregabalin. On placebo, average work-rate for FM-only patients was 332 ± 58.7 kcal/hr while average work-rate was 252 ± 52.7 in CFS + FM patients. After pregabalin treatment, average work-rate was 328 ± 69.4 and 282 ± 56.6 kcal/hr for FM-only and CFS + FM patients, respectively. Data from these two groups were combined for subsequent analyses.

3.2. Descriptive Characteristics. A total of 20 patients (9 FM and 11 CFS + FM) volunteered to participate in the study. One FM patient refused to discontinue the original treatment and thus did not complete the second arm (placebo phase) of the protocol; this subject was excluded from analysis. Eighteen healthy controls served as a comparison group for the exercise task. As shown in Table 1, there were no significant differences for age or body mass index (BMI), between controls and all patients, or between pregabalin responders and nonresponders ($p > 0.27$). All groups were composed mostly of females.

Of the 19 patients completing both treatments, 6 scored 0 (not at all satisfied) on the first item of the "Effects of Study Medication" questionnaire and were classified as nonresponders. One patient who scored this item as 1 (somewhat satisfied) was also classified as a nonresponder based on the number of symptoms that got worse versus better on pregabalin (6 versus 3) while reporting 0 symptoms getting worse or better on placebo. Therefore, 12 were classified as pregabalin responders and 7 as nonresponders (see Table 2). Importantly, 6 of the FM patients and 6 of the CFS + FM patients were classified as pregabalin responders, while 2 FM and 5 CFS + FM patients were nonresponders. Thus, the FM and the CFS + FM patient groups had similar percentages of pregabalin responders (Fisher's Exact Test $p = 0.633$). Patients with orthostatic intolerance were also present in both responder and nonresponder groups (Table 1).

3.3. Effects of Pregabalin versus Placebo in Responders versus Nonresponders. Responders reported significantly higher treatment satisfaction and significantly more symptoms that improved during the pregabalin condition compared to placebo ($p < 0.01$, Table 2). All responders reported decreased pain, including muscle and joint pain, back pain, and headaches, and the majority also noted improved ability to do chores, total energy, and sleep, as well as decreased postexertional malaise. Additionally, responders reported significantly more symptoms that worsened while on placebo.

Nonresponders reported significantly lower treatment satisfaction during the pregabalin condition ($p < 0.05$) and mixed symptom responses during both conditions. Importantly, nonresponders reported more negative symptom responses while taking pregabalin compared to placebo, although this difference was only borderline significant ($p = 0.06$). Also, two nonresponders reported decreased muscle and joint pain while taking pregabalin, but their many negative symptoms outweighed the beneficial effects. The most common symptoms that became worse during pregabalin treatment were light-headedness (3 responders and 3 nonresponders) and mental fog (0 responders and 5 nonresponders).

3.4. Subjective Responses during and after Exercise. Average exercise work-rate did not differ between healthy controls and patients on either treatment ($p > 0.11$) (Table 3), indicating that the absolute intensity of the exercise task was equivalent among groups. This also suggests that underlying fitness levels were similar for patients and controls.

TABLE 1: Participant descriptive characteristics.

	Controls (n = 18)	All patients (n = 19)	Responders (n = 12)	Nonresponders (n = 7)
Age (yrs)	40.8 ± 2.8	43.4 ± 2.9	41.7 ± 3.2	46.3 ± 5.6
BMI (kg/m^2)	27.7 ± 1.7	27.6 ± 1.4	28.9 ± 1.7	25.4 ± 2.4
Sex (M/F)	1/17	1/18	0/12	1/6
Dx (CFS + FM/FM)	na	11/8	6/6	5/2
Orthostasis	na	9	5	4

BMI: body mass index; Dx (CFS + FM/FM): proportion of patients with CFS + FM relative to FM only; Orthostasis: number of patients with orthostatic intolerance as determined by a score of 5 or greater on the Mayo Clinic Self-Report Orthostatic Grading Scale. Values are mean ± SE.

TABLE 2: Perception of treatment satisfaction and most commonly reported symptom (Sx) changes in responders and nonresponders during placebo and pregabalin conditions.

(a)

	Responders (n = 12)			Nonresponders (n = 7)		
	Pregabalin	Placebo	Preg versus Plac	Pregabalin	Placebo	Preg versus Plac
Satisfaction	2.5 ± 0.37	0.3 ± 0.25	**<0.001**	0.1 ± 0.14	1.6 ± 0.57	**0.039**
# Sx improved	7.2 ± 1.35	1.3 ± 0.91	**<0.001**	1.0 ± 0.53	4.3 ± 2.11	0.106
# Sx worse	1.8 ± 0.52	6.4 ± 1.38	**0.002**	3.7 ± 0.99	1.9 ± 0.63	0.064

(b)

	Responders (n = 12)		Nonresponders (n = 7)	
	Improved	Worse	Improved	Worse
		Placebo condition		
≥50%	0	Sleep (7) Physical fatigue (7) Ability to do chores (7) Total energy (6) Muscle pain (6) Mental fog (6)	0	0
25–49%	0	Need for bed rest (5) Headaches (4) PEM (3) Sensitivity to noise (3) Ability to relax (3)	Mental fog (3) Pain (3) Ability to do chores (2) Sleep (2) Need for bed rest (2) Anxiety (2) Depression (2) Back pain (2) Ability to relax (2) Sensitivity to noise (2)	Sleep (2) Physical fatigue (2) Light-headedness (2)
		Pregabalin condition		
≥50%	Muscle pain (10) PEM (8) Ability to do chores (8) Total energy (7) Sleep (7)	0	0	Mental Fog (5)
25–49%	Physical fatigue (5) Mental fog (4) Back pain (4) Headaches (4) Depression (4) Ability to relax (4) Need for bed rest (4)	Weight gain (3) Light-headedness (3)	Pain (2) Sleep (2) Total energy (2)	Light-headedness (3) Anxiety (2) Depression (2) Headaches (2) Blurred vision (2)

Satisfaction was rated on a 0-to-4 scale, where 0 means "not at all" and 4 means "very much."
Sx: number of symptoms reported by participants; values are mean ± SE.
≥50% refers to symptoms that were reported in at least 50% of the group.
25–49% refers to symptoms that were reported in 25–49% of the group.
PEM: postexertional malaise.

TABLE 3: Exercise task variables (mean ± SE) during pregabalin and placebo conditions in patients and healthy controls.

	Controls (n = 18)	All patients (n = 19) Pregabalin	Placebo	All patients, p value Preg versus Con	Plac versus Con	Preg versus Plac
WR (kcal/hr)	318 ± 11.6	301 ± 14.9	286 ± 15.4	0.387	0.109	0.114
RPE	3.4 ± 0.3	4.1 ± 0.4	4.9 ± 0.4	0.172	**0.011**	**0.049**
HR (bpm)	127 ± 2.1	115 ± 2.5	122 ± 3.6	**0.001**	0.276	**0.024**
HR (% PMHR)	71 ± 0.7	65 ± 1.2	69 ± 1.8	**<0.001**	0.404	**0.029**
SBP (mm Hg)	142 ± 3.7	142 ± 3.8	153 ± 3.7	0.926	**0.031**	**0.017**
DBP (mm Hg)	86 ± 2.3	88 ± 2.6	91 ± 2.2	0.676	0.086	0.136
HR/WR	41 ± 1.5	40 ± 1.8	45 ± 3.2	0.606	0.219	**0.034**
SBP/WR	46 ± 2.3	49 ± 2.6	57 ± 3.4	0.345	**0.013**	**0.002**
DBP/WR	28 ± 1.2	30 ± 1.8	34 ± 2.3	0.229	**0.020**	**0.037**

WR: work-rate; RPE: rating of perceived exertion; HR: heart rate; PMHR: age-predicted maximal heart rate; SBP: systolic blood pressure; DBP: diastolic blood pressure; HR/WR, SBP/WR, and DBP/WR: values expressed relative to exercise work-rate (kcal/hr) multiplied by 100; Preg: pregabalin; Plac: placebo.

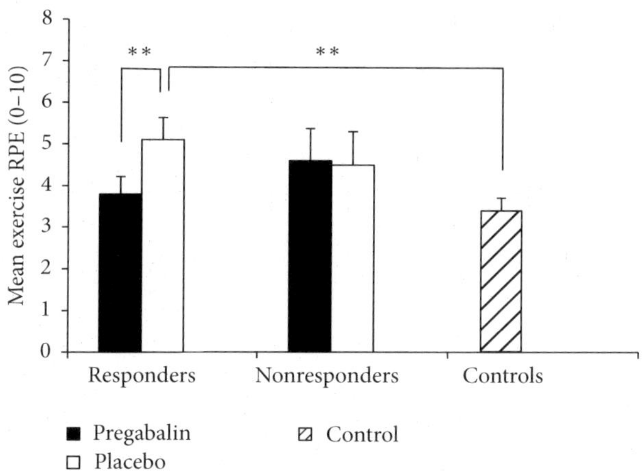

FIGURE 1: Rating of perceived exertion (RPE) in pregabalin responders, nonresponders, and controls. ** indicates significant difference, $p < 0.01$.

3.4.1. Rating of Perceived Exertion (RPE). When comparing all patients to controls, we observed that patients on placebo reported significantly higher average RPE during exercise compared to healthy controls ($p = 0.011$). In patients, average exercise RPE was significantly lower during the pregabalin condition compared to the placebo condition ($p < 0.049$, Table 3). Analysis of responders versus nonresponders showed that only responders had lower RPE during pregabalin treatment compared to placebo ($p = 0.003$). These ratings in responders on pregabalin were also similar to the RPE ratings of controls ($p = 0.459$, Figure 1). Conversely, for responders during placebo treatment, RPE was significantly higher than controls ($p = 0.006$). The nonresponders exhibited no treatment difference for RPE (pregabalin versus placebo, $p = 0.842$, Figure 1). All but one of the responders showed decreases in RPE during pregabalin treatment (Figure 2(a)), while only two of the seven nonresponders reported lower RPE while on pregabalin (Figure 2(b)).

3.4.2. Ratings of Fatigue and Pain. The patient group as a whole exhibited no treatment differences (pregabalin versus placebo) for physical fatigue, mental fatigue, or pain. When considered separately, responders had lower scores when on pregabalin versus placebo for mental fatigue ($p = 0.030$), physical fatigue ($p = 0.009$), and pain ($p = 0.001$, Figure 3). In nonresponders, mental fatigue was significantly higher during the pregabalin condition versus placebo ($p = 0.030$). Physical fatigue and pain in nonresponders also trended toward worsening with pregabalin versus placebo ($p = 0.098$ and 0.175, resp., Figure 3).

3.5. Cardiovascular Responses during Exercise. During pregabalin treatment, patients as a whole had significantly lower absolute HR and relative HR (% age-predicted maximal HR) during exercise compared to placebo ($p = 0.024$ and 0.029, resp.), despite the fact that exercise work-rate was slightly higher during the pregabalin condition (Table 3). Patients on pregabalin also had significantly lower absolute and relative exercise HR compared to controls ($p < 0.002$).

When exercise HR was expressed relative to work-rate (HR/WR), HR/WR was significantly lower during pregabalin treatment compared to placebo in the whole patient group ($p = 0.034$). There were no differences in HR/WR between controls and patients on either treatment ($p > 0.219$, Table 3). In pregabalin responders, exercise HR/WR was significantly lower during pregabalin versus placebo treatment ($p = 0.033$, Figure 4). There was no significant treatment effect for HR/WR in nonresponders ($p = 0.356$).

Analysis of all patients revealed that unadjusted SBP was significantly lower during pregabalin treatment compared to placebo ($p = 0.017$, Table 3). In addition, SBP was significantly higher in all FM patients during the placebo condition compared to controls ($p = 0.031$). Although for unadjusted DBP there were no significant treatment effects or differences between patients and controls, DBP expressed relative to exercise work-rate (DBP/WR) was significantly lower during pregabalin treatment ($p = 0.037$), as was SBP/WR ($p = 0.002$). For the whole FM patient group, both SBP/WR and DBP/WR during the placebo condition were significantly higher than controls ($p = 0.013$ and 0.020, resp., Table 3).

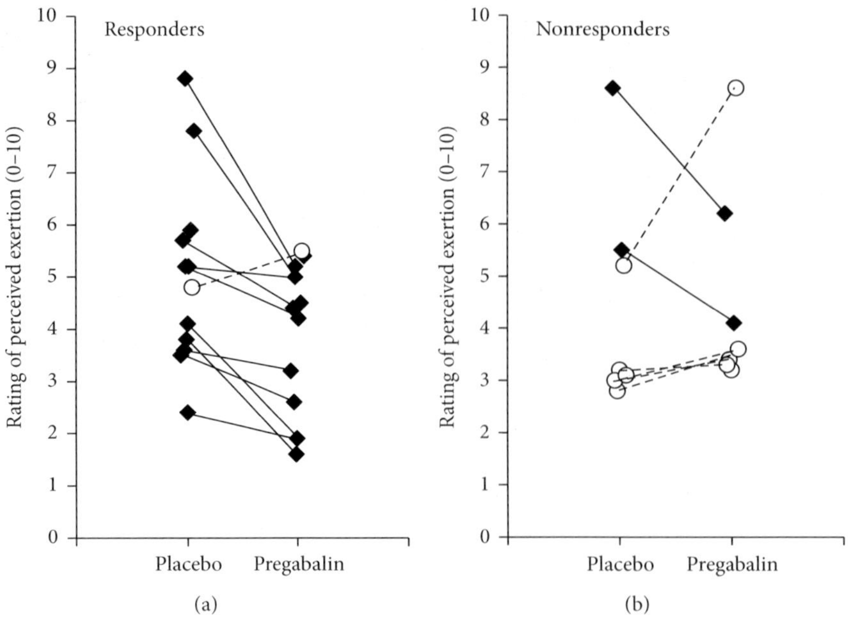

FIGURE 2: Individual ratings of perceived exertion (RPE) in pregabalin responders and nonresponders during pregabalin and placebo conditions.

Analyses of responders and nonresponders revealed that during the placebo condition SBP/WR and DBP/WR were higher than controls only in responders ($p < 0.01$, Figure 4). Pregabalin treatment significantly decreased SBP/WR and DBP/WR in responders ($p = 0.002$ and 0.027, resp., Figure 4) to levels that were similar to controls ($p > 0.261$). In nonresponders, there were no treatment effects (pregabalin versus placebo) for either SBP/WR or DBP/WR.

4. Discussion

To our knowledge, this is the first study demonstrating that pregabalin treatment (versus placebo) normalizes BP and HR responses to sustained moderate exercise in the subgroup of FM patients with a positive response to treatment. Also, pregabalin reduced these patients' exercise RPE and symptoms of pain and fatigue before and during exercise, as well as blunting their postexertional malaise for 48 hours after the task. In nonresponders, BP response was not affected, perceived exertion during exercise was not improved, and pre- and postexercise symptoms of pain and fatigue tended to worsen rather than improve with pregabalin. Strengths of this study include the randomized, double-blinded placebo-controlled crossover design and the statistical control for slight differences in exercise work-rate.

Classification of pregabalin responders was based on subjective rating of overall satisfaction and whether symptom improvements outweighed negative symptom responses. Consistent with prior research on pregabalin treatment in FM [21–24], decreased pain, including muscle and joint pain, back pain, and headaches, was the most commonly reported symptom improvement (reported by all 12 responders), with the second most common benefit being improved sleep (reported by 75% of the responders). In addition to these beneficial effects, pregabalin improved other symptoms that have not been previously studied. Specifically, several fatigue-related symptoms improved, with over 50% of responders reporting less postexertional malaise, more energy, and greater ability to do chores or have fun. Additionally, 25–49% of responders reported less physical fatigue and need for bed rest. Importantly, the presence of comorbid CFS in these FM patients was not associated with being a pregabalin nonresponder or with worsened side effects. It is possible that, in some FM patients, pregabalin has an independent beneficial effect on sensory pathways involved in fatigue pathways as well as pain.

The causes of chronic pain and fatigue in FM and CFS + FM are not well understood, but there may be common mechanisms underlying both symptoms, including increased signaling of pain and fatigue and sympathetic nervous system (SNS) dysregulation which may be a cause or effect of the increased signaling. FM has been described as a disorder characterized by enhanced SNS activity [2, 25, 26], but studies have reported both increased and blunted cardiovascular and catecholamine responses to exercise and other stressors [27, 28]. Our prior investigation noted that FM patients had lower baseline norepinephrine levels but greater blood pressure (BP) increases to postural and speech stressors than controls [29]. Blinded treatment with propranolol versus placebo normalized these SNS-related alterations and also significantly reduced pain ratings, supporting the interpretation that FM involves heightened SNS drive. Pregabalin decreases the release of several neurotransmitters including norepinephrine [30] and has been specifically linked to decreases in SNS activity and the inhibition of sympathetically maintained pain [31, 32]. This decrease in SNS activity may be an important factor in its clinical benefit for FM patients who are responders to pregabalin treatment. Our

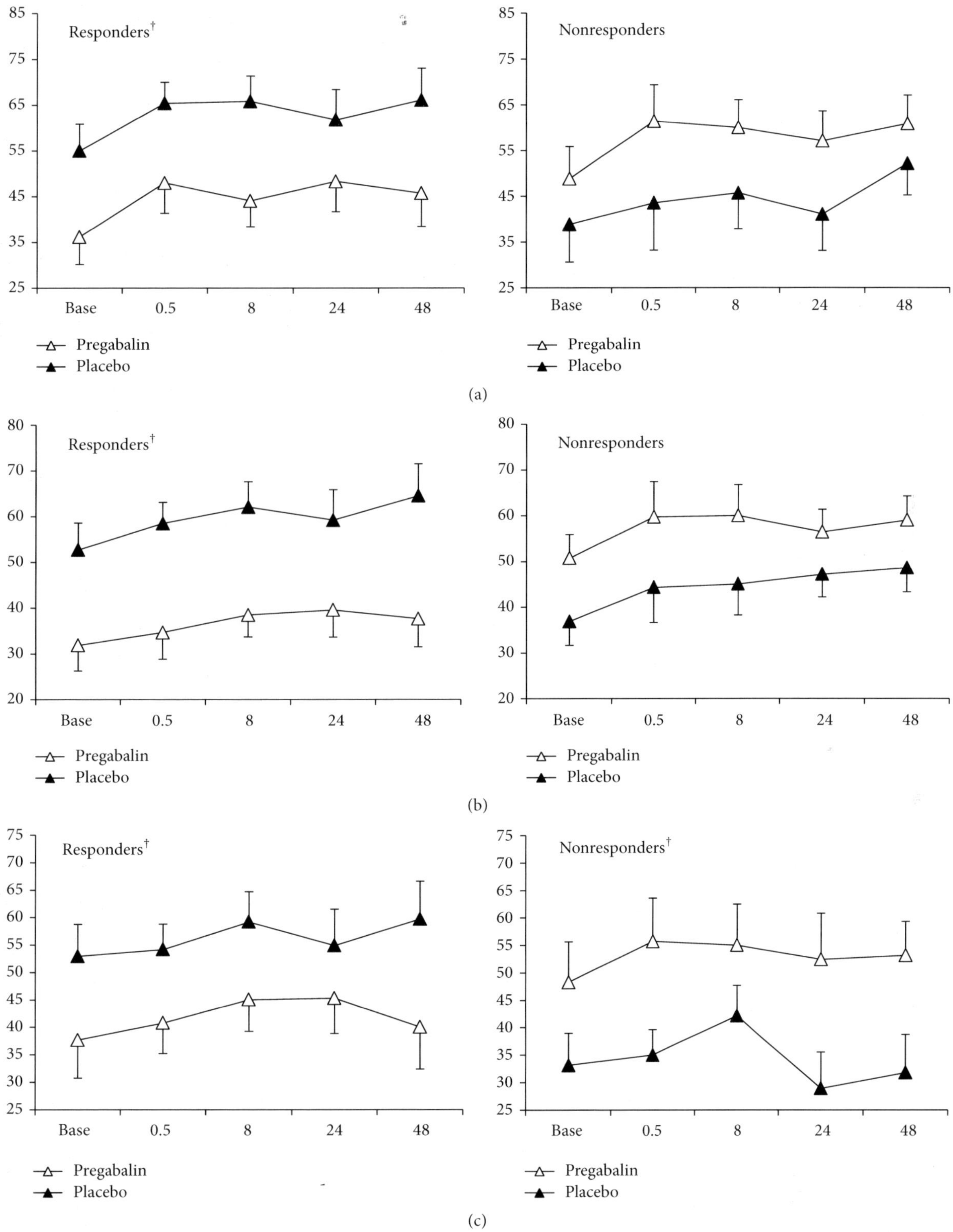

Figure 3: Subjective ratings of physical fatigue (a), pain (b), and mental fatigue (c) in responders and nonresponders during pregabalin and placebo treatments. Values are mean ± SE at baseline (preexercise) and at 0.5, 8, 24, and 48 hours after exercise. † indicates significant treatment effect across all time points, $p < 0.05$.

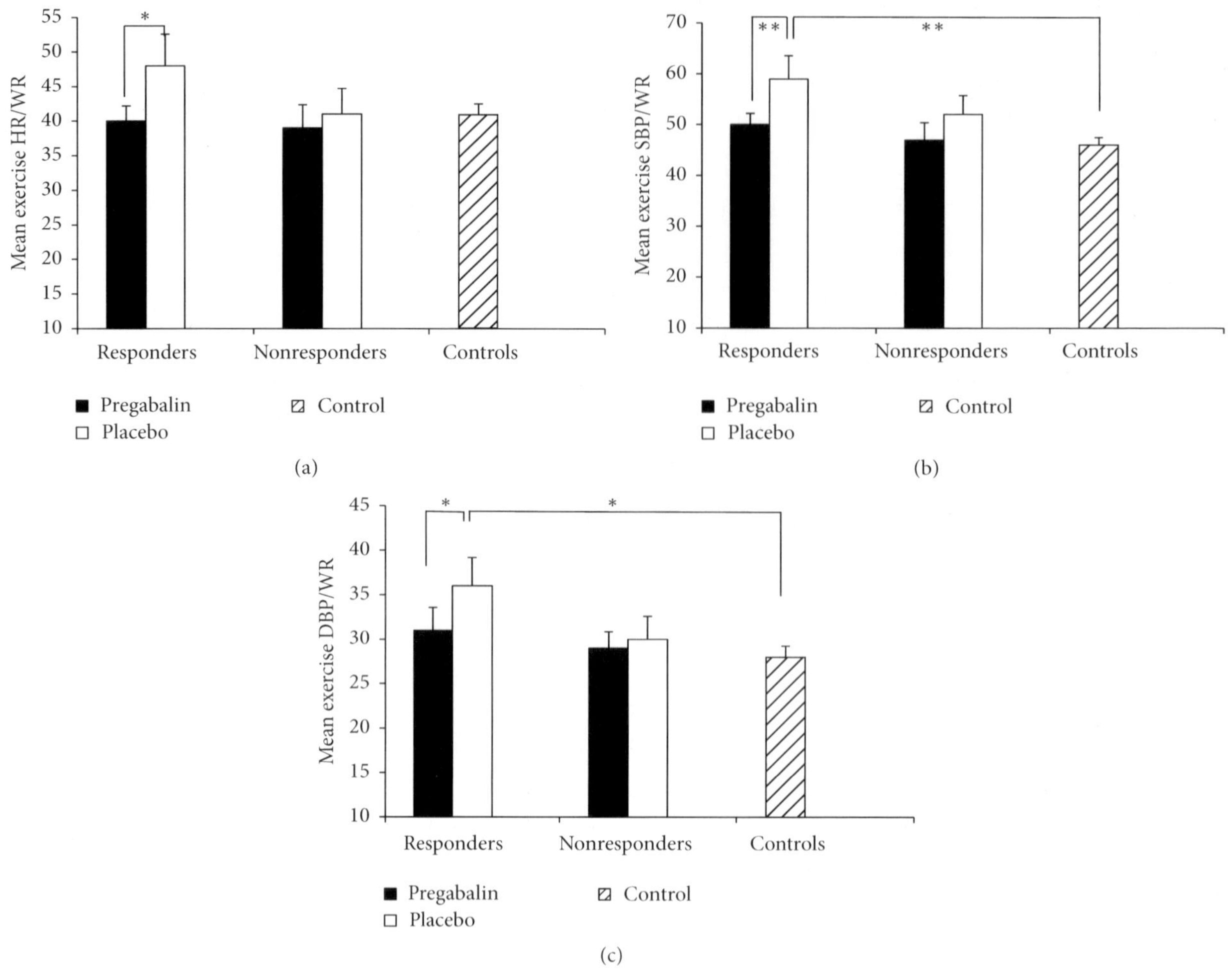

FIGURE 4: Exercise cardiovascular responses; heart rate (a), systolic blood pressure (b), and diastolic blood pressure (c) expressed relative to exercise work-rate in pregabalin responders, nonresponders, and controls. $*$ indicates significant difference, $p < 0.05$. $**$ indicates significant difference, $p < 0.01$.

research group has also identified some of the molecular receptors responsible for neuronal signaling of pain and fatigue that appear to be dysregulated in CFS and FM, especially after a moderate exercise stress [17, 18]. These receptors, including alpha- and beta-adrenergic receptors, exhibit altered expression after exercise and thus may play a role in amplifying postexertional pain and fatigue.

Our findings showed that FM patients who were nonresponders to pregabalin differed physiologically as well as symptomatically from patients who were responders. Their HR and BP responses to exercise on either treatment regimen did not differ from controls and were not altered by pregabalin. Differences in cardiovascular responses to exercise from controls that were seen in the FM patient group as a whole were subsequently found to be due to those who were responders. Thus, there may be subgroups of FM patients who do versus do not exhibit the SNS dysregulation linked to altered cardiovascular exercise responses, and this dysregulation may be associated with response to pregabalin. Furthermore, on pregabalin, the symptom profile of nonresponders (including pre- and postexercise pain, physical fatigue, and mental fatigue ratings) actually tended to worsen, although the adverse effect was significant only for mental fatigue. This suggests that different physiological systems may be the primary ones that maintain the FM pain and other symptoms in this subgroup of patients. Further research is needed to identify what processes are dysregulated in these FM patients and to clarify treatments that may be more effective in reducing their pain without increasing side effects. Our findings further suggest that pretests of SNS function in untreated FM patients may be useful as biomarkers to help target the most effective pharmacotherapy for different subgroups of FM patients.

The decreases in exercise HR and BP responses during pregabalin treatment observed in responders may be a secondary effect of decreased pain, especially pain in muscles, joints, and connective tissue that are active during such exercise. Because fibromyalgia pain is associated with elevated inflammatory and stress markers [33, 34], this secondary effect might also act through decreased SNS activity or through altered inflammatory and immune effects, both of which could influence cardiovascular reactivity at rest and during exercise.

Our observations of blunted exercise HR and BP responses are consistent with pregabalin's use during presurgical intubation during which the hemodynamic pressor response is attenuated [35]. Alterations in feedback from group III and IV sensory afferents could contribute to this response. Normally, these afferents respond to metabolites produced during exercise and influence perceptions of fatigue and pain [36] and also increase sympathetic responses [37–39].

Although our findings clearly demonstrate that not all FM patients will benefit from pregabalin treatment, those who were responders reported improvement of pain symptoms, better sleep, and lower perceived exertion during exercise. These effects may have enhanced the ability to perform daily life activities as evidenced by these patients' reports of increased energy and ability to do chores or have fun and decreased physical and mental fatigue. If these symptom improvements result in less sedentary activity and participation in more active pursuits, health and quality of life could be improved. Although both aerobic and strength training regimens are among the best documented nonpharmacological interventions to reduce FM pain [10, 11], only a small percentage of FM patients are willing to undertake such training. Most patients are concerned that exercise will worsen their pain [15] which in turn may require increased bed rest and other limitations on function. Our findings suggest that FM patients who respond positively to pregabalin treatment may respond more positively to rehabilitative exercise. Potential benefits include reduced pain and perceived exertion during exercise and less postexertional worsening of pain and fatigue. Pregabalin pretreatment could thus remove a major barrier to physical training for many FM patients. This hypothesis could be directly tested by a 2-phase intervention study combining an initial phase of pregabalin versus placebo treatment with a second phase of exercise training.

Limitations. The primary weakness of this pilot study is the small sample size. This indicates the need for replication in a larger sample of people with FM and FM + CFS in order for the results to be generalizable to these populations.

5. Conclusion

FM patients who were responders to pregabalin were characterized by increased BP and HR responses to exercise compared to healthy controls. Pregabalin treatment normalized these cardiovascular responses to exercise and reduced perceived exertion in these patients. Nonresponders to pregabalin had normal exercise BP and HR responses on placebo, and these responses were not altered by pregabalin. In addition to expected benefits on pain and sleep quality, FM patients who were pregabalin responders demonstrated significant reductions in multiple fatigue-related symptoms, and the presence of comorbid CFS was *not* associated with nonresponse to pregabalin. Future research to determine whether pretreatment of FM patients with pregabalin could reduce initial postexertional symptoms and enhance success in completing an exercise training program is recommended.

Acknowledgments

This study was supported in part by an unrestricted research grant from Pfizer Pharmaceuticals (IIR WS725105) and by NIH Grant R01 AR060336.

References

[1] F. Wolfe, H. A. Smythe, M. B. Yunus et al., "The American College of Rheumatology 1990 criteria for the classification of fibromyalgia. Report of the Multicenter Criteria Committee," *Arthritis and Rheumatism*, vol. 33, no. 2, pp. 160–172, 1990.

[2] H. S. Smith, R. Harris, and D. Clauw, "Fibromyalgia: an afferent processing disorder leading to a complex pain generalized syndrome," *Pain Physician*, vol. 14, no. 2, pp. E217–E245, 2011.

[3] L. A. Aaron, M. M. Burke, and D. Buchwald, "Overlapping conditions among patients with chronic fatigue syndrome, fibromyalgia, and temporomandibular disorder," *Archives of Internal Medicine*, vol. 160, no. 2, pp. 221–227, 2000.

[4] J. A. Cole, K. J. Rothman, H. J. Cabral, Y. Zhang, and F. A. Farraye, "Migraine, fibromyalgia, and depression among people with IBS: a prevalence study," *BMC Gastroenterology*, vol. 6, article 26, 2006.

[5] K. P. White, M. Speechley, M. Harth, and T. Østbye, "Co-existence of chronic fatigue syndrome with fibromyalgia syndrome in the general population. A controlled study," *Scandinavian Journal of Rheumatology*, vol. 29, no. 1, pp. 44–51, 2000.

[6] L. J. Crofford, M. C. Rowbotham, P. J. Mease et al., "Pregabalin for the treatment of fibromyalgia syndrome: results of a randomized, double-blind, placebo-controlled trial," *Arthritis and Rheumatism*, vol. 52, no. 4, pp. 1264–1273, 2005.

[7] I. J. Russell, L. J. Crofford, T. Leon et al., "The effects of pregabalin on sleep disturbance symptoms among individuals with fibromyalgia syndrome," *Sleep Medicine*, vol. 10, no. 6, pp. 604–610, 2009.

[8] L. Arnold, P. Mease, and S. Silverman, "Pregabalin: an alpha2-delta (alpha2-delta) ligand for the management of fibromyalgia," *The American Journal of Managed Care*, vol. 16, no. 5, pp. S138–S143, 2010.

[9] M. T. Smith and B. J. Moore, "Pregabalin for the treatment of fibromyalgia," *Expert Opinion on Pharmacotherapy*, vol. 13, no. 10, pp. 1527–1533, 2012.

[10] W. M. Hooten, W. Qu, C. O. Townsend, and J. W. Judd, "Effects of strength vs aerobic exercise on pain severity in adults with fibromyalgia: a randomized equivalence trial," *Pain*, vol. 153, no. 4, pp. 915–923, 2012.

[11] E. Nüesch, W. Häuser, K. Bernardy, J. Barth, and P. Jüni, "Comparative efficacy of pharmacological and non-pharmacological interventions in fibromyalgia syndrome: network meta-analysis," *Annals of the Rheumatic Diseases*, vol. 72, no. 6, pp. 955–962, 2013.

[12] M. B. Gavi, D. V. Vassalo, F. T. Amaral et al., "Strengthening exercises improve symptoms and quality of life but do not

change autonomic modulation in fibromyalgia: a randomized clinical trial," *PLoS ONE*, vol. 9, no. 3, Article ID e90767, 2014.

[13] D. C. Ang, A. S. Kaleth, S. Bigatti et al., "Research to encourage exercise for fibromyalgia (REEF): use of motivational interviewing, outcomes from a randomized-controlled trial," *Clinical Journal of Pain*, vol. 29, no. 4, pp. 296–304, 2013.

[14] Y. van Eijk-Hustings, M. Kroese, F. Tan, A. Boonen, M. Bessems-Beks, and R. Landewé, "Challenges in demonstrating the effectiveness of multidisciplinary treatment on quality of life, participation and health care utilisation in patients with fibromyalgia: a randomised controlled trial," *Clinical Rheumatology*, vol. 32, no. 2, pp. 199–209, 2013.

[15] J. Nijs, N. Roussel, J. Van Oosterwijck et al., "Fear of movement and avoidance behaviour toward physical activity in chronic-fatigue syndrome and fibromyalgia: state of the art and implications for clinical practice," *Clinical Rheumatology*, vol. 32, no. 8, pp. 1121–1129, 2013.

[16] M. Meeus, L. Hermans, K. Ickmans et al., "Endogenous pain modulation in response to exercise in patients with rheumatoid arthritis, patients with chronic fatigue syndrome and comorbid fibromyalgia, and healthy controls: a double-blind randomized controlled trial," *Pain Practice*, vol. 15, no. 2, pp. 98–106, 2015.

[17] A. R. Light, L. Bateman, D. Jo et al., "Gene expression alterations at baseline and following moderate exercise in patients with Chronic Fatigue Syndrome and Fibromyalgia Syndrome," *Journal of Internal Medicine*, vol. 271, no. 1, pp. 64–81, 2012.

[18] A. T. White, A. R. Light, R. W. Hughen, T. A. Vanhaitsma, and K. C. Light, "Differences in metabolite-detecting, adrenergic, and immune gene expression after moderate exercise in patients with chronic fatigue syndrome, patients with multiple sclerosis, and healthy controls," *Psychosomatic Medicine*, vol. 74, no. 1, pp. 46–54, 2012.

[19] K. Fukuda, S. E. Straus, I. Hickie, M. C. Sharpe, J. G. Dobbins, and A. Komaroff, "The chronic fatigue syndrome: a comprehensive approach to its definition and study," *Annals of Internal Medicine*, vol. 121, no. 12, pp. 953–959, 1994.

[20] B. J. Noble, G. A. V. Borg, I. Jacobs, R. Ceci, and P. Kaiser, "A category-ratio perceived exertion scale: relationship to blood and muscle lactates and heart rate," *Medicine and Science in Sports and Exercise*, vol. 15, no. 6, pp. 523–528, 1983.

[21] L. Pauer, A. Winkelmann, P. Arsenault et al., "An international, randomized, double-blind, placebo-controlled, phase III trial of pregabalin monotherapy in treatment of patients with fibromyalgia," *Journal of Rheumatology*, vol. 38, no. 12, pp. 2643–2652, 2011.

[22] A. G. Bushmakin, J. C. Cappelleri, A. B. Chandran, and G. Zlateva, "Evaluation of the fibromyalgia impact questionnaire at baseline as a predictor for time to pain improvement in two clinical trials of pregabalin," *International Journal of Clinical Practice*, vol. 67, no. 1, pp. 52–59, 2013.

[23] E. Choy, D. Marshall, Z. L. Gabriel, S. A. Mitchell, E. Gylee, and H. A. Dakin, "A systematic review and mixed treatment comparison of the efficacy of pharmacological treatments for fibromyalgia," *Seminars in Arthritis and Rheumatism*, vol. 41, no. 3, pp. 335–345.e6, 2011.

[24] T. Roth, L. M. Arnold, D. Garcia-Borreguero, M. Resnick, and A. G. Clair, "A review of the effects of pregabalin on sleep disturbance across multiple clinical conditions," *Sleep Medicine Reviews*, vol. 18, no. 3, pp. 261–271, 2014.

[25] P. Sarzi-Puttini, F. Atzeni, A. Diana, A. Doria, and R. Furlan, "Increased neural sympathetic activation in fibromyalgia syndrome," *Annals of the New York Academy of Sciences*, vol. 1069, pp. 109–117, 2006.

[26] L.-A. Martínez-Martínez, T. Mora, A. Vargas, M. Fuentes-Iniestra, and M. Martínez-Lavín, "Sympathetic nervous system dysfunction in fibromyalgia, chronic fatigue syndrome, irritable bowel syndrome, and interstitial cystitis: a review of case-control studies," *Journal of Clinical Rheumatology*, vol. 20, no. 3, pp. 146–150, 2014.

[27] S. Becker and P. Schweinhardt, "Dysfunctional neurotransmitter systems in fibromyalgia, their role in central stress circuitry and pharmacological actions on these systems," *Pain Research and Treatment*, vol. 2012, Article ID 741746, 10 pages, 2012.

[28] P. Kulshreshtha and K. K. Deepak, "Autonomic nervous system profile in fibromyalgia patients and its modulation by exercise: a mini review," *Clinical Physiology and Functional Imaging*, vol. 33, no. 2, pp. 83–91, 2013.

[29] K. C. Light, E. E. Bragdon, K. M. Grewen, K. A. Brownley, S. S. Girdler, and W. Maixner, "Adrenergic dysregulation and pain with and without acute beta-blockade in women with fibromyalgia and temporomandibular disorder," *Journal of Pain*, vol. 10, no. 5, pp. 542–552, 2009.

[30] K. D. Micheva, C. P. Taylor, and S. J. Smith, "Pregabalin reduces the release of synaptic vesicles from cultured hippocampal neurons," *Molecular Pharmacology*, vol. 70, no. 2, pp. 467–476, 2006.

[31] D. W. Han, T. D. Kweon, J. S. Lee, and Y.-W. Lee, "Antiallodynic effect of pregabalin in rat models of sympathetically maintained and sympathetic independent neuropathic pain," *Yonsei Medical Journal*, vol. 48, no. 1, pp. 41–47, 2007.

[32] R. E. Harris, V. Napadow, J. P. Huggins et al., "Pregabalin rectifies aberrant brain chemistry, connectivity, and functional response in chronic pain patients," *Anesthesiology*, vol. 119, no. 6, pp. 1453–1464, 2013.

[33] M. E. Bote, J. J. Garcia, M. D. Hinchado, and E. Ortega, "Fibromyalgia: anti-inflammatory and stress responses after acute moderate exercise," *PLoS ONE*, vol. 8, no. 9, Article ID e74524, 2013.

[34] R. P. da Cunha Ribeiro, H. Roschel, G. G. Artioli et al., "Cardiac autonomic impairment and chronotropic incompetence in fibromyalgia," *Arthritis Research and Therapy*, vol. 13, no. 6, article R190, 2011.

[35] B. Rastogi, K. Gupta, P. K. Gupta, S. Agarwal, M. Jain, and H. Chauhan, "Oral pregabalin premedication for attenuation of haemodynamic pressor response of airway instrumentation during general anaesthesia: a dose response study," *Indian Journal of Anaesthesia*, vol. 56, no. 1, pp. 49–54, 2012.

[36] K. A. Pollak, J. D. Swenson, T. A. Vanhaitsma et al., "Exogenously applied muscle metabolites synergistically evoke sensations of muscle fatigue and pain in human subjects," *Experimental Physiology*, vol. 99, no. 2, pp. 368–380, 2014.

[37] M. Amann, S. Runnels, D. E. Morgan et al., "On the contribution of group III and IV muscle afferents to the circulatory response to rhythmic exercise in humans," *Journal of Physiology*, vol. 589, no. 15, pp. 3855–3866, 2011.

[38] M. P. Kaufman and S. G. Hayes, "The exercise pressor reflex," *Clinical Autonomic Research*, vol. 12, no. 6, pp. 429–439, 2002.

[39] M. P. Kaufman, "The exercise pressor reflex in animals," *Experimental Physiology*, vol. 97, no. 1, pp. 51–58, 2012.

2

Preemptive Analgesia in Total Knee Arthroplasty: Comparing the Effects of Single Dose Combining Celecoxib with Pregabalin and Repetition Dose Combining Celecoxib with Pregabalin

Andri M. T. Lubis,[1] Rangga B. V. Rawung,[1] and Aida R. Tantri[2]

[1]*Department of Orthopaedic and Traumatology, Cipto Mangunkusumo National Central Hospital and Faculty of Medicine, Universitas Indonesia, Jalan Diponegoro No. 71, Central Jakarta, Jakarta 10430, Indonesia*
[2]*Department of Anesthesiology and Intensive Care, Cipto Mangunkusumo National Central Hospital and Faculty of Medicine, Universitas Indonesia, Jalan Diponegoro No. 71, Central Jakarta, Jakarta 10430, Indonesia*

Correspondence should be addressed to Rangga B. V. Rawung; petrus.aprianto.1989@gmail.com

Academic Editor: Steve McGaraughty

Acute pain is the most common early complication after total knee arthroplasty causing delayed mobilization and increased demands of morphine, leading to higher operative cost. Several studies have assessed the effectiveness, side-effects, and ease of use of various analgesics. Preemptive analgesia with combined celecoxib and pregabalin has been reported to yield positive outcomes. In this randomized, double-blind controlled clinical trial, 30 subjects underwent surgery for total knee arthroplasty using 15-20mg bupivacaine 5% epidural anesthesia. All subjects were divided into three groups. Group 1 was given celecoxib 400mg and pregabalin 150mg 1 hour before the operation, Group 2 was given celecoxib 200mg and pregabalin 75mg twice daily starting from 3 days before the operation, and Group 3 was given a placebo. The outcome was measured with Visual Analog Scale, knee range of motion, and postoperative mobilization. There was a significant difference in postoperative morphine usage between the groups that were administered with preemptive analgesia and the placebo group, but no significant difference was found between Group 1 and Group 2 that were given preemptive analgesia at different doses. ROM and postoperative mobilization were not significantly different among the three groups. Two patients in the first group, one patient in the second group, and one patient in the third group developed nausea. Preemptive analgesia is proven to reduce postoperative usage of morphine independent of the dosage. We recommend the use of combined celecoxib and pregabalin as preemptive analgesia after the total knee arthroplasty procedure. This trial is registered with NCT03523832 (ClinicalTrials.gov).

1. Introduction

Total knee arthroplasty (TKA) is one of the most common operation procedures in the orthopedic field [1]. Several studies have proved that the TKA procedure increases patient Quality of Life [2, 3]. Crowder et al. [4] reported that, after 10 years of follow-up, 99% of the patients that underwent the TKA procedure showed good functional outcome. The TKA procedure is indicated for patients experiencing chronic pain caused by severe joint damage. Although this procedure frequently yields positive clinical outcomes, complications during and after surgery can occur [5].

Acute pain following TKA is reported as one of the most common complications of the procedure [6, 7]. Several factors may contribute to the emerging pain sensation, such as infection, inflammatory response to the procedure, and race [8]. Effective postoperative pain management is crucial to promote recovery and to prevent complications. Although the mainstay of postoperative pain management has been opioid based, the consequent increase in demand of opioid use and the associated increase of opioid side-effects impede the rehabilitation process and increase the hospital length of stay, which in turn increases treatment cost and impacts patient satisfaction [8, 9].

The prevalent use of multimodal analgesia both intra-operatively and postoperatively has been described recently [10, 11]. Multimodal analgesia is a rational approach to pain management since no single analgesia targets all types of pain [12]. Epidurals, peripheral nerve blocks, and local articular injections have been reported to give good results; however they are associated with many side-effects such as headache, hypotension, neurologic bladder, and contralateral numbness [13, 14]. Patient Control Analgesia (PCA) using morphine is also reported to reduce postoperative acute pain, but it is associated with side-effects such as nausea and vomiting [15, 16].

Preemptive analgesia is intended to help cope with the pain sensation before the operative procedure. The aim of this therapy is to prevent central pain sensitization through the inhibition of pain stimuli and afferent signaling from the operation site [17–19]. A literature review by Katz and Clarke demonstrates the benefits of preemptive analgesia in various surgical procedures [20]. Decreasing pain sensation and lower postoperative analgesia usage was described in 60% of the cases in a study by Lee et al. [12]. Many preemptive analgesics can be taken postoperatively, such as nonsteroidal anti-inflammatory drugs (NSAIDs), N-methyl-d-aspartate (NMDAs), local anesthesia, and systemic antiepileptic drugs [12].

The use of oral preemptive analgesia is associated with positive outcomes [21]. Celecoxib (an oral NSAID) and pregabalin (an antiallodynic and antihyperalgesic) can be used as preemptive analgesia as their synergic effects may inhibit pain stimuli in different ways. Celecoxib has a better analgesic effect with lower rate of side effect compared to ibuprofen, and pregabalin has a similar analgesic effect with a lower rate of side-effects compared to gabapentin [22, 23]. A study by Niruthisard et al. showed that the combination of celecoxib and pregabalin taken 1 hour before the TKA procedure helps decrease pain during motion and postoperative anxiety [24]. Despite these promising effects, research on the repetitive dose of preemptive analgesia in the TKA procedure is limited. The aim of this study was to compare the therapeutic effect of single dose and repetitive dose of combined celecoxib and pregabalin.

2. Materials and Methods

All procedures undertaken in this study have been approved by The Ethical Committee of Faculty of Medicine Universitas Indonesia no. 851/UN2.F1/ETIK/2015. Verbal and written informed consent were obtained before the study. The study was carried out in accordance with the approved guidelines.

This study used a double-blind control clinical trial design conducted between July 2015 and December 2016. The sample size of this study was calculated based on formula of mean difference between unpaired numeric data in analytic research design. The sample size of 10 patients per group was adequate.

$$n = 2\left[\frac{\left(Z_{\alpha - Z_{\alpha}}\right)\sigma}{\mu_1 - \mu_2}\right]^2$$
$$n = 2\left[\frac{\left(1.96_{-(-0.84)}\right)126}{160}\right]^2 = 9{,}7 \quad \simeq \mathbf{10\ subjects} \tag{1}$$

Patients were included if they met the following eligibility criteria: patients who (1) are aged between 55 and 80 years who visited the orthopedic polyclinic, (2) underwent the TKA procedure, (3) have osteoarthritis, and (4) consumed a pain killer and anti-inflammatory drug routinely. Patients who met all of the aforementioned criteria were consecutively enrolled into the study. Patients were excluded if they had (1) a psychiatric disorder, (2) history of renal disease (3) history of chronic neuropathy, having knee arthritis caused by rheumatoid arthritis and infection, (4) diabetes and obesity, (5) coagulopathy, and (6) severe pain that needed immediate analgesia.

The eligible subjects of the study were collected by consecutive sampling. The tested subjects were randomly allocated into three groups: Group 1: patients administered with a single dose of celecoxib 400 mg and pregabalin 150 mg, Group 2: patients administered with a repetitive dose of celecoxib 200 mg and pregabalin 75 mg twice daily for 3 days before the operation, and Group 3: patients taking a placebo. This study used 3 groups to compare repetitive dose of oral preemptive analgesia with the more common preemptive analgesia treatment of single dose combining celecoxib with pregabalin and control group. Currently no research had been done to analyze the effect of repetitive dose of preemptive analgesia in TKA procedure according to mechanism of administration, dosage, and efficacy.

This study used block randomization with the size of 3 according to each group. Block randomization was used to reduce bias and achieve balance in the allocation of participants to treatment arms, especially when the sample size is small (10 samples). This method increases the probability that each arm will contain an equal number of individuals by sequencing participant assignments by block. Allocation proceeds by randomly selecting one of the orderings and assigning the next block of participants to study groups according to the specified sequence. The double-blind design in this study included blinding of orthopedic surgeon, anesthetic operator, medical team giving the drugs, and the patients.

All surgeries were performed by an experienced orthopedic surgeon. All groups underwent the same procedure for epidural anesthesia with 15-20 mg bupivacaine 5% before the TKA procedure. Two hours after the procedure, postoperative analgesia, which consisted of paracetamol 1000 mg + PCA morphine 2 mg/kgBW with maximal dose of 6 mg/hr and 5 minutes' interval, was administered.

The efficacy of preemptive analgesia among the groups was measured during the postoperative follow-up using the outcome parameters listed below. All side-effects of postoperative therapy were monitored and treated.

Table 1: The characteristics of the patients.

No	Variable	Group 1 (N=10)	Group 2 (N=10)	Group 3 (N=10)
1	Gender	Man (3) Woman (7)	Man (3) Woman (7)	Man (1) Woman (9)
2	Age (years)	66.1 ± 7.79	65.9 ± 5.82	68.2 ± 6.35

2.1. Outcome Parameters

2.1.1. Total Morphine Consumption. This was the primary outcome parameter to measure the efficacy of the preemptive analgesia of combined celecoxib and pregabalin. In this study, morphine was administered by patient control analgesia (PCA). Total morphine consumption was measured postoperatively for 3 days.

2.1.2. Postoperative Pain. The acute pain is measured and evaluated by Visual Analog Scale (VAS) every morning before the patients began their rehabilitation program. This parameter is measured from the first day until the third postoperative day (0-24 hours, 25-48 hours, and 49-72 hours).

2.1.3. Knee Functional Outcome. The knee range of motion was measured in the morning from the first day until the third postoperative day. The patient was asked to actively move the knee joint, and the knee angle was measured by goniometer.

2.1.4. Mobilization. The patient was expected to be able to sit on the first day, stand on the second day, and walk on the third day in the postoperative period.

2.2. Statistical Analysis. The outcomes of this research were numerically expressed and the differences among the three groups were measured within the first day until the third postoperative day.

Statistical analysis was performed with SPSS software version 20 (SPSS Inc., Chicago, IL, USA). The normality of distribution for numeric variables was assessed by the Shapiro-Wilk test. Accordingly, categorical variables are presented as means with SD or medians with interquartile range (95% CI). Data were tested using a one-way ANOVA if the data were normally distributed and with the Kruskal-Wallis test if they were not normally distributed. Any significant difference found by the one-way ANOVA was then analyzed by the Bonferroni post hoc test to assess the significance of each group.

3. Results and Discussion

A total of thirty subjects were included in this study. Each group consisted of ten randomized subjects. The characteristics of the patients are described in Table 1.

3.1. Total Morphine Consumption. There was a significant difference in the total morphine consumption among the 3 groups ($p<0.001$). The results of morphine consumption measurement are summarized in Table 2.

The post hoc Bonferroni test concluded a significant difference in the total morphine consumed between the first and third group ($p<0.001$), as well as between the second and the third group ($p<0.001$), but there were no significant differences between the first and the second group.

3.2. Postoperative Pain. Postoperative pain was measured with VAS. The measurement was done on the first day until the third day. The VAS within each group generally decreased from Day 1 until Day 3. Significant differences in VAS scores between the three groups were observed ($p<0.001$) on the first day, second day, and the third day. The third group showed higher score of VAS than the first and the second group. The VAS measurement among the groups evaluated from the first until third day can be seen on Table 3.

The post hoc Bonferroni test concluded a significant difference of total morphine consumption between the first and third group ($p<0.001$) and between the second and the third group ($p<0.001$), but there were no significant differences between the first and the second group.

3.3. Knee Functional Outcome. The range of motion in all groups improved from Day 1 until Day 3. There was no significant difference in ROM among all groups on the first day ($p=0.886$), on the second day ($p=0.131$), and on the third day ($p=0.011$). Nevertheless, the clinical outcome of knee measurement using goniometer showed daily improvement in ROM. Knee functional outcome measurement among the groups after undergoing TKA procedure can be seen on Table 4.

3.4. Mobilization. Almost all of the subjects from each group were able to sit on the first day, stand on the second day, and walk on the third day. There was no significant difference among the groups ($p=1.00$). Mobilization measurement among the groups after undergoing TKA procedure can be seen on Table 5.

Osteoarthritis often affects geriatric patients. Its incidence is impacted by age as well as gender, wherein females are more affected than men [25]. These demographic characteristics were also found in our patient sample. As more than half of the patients undergoing TKA are either late adult or geriatric, higher rates of complications can be expected. It follows that intensive evaluation is often required when using analgesia [26, 27]. In our study, the use of morphine was significantly lower in the groups that received preemptive analgesia regardless of the duration compared to the placebo group. Our findings are in line with a previous study conducted by Lee et al. [28] and Huang Yu et al. [29] which found that the use of celecoxib (400 mg) combined with pregabalin (150 mg) given 1 hour prior to the TKA procedure lowered the use of morphine and postoperative pain. However, our study found no significant difference in the time of administration of the preemptive analgesia combination (1 hour or 72 hours) prior to the procedure.

In terms of efficacy, we found that VAS in the groups that were taking preemptive analgesia was lower than the placebo group. Similar results have been described by Buvanendran et al. [19] and Carmichael et al. [30] who found that the use

TABLE 2: Total morphine consumption (PCA) among the groups after undergoing TKA procedure.

	Group 1 (1 hr preemptive analgesia) N=10	Group 2 (72 hrs preemptive analgesia) N=10	Group 3 (Placebo) N=10	P value*
Morphine (PCA)	10.60(2.675)	9.90(1.524)	30.20(5.308)	<0.001

The data were normally distributed.
The p value was measured using ANOVA parametric test.

TABLE 3: VAS measurement among the groups after undergoing TKA procedure evaluated from the first day until the third day.

	VAS D-1 N=10	VAS D-2 N=10	VAS D-3 N=10	P value*
Group 1 (1 hr preemptive analgesia)	2 (2-3)	1 (1-2)	1 (1-2)	<0.001
Group 2 (72 hrs preemptive analgesia)	2.5 (2-3)	2 (1-2)	1.2 (1-2)	0.001
Group 3 (Placebo)	4(2-5)	3 (2-4)	3 (2-3)	0.001

The data were not normally distributed.
The p value was measured using Kruskal-wallis nonparametric test.

TABLE 4: Knee functional outcome measurement among the groups after undergoing TKA procedure evaluated from the first day until the third day.

	ROM D-1 N=10	ROM D-2 N=10	ROM D-3 N=10
Group 1 (1 hr preemptive analgesia)	15 (10-30)	60 (15-60)	90 (60-90)
Group 2 (72 hrs preemptive analgesia)	15 (15-20)	30 (30-60)	60 (45-90)
Group 3 (Placebo)	15(15-20)	30 (30-60)	60 (60-90)
p-value	0.886	0.131	0.011

The data were not normally distributed.
The p value was measured using Kruskal-wallis nonparametric test.

TABLE 5: Mobilization measurement among the groups after undergoing TKA procedure evaluated from the first day until the third day.

	Motion D-1 (sitting) N=10	Motion D-2 (standing) N=10	Motion D-3 (walking) N=10	p value*
Group 1 (1 hr preemptive analgesia)	9(90%)	8 (80 %)	10 (100%)	<0.001
Group 2 (72 hrs preemptive analgesia)	8 (80%)	7 (70 %)	7 (70%)	0.001
Group 3 (Placebo)	9 (90%)	7 (70%)	8 (80%)	0.001

The data were not normally distributed
The p value was measured using Kruskal-wallis non-parametric test.

of repetitive doses of celecoxib and pregabalin succeeded in lowering acute and chronic postoperative pain. Although we did not measure the outcome of chronic pain among the treatment groups, it was found that, in general, the VAS score decreased from Day 1 to Day 3 and significantly differed from the group that used either a single dose or a repetitive dose of preemptive analgesia compared to the placebo group. Other confounding factors such as race, gender, and the method of VAS measurement warrant further consideration in future studies.

The rehabilitation program is an important aspect of postoperative recovery. It has been reported that early mobilization following the TKA procedure results in a better outcome such as lower morbidity and hospital length of stay [31]. It follows that ROM assessment is important to ensure early mobilization of patients. The fact that ROM is directly affected by pain implies that lowering postoperative pain with preemptive analgesia will increase ROM and early mobilization rate of the patients. In this study, ROM was found to improve day to day, but no significant difference was observed in ROM between subjects that were given preemptive analgesia compared to placebo group. According to Miner et al. [31] and Jacobsen et al. [32], the use of ROM as the outcome parameter after the TKA procedure is still controversial. Their studies report that many factors like knee soft tissue, knee alignment, knee muscle strength, psychological condition, preoperative ROM, and operative procedure impact the postoperative ROM. The result of our study supports the fact that ROM is not only affected by pain but also affected by multifactorial aspects that have not been studied in our research.

Preemptive analgesia is expected to permit the early mobilization of postoperative patients. Early mobilization reduces complications like DVT which can be avoided and promotes the healing process, which in turn improves functional outcomes [33, 34]. In this study, we did not find any significant differences in the mobilization period among the 3 groups. Bade reported that preoperative mobilization directly affected postoperative mobilization outcome. Many factors may affect postoperative mobilization, such as age, comorbidities, muscle strength, and psychological factors. The result of our study supported the fact that patient mobility is not only affected by postoperative pain and suggests the possibility that preemptive analgesia only lowers static postoperative pain, not lowering the pain sensation during mobilization.

Our study found that the side-effects were dose dependent and often emerged in patients using the celecoxib combination with pregabalin for prolonged periods. Buvanendran [19] reported that patients administered with 300 mg pregabalin 1 hour postoperatively experienced sedation, confusion, and dry mouth side-effects. Lee et al. [28] compared the use of the 400mg celecoxib and 150 mg pregabalin combination with 400mg celecoxib alone and found that the side-effects emerged in the combination group. In our study, we found that 2 subjects in first group, 1 subject in second group, and 1 subject in third group experienced nausea.

4. Conclusions

Preemptive analgesia treatments with the combination of celecoxib and pregabalin are effective in decreasing the acute pain sensation after the TKA procedure independent of the dose and repetition. This combination of preemptive analgesia is ineffective in decreasing pain sensation during motion. In this study, the use of combination of celecoxib and pregabalin did not show any significant side-effects.

Acknowledgments

The authors would like to express our deep gratitude to all contributors.

References

[1] G. Hawker, J. Wright, P. Coyte et al., "Health-related quality of life after knee replacement," *The Journal of Bone & Joint Surgery*, vol. 80, no. 2, pp. 163–173, 1998.

[2] S. T. Lovald, K. L. Ong, E. C. Lau, J. K. Schmier, K. J. Bozic, and S. M. Kurtz, "Mortality, Cost, and Health Outcomes of Total Knee Arthroplasty in Medicare Patients," *The Journal of Arthroplasty*, vol. 28, no. 3, pp. 449–454, 2013.

[3] C. J. M. Bachmeier, L. M. March, M. J. Cross et al., "A comparison of outcomes in osteoarthritis patients undergoing total hip and knee replacement surgery," *Osteoarthritis and Cartilage*, vol. 9, no. 2, pp. 137–146, 2001.

[4] A. R. Crowder, G. P. Duffy, and R. T. Trousdale, "Long-term results of total knee arthroplasty in young patients with rheumatoid arthritis," *The Journal of Arthroplasty*, vol. 20, no. 3, pp. 12–16, 2005.

[5] G. J. Crockarell J, "No Title," in *in Campbells operation orthopaedics, , Elsevier Mobsy*, p. 256, 11th edition, 2013.

[6] V. A. Brander, S. D. Stulberg, A. D. Adams et al., "Ranawat Award Paper: Predicting Total Knee Replacement Pain," *Clinical Orthopaedics and Related Research*, vol. 416, pp. 27–36, 2003.

[7] S. Tsukada, M. Wakui, and A. Hoshino, "Pain Control After Simultaneous Bilateral Total Knee Arthroplasty," *The Journal of Bone and Joint Surgery-American Volume*, vol. 97, no. 5, pp. 367–373, 2015.

[8] D. P. Williams, S. O'Brien, E. Doran et al., "Early postoperative predictors of satisfaction following total knee arthroplasty," *The Knee*, vol. 20, no. 6, pp. 442–446, 2013.

[9] K. K. Society, "Guidelines for the Management of Postoperative Pain after Total Knee Arthroplasty," *Knee Surgery & Related Research*, vol. 24, no. 4, pp. 201–207, 2012.

[10] J. D. Lamplot, E. R. Wagner, and D. W. Manning, "Multimodal pain management in total knee arthroplasty: a prospective randomized controlled trial," *The Journal of Arthroplasty*, vol. 29, no. 2, pp. 329–334, 2014.

[11] T. Sandhu, S. Paiboonworachat, and W. Ko-Iam, "Effects of preemptive analgesia in laparoscopic cholecystectomy: a double-blind randomized controlled trial," *Surgical Endoscopy*, vol. 25, no. 1, pp. 23–27, 2011.

[12] B. H. Lee, J.-O. Park, K.-S. Suk, T.-H. Kim, H.-M. Lee, M.-S. Park et al., "Pre-emptive and multi-modal perioperative pain management may improve quality of life in patients undergoing spinal surgery," *Pain Physician*, vol. 16, no. 3, pp. 217–226, 2013.

[13] T. H. Mahoney M, P. Noble, and J. Davidson, "No Title," *Clin Orthop Relat Res*, vol. 260, no. 30, p. 7, 1990.

[14] E. F. Hurley RW, "Preemptive and Preventive Analgesia," in *Essentials of Pain Medicine*, pp. 200–205, Elsevier Inc., 3 edition, 2011.

[15] D. M. Anastase, S. Cionac Florescu, A. M. Munteanu, T. Ursu, and C. I. Stoica, "Analgesic techniques in hip and knee arthroplasty: From the daily practice to evidence-based medicine," *Anesthesiology Research and Practice*, vol. 2014, 2014.

[16] B. J. Morris and H. R. Mir, "The Opioid Epidemic," *Journal of the American Academy of OrthopaedicSurgeons* , vol. 23, no. 5, pp. 267–271, 2015.

[17] X. Jianda, Q. Yuxing, G. Yi, Z. Hong, P. Libo, and Z. Jianning, "Impact of Preemptive Analgesia on inflammatory responses and Rehabilitation after Primary Total Knee Arthroplasty: A Controlled Clinical Study," *Scientific Reports*, vol. 6, 2016.

[18] S. Hariharan, H. Moseley, A. Kumar, and S. Raju, "The effect of preemptive analgesia in postoperative pain relief—a prospective double-blind randomized study," *Pain Medicine*, vol. 10, no. 1, pp. 49–53, 2009.

[19] A. Buvanendran and J. S. Kroin, "Multimodal analgesia for controlling acute postoperative pain," *Current Opinion in Anaesthesiology*, vol. 22, no. 5, pp. 588–593, 2009.

[20] J. Katz, H. Clarke, and Z. Seltzer, "Preventive analgesia: quo vadimus?" *Anesthesia & Analgesia*, vol. 113, no. 5, pp. 1242–1253, 2011.

[21] K. H. Fibel, H. J. Hillstrom, and B. C. Halpern, "State-of-the-Art management of knee osteoarthritis," *World Journal of Clinical Cases*, vol. 3, no. 2, pp. 89–101, 2015.

[22] A. C. Gordo, C. Walker, B. Armada, and D. Zhou, "Efficacy of celecoxib versus ibuprofen for the treatment of patients with osteoarthritis of the knee: A randomized double-blind, non-inferiority trial," *Journal of International Medical Research*, vol. 45, no. 1, pp. 59–74, 2017.

[23] M. Dauri, S. Faria, A. Gatti, L. Celidonio, R. Carpenedo, and A. F. Sabato, "Gabapentin and pregabalin for the acute post-operative pain management. A systematic-narrative review of

the recent clinical evidences," *Current Drug Targets*, vol. 10, no. 8, pp. 716–733, 2009.

[24] S. Niruthisard, A. Earsakul, P. Bunburaphong et al., "Preoperative pregabalin and/or celecoxib for pain management after total knee arthroplasty under intrathecal morphine: A randomized controlled trial," *Asian Biomedicine*, vol. 7, no. 4, pp. 578–585, 2013.

[25] B. Heidari, "Knee osteoarthritis prevalence, risk factors, pathogenesis and features: Part I," *Caspian Journal of Internal Medicine*, vol. 2, no. 2, pp. 205–212, 2011.

[26] M. H. Gonzalez and A. O. Mekhail, "The failed total knee arthroplasty: evaluation and etiology.," *Journal of the American Academy of Orthopaedic Surgeons*, vol. 12, no. 6, pp. 436–446, 2004.

[27] H. Lundblad, A. Kreicbergs, and K. Å. Jansson, "Prediction of persistent pain after total knee replacement for osteoarthritis," *The Journal of Bone & Joint Surgery (British Volume)*, vol. 90, no. 2, pp. 166–171, 2008.

[28] J. K. Lee, K.-S. Chung, and C. H. Choi, "The effect of a single dose of preemptive pregabalin administered with cox-2 inhibitor: a trial in total knee arthroplasty," *The Journal of Arthroplasty*, vol. 30, no. 1, pp. 38–42, 2015.

[29] Y.-M. Huang, C.-M. Wang, C.-T. Wang, W.-P. Lin, L.-C. Horng, and C.-C. Jiang, "Perioperative celecoxib administration for pain management after total knee arthroplasty - A randomized, controlled study," *BMC Musculoskeletal Disorders*, vol. 9, article no. 77, 2008.

[30] N. M. E. Carmichael, J. Katz, H. Clarke et al., "An Intensive Perioperative Regimen of Pregabalin and Celecoxib Reduces Pain and Improves Physical Function Scores Six Weeks after Total Hip Arthroplasty: A Prospective Randomized Controlled Trial," *Pain Research & Management*, vol. 18, Article ID 258714, 6 pages, 2013.

[31] A. L. Miner, E. A. Lingard, E. A. Wright et al., "Knee range of motion after total knee arthroplasty: how important is this as an outcome measure?" *The Journal of Arthroplasty*, vol. 18, no. 3, pp. 286–294, 2003.

[32] T. L. Jakobsen, M. Christensen, S. S. Christensen, M. Olsen, and T. Bandholm, "Reliability of knee joint range of motion and circumference measurements after total knee arthroplasty: Does tester experience matter?" *Physiotherapy Research International*, vol. 15, no. 3, pp. 126–134, 2010.

[33] S. Chandrasekaran, S. K. Ariaretnam, J. Tsung, and D. Dickison, "Early mobilization after total knee replacement reduces the incidence of deep venous thrombosis," *ANZ Journal of Surgery*, vol. 79, no. 7-8, pp. 526–529, 2009.

[34] B. C. Mears SC and PK. Edwards, "How to decrease length of hospital stay after total knee replacement," *Journal of Surgical Orthopaedic Advances*, vol. 25, no. 1, pp. 2–7, 2016.

3

Morphine versus Hydromorphone: Does Choice of Opioid Influence Outcomes?

Padma Gulur, Katharine Koury, Paul Arnstein, Hang Lee, Patricia McCarthy, Christopher Coley, and Elizabeth Mort

Massachusetts General Hospital, Boston, MA, USA

Correspondence should be addressed to Padma Gulur; pgulur@yahoo.com

Academic Editor: Anna Maria Aloisi

Morphine has traditionally been considered the first line agent for analgesia in hospitals; however, in the last few years there has been a shift towards the use of hydromorphone as a first line agent. We conducted a hospital population based observational study to evaluate the increasing use of hydromorphone over morphine in both medical and surgical populations. Additionally, we assessed the effect of this trend on three key outcomes, including adverse events, length of stay, and readmission rates. We evaluated data from the University Health Systems Consortium. Data from 38 hospitals from October 2010 to September 2013 was analyzed for patients treated with either hydromorphone or morphine. The use of morphine steadily decreased while use of hydromorphone increased in both medical and surgical groups. Rescue drugs were used more frequently in patients treated with hydromorphone in comparison to patients treated with morphine ($p < 0.01$). Patients receiving morphine tended to stay in the hospital for almost one day longer than patients receiving hydromorphone. However, 30-day all cause readmission rates were significantly higher in patients treated with hydromorphone ($p < 0.01$). Our study highlights that the choice of hydromorphone versus morphine may influence outcomes. There are implications related to resource utilization and these outcomes.

1. Introduction

In 2001, it was reported that approximately 9 in 10 Americans frequently experience pain [1]. In the United States, it has been estimated that 100 million adults suffer from chronic pain alone [2]. As a result, arguments for the undertreatment of pain in the United States have led to several outcomes. The American Pain Society (APS) released guidelines in 1995, which stated that the first step towards improving pain management is assessment and recording of patients' pain reports [3]. The Joint Commission addressed the common practice of suboptimal pain management in 2001 by requiring professionals to ask patients about their pain, treat it when necessary, and evaluate the effects of therapy rendered [4]. At about the same time, the Veterans Administration rolled out a Quality Improvement initiative calling for pain the be treated as the fifth vital sign [5]. Both of these initiatives, confronting the undertreatment of pain, contributed to practice changes that increased awareness on the importance of treating pain. These changes are notable considering that Fox and colleagues stated that the most common symptom that motivates people to seek health care is pain [6]. In turn, there have been unprecedented increases in opioid production and prescription in attempt to manage pain in the United States [5, 7]. Specifically, 80% of the worldwide opioid supply is consumed by Americans, who make up less than 5% of the world's total population [8].

An interesting national trend appears to be the increasing use of hydromorphone compared to morphine. Some evidence in the literature has supported this change [9–11]. This is supported by the US aggregate production data of opioids, which shows a 261.52% increase in hydromorphone production compared to a 190.19% increase in morphine production from 2003 to 2013 [12]. The increase in production and therapeutic use of opioids has paralleled an alarming increase in the diversion, misuse, and development of addiction disorders to prescription opioids. Hydromorphone use, in particular, may contribute to these threats to public health given a faster onset of action and greater euphoric effects when compared to morphine [13].

Morphine is a benzylisoquinoline alkaloid which acts as a potent μ-opioid receptor agonist [14–16]. Morphine is metabolized by glucuronidation into morphine-3-glucuronide (M3G) and morphine-6-glucuronide (M6G) which are active metabolites.

Hydromorphone is a semisynthetic opioid agonist which also acts as a potent μ-opioid receptor agonist and is synthesized somewhat easily by modifying morphine [14]. In comparison to morphine, hydromorphone has a shorter half-life and a greater impact on sedation [13]. Hydromorphone does not form an active 6-glucuronide metabolite; however, it does have the 3-glucoronide metabolite (H3G) which has been shown to have neurotoxic side effects [17, 18].

Studies have shown that morphine and hydromorphone at equianalgesic doses are very similar and there is no difference in side effect profile [10, 15, 19]. The street value of hydromorphone is higher than morphine, which is an indicator of its likability and recreational use potential [13]. Clinical practice drives the prescription drug abuse epidemic. Hence there is increasing national and international concern regarding the use of hydromorphone [20–23].

The purpose of our study was to evaluate the increasing use of hydromorphone over morphine for analgesia in hospitals. Further, we looked at the impact of this trend on outcome measures such as opioid related adverse events, length of stay, and readmission rates.

2. Methods

This hospital population based observational study evaluated data collected from the University Health Systems Consortium (UHC) Clinical Data Base/Resource Manager (CDB/RM). This is an alliance of 118 academic medical centers and 298 of their affiliated hospitals. It accounts for more than 90% of the not for profit academic medical centers in the United States. The UHC CDB/RM is a comparative database with patient level all-payer hospital UB-92 and discharge abstract data from these academic centers and their affiliates. Approval for the use of UHC hospital level data was waived from the Institutional Review Board at Massachusetts General Hospital as this data analysis did not meet the definition of human subjects' research.

The study period was from October 2010 to September 2013. Hospitals with over 500 beds that had reported data for all of our fields of interest during the study period were included. UHC currently has 74 hospitals with over 500 beds in the CDB/RM. Hospitals with incomplete data were excluded. 38 hospitals met all the criteria for inclusion. We collected this data using the UHC CDB/RM 2012 Risk Adjustment Model.

We queried the database for patients, of all ages, who had received either morphine or hydromorphone during their hospital stays but not both drugs (single treatment). If a patient was hospitalized more than once and received either hydromorphone or morphine, then that patient was included again in this data. The APR-DRG (all patient refined-diagnosis related groups) severity of illness (SOI) was collected for our cohorts to help us compare the groups.

We collected outcome data on length of stay, which does not include emergency department time. Additionally, we gathered data on 30-day all cause readmission rates and adverse events. For the purposes of this study, adverse events were defined as the use of a rescue drug (naloxone) during an episode of care. Specifically, naloxone administration on the same day, at any time after the patient received an opioid, was considered an adverse event.

Statistical comparisons of the rates of rescue drug use and 30-day readmission were performed by Chi-square test and 95% confidence intervals, which were constructed by using normal approximation. The 95% confidence intervals of mean lengths of stay were obtained by using normal approximation, and the test was made by independent samples t-test.

3. Results

3.1. Demographics. Averages for demographics were calculated across all three years for patients treated with morphine or hydromorphone. The average age for patients treated with morphine was 49.5 years in comparison to 52.5 years for patients treated with hydromorphone ($p = 0.995$). Of patients treated with hydromorphone, 52.8% were female and 47.2% were male in comparison to patients treated with morphine, 55.4% of which were female and 44.6% were male. Additionally, race was calculated for this population and the majority of patients treated with hydromorphone or morphine were white, 70.8% and 59.8% of each group, respectively.

3.2. Medical and Surgical Groups. Over the three years, 628,910 patients were treated with hydromorphone and 751,692 patients were treated with morphine. These patients were further grouped by medical or surgical admissions and this formed our cohort. In the medical cohort, 217,521 patients were treated with hydromorphone and 395,354 were treated with morphine. In the surgical cohort, 411,389 patients were treated with hydromorphone and 356,338 patients were treated with morphine.

3.3. Use of Hydromorphone and Morphine. Over the three-year study period, the use of morphine steadily decreased while use of hydromorphone increased in both medical and surgical groups. Specifically, we found that hydromorphone use increased by 22% in surgical patients and by 17% in medical patients. On the other hand, morphine use decreased by 22% in surgical patients and by 6% in medical patients. A noteworthy change occurred over the study period as hydromorphone overtook morphine as the more commonly used analgesic in surgical patients (see Figure 1).

3.4. Severity of Illness (SOI) of the Cohort. APR-DRG SOI is used to evaluate patient complexity and hospital resource use. SOI is classified into minor, moderate, major, and extreme.

We compared the hydromorphone and morphine groups within the medical and surgical cohorts for their APR-DRG SOI compositions. In the medical cohort, for patients treated with morphine, 49.7% of patients were in the mild

TABLE 1: Severity of Illness.

Drug	Medical		Surgical	
	Minor/moderate	Major/extreme	Minor/moderate	Major/extreme
Hydromorphone	50.69%	49.31%	75.37%	24.62%
Morphine	49.70%	50.30%	74.04%	25.96%
p value	<0.01	<0.01	<0.01	<0.01

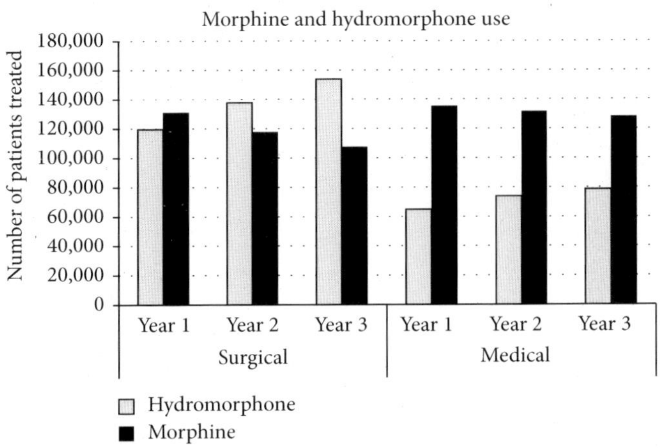

*Year 1: Oct. 2010–Sept. 2011, year 2: Oct. 2011–Sept. 2012 and year 3: Oct. 2012–Sept. 2013

FIGURE 1: Morphine and hydromorphone use.

and moderate classes and 50.3% of patients were in the major and extreme classes; in turn, for patients treated with hydromorphone, 50.69% patients were in the mild and moderate classes and 49.31% of patients were in the major and extreme classes ($p < 0.01$). In the surgical cohort, for patients treated with morphine, 75.37% of patients were in the mild and moderate classes and 24.62% of patients were in the major and extreme classes; in turn, for patients treated with hydromorphone, 74.04% of patients were in the mild and moderate classes and 25.96% of patients were in the major and extreme classes ($p < 0.01$) (see Table 1).

3.5. Adverse Events/Rescue Drug Use. Our results show that rescue drugs are used more often in patients treated with hydromorphone than patients treated with morphine. In patients treated with hydromorphone, rescue drug use was 0.25% higher in the medical group and 0.63% higher in the surgical group ($p < 0.01$) (see Table 2).

3.6. Length of Stay. The data on length of stay (LOS), which was measured in days, showed that patients receiving morphine were in the hospital longer than patients receiving hydromorphone. In patients treated with morphine, we found that the average LOS was 0.88 days longer in the medical group and 0.62 days longer in the surgical group ($p < 0.01$) (see Table 2).

3.7. 30-Day Readmission. The data shows that the 30-day readmission rate was greater amongst patients receiving hydromorphone when compared to patients receiving morphine. In patients treated with hydromorphone, the all cause 30-day readmission rate was 1.37% higher in the surgical group and 3.41% higher in the medical group ($p < 0.01$) (see Table 2).

4. Discussion

In comparing our hydromorphone and morphine groups by APR-DRG SOI, we found a slightly higher percentage of sicker patients in the morphine group compared to the hydromorphone group in both the medical and surgical cohorts ($p < 0.01$). This was statistically different; however, the clinical relevance of a 1% difference in this large population based observational study is not immediately apparent.

The results show that rescue drug use is higher in patients treated with hydromorphone compared to morphine. The main pharmacodynamic difference between hydromorphone and morphine is potency, such that hydromorphone is five to ten times more potent than morphine [10, 15, 24]. Hydromorphone crosses the blood brain barrier faster, resulting in quicker onset and peak of analgesic activity. A study of nonsurgical patients admitted to 288 hospitals in the United States showed that patients prescribed hydromorphone received nearly triple the strength of opioid when compared to patients prescribed morphine [25]. This may help explain the greater use of naloxone among hydromorphone patients found in this study [13]. Adverse events, as defined in our study by rescue drug use, have been directly implicated in increasing healthcare costs [26].

Patients treated with morphine remained in the hospital for a little under one day longer when compared to patients treated with hydromorphone. However, 30-day all cause readmission rates were significantly higher in patients treated with hydromorphone in both the medical and surgical cohorts ($p < 0.01$). Historically, shorter LOS has been equated with lower costs [27]. However, higher readmission rates, which would imply premature discharges, have significant reimbursement implications. In the new hospital value-based purchasing program, reimbursement rates to institutions can be adversely affected by costs incurred when patients are readmitted to the hospital within 30 days after discharge. This could translate to a 2% reduction in total Medicare payments to a hospital in 2014 and a 3% reduction in 2015 [28].

Limitations of our study include the observational nature of the study and the lack of risk adjustments between the groups. Of interest, however, in both medical and surgical study groups, there were more patients treated with morphine

Table 2: Outcomes by medical surgical and hydromorphone and morphine.

Outcome	30-day readmission rate		Length of stay		Rescue drug use	
Group	Surgical [95% CI]	Medical [95% CI]	Surgical [95% CI]	Medical [95% CI]	Surgical [95% CI]	Medical [95% CI]
Hydromorphone	4.88% [4.82%–4.95%]	10.15% [10.02%–10.27%]	6.21 [6.20–6.23]	5.68 [5.66–5.69]	2.19% [2.14%–2.23%]	1.11% [1.07%–1.16%]
Morphine	3.51% [3.45%–3.57%]	6.54% [6.46%–6.62%]	6.83 [6.81–6.85]	6.56 [6.54–6.58]	1.56% [1.52%–1.60%]	0.86% [0.83%–0.89%]
p value	<0.01	<0.01	<0.01	<0.01	<0.01	<0.01

alone who were admitted in the severe and extreme severity of illness categories than those treated with hydromorphone. While this may explain that patients treated with morphine stayed in the hospital longer, the higher rescue drug use and readmission rates in patients treated with hydromorphone alone are not in keeping with this observation. In addition, there are limitations with using 30-day all cause readmission rates because unrelated diseases or acute conditions that may be the cause of an additional hospitalization may be lumped together. Lastly, UHC uses billing data, which has inherent limitations as well. For example, we are unable to differentiate patients that received patient-controlled analgesia in comparison to an intravenous bolus.

The increasing use of hydromorphone over morphine does not appear to be supported by recent literature. Our study highlights that the choice of hydromorphone versus morphine may well influence outcomes such as rescue drug use/rate of adverse events, length of stay, and readmission rates. Further research in risk adjusted models may help further delineate these observations. Specifically, data on the underlying diseases of the patient populations could help provide insight into the relative risk for these patients.

Acknowledgment

The authors acknowledge Robert Hallisey, Pharm.D.

References

[1] The Joint Commission on Accreditation of Healthcare Organizations and The National Pharmaceutical Council, *Pain: Current Understanding of Assessment, Management, and Treatments*, National Pharmaceutical Council, 2001, http://www.npcnow.org/system/files/research/download/Pain-Current-Understanding-of-Assessment-Management-and-Treatments.pdf.

[2] Institute of Medicine Report from the Committee on Advancing Pain Research-Care and Education, *Relieving Pain in America, A Blueprint for Transforming Prevention, Care, Education and Research*, The National Academies Press, Washington, DC, USA, 2011, http://books.nap.edu/openbook.php?record_id=13172&page=1.

[3] APS, "American Pain Society guidelines," 1995.

[4] J. L. Dahl and D. B. Gordon, "Joint Commission pain standards: a progress report," *APS Bulletin*, vol. 12, no. 6, pp. 1–8, 2002.

[5] R. A. Mularski, F. White-Chu, D. Overbay, L. Miller, S. M. Asch, and L. Ganzini, "Measuring pain as the 5th vital sign does not improve quality of pain management," *Journal of General Internal Medicine*, vol. 21, no. 6, pp. 607–612, 2006.

[6] C. D. Fox, D. Berger, P. G. Fine et al., "Pain assessment and treatment in the managed care environment. A position statement from the American Pain Society," *The Case Manager*, vol. 11, no. 5, pp. 50–53, 2000.

[7] H. Vila Jr., R. A. Smith, M. J. Augustyniak et al., "The efficacy and safety of pain management before and after implementation of hospital-wide pain management standards: Is patient safety compromised by treatment based solely on numerical pain ratings?" *Anesthesia and Analgesia*, vol. 101, no. 2, pp. 474–480, 2005.

[8] L. Manchikanti, "Prescription drug abuse: what is being done to address this new drug epidemic? Testimony before the subcommittee on criminal justice, drug policy and human resources," *Pain Physician*, vol. 9, no. 4, pp. 287–321, 2006.

[9] A. K. Chang, P. E. Bijur, R. H. Meyer, M. K. Kenny, C. Solorzano, and E. J. Gallagher, "Safety and efficacy of hydromorphone as an analgesic alternative to morphine in acute pain: a randomized clinical trial," *Annals of Emergency Medicine*, vol. 48, no. 2, pp. 164–172, 2006.

[10] L. Felden, C. Walter, S. Harder et al., "Comparative clinical effects of hydromorphone and morphine: a meta-analysis," *British Journal of Anaesthesia*, vol. 107, no. 3, pp. 319–328, 2011.

[11] D. Hong, P. Flood, and G. Diaz, "The side effects of morphine and hydromorphone patient-controlled analgesia," *Anesthesia and Analgesia*, vol. 107, no. 4, pp. 1384–1389, 2008.

[12] US Department of Justice, *Quotas*, US Department of Justice, Drug Enforcement Administration, Springfield, Va, USA, 2012, http://www.deadiversion.usdoj.gov/quotas/index.html.

[13] E. O. Bryson, "The anesthetic implications of illicit opioid abuse," *International Anesthesiology Clinics*, vol. 49, no. 1, pp. 67–78, 2011.

[14] T. Ogura and T. D. Egan, "Opioid agonists and antagonists," in *Physiology and Pharmacology for Anesthesia: Foundations and Clinical Application*, H. C. Hemmings and T. D. Egan, Eds., pp. 253–271, Elsevier, Philadelphia, Pa, USA, 2013.

[15] C. Quigley, "Hydromorphone for acute and chronic pain (review)," *Cochrane Database of Systematic Reviews (Online)*, no. 1, Article ID CD003447, 2002.

[16] P. A. Glare and T. D. Walsh, "Clinical pharmacokinetics of morphine," *Therapeutic Drug Monitoring*, vol. 13, no. 1, pp. 1–23, 1991.

[17] H. F. Hill, B. A. Coda, A. Tanaka, and R. Schaffer, "Multiple-dose evaluation of intravenous hydromorphone pharmacokinetics in normal human subjects," *Anesthesia & Analgesia*, vol. 72, no. 3, pp. 330–336, 1991.

[18] A. W. E. Wright, L. E. Mather, and M. T. Smith, "Hydromorphone-3-glucuronide: a more potent neuro-excitant than its structural analogue, morphine-3-glucuronide," *Life Sciences*, vol. 69, no. 4, pp. 409–420, 2001.

[19] E. C. Mcnaughton, R. A. Black, M. G. Zulueta, S. H. Budman, and S. F. Butler, "Measuring online endorsement of prescription opioids abuse: an integrative methodology," *Pharmacoepidemiology and Drug Safety*, vol. 21, no. 10, pp. 1081–1092, 2012.

[20] Commonwealth of Massachusetts Board of Registration in Medicine—Quality and Patient Safety Division, "Review of Safety and Quality Reviews Involving Hydromorphone," September 2012, http://www.mass.gov/eohhs/docs/borim/physicians/pca-notifications/dilaudid-advsory.pdf.

[21] Commonwealth of Massachusetts Board of Registration in Medicine—Patient Care Assessment Division, *Hydromorphone Patient Safety Concerns with Hydromorphone versus Morphine*, Commonwealth of Massachusetts Board of Registration in Medicine, Wakefield, Mass, USA, 2007.

[22] Pennsylvania Patient Safety Authority, "Adverse drug events with hydromorphone: how preventable are they?" *Pennsylvania Patient Safety Advisory*, vol. 7, no. 3, pp. 69–75, 2010.

[23] ISMP Canada, "Hydromorphone remains a high-alert drug," *Ontario Critical Incident Learning*, no. 2, pp. 1–2, 2013.

[24] I. Nathanson and E. Daland, "Use of dilaudid in treating patients with cancer," *The New England Journal of Medicine*, vol. 59, pp. 313–316, 1935.

[25] S. J. Herzig, M. B. Rothberg, M. Cheung, L. H. Ngo, and E. R. Marcantonio, "Opioid utilization and opioid-related adverse events in nonsurgical patients in US hospitals," *Journal of Hospital Medicine*, vol. 9, no. 2, pp. 73–81, 2014.

[26] G. M. Oderda, T. J. Gan, B. H. Johnson, and S. B. Robinson, "Effect of opioid-related adverse events on outcomes in selected surgical patients," *Journal of Pain & Palliative Care Pharmacotherapy*, vol. 27, no. 1, pp. 62–70, 2013.

[27] J. F. Whiting, J. Martin, E. Zavala, and D. Hanto, "The influence of clinical variables on hospital costs after orthotopic liver transplantation," *Surgery*, vol. 125, no. 2, pp. 217–222, 1999.

[28] C. Chen and D. Clay Ackerly, "Beyond ACOs and bundled payments medicare's shift toward accountability in fee-for-service," *The Journal of the American Medical Association*, vol. 311, no. 7, pp. 673–674, 2014.

4

Vitamin D and Pain: Vitamin D and Its Role in the Aetiology and Maintenance of Chronic Pain States and Associated Comorbidities

Edward A. Shipton and Elspeth E. Shipton

Department of Anaesthesia, University of Otago, Christchurch, Corner of Riccarton and Hagley Avenues, Christchurch 8042, New Zealand

Correspondence should be addressed to Edward A. Shipton; shiptonea@xtra.co.nz

Academic Editor: Giustino Varrassi

The emergence of new data suggests that the benefits of Vitamin D extend beyond healthy bones. This paper looks at Vitamin D and its role in the aetiology and maintenance of chronic pain states and associated comorbidities. The interfaces between pain and Vitamin D and the mechanisms of action of Vitamin D on pain processes are explored. Finally the association between Vitamin D and pain comorbidities such as sleep and depression is investigated. The paper shows that Vitamin D exerts anatomic, hormonal, neurological, and immunological influences on pain manifestation, thereby playing a role in the aetiology and maintenance of chronic pain states and associated comorbidities. More research is necessary to determine whether Vitamin D is useful in the treatment of various pain conditions and whether or not the effect is limited to patients who are deficient in Vitamin D.

1. Introduction

A recent surge of published data on the proven or potential effects of Vitamin D has raised much interest in the medical community. The primary role of Vitamin D is the regulation of serum calcium levels within a narrow range. Vitamin D plays an essential role in bone formation, maintenance, and remodelling, as well as in muscle function. However, the emergence of new data suggests that the benefits of Vitamin D extend beyond healthy bones. Of great interest is the role it could play in optimising neuromuscular functioning, reducing inflammation, and decreasing the risk of many chronic illnesses; these include a variety of cancers, autoimmune diseases, infectious diseases, and cardiovascular diseases [1–5]. Research has shown that Vitamin D exerts anatomic, hormonal, neurological, and immunological influences on pain manifestation, thereby playing a role in the aetiology and maintenance of chronic pain states and associated comorbidity [1, 6–8].

2. Vitamin D

2.1. Synthesis, Absorption, and Metabolism of Vitamin D. Chemically, Vitamin D is a fat soluble secosteroid (i.e., a steroid in which one of the bonds in the steroid rings is broken). There are various forms of Vitamin D; the most common forms are Vitamin D_3 (cholecalciferol) and Vitamin D_2 (ergocalciferol). Both are collectively known as calciferol. Although it is called a vitamin, Vitamin D is really a hormone as it can be produced endogenously by humans. In the skin, 7-dehydrocholesterol is converted to pre-Vitamin D_3 by a narrow band of solar ultraviolet radiation (290–320 nm) that undergoes isomerisation in a temperature-dependent manner to Vitamin D_3. Ten thousand to 20,000 IU of Vitamin D can be produced in 30 minutes of whole-body exposure to sunlight. This endogenously produced Vitamin D enters the blood and binds with Vitamin D binding protein (DBP), facilitating transportation to the liver [1, 5]. Vitamin D can also be obtained from a limited number of dietary sources.

Vitamin D_2 (ergocalciferol) is produced by some kinds of plants and animals when ergosterol is altered by ultraviolet irradiation. However, few foods have naturally occurring substantial Vitamin D_2 levels to make this a significant source of Vitamin D in humans.

Vitamin D from the skin and diet is hydroxylated in the liver by one of several cytochrome P450 enzymes to the prehormone 25-hydroxy Vitamin D [calcidiol, or 25(OH)D] that is encoded by the gene CYP27A1 [2, 5, 9]. Most circulating 25(OH)D and the active form of Vitamin D, namely, 1,25-dihydroxyvitamin D [$1,25(OH)_2D$], are transported in the blood bound to Vitamin D binding protein (DBP) (80–90%) and to albumin (10–20%); only a small fraction remains free or unbound [10]. The 25(OH)D can be taken up by one of two mechanisms, namely, diffusion of free 25(OH)D across cell membranes throughout the body or a DBP receptor mediated endocytosis by the coreceptors megalin and cubulin [5]. It appears that endocytic transportation may be influenced by certain pathological and physiological determinants [11–13]. The amount of DBP and its effect on free versus bound 25(OH)D could inversely influence the available free 25(OH)D for uptake [5]. The primary determinant of how long a Vitamin D metabolite will stay in circulation is its affinity for DBP [14]. Further research is needed to understand the regulation of mobilization of 25(OH)D from lipid storage pools relative to health outcomes.

However, Vitamin D can also be hydroxylated to 25(OH)D in all tissues of the body, achieving autocrine production of 25(OH)D in these tissues [14]. 25(OH)D is then further metabolised in the kidneys and possibly in a wide variety of extrarenal tissues by the enzyme 25-hydroxyvitamin D-1α-hydroxylase (CYP27B1) to its active form, namely, 1,25-dihydroxyvitamin D [$1,25(OH)_2D_3$]. Vitamin D exerts its effects by modulating gene expression after binding to VDR. There appear to be potential genetic polymorphisms in key genes with Vitamin D exposure that can influence bioavailability, transport, and distribution in lipid storage pools, metabolism, and action of Vitamin D [5].

3. Pain

Pain is part of the human condition. Pain is defined by the International Association for the Study of Pain (IASP) as "an unpleasant sensory and emotional experience associated with actual or potential tissue damage, or described by the patient in terms of such damage" [15]. Pain is essentially a subjective perceptual experience. Pain originates in the nociceptors of the nervous system but the experience of pain is perceived in the conscious brain. It is influenced by a complex interaction of behavioural, environmental, biological, and societal factors.

There are two broad categories of pain, namely, acute nociceptive pain which acts as an early warning sign and pathological persistent pain, which is essentially an ongoing false alarm [16, 17].

Acute pain is a sensation that is elicited after strong stimulation of tissues in the body. Nociception relates to the biochemical and neural changes that occur in response to a noxious stimulus [18]. This stimulation causes action potentials in primary sensory neurones known as nociceptors. These nociceptors are activated by high-threshold stimuli (mechanical, thermal, chemical, or electrical) to transmit excitatory signals to the sensory cell bodies in the dorsal root ganglion (DRG) along the dorsal roots and subsequently into the spinal cord [16, 19]. In the spinal cord, these primary sensory nerve fibres release neurotransmitters such as amino acids (glutamate) and neuropeptides (such as substance P and calcitonin gene related peptide) that activate second-order neurones. The second-order neurones relay information via specific tracts that reach the thalamus where the sensation of pain occurs. Third-order neurones connecting the thalamus to the somatosensory cortex are activated, resulting in the perception of pain [16, 20].

Nociceptors are present in most tissues in the body, including skin, muscle, joints, and viscera. There are predominantly two types of nociceptors involved in the pain pathway, namely, C fibres and A-delta fibres. The thin, myelinated A-delta fibres are fast transmitting; they are activated by both mechanical and thermal stimuli [18]. The unmyelinated C fibres respond to chemical, thermal, and mechanical stimuli. C fibres in the viscera are notable in that they respond to noxious stimuli such as the stretching of hollow organs.

The International Association for the Study of Pain (IASP) defines chronic pain as "pain that has persisted beyond normal tissue healing time." This is taken (in absence of other criteria) to be 3 months [21]. However, some chronic pain disorders are characterised by recurrent short acute episodes and exacerbations such as trigeminal neuralgia and rheumatoid arthritis.

Chronic pain can be produced after tissue damage (or inflammation), after nerve damage, and after alteration of normal neural function. Chronic persistent pain leads to chemical, functional, and anatomical changes throughout the nervous system (in the periphery, spinal cord, and brain) [22–24]. The concept of neuroplasticity (the ability of the brain to change its structure and function) can be a positive adaptation to loss of function; in the case of pain, it appears maladaptive [25]. Persistent pain alters the nervous system to produce spontaneous pain that arises without any apparent peripheral stimulus as well as a hypersensitivity to peripheral stimuli [16, 17, 26]. Pain hypersensitivity can result in hyperalgesia (the exaggerated and prolonged response to noxious stimulation) and allodynia (pain resulting from a stimulus that is normally nonpainful) [27]. The reduced descending inhibition in the central nervous system (CNS) results in more peripheral noxious signals getting through to the brain resulting in an increased experience of pain [28].

The transition from acute to chronic pain is not well understood and appears to be multifactorial [29]. Nociceptive pain usually (but not always) reduces with healing. While persistent pain is often due to obvious nerve damage (e.g., injury or cancer), there are many instances when no physical pathology can be objectively verified, such as in fibromyalgia syndrome and in headaches. In general, chronic pain may involve a combination of nociceptive and neuropathic mechanisms, as well as some form of central sensitization and learnt response. The concept of central sensitization is becoming more widely recognised, whereby changes occurring within the nervous system result in previously nonnoxious stimuli being perceived as painful, a lowering of the threshold for pain generation, and an increase in the duration, amplitude, and spatial distribution of pain [23]. In addition, central sensitization initiates the interrelationship between many pain problems such as fibromyalgia, irritable bowel, low back pain, and chronic daily headache [30]. Inflammatory and nerve injury are involved in the aetiology of many chronic pain syndromes like osteoarthritis, diabetic neuropathy, or postherpetic neuralgia, but only a small proportion of those subjected to such injuries actually develop chronic pain, and the degree of pain severity can vary significantly between patients [31].

Evidence from large scale studies in Europe, North America, and Australasia has shown that about one in five of the adult population experiences chronic moderate to severe pain with other estimates indicating the prevalence of chronic pain to be closer to 20–25% [32–34]. The incidence of chronic pain can be higher in at-risk groups such as the elderly and the immune-compromised [35, 36]. The rate of persistent severe pain among all residents of United States nursing homes in 1999 was found to be 14.7%, with 41.2% of residents in pain at first assessment experiencing severe pain 60 to 180 days later [37].

The prevalence of chronic pain is projected to increase as the population ages (from around 3.2 million Australians in 2007 to 5.0 million by 2050) [38]. Life-style changes leading to obesity and inactivity will also contribute to increased level of pain in developed countries.

4. Interfaces of Pain and Vitamin D

Clinical research in the area of chronic pain and Vitamin D deficiency remains limited. There is a dearth of large double blind randomised controlled studies. However, there is enough evidence showing the potential of Vitamin D to exert anatomic and physiological influences on pain manifestation, thereby playing a role in the aetiology and maintenance of chronic pain states and associated comorbidity [1, 6]. Persistent pain is associated with Vitamin D-related bone demineralization, myopathy, and musculoskeletal pain. Pain pathways associated with cortical, immunological, hormonal, and neuronal changes are potentially also influenced by Vitamin D levels.

Vitamin D levels have been found to be low in certain groups of patients with various pain states (Box 1) [39–43]. Studies of Vitamin D supplementation in patients with known Vitamin D deficiency have shown mixed results in chronic pain patients regarding improved pain scores (Box 1) [6, 9, 44–51]. The prevalence of a variety of pain states at particular latitudes has been linked to low levels of Vitamin D [52–54]. Seasonal variations correspond with varying pain levels as well [6]. Vitamin D deficiency has been associated with headache, abdominal, knee, and back pain, persistent musculoskeletal pain, costochondritic chest pain, and failed back syndrome and with fibromyalgia [6, 45, 53–59].

Long-term Vitamin D deficiencies have been linked to a weakened immune system and to chronic inflammation [2–4, 60]. Chronic inflammation, in turn, leads to debilitating health conditions; many of these are characterised by pain as the disabling symptom [60]. Serum Vitamin D deficiency [25(OH)D] is considered a risk factor for type 1 diabetes, multiple sclerosis, and especially autoimmune rheumatic diseases (ARD) (Box 1). The severity of systemic lupus erythematosus and rheumatoid arthritis has been associated with serum Vitamin D deficiency [61, 62].

Vitamin D deficiency has been linked to other diseases that present with pain as a symptom. Cystic fibrosis patients experience chronic pain in a variety of sites (head, sinuses, back, and chest) [63]. Individuals with cystic fibrosis are at risk of Vitamin D deficiency due to limited sun exposure and malabsorption. Low bone density and osteopaenia appear to contribute to chronic pain in cystic fibrosis patients and are potentially related to low $25(OH)_2D_3$ levels [63, 64].

Gender differences may be related to Vitamin D deficiency associated with chronic pain. In one large study, prevalence of chronic widespread pain varied by 25(OH)D concentration in women but not in men [40]. Racial differences in experimental pain are mediated by differences in the Vitamin D levels [65]. Vitamin D deficiency may be a risk factor for increased knee osteoarthritis pain in black Americans.

Individuals suffering from chronic pain usually experience other comorbidities such as sleep, anxiety, and mood disorders. These conditions can impact on the patient's quality of life to a significant extent, resulting in loss of employment and/or withdrawal from social life. Adequate levels of Vitamin D have been associated with improved quality of life indicators [48, 66–68]. Significant improvements in assessment of sleep, pain levels, well-being, and various aspects of quality of life with Vitamin D supplementation have been shown [48, 66–69].

4.1. Pain Associated with Vitamin D-Related Bone Demineralization. In the absence of bone mineralisation due to Vitamin D deficiency, weight-bearing growing bones (arms and legs) of infants and children become bowed. In infants, rickets may result in delayed closing of the fontanelles and in rib cage deformities [3]. Subtle evidence of rickets in children includes leg pain, delayed age for standing and walking, and delayed growth.

Adult bones undergo a constant state of remodeling. Decreased levels of 25(OH)D facilitate osteoclast genesis with consequent increased bone resorption [9]. Inadequate mineralisation of the collagen matrix due to low calcium and phosphate levels results in osteomalacia. Bone pain and proximal muscle weakness with gait instability are characteristic of osteomalacia [3, 9]. Decreased levels of 25(OH)D have been shown to be directly related to low bone density in the hip [9, 70].

4.2. Pain Associated with Vitamin D Deficiency and Muscle Weakness. Vitamin D deficiency causes muscle weakness and pain in children and adults. Individuals with chronic low back pain have been found to have weaker gluteus medius muscles than control subjects without back pain [71]. The incidence of low back pain is associated with isometric and isokinetic trunk extensor weakness, whereas low back pain severity is

(i) Headache
(ii) Cancer pain
(iii) Persistent musculoskeletal pain and weakness (rickets, osteomalacia, osteopaenia, cystic fibrosis, back pain, knee pain, and costochondritic chest pain)
(iv) Fibromyalgia
(v) Abdominal pain
(vi) Pain associated with ischaemia (sickle cell disease and coronary artery disease)
(vii) Inflammatory pain (rheumatoid arthritis and systemic lupus erythematosus)
(viii) Neuropathic pain (diabetic neuropathy, post herpetic neuropathy, and multiple sclerosis)

Box 1: Interfaces of Vitamin D deficiency and types of persistent pain.

associated with isokinetic trunk extensor and flexor weakness and isometric trunk extensor and flexor weakness [72].

Vitamin D has an important role in the regulation of serum calcium concentration and in muscle protein synthesis. Vitamin D increases the serum calcium level that is essential for muscle contraction; protein synthesis affects muscle growth [73]. This process is mediated by the nuclear vitamin D receptor (VDR) and by a variety of nongenomic effects [74]. VDRs are found in muscle tissue. Vitamin D improves musculoskeletal function by exerting a direct effect on the muscle tissue itself [75, 76]. Vitamin D deficiency primarily affects the faster and stronger type 2 muscle fibres. This may explain why supplementation with Vitamin D improves proximal muscle strength. Hypovitaminosis D impairs neuromuscular coordination, as measured by body sway. It increases the risk of falling and painful fractures related to falls in the elderly [73, 74, 77–80]. It has been postulated that there is a genetic predisposition to the decline in strength in elderly women that is linked to the VDR [81].

Musculoskeletal pain related to osteomalacia may probably be due to spongy matrix formation under the periosteal membranes caused by demineralization of the bone [82]. This gelatin-like collagen matrix can expand when it becomes hydrated; it causes outward pressure on periosteal tissues that are richly innervated with sensory pain fibres. This pressure results in a throbbing, aching bone pain [82].

4.3. Mechanisms of Action of Vitamin D on Pain Processes. There are a number of mechanisms involved in the development of neuropathic pain after peripheral nerve damage (Box 2). These include ectopic excitability of sensory neurones, altered gene expression of sensory neurones, and sensitisation of neurones in the dorsal horn of the spinal cord [27]. These mechanisms are influenced by a number of biological and psychosocial factors. Neurotransmitters such as glutamate, substance P, serotonin, and gamma-aminobutyric acid (GABA) as well as glial inflammation are central to the excitatory and inhibitory influences on pain.

Inflammatory pain and neuropathic pain may depend on the action of diverse cytokines and other molecules; these include eicosanoids, endorphins, calcitonin-gene-related peptides (CGRP), and transcription factors. Because steroid compounds (including hormonal steroids, neurosteroids, and synthetic analogues of neuroactive steroids) control the plasticity of the nervous system, these compounds are of particular interest in the modulation of pain [83].

4.3.1. Vitamin D as a Neuroactive Steroid. Vitamin D can modulate neuronal excitability similar to that of other neuroactive steroids (Box 2) [84]. This includes spontaneous regular firing, action potential duration, intrinsic excitability, and sensitivity to neurotransmitters as well as to neurotransmitter receptors such as GABA receptor and N-methyl-D-aspartate (NMDA) receptor [85–87]. Steroid hormones influence the electrical activity of many neurones and effectors by regulating transcription of their ion channels and neurotransmitter receptors, or by modulating the activity of their channels and receptors through second messenger-coupled membrane receptors [85]. Vitamin D as a neuroactive steroid activates a variety of signal transduction systems. These include calcium ion influx, the release of calcium ions from intracellular stores, the modulation of adenylate cyclase, phospholipase C (PLC), protein kinase C, protein kinase D, the mitogen-activated protein (MAP) kinases, and the rapidly accelerated fibrosarcoma (Raf) kinase pathways [88]. As a steroid, Vitamin D modulates brain neurotransmitters (acetylcholine, dopamine, and serotonin) as well [84].

4.3.2. Vitamin D and Neurotrophins. Vitamin D upregulates the synthesis of neurotrophins such as neural growth factor (NGF), neurotrophin 3 (NT3), and glial cell line-derived neurotrophic factor (GDNF), whereas neurotrophin 4 (NT4) is downregulated (Box 2) [89–92]. Through this system, Vitamin D can potentially affect the development, maintenance, and survival of neurones. NGF is a well-established inflammatory mediator. It has direct effects on the sensory nerve endings causing hypersensitivity, amplification of sensory input signals, and enhanced innervation of injured tissue [93–95]. In the diabetic neuropathic pain model, Vitamin D supplementation has been shown to increase NGF production and prevent neurotrophic deficits [91]. There is some evidence that Vitamin D exercises a neuroprotective function by attenuating the effects of glucocorticoids and by modulating neuronal calcium ion homeostasis [96, 97].

VDRs have been localised in neurones and in glial cells [98]. Genes encoding the enzymes involved in the metabolism of Vitamin D are expressed in brain cells [98]. It has been suggested that the local synthesis of $1, 25(OH)_2D_3$

(i) Vitamin D as a neuroactive steroid modulates neuronal excitability and brain neurotransmitters and activates a variety of signal transduction systems
(ii) Vitamin D influences prostaglandin action by inhibiting COX-2 expression and by stimulating 15-prostaglandin dehydrogenase (15-PGDH) expression that degrades prostaglandins that would have lowered the firing threshold of sensory neurones
(iii) Vitamin D inhibits synthesis of nitric oxide synthase (iNOS), the enzyme that produces nitric oxide (NO, a neurotransmitter involved in nociceptive process that contributes to development of central sensitization) in macrophages that activate microglia and astrocytes
(iv) VDR, 1α-hydroxylase, and vitamin D binding protein in the hypothalamus are suggested as mechanism by which Vitamin D deficiency is implicated in pathophysiology of various primary headache disorders
(v) Vitamin D upregulates synthesis of neurotrophins affecting development, maintenance, and survival of neurones
(vi) Vitamin D affects a number of inflammatory pathways associated with chronic pain by upregulating transforming growth factor beta 1 (TGF-β1) in astrocytes and microglia that suppresses activity of various cytokines
(vii) Vitamin D suppresses tumour necrosis factor alpha (TNF-α) and macrophage colony-stimulating factor (M-CSF) in astrocytes and microglia and inhibits pain pathways
(viii) Vitamin D inhibits T-helper cell over activity and plays an important role in preventing autoimmune diseases

Box 2: Mechanisms of action of Vitamin D on pain processes.

by microglia could stimulate an antitumour response; this is because 1,25$(OH)_2D_3$ causes cell death and redifferentiation programs in glioma cells [92].

In other circumstances, microglia contribute to neuropathic pain after peripheral nerve injury [93, 99–101]. Vitamin D plays a fundamental role in astrocyte detoxification pathways, thereby exerting a neuroprotective effect [90]. Vitamin D increases the synthesis of several neurotrophins in astrocytes; these include NGF, NT3, and GDNF and γ-glutamyl transpeptidase (another mechanism involved in neuroprotection) [92].

4.3.3. Vitamin D and Prostaglandins. Vitamin D influences prostaglandin action by inhibiting COX-2 expression and by stimulating 15-prostaglandin dehydrogenase (15-PGDH) expression [102]. The enzyme 15-PGDH degrades prostaglandins and inhibits prostaglandin-E2 receptor (PGE2) subtypes and prostaglandin-F2 alpha receptor subtypes (Box 2) [102]. Prostaglandins have a direct effect on sensory neurones by lowering the firing threshold, increasing the number of action potentials elicited by a depolarizing stimulus, and enhancing SP and CGRP release [103]. Prostaglandins mediate neuropathic pain in the spinal cord via PGE2 depolarising wide dynamic range neurones [27].

4.3.4. Vitamin D Effects on Inflammatory Pathways. Vitamin D is known to affect a number of inflammatory pathways associated with the development and persistence of chronic pain (Box 2). Vitamin D upregulates transforming growth factor beta 1 (TGF-β1) and interleukin-4 (IL-4) found in astrocytes and microglia [92]. TGF-β1 suppresses the activity of various cytokines, namely, interferon-γ, TNF-α, and various T cells such as interleukin-1 (IL-1) and interleukin-2 (IL-2). It can downregulate the activity of immune cells through suppression of cytokine receptors (such as the IL-2 receptor) [104].

Vitamin D suppresses TNF-α and macrophage colony-stimulating factor (M-CSF) in astrocytes and microglia [92]. TNF-α has been convincingly implicated at both peripheral and central levels of sensitization [105]. M-CSF is a cytokine that stimulates proliferation, differentiation, and survival of monocytes and macrophages. Macrophages can release many inflammatory mediators, including proinflammatory cytokines, particularly TNF-α and interleukin-1-beta (IL-1β), NGF, NO (nitric oxide), and prostanoids [93]. By limiting M-CSF, Vitamin D has the potential to inhibit pain pathways.

4.3.5. Vitamin D and Nitric Oxide Synthase. Vitamin D has also been found to inhibit the synthesis of nitric oxide synthase (iNOS), the enzyme that produces nitric oxide (NO), in macrophages that activates microglia and astrocytes at both protein and m-RNA levels (Box 2) [106]. NO is an important neurotransmitter involved in the nociceptive process; in the dorsal horn of the spinal cord, it contributes to the development of central sensitization [107]. Astrocytes play a pivotal role in central nervous system (CNS) detoxification pathways, where glutathione (GSH) is involved in the elimination of nitric oxide. The activity of gamma-glutamyl transpeptidase (gamma-GT), an enzyme of central significance in GSH metabolism, has been shown to be regulated by 1,25-dihydroxyvitamin D_3 [1,25$(OH)_2D_3$] causes cell death [108]. The inhibition of iNOS by Vitamin D is a potential mechanism for reducing pain and neuronal damage after injury or in diseases such as ischaemia, Parkinson's disease, and acquired immune-deficiency syndrome (AIDS) [92, 93].

4.3.6. Vitamin D and T-Helper Cells. Several immune cell types contribute to peripheral neuropathy and to the development of neuropathic pain. Mast cells are released by injured nerves; they appear to reduce the recruitment of neutrophils and monocytes into the injured nerve, potentially reducing the release of chemokines and other mediators. Vitamin D downregulates neutrophil function [109]. Neutrophils produce various inflammatory factors (lipoxygenase products, nitric oxide, and cytokines) [93]. High levels of neutrophils are released after tissue injury and are linked to the development of symptoms of neuropathic pain [110]. The hyperalgesic actions of NGF appear to be partly dependent on neutrophil accumulation [93]. Vitamin D inhibits T-helper cell overactivity and plays an important role in the prevention of autoimmune diseases (Box 2) [111].

4.3.7. Vitamin D Receptor (VDR) and 1α-Hydroxylase. VDR and 1α-hydroxylase [the enzyme that converts 25(OH)D by hydroxylation to the active $1,25(OH)_2D_3$] are found in many areas of the human central nervous system. These include the prefrontal cortex, amygdala, raphe, substantia gelatinosa, cerebellum, hippocampus, cingulate gyrus, substantia nigra, thalamus, and hypothalamus [84]. Both the receptor and the enzyme have been demonstrated in neuronal and glial cells as well [112]. In the rat model, Vitamin D binding protein has been found in axonal projections in the lateral hypothalamus [113]. The presence of VDRs, 1α-hydroxylase, and Vitamin D binding protein in the hypothalamus is suggested as the mechanism by which Vitamin D deficiency is implicated in the pathophysiology of various primary headache disorders (Box 2) [52].

5. Vitamin D Associated with Pain Comorbidities (Sleep and Depression)

Anatomical and the functional colocalization of central serotonergic, noradrenergic, and dopaminergic systems involved in pain, sleep, Vitamin D, and depression also tend to point to some interconnectivity (Box 3). The enzyme 1 alpha-hydroxylase which converts 25-OHD to the active Vitamin D is present in the hypothalamus, cerebellum, and substantia nigra, areas that are also associated with depression. VDRs are widespread in the human central nervous system, including neurones and glia in many areas of the cingulated cortex and hippocampus, which have been implicated in the pathophysiology of depression [114]. Vitamin D receptors are also present in the anterior and posterior hypothalamus, substantia nigra, midbrain periaqueductal gray (PAG), raphe nuclei, and the nuclei reticularis pontis oralis and caudalis. These same areas play a role in the initiation and maintenance of sleep. Vitamin D's effects on these brain areas may be linked to sleep modulation [115].

There appears to be considerable overlap in the effects of sleep, pain, depression, and Vitamin D on the immune system. Vitamin D could be linked to depression, sleep, and chronic pain by mediating effects of immune cells such as astrocytes and macrophages (Box 3) [90, 92]. Vitamin D directly affects T cell responses inhibiting the production of IL-2, interleukin-17 (IL-17), and interleukin-21 (IL-21) and by stimulating interleukin-4 (IL-4) production [116].

Chronic sleep loss impairs immune function. This results in increases in proinflammatory mediators such as cytokines and chemokines [117, 118]. Cytokines (especially IL-1beta and TNF-α) are implicated in the regulation of sleep and modulation of sleep architecture and appear to be involved in circadian regulation of sleep [118–121].

There are suggestions of a bidirectional feedback loop between sleep and cytokine expression [118]. Insufficient sleep quantity may facilitate or exacerbate pain through elevations of interleukin-6 (IL-6) [122]. In disorders where sleep disturbances are common, insufficient sleep quantity itself may establish and maintain its cooccurrence with pain and with increased inflammation [122]. Vitamin D deficiency could contribute to poor quality sleep or symptoms of impaired wakefulness by inducing a relative elevation of circulating TNF-α and nuclear factor kappa-light-chain-enhancer of activated B cells (NFκB), both of which can result in subjective feeling of sleepiness [123].

Patients with depressive symptoms and with pain disorders display enhanced cytokine levels. These include IL-6, C-reactive protein (CRP), IL-1B, and TNF-α [124]. Major depression may be accompanied by systemic immune activation or an inflammatory response with involvement of phagocytic (monocytes, neutrophils) cells, T cell activation, increased prostaglandin secretion, and increased production of IL-1β and IL-6 by peripheral blood mononuclear cells [125]. Cytokines also play a central role in the generation and transmission of pain with increased levels of TNF-α and IL-1, IL-2, and IL-6, and decreased levels of IL-4 and IL-10 [126, 127]. Cytokines have been shown to modulate the central metabolism of serotonin and dopamine [128].

IL-1 stimulates the synthesis and/or release of growth hormone releasing hormone, prostaglandin-D_2, adenosine, and nitric oxide. These are substances that are implicated in regulation of non-REM sleep [117]. Vitamin D has been shown to downregulate these substances [106]. Vitamin D, chronic pain, sleep, and depression are intimately linked to the nervous, endocrine, metabolic, and immune systems of the body and their mediators. These mediators include neurotransmitters, neuropeptides, hormones, and cytokines [117, 119, 129].

There are four key neurotransmitters involved in Vitamin D, pain, and depression, namely, serotonin, noradrenaline, substance P, and dopamine. Serotonin levels are typically low in depressed patients [130, 131]. Serotonin can have pronociceptive or antinociceptive effects, depending on the receptor subtype and location in the central nervous system. Serotonin can be pronociceptive in the periphery, whereas the primary antinociceptive effects of serotonin are thought to occur via receptors located centrally in the descending antinociceptive pathways [132].

Chronic sleep loss has also been shown to have an effect on a variety of neurotransmitters involved in sleep regulation via increase in IL-1 [117]. IL-1 inhibits acetylcholine release and can potentiate or inhibit the effects of glutamate and has been linked to the stimulation of adenosine and monoamine release, thereby playing a role in sleep homeostasis [117, 119]. IL-1 and TNF also interact with the serotonin system to enhance non-REM sleep [133]. IL-1 reduces the firing rate of wake-active serotonergic neurones by potentiating the inhibitory effects of gamma-aminobutyric acid (GABA) [134]. IL-1 in the preoptic area (POA) of the hypothalamus and the adjoining magnocellular basal forebrain (BF) appears to be controlled by corticosteroids released into the blood by the adrenal cortex. Corticosteroid levels depend on the activity of the hypothalamic–pituitary–adrenal axis that is stimulated by the activation of the serotonin pathway [117]. As mentioned previously, IL-1 and TNF have a direct action sensitising nociceptors, enhancing excitatory currents, and reducing inhibitory pain pathways [135].

(i) Anatomical colocalization and functional interaction of central serotonergic, noradrenergic, and dopaminergic systems.
(ii) Inhibition or potentiation of other neurotransmitters such as substance P, acetylcholine, glutamate, adenosine, GABA, and monoamine.
(iii) Mediation of immune cells such as astrocytes, macrophages, and phagocytic (monocytes, neutrophils) cells.
(iv) Immune system modulation of proinflammatory mediators such as cytokines and chemokines, especially IL-1beta and TNF-α, and including NFκB, IL-2, IL-6, and CRP.
(v) Immune system modulation of T cell responses inhibiting the production of IL-2, IL-17, and IL-21, and by stimulating IL-4 and IL-10 production.
(vi) Immune system modulation via synthesis and/or release of growth hormone releasing hormone, prostaglandin-D_2, adenosine, and NO.
(vii) Influence on the hypothalamus–pituitary–adrenal axis and corticosteroid levels

Box 3: Potential interfaces of Vitamin D, pain, sleep, and depression.

Dopamine is integral to the regulation of sleep and wake [136, 137]. Dopamine has been shown to moderate motivation and reward-related behaviour that are typically disrupted in depression [138]. Dopamine also appears to have an antinociceptive effect at both spinal and supraspinal levels. It has an important role in descending inhibition of pain pathways [139].

The reduced synthesis of dopamine in the nucleus accumbens during prolonged exposure to unavoidable stress results in the development of persistent hyperalgesia [140]. Low dopamine levels have been associated with painful symptoms related to fibromyalgia as well [139].

It has also been suggested that serotonergic raphe cells involved in alertness become dysregulated during chronic pain and contribute to sleep disruption and sleep loss [136, 141]. Sleep deprivation has been shown in preclinical studies to dysregulate endogenous opioid systems and reduce the analgesic efficacy of mu-opioid receptor agonists, thereby modulating pain systems [142, 143]. Acetylcholine, adenosine, and GABA are all known to modulate sleep and pain [144]. The pontine reticular formation plays a key role in rapid eye movement (REM) sleep generation and may regulate central-pain processing mechanisms [144, 145].

Depressed patients showed reduced cerebrospinal fluid levels of noradrenaline [146]. Noradrenaline primarily has an antinociceptive effect on the alpha-2 adrenoreceptors in the descending pain pathways centrally by reducing the sensitivity of the dorsal horn neurones to noxious stimuli [147]. However, like serotonin, noradrenaline can also have a lesser pronociceptive effect on the periphery in sympathetically mediated pain [148].

Substance P has been shown to be an important neurotransmitter in pain and depression [149]. Raised cerebral spinal fluid (CSF) levels of substance P have been found in patients with depression [124]. Substance P contributes to central sensitization in persistent pain [149, 150]. Since substance P has been found to be to be present in central serotonergic, noradrenergic, and dopaminergic systems, researchers believe that it may be an important modulator in depression and pain [124].

Proinflammatory cytokines potently activate the hypothalamus–pituitary–adrenal axis [151]. This effect is usually attributed to increased production of corticotrophin-releasing factor (CRF) [151]. CRF appears to have an important role in both depression and pain. Raised levels of CRF have been linked to melancholic depression [152]. CRF has also been shown to be antinociceptive in the central nervous system as well as in the periphery [153]. A hyperactive hypothalamus–pituitary–adrenal (HPA) axis is often associated with clinical depression [151]. Vitamin D modulates this axis by regulating adrenaline, noradrenaline, and dopamine production through VDRs in the adrenal cortex and protects against the depletion of dopamine and serotonin centrally.

6. Conclusion

In summary, low Vitamin D levels are implicated in various chronic pain conditions. Research has shown that Vitamin D exerts anatomic, hormonal, neurological, and immunological influences on pain manifestation, thereby playing a role in the aetiology and maintenance of chronic pain states and associated comorbidity [1, 6–8]. More research is necessary to determine whether Vitamin D is useful in the treatment of various pain conditions and whether or not the effect is limited to patients who are deficient in Vitamin D [43].

References

[1] M. F. Holick, "Vitamin D deficiency," *The New England Journal of Medicine*, vol. 357, no. 3, pp. 266–281, 2007.

[2] K. K. Deeb, D. L. Trump, and C. S. Johnson, "Vitamin D signalling pathways in cancer: potential for anticancer therapeutics," *Nature Reviews Cancer*, vol. 7, no. 9, pp. 684–700, 2007.

[3] T. D. Thacher and B. L. Clarke, "Vitamin D insufficiency," *Mayo Clinic Proceedings*, vol. 86, no. 1, pp. 50–60, 2011.

[4] K. L. Munger, L. I. Levin, B. W. Hollis, N. S. Howard, and A. Ascherio, "Serum 25-hydroxyvitamin D levels and risk of multiple sclerosis," *Journal of the American Medical Association*, vol. 296, no. 23, pp. 2832–2838, 2006.

[5] P. M. Brannon, "Key questions in Vitamin D research," *Scandinavian Journal of Clinical and Laboratory Investigation Supplementum*, vol. 243, pp. 154–162, 2012.

[6] G. A. Plotnikoff and J. M. Quigley, "Prevalence of severe hypovitaminosis D in patients with persistent, nonspecific musculoskeletal pain," *Mayo Clinic Proceedings*, vol. 78, no. 12, pp. 1463–1470, 2003.

[7] M. Cutolo, S. Paolino, A. Sulli, V. Smith, C. Pizzorni, and B. Seriolo, "Vitamin D, steroid hormones, and autoimmunity," *Annals of the New York Academy of Sciences*, vol. 1317, no. 1, pp. 39–46, 2014.

[8] C. A. S. Jesus, D. Feder, and M. F. P. Peres, "The role of vitamin D in pathophysiology and treatment of fibromyalgia," *Current Pain and Headache Reports*, vol. 17, no. 8, p. 355, 2013.

[9] J. S. Adams and M. Hewison, "Update in vitamin D," *The Journal of Clinical Endocrinology and Metabolism*, vol. 95, no. 2, pp. 471–478, 2010.

[10] J. Zerwekh, "Blood biomarkers of vitamin D status 1, 2, 3, 4," *The American Journal of Clinical Nutrition*, vol. 87, no. 4, pp. 1087S–1091S, 2008.

[11] O. A. Gressner, B. Lahme, and A. M. Gressner, "Gc-globulin (vitamin D binding protein) is synthesized and secreted by hepatocytes and internalized by hepatic stellate cells through Ca^{2+}-dependent interaction with the megalin/gp330 receptor," *Clinica Chimica Acta*, vol. 390, no. 1-2, pp. 28–37, 2008.

[12] G. J. Atkins, P. H. Anderson, D. M. Findlay et al., "Metabolism of vitamin D3 in human osteoblasts: evidence for autocrine and paracrine activities of 1 alpha, 25-dihydroxyvitamin D3," *Bone*, vol. 40, no. 6, pp. 1517–1528, 2007.

[13] T. E. Willnow and A. Nykjaer, "Cellular uptake of steroid carrier proteins—mechanisms and implications," *Molecular and Cellular Endocrinology*, vol. 316, no. 1, pp. 93–102, 2010.

[14] B. W. Hollis and C. L. Wagner, "The role of the parent compound vitamin D with respect to metabolism and function: why clinical dose intervals can affect clinical outcomes," *Journal of Clinical Endocrinology and Metabolism*, vol. 98, no. 12, pp. 4619–4628, 2013.

[15] H. Merskey and N. Bogduk, *Classification of Chronic Pain: Descriptions of Chronic Pain Syndromes and Definitions of Pain Terms*, IASP Press, Seattle, Wash, USA, 2nd edition, 1994.

[16] A. Basbaum, C. Bushnell, and M. Devor, "Pain: basic mechanisms," in *Pain 2005: An Updated Review: Refresher Course Syllabus*, D. Justins, Ed., pp. 3–12, IASP Press, Seattle, Wash, USA, 2005.

[17] C. J. Woolf and Q. Ma, "Nociceptors-noxious stimulus detectors," *Neuron*, vol. 55, no. 3, pp. 353–364, 2007.

[18] P. Suchdev, "Pathophysiology of pain," in *Manual of Pain Management*, C. Warfield and H. Fausett, Eds., pp. 6–10, Lippincott Williams & Wilkins, Philadelphia, Pa, USA, 2nd edition, 2002.

[19] F. Porrec, "Nociceptors, the spinal dorsal horn, and descending modulation," in *Pain 2012: Refresher Courses, 14th World Congress on Pain*, I. Tracey, Ed., pp. 3–14, IASP Press, Seattle, DC, USA, 2012.

[20] T. W. Vanderah, "Pathophysiology of pain," *The Medical Clinics of North America*, vol. 91, no. 1, pp. 1–12, 2007.

[21] International Association for the Study of Pain, "Classification of chronic pain," *Pain*, supplement 3, pp. S1–S226, 1986.

[22] F. Seifert and C. Maihöfner, "Functional and structural imaging of pain-induced neuroplasticity," *Current Opinion in Anaesthesiology*, vol. 24, no. 5, pp. 515–523, 2011.

[23] A. Latremoliere and C. J. Woolf, "Central sensitization: a generator of pain hypersensitivity by central neural plasticity," *Journal of Pain*, vol. 10, no. 9, pp. 895–926, 2009.

[24] H. Flor, T. Elbert, S. Knecht et al., "Phantom-limb pain as a perceptual correlate of cortical reorganization following arm amputation," *Nature*, vol. 375, no. 6531, pp. 482–484, 1995.

[25] P. J. Siddall, "Neuroplasticity and pain: what does it all mean?" *Medical Journal of Australia*, vol. 198, no. 4, pp. 177–178, 2013.

[26] C. Stein, "Opioids, sensory systems and chronic pain," *European Journal of Pharmacology*, vol. 716, no. 1–3, pp. 179–187, 2013.

[27] G. Moalem and D. J. Tracey, "Immune and inflammatory mechanisms in neuropathic pain," *Brain Research Reviews*, vol. 51, no. 2, pp. 240–264, 2006.

[28] P. J. Siddall and M. J. Cousins, "Persistent pain as a disease entity: implications for clinical management," *Anesthesia and Analgesia*, vol. 99, no. 2, pp. 510–520, 2004.

[29] E. A. Shipton, "The transition from acute to chronic post surgical pain," *Anaesthesia and Intensive Care*, vol. 39, no. 5, pp. 824–836, 2011.

[30] C. J. Woolf, "Central sensitization: Implications for the diagnosis and treatment of pain," *Pain*, vol. 152, no. 3, pp. S2–S15, 2011.

[31] I. Belfer, "Nature and nurture of human pain," *Scientifica*, vol. 2013, Article ID 415279, 19 pages, 2013.

[32] F. M. Blyth, L. M. March, A. J. M. Brnabic, L. R. Jorm, M. Williamson, and M. J. Cousins, "Chronic pain in Australia: a prevalence study," *Pain*, vol. 89, no. 2-3, pp. 127–134, 2001.

[33] H. Breivik, B. Collett, V. Ventafridda, R. Cohen, and D. Gallacher, "Survey of chronic pain in Europe: prevalence, impact on daily life, and treatment," *European Journal of Pain*, vol. 10, no. 4, pp. 287–333, 2006.

[34] D. Hoy, C. Bain, G. Williams et al., "A systematic review of the global prevalence of low back pain," *Arthritis and Rheumatism*, vol. 64, no. 6, pp. 2028–2037, 2012.

[35] A. Abdulla, N. Adams, M. Bone et al., "Guidance on the management of pain in older people," *Age and Ageing*, vol. 42, supplement 1, pp. 1–57, 2013.

[36] P. M. Grace, M. R. Hutchinson, S. F. Maier, and L. R. Watkins, "Pathological pain and the neuroimmune interface," *Nature Reviews Immunology*, vol. 14, no. 4, pp. 217–231, 2014.

[37] J. M. Teno, S. Weitzen, T. Wetle, and V. Mor, "Persistent pain in nursing home residents," *The Journal of the American Medical Association*, vol. 285, no. 16, p. 2081, 2081.

[38] *Economics A. The High Price of Pain: The Economic Impact of Persistent Pain in Australia*, MBF Foundation, 2007.

[39] P. L. Kaza and T. Moulton, "Severe vitamin D deficiency in a patient with sickle cell disease: a case study with literature review," *Journal of Pediatric Hematology/Oncology*, vol. 36, no. 4, pp. 293–296, 2014.

[40] K. Atherton, D. J. Berry, T. Parsons, G. J. Macfarlane, C. Power, and E. Hyppönen, "Vitamin D and chronic widespread pain in a white middle-aged British population: evidence from a cross-sectional population survey," *Annals of the Rheumatic Diseases*, vol. 68, no. 6, pp. 817–822, 2009.

[41] S. Straube, S. Derry, R. A. Moore, and H. J. McQuay, "Vitamin D for the treatment of chronic painful conditions in adults," *The Cochrane Database of Systematic Reviews*, no. 1, Article ID CD007771, 2010.

[42] J. Bartley, "Prevalence of vitamin D deficiency among patients attending a multidisciplinary tertiary pain clinic," *New Zealand Medical Journal*, vol. 121, no. 1286, pp. 57–62, 2008.

[43] M. Z. Erkal, J. Wilde, Y. Bilgin et al., "High prevalence of vitamin D deficiency, secondary hyperparathyroidism and generalized bone pain in Turkish immigrants in Germany: identification of risk factors," *Osteoporosis International*, vol. 17, no. 8, pp. 1133–1140, 2006.

[44] P. J. van Veldhuizen, S. A. Taylor, S. Williamson, and B. M. Drees, "Treatment of vitamin D deficiency in patients with metastatic prostate cancer may improve bone pain and muscle strength," *Journal of Urology*, vol. 163, no. 1, pp. 187–190, 2000.

[45] A. Lotfi, A. M. Abdel-Nasser, A. Hamdy, A. A. Omran, and M. A. El-Rehany, "Hypovitaminosis D in female patients with chronic low back pain," *Clinical Rheumatology*, vol. 26, no. 11, pp. 1895–1901, 2007.

[46] S. Al Faraj and K. Al Mutairi, "Vitamin d deficiency and chronic low back pain in Saudi Arabia," *Spine*, vol. 28, no. 2, pp. 177–179, 2003.

[47] G. de Torrenté de la Jara, A. Pécoud, and B. Favrat, "Female asylum seekers with musculoskeletal pain: the importance of diagnosis and treatment of hypovitaminosis D," *BioMedical Central Family Practice*, vol. 7, article 4, 2006.

[48] W. Huang, S. Shah, Q. Long, A. K. Crankshaw, and V. Tangpricha, "Improvement of pain, sleep, and quality of life in chronic pain patients with vitamin D supplementation," *Clinical Journal of Pain*, vol. 29, no. 4, pp. 341–347, 2013.

[49] J. Iwamoto, T. Takeda, S. Ichimura, K. Matsu, and M. Uzawa, "Effects of cyclical etidronate with alfacalcidol on lumbar bone mineral density, bone resorption, and back pain in postmenopausal women with osteoporosis," *Journal of Orthopaedic Science*, vol. 8, no. 4, pp. 532–537, 2003.

[50] G. de Torrenté de la Jara, A. Pécoud, and B. Favrat, "Musculoskeletal pain in female asylum seekers and hypovitaminosis D_3," *British Medical Journal*, vol. 329, no. 7458, pp. 156–157, 2004.

[51] P. Lee and R. Chen, "Vitamin D as an analgesic for patients with type 2 diabetes and neuropathic pain," *Archives of Internal Medicine*, vol. 168, no. 7, pp. 771–772, 2008.

[52] S. Prakash, N. C. Mehta, A. S. Dabhi, O. Lakhani, M. Khilari, and N. D. Shah, "The prevalence of headache may be related with the latitude: a possible role of Vitamin D insufficiency?" *The Journal of Headache and Pain*, vol. 11, no. 4, pp. 301–307, 2010.

[53] M. Saps, C. Blank, S. Khan et al., "Seasonal variation in the presentation of abdominal pain," *Journal of Pediatric Gastroenterology and Nutrition*, vol. 46, no. 3, pp. 279–284, 2008.

[54] D. D. Mitsikostas, D. Tsaklakidou, N. Athanasiadis, and A. Thomas, "The prevalence of headache in Greece: correlations to latitude and climatological factors," *Headache*, vol. 36, no. 3, pp. 168–173, 1996.

[55] Q. Y. Zeng, R. Chen, Z. Y. Xiao et al., "Low prevalence of knee and back pain in southeast China; the Shantou COPCORD study," *The Journal of Rheumatology*, vol. 31, no. 12, pp. 2439–2443, 2004.

[56] H. Glerup, K. Mikkelsen, L. Poulsen et al., "Commonly recommended daily intake of vitamin D is not sufficient if sunlight exposure is limited," *Journal of Internal Medicine*, vol. 247, no. 2, pp. 260–268, 2000.

[57] D. S. Arvold, M. J. Odean, M. P. Dornfeld et al., "Corelation of symptoms with vitamin D deficiency and symptom response to cholecalciferol treatment: a randomized controlled trial," *Endocrine Practice*, vol. 15, no. 3, pp. 203–212, 2009.

[58] R. C. Oh and J. D. Johnson, "Chest pain and costochondritis associated with vitamin D deficiency: a report of two cases," *Case Reports in Medicine*, vol. 2012, Article ID 375730, 3 pages, 2012.

[59] S. Waikakul, "Serum 25-hydroxy-calciferol level and failed back surgery syndrome," *Journal of Orthopaedic Surgery (Hong Kong)*, vol. 20, no. 1, pp. 18–22, 2012.

[60] B. N. Ames, "Low micronutrient intake may accelerate the degenerative diseases of aging through allocation of scarce micronutrient by triage," *Proceedings of the National Academy of Sciences of the United States of America*, vol. 103, no. 47, pp. 17589–17594, 2006.

[61] L. L. Ritterhouse, S. R. Crowe, T. B. Niewold et al., "Vitamin D deficiency is associated with an increased autoimmune response in healthy individuals and in patients with systemic lupus erythematosus," *Annals of the Rheumatic Diseases*, vol. 70, no. 9, pp. 1569–1574, 2011.

[62] K. Gopinath and D. Danda, "Supplementation of 1,25 dihydroxy vitamin D_3 in patients with treatment naive early rheumatoid arthritis: a randomised controlled trial," *International Journal of Rheumatic Diseases*, vol. 14, no. 4, pp. 332–339, 2011.

[63] M. Hayes, M. Yaster, J. A. Haythornthwaite et al., "Pain is a common problem affecting clinical outcomes in adults with cystic fibrosis," *Chest*, vol. 140, no. 6, pp. 1598–1603, 2011.

[64] N. E. West, N. Lechtzin, C. A. Merlo et al., "Appropriate goal level for 25-hydroxyvitamin D in cystic fibrosis," *Chest*, vol. 140, no. 2, pp. 469–474, 2011.

[65] T. L. Glover, B. R. Goodin, A. L. Horgas et al., "Vitamin D, race, and experimental pain sensitivity in older adults with knee osteoarthritis," *Arthritis & Rheumatism*, vol. 64, no. 12, pp. 3926–3935, 2012.

[66] G. Högberg, S. A. Gustafsson, T. Hällström, T. Gustafsson, B. Klawitter, and M. Petersson, "Depressed adolescents in a case-series were low in vitamin D and depression was ameliorated by vitamin D supplementation," *Acta Paediatrica*, vol. 101, no. 7, pp. 779–783, 2012.

[67] S. Basaran, R. Guzel, I. Coskun-Benlidayi, and F. Guler-Uysal, "Vitamin D status: effects on quality of life in osteoporosis among Turkish women," *Quality of Life Research*, vol. 16, no. 9, pp. 1491–1499, 2007.

[68] R. Vieth, S. Kimball, A. Hu, and P. G. Walfish, "Randomized comparison of the effects of the vitamin D3 adequate intake versus 100 mcg (4000 IU) per day on biochemical responses and the wellbeing of patients," *Nutrition Journal*, vol. 3, article 8, 2004.

[69] V. Kunadian, G. A. Ford, B. Bawamia, W. Qiu, and J. E. Manson, "Vitamin D deficiency and coronary artery disease: a review of the evidence," *American Heart Journal*, vol. 167, no. 3, pp. 283–291, 2014.

[70] H. A. Bischoff-Ferrari, D. P. Kiel, B. Dawson-Hughes et al., "Dietary calcium and serum 25-hydroxyvitamin D status in relation to BMD among U.S. adults," *Journal of Bone and Mineral Research*, vol. 24, no. 5, pp. 935–942, 2009.

[71] T. Penney, M. Ploughman, M. W. Austin, D. G. Behm, and J. M. Byrne, "Determining the activation of gluteus medius and the validity of the single leg stance test in chronic non-specific low back pain," *Archives of Physical Medicine and Rehabilitation*, vol. 95, no. 10, pp. 1969–1976, 2014.

[72] K. H. Cho, J. W. Beom, T. S. Lee, J. H. Lim, T. H. Lee, and J. H. Yuk, "Trunk muscles strength as a risk factor for nonspecific low back pain: a pilot study," *Annals of Rehabilitation Medicine*, vol. 38, no. 2, pp. 234–240, 2014.

[73] H. A. Bischoff, H. B. Stähelin, W. Dick et al., "Effects of vitamin D and calcium supplementation on falls: a randomized controlled trial," *Journal of Bone and Mineral Research*, vol. 18, no. 2, pp. 343–351, 2003.

[74] M. Pfeifer, B. Begerow, and H. W. Minne, "Vitamin D and muscle function," *Osteoporosis International*, vol. 13, no. 3, pp. 187–194, 2002.

[75] R. U. Simpson, G. A. Thomas, and A. J. Arnold, "Identification of 1,25-dihydroxyvitamin: D3 receptors and activities in muscle," *The Journal of Biological Chemistry*, vol. 260, no. 15, pp. 8882–8891, 1985.

[76] H. A. Bischoff, M. Borchers, F. Gudat et al., "In situ detection of 1,25-dihydroxyvitamin D_3 receptor in human skeletal muscle tissue," *The Histochemical Journal*, vol. 33, no. 1, pp. 19–24, 2001.

[77] O. H. Sørensen, B. Lund, B. Saltin et al., "Myopathy in bone loss of ageing: improvement by treatment with 1α-hydroxycholecalciferol and calcium," *Clinical Science*, vol. 56, no. 2, pp. 157–161, 1979.

[78] M. Pfeifer, B. Begerow, H. W. Minne et al., "Vitamin D status, trunk muscle strength, body sway, falls, and fractures among 237 postmenopausal women with osteoporosis," *Experimental and Clinical Endocrinology & Diabetes*, vol. 109, no. 2, pp. 87–92, 2001.

[79] K. E. Broe, T. C. Chen, J. Weinberg, H. A. Bischoff-Ferrari, M. F. Holick, and D. P. Kiel, "A higher dose of vitamin D reduces the risk of falls in nursing home residents: a randomized, multiple-dose study," *Journal of the American Geriatrics Society*, vol. 55, no. 2, pp. 234–239, 2007.

[80] L. Flicker, K. Mead, C. Nowson et al., "Risk factors for falls in older women in residential care in Australia," *Journal of Bone and Mineral Research*, vol. 16, supplement 1, p. S170, 2001.

[81] P. Geusens, C. Vandevyver, J. Vanhoof, J.-J. Cassiman, S. Boonen, and J. Raus, "Quadriceps and grip strength are related to vitamin D receptor genotype in elderly nonobese women," *Journal of Bone and Mineral Research*, vol. 12, no. 12, pp. 2082–2088, 1997.

[82] L. M. Shinchuk and M. F. Holick, "Vitamin D and rehabilitation: improving functional outcomes," *Nutrition in Clinical Practice*, vol. 22, no. 3, pp. 297–304, 2007.

[83] D. A. Fernandes de Abreu, D. Eyles, and F. Féron, "Vitamin D, a neuro-immunomodulator: implications for neurodegenerative and autoimmune diseases," *Psychoneuroendocrinology*, vol. 34, supplement 1, pp. S265–S277, 2009.

[84] A. V. Kalueff and P. Tuohimaa, "Neurosteroid hormone vitamin D and its utility in clinical nutrition," *Current Opinion in Clinical Nutrition and Metabolic Care*, vol. 10, no. 1, pp. 12–19, 2007.

[85] H. H. Zakon, "The effects of steroid hormones on electrical activity of excitable cells," *Trends in Neurosciences*, vol. 21, no. 5, pp. 202–207, 1998.

[86] F.-S. Wu, T. T. Gibbs, and D. H. Farb, "Pregnenolone sulfate: a positive allosteric modulator at the N-methyl-D-aspartate receptor," *Molecular Pharmacology*, vol. 40, no. 3, pp. 333–336, 1991.

[87] A. G. Mensah-Nyagan, L. Meyer, V. Schaeffer, C. Kibaly, and C. Patte-Mensah, "Evidence for a key role of steroids in the modulation of pain," *Psychoneuroendocrinology*, vol. 34, supplement 1, pp. S169–S177, 2009.

[88] C. Carlberg and M. J. Campbell, "Vitamin D receptor signaling mechanisms: integrated actions of a well-defined transcription factor," *Steroids*, vol. 78, no. 2, pp. 127–136, 2013.

[89] I. Neveu, P. Naveilhan, F. Jehan et al., "1,25-dihydroxyvitamin D_3 regulates the synthesis of nerve growth factor in primary cultures of glial cells," *Molecular Brain Research*, vol. 24, no. 1–4, pp. 70–76, 1994.

[90] J. Brown, J. I. Bianco, J. J. McGrath, and D. W. Eyles, "1,25-Dihydroxyvitamin D_3 induces nerve growth factor, promotes neurite outgrowth and inhibits mitosis in embryonic rat hippocampal neurons," *Neuroscience Letters*, vol. 343, no. 2, pp. 139–143, 2003.

[91] S. Riaz, M. Malcangio, M. Miller, and D. R. Tomlinson, "A vitamin D_3 derivative (CB1093) induces nerve growth factor and prevents neurotrophic deficits in streptozotocin-diabetic rats," *Diabetologia*, vol. 42, no. 11, pp. 1308–1313, 1999.

[92] E. Garcion, N. Wion-Barbot, C. N. Montero-Menei, F. Berger, and D. Wion, "New clues about vitamin D functions in the nervous system," *Trends in Endocrinology and Metabolism*, vol. 13, no. 3, pp. 100–105, 2002.

[93] F. Marchand, M. Perretti, and S. B. McMahon, "Role of the immune system in chronic pain," *Nature Reviews Neuroscience*, vol. 6, no. 7, pp. 521–532, 2005.

[94] L. McKelvey, G. D. Shorten, and G. W. O'Keeffe, "Nerve growth factor-mediated regulation of pain signalling and proposed new intervention strategies in clinical pain management," *Journal of Neurochemistry*, vol. 124, no. 3, pp. 276–289, 2013.

[95] C. J. Woolf, "Phenotypic modification of primary sensory neurons: the role of nerve growth factor in the production of persistent pain," *Philosophical Transactions of the Royal Society B: Biological Sciences*, vol. 351, no. 1338, pp. 441–448, 1996.

[96] L. R. Harms, T. H. J. Burne, D. W. Eyles, and J. J. McGrath, "Vitamin D and the brain," *Best Practice & Research: Clinical Endocrinology & Metabolism*, vol. 25, no. 4, pp. 657–669, 2011.

[97] L. D. Brewer, V. Thibault, K.-C. Chen, M. C. Langub, P. W. Landfield, and N. M. Porter, "Vitamin D hormone confers neuroprotection in parallel with downregulation of L-type calcium channel expression in hippocampal neurons," *Journal of Neuroscience*, vol. 21, no. 1, pp. 98–108, 2001.

[98] S. J. Kiraly, M. A. Kiraly, R. D. Hawe, and N. Makhani, "Vitamin D as a neuroactive substance: review," *TheScientificWorldJournal*, vol. 6, pp. 125–139, 2006.

[99] R. S. Griffin, M. Costigan, G. J. Brenner et al., "Complement induction in spinal cord microglia results in anaphylatoxin C5a-mediated pain hypersensitivity," *Journal of Neuroscience*, vol. 27, no. 32, pp. 8699–8708, 2007.

[100] M. Tsuda, K. Inoue, and M. W. Salter, "Neuropathic pain and spinal microglia: a big problem from molecules in 'small' glia," *Trends in Neurosciences*, vol. 28, no. 2, pp. 101–107, 2005.

[101] M. Hewison, "Vitamin D and the immune system: new perspectives on an old theme," *Endocrinology and Metabolism Clinics of North America*, vol. 39, no. 2, pp. 365–379, 2010.

[102] D. Feldman, A. Krishnan, J. Moreno, S. Swami, D. M. Peehl, and S. Srinivas, "Vitamin D inhibition of the prostaglandin pathway as therapy for prostate cancer," *Nutrition Reviews*, vol. 65, no. 8, part 2, pp. S113–S115, 2007.

[103] J. D. Richardson and M. R. Vasko, "Cellular mechanisms of neurogenic inflammation," *The Journal of Pharmacology and Experimental Therapeutics*, vol. 302, no. 3, pp. 839–845, 2002.

[104] J. J. Letterio and A. B. Roberts, "Regulation of immune responses by TGF-beta," *Annual Review of Immunology*, vol. 16, pp. 137–161, 1998.

[105] L. Leung and C. M. Cahill, "TNF-α and neuropathic pain—a review," *Journal of Neuroinflammation*, vol. 7, article 27, 2010.

[106] H. F. Deluca and M. T. Cantorna, "Vitamin D: its role and uses in immunology," *The FASEB Journal*, vol. 15, no. 14, pp. 2579–2585, 2001.

[107] Y. Cury, G. Picolo, V. P. Gutierrez, and S. H. Ferreira, "Pain and analgesia: the dual effect of nitric oxide in the nociceptive system," *Nitric Oxide*, vol. 25, no. 3, pp. 243–254, 2011.

[108] E. Garcion, L. Sindji, G. Leblondel, P. Brachet, and F. Darcy, "1, 25-dihydroxyvitamin D_3 regulates the synthesis of gamma-glutamyl transpeptidase and glutathione levels in rat primary astrocytes," *Journal of Neurochemistry*, vol. 73, no. 2, pp. 859–866, 1999.

[109] K. Takahashi, Y. Nakayama, H. Horiuchi et al., "Human neutrophils express messenger RNA of vitamin D receptor and respond to 1alpha,25-dihydroxyvitamin D3," *Immunopharmacology and Immunotoxicology*, vol. 24, no. 3, pp. 335–347, 2002.

[110] N. M. Perkins and D. J. Tracey, "Hyperalgesia due to nerve injury: role of neutrophils," *Neuroscience*, vol. 101, no. 3, pp. 745–757, 2000.

[111] J. Lemire, "1,25-dihydroxyvitamin D_3—a hormone with immunomodulatory properties," *Zeitschrift für Rheumatologie*, vol. 59, supplement 1, pp. 24–27, 2000.

[112] D. W. Eyles, S. Smith, R. Kinobe, M. Hewison, and J. J. McGrath, "Distribution of the vitamin D receptor and 1α-hydroxylase in human brain," *Journal of Chemical Neuroanatomy*, vol. 29, no. 1, pp. 21–30, 2005.

[113] G. F. Jirikowski, U. W. Kauntzer, A. E. E. Dief, and J. D. Caldwell, "Distribution of vitamin D binding protein expressing neurons in the rat hypothalamus," *Histochemistry and Cell Biology*, vol. 131, no. 3, pp. 365–370, 2009.

[114] R. E. S. Anglin, Z. Samaan, and S. D. Walter, "Vitamin D deficiency and depression in adults: systematic review and meta-analysis," *British Journal of Psychiatry*, vol. 202, no. 2, pp. 100–107, 2013.

[115] S. C. Gominak and W. E. Stumpf, "The world epidemic of sleep disorders is linked to vitamin D deficiency," *Medical Hypotheses*, vol. 79, no. 2, pp. 132–135, 2012.

[116] F. Baeke, T. Takiishi, H. Korf, C. Gysemans, and C. Mathieu, "Vitamin D: modulator of the immune system," *Current Opinion in Pharmacology*, vol. 10, no. 4, pp. 482–496, 2010.

[117] L. Imeri and M. R. Opp, "How (and why) the immune system makes us sleep," *Nature Reviews Neuroscience*, vol. 10, no. 3, pp. 199–210, 2009.

[118] L. Clevenger, A. Schrepf, D. Christensen et al., "Sleep disturbance, cytokines, and fatigue in women with ovarian cancer," *Brain, Behavior, and Immunity*, vol. 26, no. 7, pp. 1037–1044, 2012.

[119] M. R. Opp, "Cytokines and sleep," *Sleep Medicine Reviews*, vol. 9, no. 5, pp. 355–364, 2005.

[120] M. Opp, J. Born, and M. Irwin, "Sleep and the immune system," in *Psychoneuroimmunology*, R. Ader, Ed., pp. 579–618, Elsevier Academic Press, Burlington, Mass, USA, 2007.

[121] J. M. Krueger, F. J. Obál, J. Fang, T. Kubota, and P. Taishi, "The role of cytokines in physiological sleep regulation," *Annals of the New York Academy of Sciences*, vol. 933, pp. 211–221, 2001.

[122] M. Haack, E. Sanchez, and J. M. Mullington, "Elevated inflammatory markers in response to prolonged sleep restriction are associated with increased pain experience in healthy volunteers," *Sleep*, vol. 30, no. 9, pp. 1145–1152, 2007.

[123] D. E. McCarty, A. Reddy, Q. Keigley, P. Y. Kim, and A. A. Marino, "Vitamin D, race, and excessive daytime sleepiness," *Journal of Clinical Sleep Medicine*, vol. 8, no. 6, pp. 693–697, 2012.

[124] K. Chopra and V. Arora, "An intricate relationship between pain and depression: clinical correlates, coactivation factors and therapeutic targets," *Expert Opinion on Therapeutic Targets*, vol. 18, no. 2, pp. 159–176, 2014.

[125] M. I. Maes, "Evidence for an immune response in major depression: a review and hypothesis," *Progress in Neuro-psychopharmacology and Biological Psychiatry*, vol. 19, no. 1, pp. 11–38, 1995.

[126] G. J. Summer, E. A. Romero-Sandoval, O. Bogen, O. A. Dina, S. G. Khasar, and J. D. Levine, "Proinflammatory cytokines mediating burn-injury pain," *Pain*, vol. 135, no. 1-2, pp. 98–107, 2008.

[127] N. Üçeyler, T. Eberle, R. Rolke, F. Birklein, and C. Sommer, "Differential expression patterns of cytokines in complex regional pain syndrome," *Pain*, vol. 132, no. 1-2, pp. 195–205, 2007.

[128] C. L. Raison, L. Capuron, and A. H. Miller, "Cytokines sing the blues: Inflammation and the pathogenesis of depression," *Trends in Immunology*, vol. 27, no. 1, pp. 24–31, 2006.

[129] Y. Dowlati, N. Herrmann, W. Swardfager et al., "A meta-analysis of cytokines in major depression," *Biological Psychiatry*, vol. 67, no. 5, pp. 446–457, 2010.

[130] I. J. Russell, H. Vaeroy, M. Javors, and F. Nyberg, "Cerebrospinal fluid biogenic amine metabolites in fibromyalgia/fibrositis syndrome and rheumatoid arthritis," *Arthritis and Rheumatism*, vol. 35, no. 5, pp. 550–556, 1992.

[131] J. J. Mann and K. M. Malone, "Cerebrospinal fluid amines and higher-lethality suicide attempts in depressed inpatients," *Biological Psychiatry*, vol. 41, no. 2, pp. 162–171, 1997.

[132] L. C. Campbell, D. J. Clauw, and F. J. Keefe, "Persistent pain and depression: a biopsychosocial perspective," *Biological Psychiatry*, vol. 54, no. 3, pp. 399–409, 2003.

[133] A. J. Dunn, "Effects of cytokines and infections on brain neurochemistry," *Clinical Neuroscience Research*, vol. 6, no. 1-2, pp. 52–68, 2006.

[134] D. Brambilla, S. Franciosi, M. R. Opp, and L. Imeri, "Interleukin-1 inhibits firing of serotonergic neurons in the dorsal raphe nucleus and enhances GABAergic inhibitory postsynaptic potentials," *European Journal of Neuroscience*, vol. 26, no. 7, pp. 1862–1869, 2007.

[135] A. Ellis and D. L. H. Bennett, "Neuroinflammation and the generation of neuropathic pain," *British Journal of Anaesthesia*, vol. 111, no. 1, pp. 26–37, 2013.

[136] P. H. Finan, B. R. Goodin, and M. T. Smith, "The association of sleep and pain: an update and a path forward," *Journal of Pain*, vol. 14, no. 12, pp. 1539–1552, 2013.

[137] S. González, D. Moreno-Delgado, E. Moreno et al., "Circadian-related heteromerization of adrenergic and dopamine D4 receptors modulates melatonin synthesis and release in the pineal gland," *PLoS Biology*, vol. 10, no. 6, Article ID e1001347, 2012.

[138] C. A. Naranjo, L. K. Tremblay, and U. E. Busto, "The role of the brain reward system in depression," *Progress in Neuro-Psychopharmacology and Biological Psychiatry*, vol. 25, no. 4, pp. 781–823, 2001.

[139] P. B. Wood, "Role of central dopamine in pain and analgesia," *Expert Review of Neurotherapeutics*, vol. 8, no. 5, pp. 781–797, 2008.

[140] P. B. Wood, "Stress and dopamine: implications for the pathophysiology of chronic widespread pain," *Medical Hypotheses*, vol. 62, no. 3, pp. 420–424, 2004.

[141] H. Foo and P. Mason, "Brainstem modulation of pain during sleep and waking," *Sleep Medicine Reviews*, vol. 7, no. 2, pp. 145–154, 2003.

[142] D. C. Nascimento, M. L. Andersen, D. C. Hipólide, J. N. Nobrega, and S. Tufik, "Pain hypersensitivity induced by paradoxical sleep deprivation is not due to altered binding to brain μ-opioid receptors," *Behavioural Brain Research*, vol. 178, no. 2, pp. 216–220, 2007.

[143] O. E. Ukponmwan, J. Rupreht, and M. R. Dzoljic, "REM sleep deprivation decreases the antinociceptive property of enkephalinase-inhibition, morphine and cold-water-swim," *General Pharmacology*, vol. 15, no. 3, pp. 255–258, 1984.

[144] H. A. Baghdoyan, "Hyperalgesia induced by REM sleep loss: a phenomenon in search of a mechanism," *Sleep*, vol. 29, no. 2, pp. 137–139, 2006.

[145] A. M. Kshatri, H. A. Baghdoyan, and R. Lydic, "Cholinomimetics, but not morphine, increase antinociceptive behavior from pontine reticular regions regulating rapid-eye-movement sleep," *Sleep*, vol. 21, no. 7, pp. 677–685, 1998.

[146] P. L. Delgado, "Depression: the case for a monoamine deficiency," *The Journal of Clinical Psychiatry*, vol. 61, no. 6, pp. 7–11, 2000.

[147] H. L. Fields and A. I. Basbaum, "Central nervous system mechanisms of pain modulation," in *Textbook of Pain*, P. Wall and R. Melzack, Eds., pp. 243–257, Churchill Livingstone, New York, NY, USA, 1994.

[148] J. Levine and Y. Taiwo, "Inflammatory pain," in *Textbook of Pain*, P. Wall and R. Melzack, Eds., pp. 45–56, Churchill Livingstone, New York, NY, USA, 1994.

[149] P. M. Dougherty and W. D. Willis, "Enhanced responses of spinothalamic tract neurons to excitatory amino acids accompany capsaicin-induced sensitization in the monkey," *Journal of Neuroscience*, vol. 12, no. 3, pp. 883–894, 1992.

[150] D. J. Claliw, "The pathogenesis of chronic pain and fatigue syndromes, with special reference to fibromyalgia," *Medical Hypotheses*, vol. 44, no. 5, pp. 369–378, 1995.

[151] R. Dantzer, J. C. O'Connor, G. G. Freund, R. W. Johnson, and K. W. Kelley, "From inflammation to sickness and depression: when the immune system subjugates the brain," *Nature Reviews. Neuroscience*, vol. 9, no. 1, pp. 46–56, 2008.

[152] J. W. Kasckow, D. Baker, and T. D. Geracioti Jr., "Corticotropin-releasing hormone in depression and post-traumatic stress disorder," *Peptides*, vol. 22, no. 5, pp. 845–851, 2001.

[153] M. Schäfer, S. A. Mousa, Q. Zhang, L. Carter, and C. Stein, "Expression of corticotropin-releasing factor in inflamed tissue is required for intrinsic peripheral opioid analgesia," *Proceedings of the National Academy of Sciences of the United States of America*, vol. 93, no. 12, pp. 6096–6100, 1996.

5

A Small Randomized Controlled Pilot Trial Comparing Mobile and Traditional Pain Coping Skills Training Protocols for Cancer Patients with Pain

Tamara J. Somers,[1] Sarah A. Kelleher,[1] Kelly W. Westbrook,[2] Gretchen G. Kimmick,[2] Rebecca A. Shelby,[1] Amy P. Abernethy,[3] and Francis J. Keefe[1]

[1] *Department of Psychiatry and Behavioral Sciences, Duke University Medical Center, Durham, NC, USA*
[2] *Department of Internal Medicine, Duke Cancer Institute, Duke University Medical Center, Durham, NC, USA*
[3] *Duke University School of Medicine, Durham, NC, USA*

Correspondence should be addressed to Tamara J. Somers; tamara.somers@duke.edu

Academic Editor: Stefan Evers

Psychosocial pain management interventions are efficacious for cancer pain but are underutilized. Recent advances in mobile health (mHealth) technologies provide new opportunities to decrease barriers to access psychosocial pain management interventions. The objective of this study was to gain information about the accessibility and efficacy of mobile pain coping skills training (mPCST) intervention delivered to cancer patients with pain compared to traditional in-person pain coping skills training intervention. This study randomly assigned participants ($N = 30$) to receive either mobile health pain coping skills training intervention delivered via Skype or traditional pain coping skills training delivered face-to-face (PCST-trad). This pilot trial suggests that mPCST is feasible, presents low burden to patients, may lead to high patient engagement, and appears to be acceptable to patients. Cancer patients with pain in the mPCST group reported decreases in pain severity and physical symptoms as well as increases in self-efficacy for pain management that were comparable to changes in the PCST-trad group (p's < 0.05). These findings suggest that mPCST, which is a highly accessible intervention, may provide benefits similar to an in-person intervention and shows promise for being feasible, acceptable, and engaging to cancer patients with pain.

1. Introduction

In patients with cancer, persistent pain is related to poor physical functioning, increased physical symptoms, and low overall health-related quality of life [1, 2]. High pain level in cancer patients also is associated with decreased survival time and can be a significant predictor of survival time [3, 4]. Patients with cancer report pain to be their most distressing symptom [5, 6]. While psychosocial pain management interventions have shown efficacy for cancer patients, patient access to such interventions is a significant challenge. Most psychosocial pain management interventions are delivered through in-person sessions at large tertiary medical centers. For patients with cancer and pain, there are several barriers to in-person sessions [7].

Mobile health (mHealth) technology advances may decrease a number of the barriers to psychosocial cancer pain interventions. First, patients with chronic diseases report being too busy or not having enough time to attend in-person sessions; mHealth technology can make intervention delivery available at a time and place convenient for the patient [8]. Second, patients with chronic disease report not feeling well, emotional distress, and problems with transportation (e.g., cost) as barriers to accessing psychosocial interventions [8, 9]; mHealth technology decreases the physical burdens associated with in-person appointments and can eliminate cost of travel. Third, patients report that attributes of an acceptable intervention include convenience, appropriateness, and effectiveness of the intervention [10–12]; mHealth technologies can be used to increase the availability of

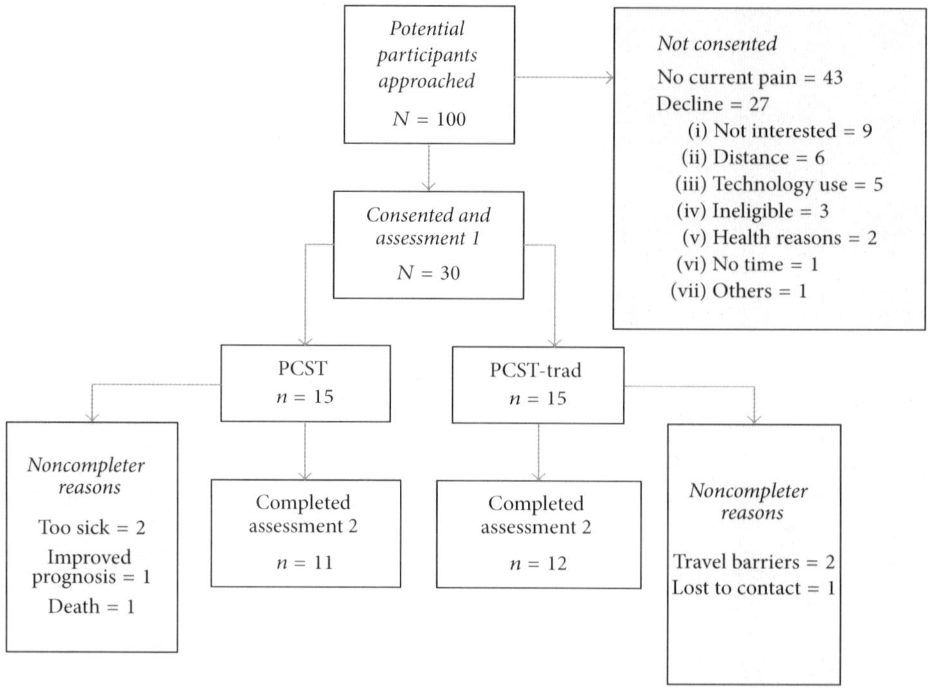

Figure 1

interventions that are convenient, acceptable to patients, and effective.

We recently conducted a single-arm pilot trial that examined the feasibility, acceptability, and value of mHealth psychosocial pain management intervention—mobile pain coping skills training (mPCST) [13]. In this trial ($N = 25$), breast, lung, prostate, and colorectal cancer patients with pain participated in a four-session mPCST protocol using video conferencing on a tablet computer while in their home environment. Feasibility was demonstrated by a high average number of intervention sessions completed (3.36 sessions out of a possible 4) and 84% overall trial completion. Participants reported mPCST to be a highly acceptable intervention using a standardized satisfaction questionnaire and 95% reported that mPCST improved their pain management. Participants receiving the mPCST intervention also reported lower levels of pain severity, physical symptoms, psychological distress, and pain catastrophizing from the period before to the period after intervention.

Building on this single-arm pilot trial, the primary objective of the current small pilot randomized controlled trial was to gain additional information about the accessibility and efficacy of mPCST delivered to cancer patients when compared to traditional in-person pain coping skills training intervention. We hypothesized the following: (1) compared to PCST-trad, mPCST would improve intervention access as assessed by feasibility (i.e., attrition, adherence, and completion time), patient's self-report of burden related to intervention, patient intervention engagement (i.e., use of skills), and self-report of a standardized acceptability scale and (2) mPCST would lead to significant decreases in pain, pain catastrophizing, physical functioning, physical symptoms, and psychological distress and despair and increases in self-efficacy for pain management comparable to PCST-trad.

2. Materials and Methods

2.1. Study Design. This small randomized controlled pilot trial randomly assigned participants ($N = 30$) to either mPCST or PCST-trad. Pre- (prior to randomization) and postintervention assessments included measures of pain, pain catastrophizing, self-efficacy for pain management, physical functioning, physical symptoms, and psychological distress and despair. Patient burden, acceptability, and engagement were also assessed after intervention. The preintervention assessment was completed with the study team at the participant's first visit and the postintervention assessment was completed one to two weeks following their final study intervention session. Participants completed both pre- and postintervention assessments using a tablet computer and were compensated \$20 per assessment for a total of \$40. All participants continued to receive their usual medical care. Institutional review board approved the study. Figure 1 provides a chart of recruitment, consent, and completion.

2.2. Participants. Participants in this study were diagnosed with breast, prostate, lung, or colorectal cancer. All participants had a clinical pain score of 3 or greater [14] (on a scale of 0 = "no pain" to 10 = "pain as bad as you can imagine") recorded in their medical record on two occasions > three weeks apart but < 12 months apart. To be included, patients had to be at least 18 years old and have a life expectancy of at least 6 months as assessed by their oncologist. Exclusion criteria included metastases to the brain, treatment for a serious psychological disorder (e.g., schizophrenia) in the last 6 months, and prior engagement in cancer pain coping skills training protocol.

2.3. Intervention Conditions

2.3.1. Mobile Health Pain Coping Skills Training. Participants randomized to this condition were provided with an iPad to take home with them to participate in mPCST videoconferencing sessions using Skype. Skype sessions were delivered by a Ph.D.-level clinical psychologist or an advanced clinical psychology student/intern closely supervised by a licensed Ph.D.-level clinical psychologist. Sessions for both the mPCST and PCST-trad conditions were conducted in an individual format and were scheduled based on patient and provider availability; however, the therapist always worked to schedule at times most convenient to the patient. mPCST Skype sessions were delivered by the therapist in the medical center to the patient in his or her own home likely increasing flexibility and ease of scheduling as mPCST patients did not have to leave their home.

Session content was based on pain coping skills training (PCST) intervention developed by Keefe et al. [15]. PCST uses cognitive-behavioral theory principles to teach patients coping skills that can enhance their pain management. The 4-session mPCST in this study was carefully designed to include pain coping skills that have shown efficacy in patients with cancer pain. In each session, participants were taught a skill intended to increase their ability to manage their pain and then given the assignment of practicing with that skill prior to the next session. Session 1 included pain education focused on the gate control theory of pain [16] to promote understanding that pain is a complex experience influenced by thoughts, feelings, and behaviors; progressive muscle relaxation (PMR) was taught as a strategy to decrease bodily tension and subjective distress. Session 2 included two skills. Activity-rest cycling was provided as a strategy to pace activities so as to gradually increase involvement in daily activities that were painful. Pleasant activity scheduling involved helping participants identify activities they enjoy that they have stopped doing due to pain (e.g., seeing friends) and set goals for new activities they may enjoy trying (e.g., walking, going out to dinner, and visiting friends). Session 3 taught the skill of cognitive restructuring which involves examining overly negative thoughts about pain (e.g., I can not do anything I used to do) that lead to negative consequences (e.g., feeling depressed, angry) and shifting negative thoughts to be more neutral or positive (e.g., I cannot do everything I used to, but I can still do some things I enjoy). Session 4 taught participants the skill of imagery for relaxation and distraction and brief applied relaxation exercise (the minirelaxation practice).

2.3.2. Traditional Pain Coping Skills Training. Participants in this condition received the same 4 sessions and content as participants in the mPCST condition, but all of the training was conducted at in-person sessions at the medical center.

2.4. Measures

2.4.1. Feasibility. We assessed feasibility by examining study attrition (i.e., study completion), adherence (i.e., completed intervention sessions and assessments), and completion time for each study condition (i.e., days from session 1 to session 4).

2.4.2. Patient Burden. Patient burden was measured by assessing 13 burden areas associated with accessing care following a cancer diagnosis. Items were selected based on information gathered from focus groups asking cancer survivors about barriers and burdens to accessing cancer care. Patients rated on a scale from 1 = "not at all" to 4 = "very much" how difficult it was to complete the study intervention sessions based on each burden. Scale 1 (Symptom Burdens) included items (factor loadings) asking about fatigue (0.73), pain (0.68), time (0.64), anxiety (0.67), feeling down or blue (0.53), and feeling stressed and overwhelmed (0.57). Scale 2 (Practical Burdens) included items on distance (0.51) and difficulties getting to session (0.98). Items asking about the cost of sessions, finding transportation to sessions, taking time off work, finding childcare, and forgetting about sessions had small factor loadings and they were dropped from analyses. The correlation between the two factor scales was $r = 0.10$ and scale reliability was 0.78 and 0.59, respectively.

2.4.3. Patient Engagement. Patient engagement was assessed at the postintervention assessment. Participants were asked how many days in the last seven days they had used each of the pain coping skills. They were also asked how often since their final intervention session they had used the pain coping skills or ideas taught on this scale 0 = "not at all" to 4 = "almost every day."

2.4.4. Patient Acceptability. Acceptability was assessed at the postintervention assessment with the Client Satisfaction Questionnaire 10-item version [17]. Sample questions include the following: "Did you get the kind of information you wanted?"; "Would you recommend this program to a friend with pain?"; and "Did this program help you to deal more effectively with the pain you experience due to cancer?"; this questionnaire contained 10 items rated from 1 = "low acceptability" to 4 = "high acceptability." Summing patient responses created scores. We also examined the individual item asking participants about the quality of the program rated 1 = "poor" to 4 = "excellent."

2.4.5. Pain Severity. Pain severity was assessed at the period before and the period after intervention with the Brief Pain Inventory (BPI) [18]. The BPI asked patients to assess their worst, least, average, and current pain, where 0 = "no pain" and 10 = "pain as bad as you can imagine." Applicable items were reference to the last 7 days. Items were averaged for the pain severity score. This measure has been recommended for use in all chronic pain clinical trials [19, 20]. Internal consistency was good in this sample (Cronbach's alpha = 0.82–0.84).

2.4.6. Pain Catastrophizing. Pain catastrophizing was assessed at the period before and the period after intervention with the 6-item pain catastrophizing scale of the Coping Strategies Questionnaire [21]. These items ask about participants' tendency to catastrophize when faced with pain and are answered on a scale of 0 = "never" to 6 = "always." Items are summed. This scale has good reliability in cancer patients

[22] and had good reliability in this sample (Cronbach's alpha = 0.90–0.93).

2.4.7. Pain Self-Efficacy. Pain self-efficacy was assessed at the period before and the period after intervention with the pain self-efficacy subscale of the Chronic Pain Self-Efficacy Scale [23]. This subscale contains 5 items that inquire about participants: certainty about degree of pain control, pain during daily activities, controlling pain during sleep, and making pain reductions without extra medication. Items were answered on a scale of 10 = "very uncertain" to 100 = "very certain." An average of the items was used as the final score. This scale has shown good reliability in cancer patients [19, 23] and evidenced fair reliability in this sample (Cronbach's alpha = 0.71–0.80).

2.4.8. Physical Functioning. Physical functioning was assessed at the period before and the period after intervention with the 4-item physical functioning scale of the Patient Care Monitor (PCM) v2 [20, 24]. The PCM has been validated against other standard symptom inventories and quality-of-life scales. Physical functioning items asked about participants' ability to run, do light physical work or fun activities, do hard physical work or fun activities, and function normally, referencing the last 7 days. Patients rate their responses: 0 = "not a problem" to 10 = "as bad as possible." Higher scores represent lower physical functioning; internal consistency was good in this sample (Cronbach's alpha = 0.83–0.84).

2.4.9. Physical Symptoms. Physical symptoms were assessed at the period before and the period after intervention with the physical symptom scale of the PCM [20, 24]. The physical symptoms subscale has five items, which ask about patients' fatigue, concentration, pain, sleepiness, and insomnia. Responses were on a scale of 0 = "not a problem" to 10 = "as bad as possible." Internal consistency in this sample was fair to good (Cronbach's alpha = 0.73–0.86).

2.4.10. Psychological Distress. Psychological distress was assessed at the period before and the period after intervention with 4 items from the PCM asking about crying or feeling like crying, being worried, feeling nervous, tense, or anxious, and feeling sad or depressed [20, 24]. Items referenced the last 7 days and were scored on a scale of 0 = "not a problem" to 10 = "as bad as possible." Internal consistency was good (Cronbach's alpha = 0.83–0.89).

2.4.11. Psychological Despair. Despair was assessed at the period before and the period after intervention with 6 items from the PCM asking about hopelessness, lost interest in people and activities, helplessness, guilt, and worthlessness [20, 24]. Items referenced the last 7 days and were scored on a scale of 0 = "not a problem" to 10 = "as bad as possible." Internal consistency was good in this sample (Cronbach's alpha = 0.85–0.91)

2.4.12. Demographic and Medical Variables. Participants' age, gender, race, cancer type, diagnosis date, and cancer stage at study entry were collected through the patients electronic medical record. Participants' marital status, education level, comorbid medical disorders, and cancer treatments in the last week were collected through patient self-report at the preintervention assessment.

2.5. Statistical Analyses. Descriptive analyses were computed for patient demographic (i.e., age, gender, race, education, and marital status) and medical variables (i.e., cancer type, months since diagnosis, cancer stage at study entry, comorbid disorders, and cancer treatments in the last week) (Table 1). We examined the rates and/or descriptive data related to attrition, adherence, completion time, patient burden, and patient engagement. t-tests were used to examine if there were group differences in days to completion, patient burden, and patient engagement. Pearson or point biserial correlations were used to examine the relationships between demographic/medical information and study variables of interest. We used repeated measures analysis of variance (ANOVA) to examine intervention related changes.

3. Results

30 participants with breast, lung, prostate, and colorectal cancer were enrolled in this trial; 15 were randomized to each condition. Participants were M = 60 (SD = 11) years old, 50% were female, 80% reported being partnered, and most participants were White (97%). Descriptive information is summarized in Table 1.

Table 2 examines the preintervention bivariate relationships between demographic/medical variables and the study variables of interest (i.e., pain intensity, pain catastrophizing, pain self-efficacy, physical functioning, physical symptoms, distress, and despair). Pain intensity was associated with age ($r = -0.43$; $p < 0.05$), suggesting that younger participants reported higher levels of pain. Psychological distress was associated with gender ($r = 0.49$; $p < 0.01$), suggesting women reported more psychological distress compared to men. Psychological despair was associated with cancer stage ($r = 0.38$; $p < 0.05$) and number of comorbid medical disorders ($r = 0.40$; $p < 0.05$). These relationships suggest that higher levels of psychological despair are associated with more advanced cancer and more comorbid disorders. Race was not examined in these analyses as the majority of participants were White (97%).

3.1. Feasibility

3.1.1. Attrition. Thirty participants were enrolled into the study and randomized. Of these 30 participants, 4 (3 mPCST, 1 PCST-trad) participants never started the study intervention. An additional 3 (1 mPCST, 2 PCST-trad) participants did not complete the second study assessment. Reasons for the 7 noncompleters included the following: cancer progression and/or less than 1-month life expectancy (2 mPCST), death (1 mPCST), improved prognosis (1 mPCST), not traveling to cancer center (1 PCST-trad), traveling too far (1 PCST-trad), and being lost to contact (1 PCST-trad). It is possible that this small trial ($N = 30$) may not have had enough participants to detect equal events such as disease progression

Table 1: Baseline demographic and medical data (N = 30).

	M	SD	%	n
Age	60	11		
Gender-female			50%	15
Marital status				
Single, widowed, divorced			21%	8
Married/life partner			79%	22
Education				
Less than high school			3%	1
High school diploma			14%	4
Some college			21%	6
Bachelor's degree or higher			62%	18
Race				
White			97%	29
Black			3%	1
Cancer type				
Breast			23%	7
Lung			23%	7
Prostate			46%	13
Colorectal			11%	3
Time since initial diagnosis (months)	41	55		
Stage at study entry				
0			3%	1
1			13%	4
2			17%	5
3			27%	8
4			40%	12
Comorbid disorders[a]				
Hypertension			39%	11
Heart disease			14%	4
Rheumatoid arthritis			4%	1
Osteoarthritis			21%	6
Diabetes			21%	6
Sciatica			8%	2
Emphysema, asthma, COPD			31%	8
Crohn's disease or irritable bowel syndrome			4%	1
Cancer treatments in last week[b]				
Chemotherapy			40%	11
Radiation			11%	3
Surgery			0%	0
Hormone therapy			30%	8
Vaccine			4%	1
Patient reported cancer therapy			28%	8

Note. [a]10 participants reported more than one comorbid disorder; [b]7 participants reported two or more treatments in the last week.

or death across groups; participants in the mPCST group were more likely to report non-study completion due to disease progression and in one case, death. Of note, disease status at study entry by group was as follows: Stage 0 (mPCST = 0, mPCST-trad = 1), Stage 1 (mPCST = 2, mPCST-trad = 2), Stage 2 (mPCST = 2, mPCST-trad = 3), Stage 3 (mPCST = 5, mPCST-trad = 3), and Stage 4 (mPCST = 6, mPCST-trad = 6). The reasons for noncompleters in the PCST-trad group may have been due to the constraints of an in-person intervention (e.g., that it is too far to travel).

3.1.2. Adherence. Participants in both conditions who completed the study (n = 23) participated in an average of 3.83 (SD = 0.65) out of 4 possible sessions. mPCST study completers (n = 11) participated in an average of 3.64 (SD = 0.92) study intervention sessions, with 9 participants completing all sessions. One mPCST participant completed only one study session but agreed to complete the follow-up assessment; another mPCST participant completed 3 out of the 4 sessions. The 12 PCST-trad study completers participated in all four study intervention sessions.

3.1.3. Intervention Completion Time. Among all study participants (n = 21) that completed all four intervention sessions, the average time from session 1 to session 4 was 46.81 (SD = 28.46) days. mPCST patients (n = 9) took an average of 29.67 (SD = 11) days and PCST-trad participants (n = 11) took an average of 59.67 (SD = 31.01) days. The average number of days to completion was significantly different between groups ($t(19) = 2.76$; $p = 0.01$).

3.2. Patient Burden. Two subscales of burdens (Symptom, Practical) to intervention participation were created and examined. All participants scored an average of M = 1.51 (SD = 0.55) on the Symptom Burden scale and M = 1.37 (SD = 0.57) on the Practical Burden scale. The reported barriers to intervention were low and there were no differences between groups. The three barriers with the highest individual averages were being tired or fatigued (M = 2.04; SD = 1.15), pain (M = 2.04; 1.14), and distance from the medical center (M = 1.61; SD = 0.84).

3.3. Patient Engagement. At the postintervention assessment, all participants reported practicing the skills over the last 7 days as follows: progressive muscle relaxation with provided audio, M = 2.43 (SD = 1.95); progressive muscle relaxation without audio, M = 3.78 (SD = 2.54); activity-rest cycling, M = 4.17 (SD = 2.72); pleasant activity planning, M = 4.09 (SD = 2.13); cognitive restructuring, M = 4.77 (SD = 2.22); imagery, M = 4.13 (SD = 2.52); and minirelaxation, M = 3.70 (SD = 2.58). Following treatment, participants reported using pain coping skills learned in the intervention on average several days a week (M = 3.26, SD = 1.05; scale 0 = "not at all" to 4 = "almost every day"). There were no group differences reported in specific pain coping skills use or all skills use (p's > 0.17).

3.4. Patient Acceptability. All participants rated the program to be highly acceptable with an average rating of 3.5 (SD = 0.59) (1 = "low acceptability" to 4 = "high acceptability"). There were no significant differences in acceptability between groups. Participants rated the pain coping skills program overall with 61% (n = 14) rating it excellent, 35% (n = 8) rating it good, and 4% (n = 1) rating it poor.

Table 2: Correlations between demographic and medical variables and study outcome variables at baseline.

	Age	Gender	Marital	Education	Race	Time diagnosed	Cancer stage	Comorbid disorders
Pain intensity	−.43*	.20	.01	−.24	−.01	−.16	.21	.30
Pain catastrophizing	−.29	.12	.27	.04	.21	−.02	.33	.36
Pain self-efficacy	.21	.06	.03	.07	.04	.07	−.05	−.02
Physical functioning	−.28	.02	.15	.17	−.13	−.16	.14	−.01
Physical symptoms	−.01	.14	−.14	−.08	.10	−.20	−.15	.26
Distress	−.23	.49**	−.11	−.21	.21	−.12	−.13	.05
Despair	−.13	.12	.05	−.11	.44*	.12	.38*	.40*

Note. * $p < 0.05$ and ** $p < 0.01$; gender code: 0 = male and 1 = female; marital code: 0 = not partnered and 1 = partnered; and race code: 0 = White and 1 = African American.

3.5. Pre- to Postintervention Changes

3.5.1. Between-Group Pre- to Postintervention Effects. There were between-group differences for pain catastrophizing ($F(1,20) = 14.23$; $p = 0.001$) and physical disability ($F(1,21) = 13.59$; $p = 0.001$). Mean scores suggest that the PCST-trad group experienced decreases in pain catastrophizing and physical disability not seen in the mPCST group. The statistics reported are for the between-groups interaction. No other pre- to postintervention differences between groups were found.

3.5.2. Main Pre- to Postintervention Effects. When examining the outcomes of interest across all participants, there were time effects for pain severity ($F(1,19) = 6.43$; $p = 0.20$), pain catastrophizing ($F(1,20) = 25.93$; $p < 0.001$), self-efficacy for pain management ($F(1,21) = 6.44$; $p = 0.02$), physical symptoms ($F(1,20) = 4.72$; $p = 0.04$), and physical disability ($F(1,21) = 5.16$; $p = 0.03$). Mean scores (Table 3) suggest all changes were in a beneficial direction. No time effects were seen for psychological distress or psychological despair.

Table 3: Comparative pre- and postintervention data ($N = 23$).

	Before intervention		After intervention	
	M	SD	M	SD
Pain intensity				
Full group	4.19	1.86	2.68	1.98
mHealth	4.53	2.12	3.32	1.89
In person	3.86	1.61	2.05	1.95
Pain catastrophizing				
Full group	1.89	1.13	1.01	0.96
mHealth	1.64	1.33	1.42	0.99
In person	2.13	0.91	0.60	0.77
Pain self-efficacy				
Full group	48.76	18.40	60.32	27.81
mHealth	46.00	20.51	51.45	25.78
In person	51.30	16.72	68.44	28.16
Physical functioning				
Full group	5.08	2.37	3.94	2.51
mHealth	4.10	2.78	4.75	2.37
In person	5.98	1.52	3.20	2.51
Physical symptoms				
Full group	3.85	1.72	2.78	2.13
mHealth	3.27	1.51	2.80	1.0
In person	4.34	1.64	2.76	2.93
Distress				
Full group	2.13	1.72	1.75	2.18
mHealth	1.70	1.26	1.23	1.21
In person	2.52	2.04	2.27	2.81
Despair				
Full group	1.24	1.48	0.95	1.71
mHealth	1.05	1.31	0.70	0.80
In person	1.43	1.66	1.21	2.32

Note. All comparisons were nonsignificant.

4. Discussion

This study used a small, randomized controlled pilot trial to begin to examine the accessibility of mobile pain coping skills training intervention when compared to traditional in-person pain coping skills training intervention. Accessibility was examined in several ways including feasibility, patient burden, patient engagement, and acceptability. Evidence from this trial suggests that mPCST is an accessible intervention for cancer patients with pain; participants completed on average 3.83 out of 4 video-conferencing sessions. mPCST was also found to be feasible, present a low burden to patients, and have high patient engagement and to be acceptable to patients. We were also interested in examining the value of mPCST by examining pre- to postintervention changes in key pain-related outcomes and comparing these changes to those obtained in patients undergoing a traditional PCST program. Cancer patients with pain in the mPCST group reported decreases in pain severity and physical symptoms as well as increases in self-efficacy for pain management that were comparable to changes in the PCST-trad group, suggesting that mPCST may provide similar benefits to an in-person intervention.

Findings regarding the accessibility of mPCST provide important information about this intervention and suggest areas of future work. First, one of the most interesting findings was the statistically significant difference in completion time between mPCST and PCST-trad. Participants in the PCST-trad condition took twice as long to complete the four-session intervention (M = 60 days) as participants in the mPCST condition (M = 30 days). The pain coping skills training protocol in this study was designed and intended to be delivered weekly over four weeks. This finding may suggest that providing cancer patients with pain the option to receive pain coping skills training intervention in their home with mobile technology may increase treatment fidelity (e.g., delivery of intervention in the timeframe intended). It may be that, in a clinical setting where providers are faced with the challenges of timing, billing, and scheduling compared to this formal research trial in which we used multiple resources to retain patients, many of the PCST-trad participants would not have completed the 4-session in-person intervention. Second, we found that study attrition in the PCST-trad condition appeared to be due to difficulties with distance to the medical center as one participant reported they could not complete sessions because they were no longer traveling to the medical center, one reported it was too far to travel, and a third was lost to contact. Attrition in the mPCST randomization group was largely due to worsening disease prognosis/death that may not have been equally represented in both groups due to the small sample size. As shown in Figure 1, almost 10% of eligible patients who declined study participation cited that distance or possible travel to the medical center was the major factor for declining participation. Third, among participants who completed the study there were no differences between groups in adherence to study sessions, reported patient burden, or patient engagement in study skills practice. Interestingly, one of the top three reported patient burdens was distance to the medical center. No significant differences between groups were found in burdens, but it would be valuable to examine this variable in a larger trial.

We found that overall participants in this trial reported pre- to postintervention improvements in pain severity, pain catastrophizing, self-efficacy for pain management, physical symptoms, and physical disability. Participants in both groups experienced similar benefits in decreased pain and increased self-efficacy for pain management. This finding is significant for two reasons. First, patients with cancer often have progression in disease and/or receive intense cancer-related treatments that can lead to increased pain levels. The fact that patients in this study reported significant decreases in pain from the period before to the period after intervention may suggest that pain coping skills training protocols can help cancer patients with pain to improve their pain and pain coping even in the face of disease progression and cancer-related treatments. Second, self-efficacy for pain management has emerged as one of the most important psychosocial constructs in predicting patients' pain and their pain-related disability. Increasing patients' self-efficacy for pain management may be particularly important as cancer patients with pain often experience persistent pain even following cancer treatment (e.g., breast cancer patients on preventative hormone medication). Interestingly, our data suggests that PCST-trad led to greater decreases in pain catastrophizing and physical disability when compared to the mPCST group. This finding may suggest that the mPCST protocol did not target these outcomes as well as a traditional in-person intervention and that further iterations of the intervention protocol should be altered to more intensely intervene in these areas.

This study is a small, randomized pilot trial and future work with larger sample sizes is necessary. This work has several limitations. This study is limited by the small sample size, multiple assessment measures, and the possibility that patients who participated may have been more open to use of mobile health technology compared to patients who dropped out or chose not to participate. Future work should examine these relationships in larger samples of patients and patients with varying comfort levels with mobile technology. Also important to note is that medical-related factors such as illness severity/progression, medication effects, and cognitive limitations may limit a patient's ability to participate meaningfully in cognitive-behavioral coping skills training protocol; future research should consider this issue and work to identify those patients who are appropriate candidates and most likely to benefit from this treatment approach. Finally, given the significant difference in time to intervention completion but the absence of difference in outcomes (e.g., pain) between groups, it will be important to consider optimal time for intervention in future trials.

5. Conclusions

This small, randomized controlled pilot trial is one of the first trials to examine the accessibility and efficacy of mPCST intervention for cancer patients with pain compared to an in-person PCST intervention. Our findings suggest that pain coping skills training intervention that capitalizes on the advantages provided by mobile technologies is accessible to cancer patients with pain and is likely to lead to improved pain, self-efficacy for pain management, and other important pain-related outcomes. More work is necessary in this area to provide definitive information on the value of mobile health behavioral pain interventions.

Competing Interests

The authors declare no competing interests.

Acknowledgments

A pilot grant awarded to the first author from the Duke Cancer Control and Population Sciences Program at the Duke Cancer Institute supported this work. The authors would like to thank all of the patients, research staff, and medical providers that made this work possible.

References

[1] C. R. Green, T. Hart-Johnson, and D. R. Loeffler, "Cancer-related chronic pain: examining quality of life in diverse cancer survivors," *Cancer*, vol. 117, no. 9, pp. 1994–2003, 2011.

[2] Q. Shi, T. G. Smith, J. D. Michonski, K. D. Stein, C. Kaw, and C. S. Cleeland, "Symptom burden in cancer survivors 1 year after diagnosis: a report from the American Cancer Society's Studies of Cancer Survivors," *Cancer*, vol. 117, no. 12, pp. 2779–2790, 2011.

[3] A. Montazeri, "Quality of life data as prognostic indicators of survival in cancer patients: an overview of the literature from 1982 to 2008," *Health and Quality of Life Outcomes*, vol. 7, article 102, 2009.

[4] S. Halabi, N. J. Vogelzang, A. B. Kornblith et al., "Pain predicts overall survival in men with metastatic castration-refractory prostate cancer," *Journal of Clinical Oncology*, vol. 26, no. 15, pp. 2544–2549, 2008.

[5] R. Swarm, A. P. Abernethy, D. L. Anghelescu et al., "Adult cancer pain," *Journal of the National Comprehensive Cancer Network*, vol. 8, no. 9, pp. 1046–1086, 2010.

[6] D. N. Levin, C. S. Cleeland, and R. Dar, "Public attitudes toward cancer pain," *Cancer*, vol. 56, no. 9, pp. 2337–2339, 1985.

[7] R. Selove, T. Kroll, M. Coppes, and Y. Cheng, "Psychosocial services in the first 30 days after diagnosis: results of a web-based survey of Children's Oncology Group (COG) member institutions," *Pediatric Blood and Cancer*, vol. 58, no. 3, pp. 435–440, 2012.

[8] L. Pfaeffli, R. Maddison, R. Whittaker et al., "A mHealth cardiac rehabilitation exerciseintervention: findings from content developmentstudies," *BMC Cardiovascular Disorders*, vol. 12, article 36, 2012.

[9] R. T. Goins, K. A. Williams, M. W. Carter, S. M. Spencer, and T. Solovieva, "Perceived barriers to health care access among rural older adults: A Qualitative Study," *Journal of Rural Health*, vol. 21, no. 3, pp. 206–213, 2005.

[10] D. S. Burns, R. B. Sledge, L. A. Fuller, J. K. Daggy, and P. O. Monahan, "Cancer patients' interest and preferences for music therapy," *Journal of Music Therapy*, vol. 42, no. 3, pp. 185–199, 2005.

[11] N. Tarrier, T. Liversidge, and L. Gregg, "The acceptability and preference for the psychological treatment of PTSD," *Behaviour Research and Therapy*, vol. 44, no. 11, pp. 1643–1656, 2006.

[12] S. Sidani, J. Miranda, D. R. Epstein, R. R. Bootzin, J. Cousins, and P. Moritz, "Relationships between personal beliefs and treatment acceptability, and preferences for behavioral treatments," *Behaviour Research and Therapy*, vol. 47, no. 10, pp. 823–829, 2009.

[13] T. J. Somers, A. P. Abernethy, S. N. Edmond et al., "A pilot study of a mobile health pain coping skills training protocol for patients with persistent cancer pain," *Journal of Pain and Symptom Management*, vol. 50, no. 4, pp. 553–558, 2015.

[14] R. C. Serlin, T. R. Mendoza, Y. Nakamura, K. R. Edwards, and C. S. Cleeland, "When is cancer pain mild, moderate or severe? Grading pain severity by its interference with function," *Pain*, vol. 61, no. 2, pp. 277–284, 1995.

[15] F. J. Keefe, S. Kashikar-Zuck, J. Opiteck, E. Hage, L. Dalrymple, and J. A. Blumenthal, "Pain in arthritis and musculoskeletal disorders: the role of coping skills training and exercise interventions," *Journal of Orthopaedic and Sports Physical Therapy*, vol. 24, no. 4, pp. 279–290, 1996.

[16] R. Melzack and P. D. Wall, "Pain mechanisms: a new theory," *Science*, vol. 150, no. 3699, pp. 971–979, 1965.

[17] C. C. Attkisson and R. Zwick, "The client satisfaction questionnaire. Psychometric properties and correlations with service utilization and psychotherapy outcome," *Evaluation and Program Planning*, vol. 5, no. 3, pp. 233–237, 1982.

[18] C. S. Cleeland and K. M. Ryan, "Pain assessment: global use of the brief pain inventory," *Annals of the Academy of Medicine Singapore*, vol. 23, no. 2, pp. 129–138, 1994.

[19] L. S. Porter, F. J. Keefe, J. Garst, C. M. McBride, and D. Baucom, "Self-efficacy for managing pain, symptoms, and function in patients with lung cancer and their informal caregivers: associations with symptoms and distress," *Pain*, vol. 137, no. 2, pp. 306–315, 2008.

[20] A. P. Abernethy, S. Y. Zafar, H. Uronis et al., "Validation of the patient care monitor (version 2.0): a review of system assessment instrument for cancer patients," *Journal of Pain and Symptom Management*, vol. 40, no. 4, pp. 545–558, 2010.

[21] A. K. Rosenstiel and F. J. Keefe, "The use of coping strategies in chronic low back pain patients: relationship to patient characteristics and current adjustment," *Pain*, vol. 17, no. 1, pp. 33–44, 1983.

[22] D. J. Fischer, D. Villines, Y. O. Kim, J. B. Epstein, and D. J. Wilkie, "Anxiety, depression, and pain: differences by primary cancer," *Supportive Care in Cancer*, vol. 18, no. 7, pp. 801–810, 2010.

[23] K. O. Anderson, B. N. Dowds, R. E. Pelletz, W. T. Edwards, and C. Peeters-Asdourian, "Development and initial validation of a scale to measure self-efficacy beliefs in patients with chronic pain," *Pain*, vol. 63, no. 1, pp. 77–83, 1995.

[24] B. Fortner, T. Okon, L. Schwartzberg, K. Tauer, and A. C. Houts, "The Cancer Care Monitor: psychometric content evaluation and pilot testing of a computer administered system for symptom screening and quality of life in adult cancer patients," *Journal of Pain and Symptom Management*, vol. 26, no. 6, pp. 1077–1092, 2003.

6

The Role of Descending Modulation in Manual Therapy and Its Analgesic Implications

Andrew D. Vigotsky[1] and Ryan P. Bruhns[2]

[1]*Kinesiology Program, Arizona State University, Phoenix, AZ 85004, USA*
[2]*College of Medicine, University of Arizona, Tucson, AZ 85724, USA*

Correspondence should be addressed to Andrew D. Vigotsky; avigotsk@asu.edu

Academic Editor: Bjorn Meyerson

Manual therapy has long been a component of physical rehabilitation programs, especially to treat those in pain. The mechanisms of manual therapy, however, are not fully understood, and it has been suggested that its pain modulatory effects are of neurophysiological origin and may be mediated by the descending modulatory circuit. Therefore, the purpose of this review is to examine the neurophysiological response to different types of manual therapy, in order to better understand the neurophysiological mechanisms behind each therapy's analgesic effects. It is concluded that different forms of manual therapy elicit analgesic effects via different mechanisms, and nearly all therapies appear to be at least partially mediated by descending modulation. Additionally, future avenues of mechanistic research pertaining to manual therapy are discussed.

1. Introduction

Manual therapy has been a component of physical rehabilitation programs since as early as 400 BC [1]. Since its inception, many variations of manual therapy techniques have been developed and marketed. Each year, upwards of $8.1 billion is spent in the US on manual therapies, including chiropractic/osteopathic manipulation and massage [2]. Despite the large annual financial expenditures on manual therapies, its mechanisms are not yet fully understood. Current research suggests that a neurophysiological response to manual therapy is responsible for clinically significant decreases in pain [3–8]. Included in the neurophysiological response is the descending pain modulation circuit, which may be a principle mechanism in the analgesic effect of manual therapies.

2. Descending Modulation of Pain

Melzack and Wall [9] were the first to explain the potential mechanisms of a central pain modulatory system, wherein the authors described the gate control theory of pain, which simply states that nonnoxious input suppresses painful output by inhibiting dorsal root nociceptors. Gate control is often triggered by touch or nonthreatening sensory input, which activates low-threshold Aβ fibers that inhibit nociceptive input from Aδ and C afferent fibers [9, 10]. However, another mechanism by which analgesia is induced is through descending modulatory circuits, wherein numerous neurotransmitters, including serotonin (5-HT), vasopressin, oxytocin, adenosine, endocannabinoids, and endogenous opioids (EOs), have been shown to act on structures such as the rostral ventromedial medulla (RVM) and periaqueductal grey (PAG) in order to modulate nociceptive circuits and pain output [11–19]. What is more, and important to consider, is that the analgesic response elicited by human touch [20] and placebo [21–27] is also mediated by EO and endocannabinoids.

β-endorphins are EO peptides that have not only been shown to have a comparable analgesic effect to morphine [28], but are 18 to 33 times more potent [29]. Diffuse noxious inhibitory control (DNIC) is the process by which afferent noxious signals are inhibited from the peripheral nervous system (PNS). Using a rat model, Le Bars et al. [30] and Le Bars et al. [31] found that neurons were inhibited by noxious stimuli (a hot bath), therein coining the term DNIC. Since then, multiple studies have suggested that EO is an underlying mechanism of DNIC [32, 33], and more recently it has been suggested that DNIC be referred to as conditioned pain modulation (CPM), by which this mechanism will be referred to herein [34]. It has been suggested that manual therapies that are nociceptive in nature are mediated by CPM [35].

Previous reviews have noted potential descending modulatory mechanisms, an endogenous opioid response, in both physical therapy [36] and physical medicine [37]; however, the neurochemical response to manual therapy and its implications for descending pain modulation, to the authors' knowledge, have not yet been thoroughly reviewed.

3. Search Methodology

In order to investigate the neurotransmitters associated with a descending inhibitory response to manual therapy, PubMed was searched using the following query: ("manual therapy" OR "acupressure" OR "neural mobilization" OR "joint manipulation" OR "joint mobilization" OR "massage" OR "manipulative" OR "spinal manipulation") AND ("vasopressin" OR "naloxone" OR "glial" OR "receptors" OR "biomarkers" OR "cannabinoid" OR "biochemical" OR "endorphin" OR "beta-endorphin" OR "oxytocin" OR "opioid" OR "opioids" OR "serotonin" OR "dopamine" OR "neurotransmitter" OR "neuropeptide" OR "antinociceptive") NOT ("labor" OR "cardiac" OR "uterus" OR "milk") in November 2015. All relevant studies and reviews that were written in English were included, with the exception of those that were retracted. Animal studies were included, as they may provide further insight into mechanisms that may not be ethical to directly measure in humans; for example, utilizing brain biopsies to observe receptor activity. The general methods and important findings pertaining to descending pain modulatory systems were described.

4. Manipulation Therapies

Through the millennia, numerous types of manipulation therapies have been developed and advocated, and have been purported to cure everything from scarlet fever and diphtheria to hearing loss [1]. However, perhaps the most widely proclaimed outcome from manipulative therapy is pain relief, which may be modulated by neurotransmitters that act on the RVM and PAG.

4.1. Osteopathic Manipulative Therapy. Degenhardt et al. [38] recruited twenty male subjects: ten with low back pain and ten without. Four osteopathic manipulative therapy (OMT) techniques (articulatory treatment system, muscle energy, soft tissue technique, and Strain-Counterstrain) were performed on areas of subjects' "somatic dysfunction," defined as "sites of muscle hypertonicity, tenderness, and joint restriction" [38]. Blood was collected prior to (baseline), 30 minutes, and 24 hours after OMT. Increases in β-endorphin and N-palmitoylethanolamide (PEA), an endogenous analog of arachidonylethanolamide (AEA), or anandamide, an endocannabinoid, were observed 30 minutes after treatment; at 24 hours, similar biomarker changes from baseline were found. Subjects with chronic low back pain presented greater biomarker alterations following OMT than the control (asymptomatic) group. However, because no true control or sham group was utilized, it is not possible to distinguish whether these changes in biomarkers were due to the placebo effect or something greater, as endocannabinoids are implicated in placebo-induced analgesia [21], though these data do show that those in pain respond differently to treatment than asymptomatic individuals.

In a blinded, randomized control trial, McPartland et al. [39] investigated the effects of OMT on plasma endocannabinoid concentrations; that is, AEA and 2-arachidonoylglycerol (2-AG). Thirty-one subjects received either an OMT treatment (biodynamic osteopathy in the cranial field) or a sham treatment. Importantly, subjects were recruited from a patient population of an osteopath who regularly uses OMT; therefore, the patients most likely believe the treatment is efficacious. No changes were observed in 2-AG concentrations in either group. In the sham group, negligible, insignificant changes in AEA were observed (17%). The OMT group experienced a 168% increase (5.02 pmol/mL) in AEA over baseline, but this increase did not achieve statistical significance; however, this difference may certainly be clinically relevant, as indicated by changes in Drug Reaction Scale (DRS) scores. These data suggest that endocannabinoids do play a role in the analgesic effect of OMT.

4.2. Spinal Manipulation. A number of studies have investigated the pain modulation mechanisms of spinal manipulation, which, as the name implies, is specific only to spinal articulation. The first to do so were Vernon et al. [40], who found a small but statistical increase in plasma β-endorphin levels in the experimental group ($n = 9$) who, following a 20-minute relaxation period, underwent a procedure intended to mobilize the upper cervical spine through "joint play maneuvers" [41], during which mild pressure is exerted dorsally on the ligamentous soft tissue of the fixed segment of the neck (the subject is lying supine). Following the introduction of pressure, a fast, low-amplitude rotary thrust is applied that brings the joint through the elastic barrier, producing an "audible or palpable release." Plasma β-endorphin levels were taken at −20, −15, +5, +15, and +30 minutes prior to and following the intervention, and effects were determined via an analysis of variance. Neither the sham group ($n = 9$), which underwent the same joint play manipulation but *without* the thrusting maneuver (only mild, oscillatory pressure was exerted on the fixed segment of the cervical spine while the head and neck underwent passive rotation), nor the control group ($n = 9$) experienced such an increase in plasma β-endorphin concentration. However, two subsequent studies demonstrated findings contradicting those of Vernon et al. [40]: Christian et al. [42] and Sanders et al. [43] both failed to find increases in plasma β-endorphin concentrations in experimental groups with respect to sham and control groups following spinal manipulation. Sanders et al. [43] drew blood samples −10, +5, and +30 minutes prior to and following the intervention and, like Vernon et al. [40], an analysis of variance was used to examine the presence of a difference of plasma β-endorphin levels across all time points. Christian et al. [42] drew three 10 mL blood samples 10 minutes apart prior to the intervention, averaged these values as a baseline, and took 10 mL blood samples five and thirty minutes following the intervention. Of note, Christian et al. [42] described a between-assay coefficient of variation of 11% for 50 pg/tube and 13% for 200 pg/tube plasma β-endorphin assays. Relevant methodological differences between the investigations of Christian et al. [42] and Vernon et al. [40] include the division of subjects into four groups by Christian et al. [42]: asymptomatic ($n = 10$) and symptomatic ($n = 10$) groups that received the experimental spinal manipulative therapy (SMT) protocol and asymptomatic ($n = 10$) and symptomatic ($n = 10$) groups that received the sham SMT procedure. Experimental and sham SMT procedures employed by Christian et al. [42] and Vernon et al. [40] were identical. Unlike the studies by Vernon et al. [40] and Sanders et al. [43], no control group was included in that of Christian et al. [42]. Methodological differences in the Sanders et al. [43] study (which included experimental, sham, and control groups each of $n = 6$) from the aforementioned two include the region of the spine considered (the lower lumbar, as opposed to the upper cervical spine), the application of light touch to the affected area in the sham group as opposed to joint play of any kind, and the population sampled. Unlike Christian et al. [42] and Vernon et al. [40], Sanders et al. [43] recruited subjects who were "naïve to chiropractic adjustive manipulation," as opposed to patients from chiropractic teaching clinics and/or students of the same chiropractic college, which helps to eliminate the potential, previously discussed effect of presuppositions harbored by the sample population. Christian et al. [42] attributed the outcome discrepancies between their data and those of Vernon et al. [40] to between-assay variation, as Vernon et al. [40] reported an 8% increase, which is less than the aforementioned between-assay coefficients of variation.

Recently, Plaza-Manzano et al. [44] compared cervical ($n = 10$) and thoracic manipulations ($n = 10$) to a control group ($n = 10$) in a single-blind, randomized study of graduate student subjects who responded to university-placed advertisements. Cervical manipulations consisted of a high-velocity, mid-range, and leftward rotary thrust about the C4 and C5 vertebrae of the supine subject. Thoracic manipulations consisted of a high-velocity, end-range force applied in the anteroposterior plane to T3-4/T4-5 articulations. Blood was collected from the cephalic vein of each subject before, immediately after, and two hours following the intervention. Both cervical and thoracic groups saw decreases in neurotensin *and* oxytocin, as well as increases in orexin A plasma concentrations following respective interventions.

Multiple reviews have also investigated the pain modulating mechanisms of spinal manipulation [6, 45] and agreed that the analgesic origins are neurophysiological in nature, occurring through some type of descending pain modulation circuit. This is due to observed analgesic effects associated with SMT, including increased pain tolerance and decreased sensitization. The exact circuit, however, is not fully understood, and it appears that different types of spinal manipulations, namely, the velocity with which and the location at which they are performed, may elicit different neurochemical responses indicative of different descending pain modulation mechanisms [46]. For further information on the neurophysiological effects of SMT, readers are directed to Vernon [45] and Pickar [6].

4.3. Knee Joint Manipulation. Skyba et al. [47] investigated the effects of knee joint manipulation in rats on monoamine, opioid, and type A γ-aminobutyric acid ($GABA_A$) receptors in the spinal cord. Knee manipulations employed consisted of the movement of the tibia on the fixed femur. For a duration of three minutes, the joint was flexed and extended across its full range of motion while the tibia was made to translate in the anteroposterior plane. One minute was allowed for rest between each of the three manipulation sessions. Using a model of capsaicin-induced hyperalgesia and the systematic introduction of $GABA_A$, opioid, α2-adrenergic, 5-$HT_{1/2}$, 5-HT_{1A}, 5-HT_{2A}, and 5-HT_3 receptor inhibitors, the authors determined that the analgesic effects of knee joint manipulation were not impacted by the spinal blockade of opioid or $GABA_A$ receptors but *were* impacted by the blockade of 5-HT_{1A} and α2-adrenergic receptors. It was therefore posited that descending inhibition following knee joint manipulation may be modulated by serotonergic and noradrenergic mechanisms. No attempt has been made to replicate these findings in humans.

5. Mobilization Therapies

5.1. Ankle Joint Mobilization. There is evidence to support that, in male, Swiss mice, ankle mobilization-induced analgesia is mediated by EO, endocannabinoidergic, and adenosinergic pathways [48–50]. All of these investigations sought to establish the effect of ankle joint mobilization (AJM) on mechanical sensitivity in mice subjected to plantar incision (PI) surgery, for the purpose of inducing an algesic response. AJM was carried out in a manner consistent with Maitland [51]; this involved the rhythmic flexion and extension of the ankle joint following fixation of the knee. The dosage regime of AJM employed is the same regime delineated by Skyba et al. [47], as discussed in the previous section. In the interest of succinctness, the convoluted methods of these investigations and some to follow will not be described in tremendous detail. Readers who are interested in study methodology are directed to each respective study. Each of the studies by Martins and others employed experimental, sham, and control groups. In order to examine the pathways by which analgesia occurred, Martins and others used the appropriate receptor antagonist; for example, naloxone, an opioid receptor antagonist, to determine the role of EO [48]. Mechanical sensitivity following AJM was assessed by measuring the frequency with which mice would withdraw the foot following the application of pressure to its ventral surface. The withdrawal frequency out of 10 pressure applications was taken as a percentage, which constituted each mouse's resultant value.

Importantly, Martins et al. [48] noted that the bottleneck in antihypersensitivity was opioid receptor availability as opposed to opioid-containing leukocytes. Although opioid receptor availability may be the bottleneck in mice, this is not necessarily true for humans. These data should be replicated in human subjects and could have large implications for those in chronic pain or those with central sensitization, as these individuals may have decreased opioid receptor availability [52] and therefore may not benefit as much from this technique.

Further research by Martins et al. [53] investigated the antihyperalgesic and neuroregenerative effects of AJM following a crush injury of the sciatic nerve in adult male Wistar rats. Six groups were studied in order to isolate the effects of AJM so as not to be confounded by the effects of anesthesia and surgery. Mechanical hyperalgesia was tested in a manner similar to the aforementioned studies by Martins and others, and cold hyperalgesia was performed by dropping acetone onto the mid-plantar hind paw. Histological analyses were performed to investigate the effects of AJM on dorsal horn glial cell activation. It was found that glial cell activation and hyperalgesia decreased following AJM. Furthermore, the AJM group had greater myelin sheath thickness. It is possible that these outcomes are related and are of relevance, being that recent research has shown that those in chronic pain exhibit greater glial cell activation [54]; therefore, despite the possibility that AJM may not work well in chronic pain patients through EO-mediated analgesia, it is possible that glial cell inhibition would produce favorable outcomes for chronic pain patients.

5.2. Mulligan's Mobilization with Movement. Paungmali and colleagues have studied Mulligan's Mobilization with Movement (MWM) in lateral epicondylalgia [55, 56]. Twenty-four subjects with unilateral chronic lateral epicondylalgia were treated with MWM on six occasions at least two days apart. No statistical decreases in hypoalgesic effects were seen over the treatment period [56]. In a follow-up study, Paungmali et al. [55] failed to antagonize the hypoalgesic effects of MWM with naloxone, an opioid antagonist, and concluded that MWM works through nonopioid methods. However, as noted by Payson and Holloway [57], naloxone by itself can produce an analgesic effect due to its inhibitory effects on inflammation and ischemia; therefore, the results of Paungmali et al. [55] should be called into question.

5.3. Neural Mobilization. Neural mobilization (NM) is a type of therapy that purports to relieve adverse neural tension, using methods such as nerve gliding and neural stretching. A systematic review put forth by Ellis and Hing [58] highlights the concerns of methodological quality behind claims of therapeutic efficacy in randomized control trials (RCTs) aimed at studying the clinical utility of neuromanipulative therapy, neurodynamic therapy, or, simply, NM. This review took into account 10 randomized clinical trials (represented by 11 publications), gleaned from the more numerous case studies and other nonblinded trials filling the pool of literature on the topic. Investigative heterogeneity in the 11 studies resulting from dissimilar patient populations considered a variety of pathologies treated and different types of NM techniques analyzed necessitated the use of a qualitative means of assessment rather than meta-analytical means. Ellis and Hing [58] reported that nine of the 11 studies were given, based on the criteria of the PEDro Scale [59], an internal validity score (IVS) of 4 or 5, indicating "moderate" methodological quality. The remaining two studies were given an IVS of 3, indicating "limited" methodological quality. None of the 11 studies satisfied the only two classification items pertaining to subject-therapist blinding. Though a majority of these investigations report a positive clinical benefit from the type of NM employed, Ellis and Hing [58] conclude that only limited evidence exists to support its use. Interestingly, some researchers (such as the next group to be discussed) assert that this noninvasive treatment method has been "*proven* to be clinically effective," at least in the reduction of pain.

Under the hypothesis that the EO system mediates the reversion of neuropathic pain following neurodynamic treatment and an earlier study suggesting that glial cells and neural growth factor may be involved in the analgesia associated with neural mobilization [60], Santos et al. [61] studied behavioral responses and immunochemical indication of EOs following NM in rats with chronic constriction injury (CCI). CCI, as described by Santos et al. [61], is an induced peripheral nerve injury wherein epineural blood flow (to the sciatic, in this case) is occluded, but not arrested, using chromic gut ligatures. Using male Wistar rats subjected to NM two weeks following CCI (experimental group, $n = 5$) and Western blot assays of the PAG, the authors examined the brains of the rats for μ-, δ-, and κ-opioid receptor expression potentially resulting from the neurodynamic intervention. The NM protocol adopted by the investigators is as follows: rats in the experimental group were anesthetized and placed on their left sides such that the side affected by the CCI (the right) could be manipulated freely; rats in the sham group were just anaesthetized. With the right knee remaining fully extended throughout the session, the investigators flexed the right hip to 70–80° (absolute) until the hamstrings produced a light resistance. At this point, the right ankle was dorsiflexed 30–45° relative to its resting position until a similar resistance (presumably from the gastrocnemius) was detected by the manipulator. Following the establishment of minimal resistance in the manipulated joints, oscillations of the right ankle, wherein the joint was dorsiflexed to 30–45° repeatedly from resting, were initiated. The oscillations were carried out every other day for two minutes, each at 20 oscillations/min with 25-second pauses between them. A total of 10 sessions were completed. Apart from the experimental group (CCI + NM), four other groups were considered. These included "naïve" control, CCI only, sham, and sham + NM groups. Researchers did not find changes in δ- or μ-opioid receptor expression following the intervention; however, κ-opioid receptor expression underwent a significant, 17% increase. These data indicate that the analgesic effects reported by those treated with neural mobilization may be mediated by EOs that act on κ-opioid receptors, such as dynorphin A and subtypes thereof.

6. Massage Therapies

Massage therapy is often sought for both pleasure and therapy. It has been proposed to work through the gate control theory of pain [62], initially described by Melzack and Wall [9]. However, Field [62] failed to note that different types of massage therapy may work via different mechanisms and did not dive deeply into possible mechanisms. More specifically, light or touch massages may activate low-threshold Aβ fibers, which inhibit nociceptive input from Aδ and C afferent fibers [9, 10]. Deeper massages, however, may elicit a CPM response due to their pronociceptive nature [35]. Therefore, a more comprehensive review of massage therapy's mechanisms is warranted.

6.1. Connective Tissue Massage. Connective tissue massage is intended to both decrease pain and increase range of motion [63]. In the interest of determining the mechanisms behind the pain relief and increases in microcirculation associated with this type of massage, Kaada and Torsteinbø [64] recruited six male and six female subjects, ranging from 23 to 61 years of age, all with a history of "myalgia and various other types of pain." Of note, the same volunteer cohort was studied in a similar investigation by the pair of authors [65]. Thirty minutes on a bed in a "thermoregulated" room was allowed for each subject to rest prior to the first of four, 9 mL blood samples being taken from the (median) cubital vein. The latter three were taken at 5, 30, and 90 minutes after massage; all were collected in chilled vacutainers containing 0.5 mL of an antiproteolytic buffer. The massage itself was performed by a physiotherapist on laterally positioned, recumbent subjects. Initially, 20 minutes of slow, 1–1.5 in. strokes was applied to the lumbosacral region, including T_{12} and subcostal strokes, giving rise to "sharp, cutting" sensations in the subjects. Following this, 10 minutes was spent treating more local areas of pain specific to each subject using the same stroke length and pressure as applied to the initially treated region. Following the termination of massage treatment and an unspecified storage time on ice (as opposed to conventional, −80°C storage temperatures), blood samples were centrifuged and processed using an assay designed specifically to detect human β-endorphin (New England Nuclear β-endorphin ^{125}I radioimmunoassay). Blood work reportedly indicated a statistical increase in plasma β-endorphin levels following connective tissue massage, similar to the *time course* observed in acupuncture and to the *magnitude* observed during exercise. These results are indicative of a CPM response, which modulates pain through descending inhibition.

6.2. Acupressure. Using naloxone in male and female Sprague-Dawley rats, Trentini et al. [66] suggested that antinociceptive effects of acupressure applied to areas of low transcutaneous resistance (<30 MΩ), that is, "acupoints," are mediated by EOs. This conclusion was derived from results obtained from two separate groups of five rats, one of which was subjected to three different trials: (1) an experimental trial in which acupressure was applied to an acupoint, (2) a sham trial in which acupressure was applied to an adjacent point of higher transcutaneous resistance, and (3) a control trial in which no acupressure was applied at all. The other group of five rats, however, was not subjected to a sham trial, but rather to three trials of acupressure at the acupoint 10 minutes after intraperitoneal injection of naloxone (0.05 mg/kg) *or* a saline substitute. No indication of exactly how many of the five rats received naloxone versus saline was provided by the authors. Assessments of antinociception consisted of tail-flick latency tests in which the distal portion of the rats' tails was subjected to a current-containing, tungsten wire heated to 75 ± 5°C. These assessments were performed 10 minutes prior, 10 minutes into, and 20 minutes following the acupressure procedure. Trentini et al. [66] found statistical increases in tail-flick latency during acupressure (10–20 min) and postacupressure (20–40 min) periods in rats injected with *saline* versus those injected with naloxone, indicating possible EO-mediated nociception resulting from acupressure at the acupoint. These results are internally substantiated by the authors' establishment of a statistically greater tail-flick latency in experimental trials as opposed to sham and control trials, which remained at or below baseline for the duration of the assessment.

Despite the findings of Trentini et al. [66], changes in plasma β-endorphin levels were not observed in follow-up research in humans [67] following the processing of blood samples collected at baseline, immediately after acupressure treatment, and one hour after acupressure treatment. Like Trentini et al. [66], Fassoulaki et al. [67] only investigated the effects of one experimental acupressure point with respect to one sham acupressure point, but rather than the chosen points being on the hind limb (as was the case in the former), the chosen acupoint and sham point in the latter investigation were both on the face of the human subjects. Thus, the effects of acupressure applied to other parts of the body on β-endorphin levels remain unclear. It is also worth noting that both groups of investigators discussed here applied experimental, sham, and control treatments on the same groups of subjects. It was specified by Fassoulaki et al. [67] that each successive treatment for their cohort was performed one day after the last; however, Trentini et al. [66] provided no such specification as to the time allowed between trials in the group of rats studied. From these equivocal data, a potential mechanism by which acupressure may produce analgesia cannot be concluded.

6.3. Conventional Massage. Regular massage, consisting of effleurage and other common techniques, has been well studied, but its effects are still not completely understood. Day et al. [68] were the first to note that there is no change in plasma β-endorphin or β-lipotropin levels following a 30-minute back massage. The possibility of oxytocinergic mechanisms in massage-like stroking in rats was investigated by Agren et al. [69], who tested withdrawal latencies from a hot plate (52°C) in addition to performing the Randall-Selitto test. The rats were injected with saline, oxytocin (1 mg/kg or 0.1 mg/kg), oxytocin antagonist, or a combination of oxytocin and its antagonist (1 mg/kg). The trunk was stroked 50–75 times in 30–45 seconds on both lateral sides, simultaneously, while alternating between ventral and dorsal sides. Withdrawal latency was then retested following massage; investigators reported that the oxytocin antagonist reversed the increases in latency of withdrawal observed in the saline group. Further research in humans (female cyclists) has also demonstrated an oxytocin response to massage [70]. Participants received a 15-minute Swedish massage of the neck and shoulders. Plasma oxytocin levels were measured prior to massage (baseline), during the massage, five minutes following the massage, and 30 minutes following the massage. A nonstatistical increase (Cohen's $d = 0.89$) in plasma oxytocin was observed five minutes after massage, which returned to baseline after 30 minutes. Bello et al. [71] also observed an acute increase in plasma oxytocin in healthy men following 20 minutes of massage applied to the shoulders, upper arms, neck, upper back, and along the spine, but this increase was similar to that observed in the "reading" control at both 15 and 30 minutes following intervention. Additionally, no changes in arginine vasopressin were observed [71]. Similar findings were also observed by Morhenn et al. [72], who compared 15 minutes of Swedish massage on the upper back to rest and found statistical increases in plasma oxytocin and statistical decreases in β-endorphin in the massage group relative to the control group. Importantly, a larger sample size was incorporated here, relative to the other studies (experimental: $n = 65$; control: $n = 30$), so the findings of Morhenn et al. [72] may be more reliable and robust when compared to those mentioned previously.

Since then, two studies have found that massage increases urine concentration of dopamine and serotonin [73, 74], suggesting that massage therapy's analgesic effects are mediated by dopaminergic and serotonergic pathways. In addition, a more recent review of the mechanisms of massage therapy noted a 28 and 31% increase in serotonin and dopamine levels, respectively [75].

The longitudinal effects of massage on select catecholamines and neuropeptides have also been investigated. Hart et al. [76] treated young women (mean age = 26) with anorexia nervosa with 30-minute massage twice per week for five weeks. Investigators observed a 72.5% increase in urine dopamine assays, while no statistical change was observed in the control group.

Corticotropin releasing factor (CRF) acts on the locus coeruleus and is associated with analgesic responses, possibly due to the role of the locus coeruleus in modulating ascending and descending pain pathways [82]. Therefore, a CRF response to massage may have analgesic implications. Lund et al. [77] investigated the effects of 30 minutes of massage therapy administered twice weekly for six weeks on urinary CRF concentrations. Increases in urinary CRF concentration were observed following the treatment period, and a nonstatistical increase was observed one month following treatment.

In a randomized-controlled trial in women with breast cancer, subjects received ten twenty-minute effleurage massage treatments over three to four weeks. These treatments were applied to either both feet and lower legs *or* both hands and lower arms. The control group received the same amount of attention but was not touched. Plasma oxytocin levels experienced no statistical changes over the course of therapy in either group; however, a 47.6% decrease in oxytocin in the massage group over the treatment period was observed [78].

Recently, Tsuji et al. [79] carried out a pilot study on the effects of mother-son massage on salivary oxytocin levels in mothers with boys with Autism Spectrum Disorder. After a single 20-minute massage session, no changes in salivary oxytocin concentrations were observed; however, dramatic increases were observed in both the mother and child after massages were given for 20 minutes per day, every day, for three months, when compared to a four-month nonmassage period. It cannot be said for certain whether such outcomes can be generalized to other populations.

Further longitudinal and acute work has been done by Rapaport et al. [81] and Rapaport et al. [80], who investigated the effects of a 45-minute massage or light touch treatment (control) in one session *and* one versus two times per week, for five weeks, on a number of neuroendocrine measures, including arginine vasopressin and oxytocin. In the acute trial, a larger decrease in arginine vasopressin was found relative to the touch group, but no statistical differences were observed for oxytocin [80]. In the longitudinal trial, neuroendocrine samples were collected at 5 minutes and 1 minute prior to the therapy sessions and at 1, 5, 10, 15, 30, and 60 minutes after the end of the session. Two analyses were performed: one that compared baseline (pre) values to the values directly following the final intervention and another that compared baseline (pre) values to the values preceding the final intervention. The latter measure is of particular interest, because it is indicative of longitudinal effects. The following Cohen's d effect sizes are presented relative to the touch (control) group. Following the final intervention, the once per week group experienced negligible effects for oxytocin (−0.14). The twice per week group, following the final intervention, noted increased levels of oxytocin (0.50). Preceding the final intervention, negligible increases in oxytocin were noted (0.05) for the once per week massage group. A large effect was observed in the twice per week group for oxytocin (0.92) following the final intervention [81].

From the aforementioned studies, it appears clear that oxytocin plays a role in the analgesic response following conventional massage therapy, but the role of other neuropeptides is unclear.

7. Future Research

Being that the analgesic effects of both human touch [20] and placebo [21–27] are mediated by an EO or endocannabinoid response, it is imperative that a placebo control group be utilized in research examining the neurochemical response to manual therapy, as placebo and touch alone are confounding variables. Future research should target therapies that have already been shown to be effective, as to prevent the wasting of resources investigating mechanisms that are not clinically meaningful and should utilize both a control and sham group. Investigators should be cautious when designing experiments that use naloxone, as it can inhibit pain via peripheral mechanisms; thus, it may not be appropriate to use with those who have low back pain [57]. Lastly, it is imperative that researchers be vigilant when interpreting the results of serum levels of EO, as they may not reflect levels seen in the brain or cerebral spinal fluid [83].

Table 1: Neurophysiological response to manual therapy variations.

Study	Subjects	Control/sham	Variation	Findings
Degenhardt et al. [38]	7 women and 3 men with (n = 10) and without (n = 10) low back pain	Light touch	OMT	↑ β-endorphins ↑ PEA
McPartland et al. [39]	Osteopathic patient population (n = 31)	Sham manipulation	OMT	↑ AEA
Vernon et al. [40]	27 healthy males	(1) Control group laid supine on a treatment table (2) Sham group received joint play maneuvers	SMT	↑ β-endorphins
Christian et al. [42]	40 male subjects who were chiropractic patients and students with and without pain	Sham (joint taken to end-range of motion)	SMT	→ β-endorphins
Sanders et al. [43]	9 males and 9 females with acute (<2 weeks) low back pain	Sham group (n = 6) received light touch at L4/L5–S1	SMT	→ β-endorphins
Plaza-Manzano et al. [44]	30 graduate school students	No treatment	SMT	↑ orexin A ↓ neurotensin ↓ oxytocin
Skyba et al. [47]	113 male Sprague-Dawley rats	(1) Vehicle w/manipulation (2) Vehicle w/anesthesia (3) Drugs w/anesthesia	Knee manipulation	Serotonin-mediated Norepinephrine-mediated Non-GABA-mediated
Martins et al. [48]	8 male Swiss mice per group	(1) Control (2) Sham	Ankle joint mobilization	EO-mediated†
Martins et al. [49]	8 male Swiss mice per group	(1) Control (2) Sham	Ankle joint mobilization	CBR-mediated†
Martins et al. [50]	8 male Swiss mice per group	(1) Control (2) Sham	Ankle joint mobilization	Adenosine-mediated†
Martins et al. [53]	8 adult male Wistar rats per group	(1) Sham (2) Sham w/anesthesia (3) Sham w/mobilization (4) Crush (5) Crush w/anesthesia	Ankle joint mobilization	↓ glial cell activation
Paungmali et al. [56]	7 females and 17 males with lateral epicondylalgia	(1) Placebo (2) Control	MWM	No increase in tolerance over treatment period
Paungmali et al. [55]	4 females and 14 males with lateral epicondylalgia	(1) Placebo (2) Control	MWM	Non-EO-mediated†
Santos et al. [61]	Male Wistar rats	(1) Control (2) Injury only (3) Sham (4) Sham w/mobilization	NM	Dynorphin-mediated
Kaada and Torsteinbø [64]	6 male and 6 female subjects with a history of myalgia		Connective tissue massage	↑ β-endorphins
Trentini et al. [66]	Male and female Sprague-Dawley rats	(1) Control (2) Placebo	Acupressure	EO-mediated†
Fassoulaki et al. [67]	4 females and 8 males without a familiarity with acupuncture	(1) Control (2) Sham	Acupressure	→ β-endorphins
Day et al. [68]	17 women and 14 men who were healthy and free of pain	Control	Conventional massage	→ β-endorphins → β-lipotropins
Agren et al. [69]	13–21 male Sprague-Dawley rats	Control	Conventional massage	Oxytocin-mediated†
Turner et al. [70]	26 nulliparous women that cycle	(1) Positive emotion (2) Negative emotion	Conventional massage	↑ oxytocin
Bello et al. [71]	14 males	Control	Conventional massage	↑ oxytocin → arginine vasopressin

Table 1: Continued.

Study	Subjects	Control/sham	Variation	Findings
Morhenn et al. [72]	50 females and 45 males	Rest	Conventional massage	↑ oxytocin ↓ β-endorphins
Hernandez-Reif et al. [73]	13 women and 11 men with >6 months low back pain	Relaxation therapy	Conventional massage	↑ dopamine ↑ serotonin
Hernandez-Reif et al. [74]	34 women with stage 1 or 2 breast cancer	Control (medical treatment only)	Conventional massage	↑ dopamine ↑ serotonin
Field et al. [75]*	Review		Conventional massage	↑ dopamine ↑ serotonin
Hart et al. [76]	Nineteen women with anorexia nervosa	Control (standard treatment only)	Conventional massage	↑ dopamine
Lund et al. [77]	19 fibromyalgia patients	Guided relaxation	Conventional massage	↑ corticotropin releasing factor
Billhult et al. [78]	32 women with breast cancer	Attention	Conventional massage	↑ oxytocin
Tsuji et al. [79]	7 Japanese boys with Autism Spectrum Disorder and their mothers	Control (no massage, crossover)	Conventional massage	↑ oxytocin
Rapaport et al. [80]	29 females and 24 males	Light touch	Conventional massage	→ oxytocin ↓ arginine vasopressin
Rapaport et al. [81]	23 females and 22 males	Light touch	Conventional massage	↑ oxytocin (acute) → oxytocin (chronic)

* denotes review; † denotes a conclusion inferred from naloxone or relevant antagonistic response.

8. Conclusion

Nearly all types of manual therapy have been shown to elicit a neurophysiological response that is associated with the descending pain modulation circuit; however, it appears that different types of manual therapy work through different mechanisms (Table 1). For example, while massage therapy appears to elicit an oxytocin response, spinal manipulation does not. It is crucial that more higher quality research be performed to better understand these mechanisms, as it can lead to a better understanding of how each therapy can be applied to drive more specific clinical research.

For some therapies, such as manipulation, a minimal amount of force may be required for an analgesic effect [84], but whether a minimum force is required for descending inhibition to occur does not seem to be the case, as touch and placebo alone can trigger a descending inhibitory response. However, this may also be treatment dependent. Being that the gate control theory of pain states that nonnoxious stimuli inhibit noxious stimuli, more aggressive therapies may be too noxious to trigger a gate control response, but not noxious enough to produce a CPM response. Thus, more research is needed to shed light on these paradoxical treatment outcomes.

Despite the large popularity and long history of manual therapy, its mechanisms are not truly understood. Understanding these mechanisms may help researchers and clinicians to choose which therapy is most appropriate for each patient or subpopulation and may also lead to more effective therapies in the future.

References

[1] E. Pettman, "A history of manipulative therapy," *Journal of Manual & Manipulative Therapy*, vol. 15, no. 3, pp. 165–174, 2007.

[2] R. L. Nahin, P. M. Barnes, B. J. Stussman, and B. Bloom, "Costs of complementary and alternative medicine (CAM) and frequency of visits to CAM practitioners: United States, 2007," *National Health Statistics Reports*, vol. 18, pp. 1–14, 2009.

[3] J. E. Bialosky, M. D. Bishop, D. D. Price, M. E. Robinson, and S. Z. George, "The mechanisms of manual therapy in the treatment of musculoskeletal pain: a comprehensive model," *Manual Therapy*, vol. 14, no. 5, pp. 531–538, 2009.

[4] R. W. Boal and R. G. Gillette, "Central neuronal plasticity, low back pain and spinal manipulative therapy," *Journal of Manipulative and Physiological Therapeutics*, vol. 27, no. 5, pp. 314–326, 2004.

[5] B. C. Clark, J. S. Thomas, S. A. Walkowski, and J. N. Howell, "The biology of manual therapies," *Journal of the American Osteopathic Association*, vol. 112, no. 9, pp. 617–629, 2012.

[6] J. G. Pickar, "Neurophysiological effects of spinal manipulation," *Spine Journal*, vol. 2, no. 5, pp. 357–371, 2002.

[7] A. Schmid, F. Brunner, A. Wright, and L. M. Bachmann, "Paradigm shift in manual therapy? Evidence for a central nervous system component in the response to passive cervical joint mobilisation," *Manual Therapy*, vol. 13, no. 5, pp. 387–396, 2008.

[8] A. Wright, "Hypoalgesia post-manipulative therapy: a review of a potential neurophysiological mechanism," *Manual Therapy*, vol. 1, no. 1, pp. 11–16, 1995.

[9] R. Melzack and P. D. Wall, "Pain mechanisms: a new theory," *Science*, vol. 150, no. 3699, pp. 971–979, 1965.

[10] V. E. Abraira and D. D. Ginty, "The sensory neurons of touch," *Neuron*, vol. 79, no. 4, pp. 618–639, 2013.

[11] M. L. Adams, D. A. Brase, S. P. Welch, and W. L. Dewey, "The role of endogenous peptides in the action of opioid analgesics," *Annals of Emergency Medicine*, vol. 15, no. 9, pp. 1030–1035, 1986.

[12] F. Benedetti, W. Thoen, C. Blanchard, S. Vighetti, and C. Arduino, "Pain as a reward: changing the meaning of pain from negative to positive co-activates opioid and cannabinoid systems," *Pain*, vol. 154, no. 3, pp. 361–367, 2013.

[13] H. L. Fields, M. M. Heinricher, and P. Mason, "Neurotransmitters in nociceptive modulatory circuits," *Annual Review of Neuroscience*, vol. 14, pp. 219–245, 1991.

[14] J. W. Little, A. Ford, A. M. Symons-Liguori et al., "Endogenous adenosine A3 receptor activation selectively alleviates persistent pain states," *Brain*, vol. 138, no. 1, pp. 28–35, 2015.

[15] T. Lundeberg, K. Uvnäs-Moberg, G. Ågren, and G. Bruzelius, "Anti-nociceptive effects of oxytocin in rats and mice," *Neuroscience Letters*, vol. 170, no. 1, pp. 153–157, 1994.

[16] P. Mason, "Central mechanisms of pain modulation," *Current Opinion in Neurobiology*, vol. 9, no. 4, pp. 436–441, 1999.

[17] X. Nadal, C. La Porta, S. A. Bura, and R. Maldonado, "Involvement of the opioid and cannabinoid systems in pain control: new insights from knockout studies," *European Journal of Pharmacology*, vol. 716, no. 1–3, pp. 142–157, 2013.

[18] M. H. Ossipov, G. O. Dussor, and F. Porreca, "Central modulation of pain," *Journal of Clinical Investigation*, vol. 120, no. 11, pp. 3779–3787, 2010.

[19] J. Sawynok, "Adenosine receptor targets for pain," *Neuroscience*, 2015.

[20] L. Lindgren, G. Westling, C. Brulin, S. Lehtipalo, M. Andersson, and L. Nyberg, "Pleasant human touch is represented in pregenual anterior cingulate cortex," *NeuroImage*, vol. 59, no. 4, pp. 3427–3432, 2012.

[21] F. Benedetti, M. Amanzio, R. Rosato, and C. Blanchard, "Nonopioid placebo analgesia is mediated by CB1 cannabinoid receptors," *Nature Medicine*, vol. 17, no. 10, pp. 1228–1230, 2011.

[22] L. Colloca, R. Klinger, H. Flor, and U. Bingel, "Placebo analgesia: psychological and neurobiological mechanisms," *Pain*, vol. 154, no. 4, pp. 511–514, 2013.

[23] F. Eippert, U. Bingel, E. D. Schoell et al., "Activation of the opioidergic descending pain control system underlies placebo analgesia," *Neuron*, vol. 63, no. 4, pp. 533–543, 2009.

[24] D. L. Morton, W. El-Deredy, and A. K. P. Jones, "Placebo analgesia: cognition or perception," in *Placebo*, vol. 225 of *Handbook of Experimental Pharmacology*, pp. 71–80, Springer, Berlin, Germany, 2014.

[25] M. D. Sauro and R. P. Greenberg, "Endogenous opiates and the placebo effect: a meta-analytic review," *Journal of Psychosomatic Research*, vol. 58, no. 2, pp. 115–120, 2005.

[26] T. D. Wager, D. J. Scott, and J.-K. Zubieta, "Placebo effects on human μ-opioid activity during pain," *Proceedings of the National Academy of Sciences of the United States of America*, vol. 104, no. 26, pp. 11056–11061, 2007.

[27] J.-K. Zubieta, J. A. Bueller, L. R. Jackson et al., "Placebo effects mediated by endogenous opioid activity on μ-opioid receptors," *Journal of Neuroscience*, vol. 25, no. 34, pp. 7754–7762, 2005.

[28] M. A. F. M. Gerrits, H. B. M. Lesscher, and J. M. van Ree, "Drug dependence and the endogenous opioid system," *European Neuropsychopharmacology*, vol. 13, no. 6, pp. 424–434, 2003.

[29] H. H. Loh, L. F. Tseng, E. Wei, and C. Hao Li, "β-endorphin is a potent analgesic agent," *Proceedings of the National Academy of Sciences of the United States of America*, vol. 73, no. 8, pp. 2895–2898, 1976.

[30] D. Le Bars, A. H. Dickenson, and J.-M. Besson, "Diffuse noxious inhibitory controls (DNIC). I. Effects on dorsal horn convergent neurones in the rat," *Pain*, vol. 6, no. 3, pp. 283–304, 1979.

[31] D. Le Bars, A. H. Dickenson, and J.-M. Besson, "Diffuse noxious inhibitory controls (DNIC). II. Lack of effect on non-convergent neurones, supraspinal involvement and theoretical implications," *Pain*, vol. 6, no. 3, pp. 305–327, 1979.

[32] D. Chitour, A. H. Dickenson, and D. Le Bars, "Pharmacological evidence for the involvement of serotonergic mechanisms in diffuse noxious inhibitory controls (DNIC)," *Brain Research*, vol. 236, no. 2, pp. 329–337, 1982.

[33] E. Kraus, D. Le Bars, and J.-M. Besson, "Behavioral confirmation of 'diffuse noxious inhibitory controls' (DNIC) and evidence for a role of endogenous opiates," *Brain Research*, vol. 206, no. 2, pp. 495–499, 1981.

[34] D. Yarnitsky, "Conditioned pain modulation (the diffuse noxious inhibitory control-like effect): its relevance for acute and chronic pain states," *Current Opinion in Anaesthesiology*, vol. 23, no. 5, pp. 611–615, 2010.

[35] S. Mense, "Neurobiological concepts of fibromyalgia—the possible role of descending spinal tracts," *Scandinavian Journal of Rheumatology. Supplement*, vol. 29, no. 113, pp. 24–29, 2000.

[36] T. Bender, G. Nagy, I. Barna, I. Tefner, É. Kádas, and P. Géher, "The effect of physical therapy on beta-endorphin levels," *European Journal of Applied Physiology*, vol. 100, no. 4, pp. 371–382, 2007.

[37] J. M. Crielaard, R. Bastin, and P. Franchimont, "The endorphin system and physical medicine," *Acta Belgica. Medica Physica*, vol. 6, no. 4, pp. 141–145, 1983.

[38] B. F. Degenhardt, N. A. Darmani, J. C. Johnson et al., "Role of osteopathic manipulative treatment in altering pain biomarkers: a pilot study," *Journal of the American Osteopathic Association*, vol. 107, no. 9, pp. 387–400, 2007.

[39] J. M. McPartland, A. Giuffrida, J. King, E. Skinner, J. Scotter, and R. E. Musty, "Cannabimimetic effects of osteopathic manipulative treatment," *Journal of the American Osteopathic Association*, vol. 105, no. 6, pp. 283–291, 2005.

[40] H. T. Vernon, M. S. Dhami, T. P. Howley, and R. Annett, "Spinal manipulation and beta-endorphin: a controlled study of the effect of a spinal manipulation on plasma beta-endorphin levels in normal males," *Journal of Manipulative and Physiological Therapeutics*, vol. 9, no. 2, pp. 115–123, 1986.

[41] A. Grice, "A biomechanical approach to cervical and dorsal adjusting," in *Modem Developments in the Principles and Practice of Chiropractic*, pp. 331–358, Appleton-Century-Crofts, New York, NY, USA, 1980.

[42] G. F. Christian, G. J. Stanton, D. Sissons et al., "Immunoreactive ACTH, β-endorphin, and cortisol levels in plasma following spinal manipulative therapy," *Spine*, vol. 13, no. 12, pp. 1411–1417, 1988.

[43] G. E. Sanders, O. Reinert, R. Tepe, and P. Maloney, "Chiropractic adjustive manipulation on subjects with acute low back pain: visual analog pain scores and plasma β-endorphin levels," *Journal of Manipulative and Physiological Therapeutics*, vol. 13, no. 7, pp. 391–395, 1990.

[44] G. Plaza-Manzano, F. Molina, R. Lomas-Vega, A. Martínez-Amat, A. Achalandabaso, and F. Hita-Contreras, "Changes in biochemical markers of pain perception and stress response after spinal manipulation," *Journal of Orthopaedic and Sports Physical Therapy*, vol. 44, no. 4, pp. 231–239, 2014.

[45] H. Vernon, "Qualitative review of studies of manipulation-induced hypoalgesia," *Journal of Manipulative and Physiological Therapeutics*, vol. 23, no. 2, pp. 134–138, 2000.

[46] C. Savva, G. Giakas, and M. Efstathiou, "The role of the descending inhibitory pain mechanism in musculoskeletal pain following high-velocity, low amplitude thrust manipulation: a review of the literature," *Journal of Back and Musculoskeletal Rehabilitation*, vol. 27, no. 4, pp. 377–382, 2014.

[47] D. A. Skyba, R. Radhakrishnan, J. J. Rohlwing, A. Wright, and K. A. Sluka, "Joint manipulation reduces hyperalgesia by activation of monoamine receptors but not opioid or GABA receptors in the spinal cord," *Pain*, vol. 106, no. 1-2, pp. 159–168, 2003.

[48] D. F. Martins, F. Bobinski, L. Mazzardo-Martins et al., "Ankle joint mobilization decreases hypersensitivity by activation of peripheral opioid receptors in a mouse model of postoperative pain," *Pain Medicine*, vol. 13, no. 8, pp. 1049–1058, 2012.

[49] D. F. Martins, L. Mazzardo-Martins, F. J. Cidral-Filho, V. M. Gadotti, and A. R. S. Santos, "Peripheral and spinal activation of cannabinoid receptors by joint mobilization alleviates post-operative pain in mice," *Neuroscience*, vol. 255, pp. 110–121, 2013.

[50] D. F. Martins, L. Mazzardo-Martins, F. J. Cidral-Filho, J. Stramosk, and A. R. S. Santos, "Ankle joint mobilization affects postoperative pain through peripheral and central adenosine A1 receptors," *Physical Therapy*, vol. 93, no. 3, pp. 401–412, 2013.

[51] G. D. Maitland, *Peripheral Manipulation*, Butterworth-Heinemann, London, UK, 1991.

[52] M. F. DosSantos, I. K. Martikainen, T. D. Nascimento et al., "Reduced basal ganglia μ-opioid receptor availability in trigeminal neuropathic pain: a pilot study," *Molecular Pain*, vol. 8, article 74, 2012.

[53] D. F. Martins, L. Mazzardo-Martins, V. M. Gadotti et al., "Ankle joint mobilization reduces axonotmesis-induced neuropathic pain and glial activation in the spinal cord and enhances nerve regeneration in rats," *Pain*, vol. 152, no. 11, pp. 2653–2661, 2011.

[54] M. L. Loggia, D. B. Chonde, O. Akeju et al., "Evidence for brain glial activation in chronic pain patients," *Brain*, vol. 138, no. 3, pp. 604–615, 2015.

[55] A. Paungmali, S. O'Leary, T. Souvlis, and B. Vicenzino, "Naloxone fails to antagonize initial hypoalgesic effect of a manual therapy treatment for lateral epicondylalgia," *Journal of Manipulative and Physiological Therapeutics*, vol. 27, no. 3, pp. 180–185, 2004.

[56] A. Paungmali, B. Vicenzino, and M. Smith, "Hypoalgesia induced by elbow manipulation in lateral epicondylalgia does not exhibit tolerance," *Journal of Pain*, vol. 4, no. 8, pp. 448–454, 2003.

[57] S. M. Payson and H. S. Holloway, "Possible complications of using naloxone as an internal opiate antagonist in the investigation of the role of endorphins in osteopathic manipulative treatment," *Journal of the American Osteopathic Association*, vol. 84, no. 1, pp. 152–156, 1984.

[58] R. F. Ellis and W. A. Hing, "Neural mobilization: a systematic review of randomized controlled trials with an analysis of therapeutic efficacy," *Journal of Manual and Manipulative Therapy*, vol. 16, no. 1, pp. 8–22, 2008.

[59] N. A. de Morton, "The PEDro scale is a valid measure of the methodological quality of clinical trials: a demographic study," *Australian Journal of Physiotherapy*, vol. 55, no. 2, pp. 129–133, 2009.

[60] F. M. Santos, J. T. Silva, A. C. Giardini et al., "Neural mobilization reverses behavioral and cellular changes that characterize neuropathic pain in rats," *Molecular Pain*, vol. 8, article 57, 2012.

[61] F. M. Santos, L. H. Grecco, M. G. Pereira et al., "The neural mobilization technique modulates the expression of endogenous opioids in the periaqueductal gray and improves muscle strength and mobility in rats with neuropathic pain," *Behavioral and Brain Functions*, vol. 10, article 19, 2014.

[62] T. Field, "Massage therapy research review," *Complementary Therapies in Clinical Practice*, vol. 20, no. 4, pp. 224–229, 2014.

[63] A. J. Threlkeld, "The effects of manual therapy on connective tissue," *Physical Therapy*, vol. 72, no. 12, pp. 893–902, 1992.

[64] B. Kaada and O. Torsteinbø, "Increase of plasma beta-endorphins in connective tissue massage," *General Pharmacology*, vol. 20, no. 4, pp. 487–489, 1989.

[65] B. Kaada and O. Torsteinbø, "Vasoactive intestinal polypeptides in connective tissue massage. With a note on VIP in heat pack treatment," *General Pharmacology*, vol. 18, no. 4, pp. 379–384, 1987.

[66] J. F. Trentini III, B. Thompson, and J. S. Erlichman, "The antinociceptive effect of acupressure in rats," *The American Journal of Chinese Medicine*, vol. 33, no. 1, pp. 143–150, 2005.

[67] A. Fassoulaki, A. Paraskeva, G. Kostopanagiotou, E. Tsakalozou, and S. Markantonis, "Acupressure on the extra 1 acupoint: the effect on bispectral index, serum melatonin, plasma beta-endorphin, and stress," *Anesthesia and Analgesia*, vol. 104, no. 2, pp. 312–317, 2007.

[68] J. A. Day, R. R. Mason, and S. E. Chesrown, "Effect of massage on serum level of β-endorphin and β-lipoprotein in healthy adults," *Physical Therapy*, vol. 67, no. 6, pp. 926–930, 1987.

[69] G. Agren, T. Lundeberg, K. Uvnäs-Moberg, and A. Sato, "The oxytocin antagonist 1-deamino-2-D-Tyr-(Oet)-4-Thr-8-Orn-oxytocin reverses the increase in the withdrawal response latency to thermal, but not mechanical nociceptive stimuli following oxytocin administration or massage-like stroking in rats," *Neuroscience Letters*, vol. 187, no. 1, pp. 49–52, 1995.

[70] R. A. Turner, M. Altemus, T. Enos, B. Cooper, and T. McGuinness, "Preliminary research on plasma oxytocin in normal cycling women: investigating emotion and interpersonal distress," *Psychiatry*, vol. 62, no. 2, pp. 97–113, 1999.

[71] D. Bello, R. White-Traut, D. Schwertz, H. Pournajafi-Nazarloo, and C. S. Carter, "An exploratory study of neurohormonal responses of healthy men to massage," *Journal of Alternative and Complementary Medicine*, vol. 14, no. 4, pp. 387–394, 2008.

[72] V. Morhenn, L. E. Beavin, and P. J. Zak, "Massage increases oxytocin and reduces adrenocorticotropin hormone in humans," *Alternative Therapies in Health and Medicine*, vol. 18, no. 6, pp. 11–18, 2012.

[73] M. Hernandez-Reif, T. Field, J. Krasnegor, and H. Theakston, "Lower back pain is reduced and range of motion increased after massage therapy," *International Journal of Neuroscience*, vol. 106, no. 3-4, pp. 131–145, 2001.

[74] M. Hernandez-Reif, G. Ironson, T. Field et al., "Breast cancer patients have improved immune and neuroendocrine functions following massage therapy," *Journal of Psychosomatic Research*, vol. 57, no. 1, pp. 45–52, 2004.

[75] T. Field, M. Hernandez-Reif, M. Diego, S. Schanberg, and C. Kuhn, "Cortisol decreases and serotonin and dopamine increase following massage therapy," *International Journal of Neuroscience*, vol. 115, no. 10, pp. 1397–1413, 2005.

[76] S. Hart, T. Field, M. Hernandez-Reif et al., "Anorexia nervosa symptoms are reduced by massage therapy," *Eating Disorders*, vol. 9, no. 4, pp. 289–299, 2001.

[77] I. Lund, T. Lundeberg, J. Carleson, H. Sönnerfors, B. Uhrlin, and E. Svensson, "Corticotropin releasing factor in urine—a possible biochemical marker of fibromyalgia. Responses to massage and guided relaxation," *Neuroscience Letters*, vol. 403, no. 1-2, pp. 166–171, 2006.

[78] A. Billhult, C. Lindholm, R. Gunnarsson, and E. Stener-Victorin, "The effect of massage on cellular immunity, endocrine and psychological factors in women with breast cancer—a randomized controlled clinical trial," *Autonomic Neuroscience*, vol. 140, no. 1-2, pp. 88–95, 2008.

[79] S. Tsuji, T. Yuhi, K. Furuhara, S. Ohta, Y. Shimizu, and H. Higashida, "Salivary oxytocin concentrations in seven boys with autism spectrum disorder received massage from their mothers: a pilot study," *Frontiers in Psychiatry*, vol. 6, article 58, 2015.

[80] M. H. Rapaport, P. Schettler, and C. Bresee, "A preliminary study of the effects of a single session of Swedish Massage on hypothalamic-pituitary-adrenal and immune function in normal individuals," *Journal of Alternative and Complementary Medicine*, vol. 16, no. 10, pp. 1079–1088, 2010.

[81] M. H. Rapaport, P. Schettler, and C. Bresee, "A preliminary study of the effects of repeated massage on hypothalamic-pituitary-adrenal and immune function in healthy individuals: a study of mechanisms of action and dosage," *Journal of Alternative and Complementary Medicine*, vol. 18, no. 8, pp. 789–797, 2012.

[82] W. R. Lariviere and R. Melzack, "The role of corticotropin-releasing factor in pain and analgesia," *Pain*, vol. 84, no. 1, pp. 1–12, 2000.

[83] H. L. Wen, W. K. K. Ho, L. Ma, G. H. Choa, and N. Ling, "The influence of electro-acupuncture on naloxone-induced morphine withdrawal: II. Elevation of immunoassayable beta-endorphin activity in the brain but not the blood," *The American Journal of Chinese Medicine*, vol. 7, no. 3, pp. 237–240, 1979.

[84] S. McLean, R. Naish, L. Reed, S. Urry, and B. Vicenzino, "A pilot study of the manual force levels required to produce manipulation induced hypoalgesia," *Clinical Biomechanics*, vol. 17, no. 4, pp. 304–308, 2002.

Association of Serum Serotonin and Pain in Patients with Chronic Low Back Pain before and after Spinal Surgery

Afshin Farhanchi,[1] Behrouz Karkhanei,[1] Negar Amani,[1] Mashhood Aghajanloo,[2] Elham Khanlarzadeh,[3] and Zahra Emami[4]

[1] *Department of Anesthesiology, Hamadan University of Medical Sciences, Hamadan, Iran*
[2] *Department of Neurosurgery, Hamadan University of Medical Sciences, Hamadan, Iran*
[3] *Department of Community Medicine, Hamadan University of Medical Sciences, Hamadan, Iran*
[4] *Bu-Ali Sina University, Hamadan, Iran*

Correspondence should be addressed to Behrouz Karkhanei; behrouzkarkhanei@yahoo.com

Academic Editor: Fabio Antonaci

Introduction. In this study we are aiming to evaluate the changes of serum serotonin and its association with pain in patients suffering from chronic low back pain before and after lumbar discectomy surgery. *Patients and Methods.* A prospective study was performed on the patients referring to the outpatient clinic in Besat hospital, Hamadan University of Medical Sciences, Hamadan, Iran, during 2016. A 2 mL fasting blood sample was collected from each patient at preoperative day 1 and postoperative day 14 and they were measured for level of serum serotonin. Besides, all patients were asked for severity of their low back pain in preoperative day 1 and postoperative day 14 and scored their pain from zero to ten using a Numerical Rating Scale. *Results.* Forty patients with the mean age of 47 ± 13 yrs/old (range 25–77) including 15 (37.5%) males were enrolled into the study. The overall mean score of preoperative pain was significantly decreased from 7.4 ± 2.18 (range 4–10) to the postoperative pain score 3.87 ± 2.92 (range 0–10) ($P < .001$). The overall levels of pre- and postoperative serum serotonin were 3.37 ± 1.27 (range 1.1–6.4) and 3.58 ± 1.32 (range .94–7.1) ng/mL, respectively, with no significant difference ($P = .09$). The levels of pre- and postoperative serum serotonin were significantly higher in males and patients older than 50 yrs/old compared to the females and patients younger than 50 yrs/old, respectively ($P = .03$ and .005, respectively). A significant inverse correlation between the postoperative levels of pain and serum serotonin was observed ($r = -.36$ and $P = .02$). *Conclusion.* A negative medium strength linear relationship may exist between the postoperative serum serotonin and low back pain.

1. Introduction

Low back pain is one the most common health care issues causing enormous financial and social costs globally. Chronic low back pain with duration of pain greater than three months is the second most frequent complaint in physician visits which is related to disability of one-fourth of working populations and significant loss of working days [1, 2]. Lumbar disk herniation is one of the most common causes of chronic low back pain due to mechanical compression of nerve roots and inflammation of intervertebral disks and sometimes surgery is indicated if medical therapy fails to control the disabling symptoms [3, 4].

Although the role of some mechanical, thermal, and chemical agents have been studied in pain regulation, the mechanism of pain induction and perception has not been completely elucidated yet [5]. Recently, serotonin has been proposed to have a role in postoperative pain modulation in both central and peripheral nervous systems. Although postoperative neuropathic pain has been reduced by using selective serotonin reuptake inhibitors (SSRIs) [6], serotonin released from mast cells and platelets due to tissue damage during surgery has been shown to result in pain induction or inhibition [7–9]. To the best of our knowledge, there is no clinical study to find the alterations of serum serotonin in patients suffering from chronic back pain in whom surgical treatment is indicated.

Table 1: The detailed data about levels of pre- and postoperative pain based on numerical rating scale.

	Pain (Numerical Rating Scale score)		
	Pre-operation	**Post-operation**	**P value**
Surgery			
Laminectomy & discectomy	7.66 ± 2.27	3.72 ± 2.82	< **.001**
Laminotomy & discectomy	7.18 ± 2.13	4 ± 3.07	< **.001**
Gender			
Male	7.66 ± 2.28	4.4 ± 3.45	**.006**
Female	7.24 ± 2.14	3.56 ± 2.58	< **.001**
Age			
< **50 yrs/old**	7.21 ± 2.11	3.64 ± 3.12	**.001**
> **50 yrs/old**	7.5 ± 2.24	4 ± 2.87	< **.001**
Cigarette smoker			
Yes	7.16 ± 2.63	6.5 ± 3.98	.63
No	7.44 ± 2.13	3.41 ± 2.49	< **.001**
Opium addict			
Yes	7.25 ± 2.36	5.25 ± 4.42	.51
No	7.41 ± 2.19	3.72 ± 2.76	< **.001**

Data are shown as mean ± standard deviation.

In this study we are aiming to evaluate the effectiveness of lumbar discectomy with either laminectomy or laminotomy surgery on chronic low back pain, changes of pre- and postoperative serum serotonin, and the association of serum serotonin and pain of the patients.

2. Patients and Methods

A prospective study was performed on the patients referring to the outpatient clinic in Besat hospital, Hamadan University of Medical Sciences, Hamadan, Iran, during 2016. Inclusion criteria were the patients suffering from chronic low back pain due to lumbar disk herniation who were candidates for surgical treatment. The pain of the patients was disabling even with full medical treatment and was associated with radiculopathy, neurologic deficit, and physical status of class two or less based on the American Society of Anesthesiology classification system. The diagnosis of lumbar disk herniation was made based on the related signs and symptoms of the patients and magnetic resonance imaging findings. Patients with major depression, neurological disorders, diabetes mellitus, and history of using antidepressant or antipsychotic medications were excluded from the study.

A 2 mL fasting blood sample was collected from each patient at preoperative day 1 and postoperative day 14 and was kept at -20°C under the same condition. All samples were measured for level of serum serotonin on the same day using Enzyme-linked immunosorbent assay kit (IBL International Immunoassays GmBH, Germany). Besides, all patients were asked for severity of their low back pain at preoperative day 1 and postoperative day 14 and scored their pain from zero to ten using a Numerical Rating Scale with score of zero indicating having no pain and ten indicating the most severe experienced pain. These data in addition to the demographics and status of smoking and opium use were recorded prospectively. All patients underwent lumbar discectomy with either laminectomy or laminotomy surgery by the same surgeon. Also, all postoperative visits were done by the same surgeon.

The approval of the Ethics Committee of Hamadan University of Medical Sciences was granted prior to patient recruitment and once the aims and procedures of the study were explained, a written informed consent was granted from all participants.

Analysis of data was performed by using the SPSS statistical software (IBM SPSS Statistics for Windows, Version 23.0, IBM Corp., Armonk, NY, USA). Data were expressed as mean ± standard deviation and were compared by using independent or paired samples t-tests. Correlation between the level of serum serotonin and the Numerical Rating Scale score was assessed by using Pearson correlation coefficient. P value less than .05 was considered statistically significant.

3. Results

Forty patients with the mean age of 47 ± 13 yrs/old (range 25–77) including 15 (37.5%) males were enrolled into the study. Laminectomy surgery alone has been performed in 18 (45%) patients while laminectomy and lumbar pedicle screw fixation has been performed in the others. Frequencies of the patients who were current cigarette smoker and opium addict were 6 (15%) and 4 (10%), respectively.

The overall mean score of preoperative pain was significantly decreased from 7.4 ± 2.18 (range 4–10) to the postoperative pain score 3.87 ± 2.92 (range 0 – 10) ($P < .001$). The detailed data about scores of pre- and postoperative pain are shown in Table 1. Moreover, the overall levels of pre- and postoperative serum serotonin were 3.37 ± 1.27 (range 1.1–6.4) and 3.58 ± 1.32 (range .94–7.1) ng/mL, respectively, with no significant difference ($P = .09$). As shown in Table 2, the levels

Table 2: The detailed data about levels of pre- and postoperative serum serotonin.

	Serum serotonin (ng/mL)		
	Pre-operation	Post-operation	P value
Surgery			
Laminectomy & discectomy	3.59 ± 1.11	3.62 ± 0.94	.84
Laminectomy & discectomy	3.19 ± 1.39	3.56 ± 1.58	.07
Gender			
Male	3.36 ± 1.05	3.79 ± 1.24	**.03**
Female	3.37 ± 1.41	3.46 ± 1.37	.59
Age			
< 50 yrs/old	3.77 ± 1.18	3.77 ± 1.33	.97
> 50 yrs/old	2.62 ± 1.11	3.23 ± 1.27	**.005**
Current cigarette smoker			
Yes	3.66 ± 0.82	4.17 ± 1.09	.1
No	3.32 ± 1.34	3.48 ± 1.34	.25
Current opium addict			
Yes	3.29 ± 1.17	3.34 ± 1.13	.63
No	3.38 ± 1.3	3.61 ± 1.35	.1

Data are shown as mean ± standard deviation.

of postoperative serum serotonin were significantly higher than the related preoperative serum serotonin just in males and patients older than 50 yrs/old, respectively ($P = .03$ and .005, respectively).

A significant inverse correlation between the postoperative levels of pain and serum serotonin was observed ($r = -.36$ and $P = .02$). However, there was no significant correlation between the preoperative levels of pain and serum serotonin ($r = .08$ and $P = .6$).

4. Discussion

In our study, pain of the patients was significantly reduced from the pre- to the postoperative period regardless of the type of surgery, age, and gender of the patients. Consistent with our data, it has been shown that there is no significant difference between lumbar discectomy surgery with either laminectomy or laminotomy in reducing low back pain [10]. However, the data about relation of age and gender of patients with postoperative outcome is debatable. Like ours, some studies suggested that outcomes of lumbar discectomy in elderly patients were comparable to the younger ones [11, 12]; however, some showed that aging would be associated with adverse outcomes in such patients [10]. Regarding gender, some previous studies, in contrast to ours, suggested that female gender might be associated with poorer outcome [13, 14]. In contrast, a recent randomized and observational study by Kerr et al. showed that gender of the patients was not a predictor of postoperative outcome [15]. Our results also show that the smokers experienced no significant improvement with their low back pain, in contrast to the nonsmokers, which is inconsistent with other studies suggesting better postoperative outcomes for nonsmokers [16, 17].

Serotonin synthesis is controlled by sex hormones; therefore, the alteration of serum serotonin can be expected by difference in ethnicity, gender, and advancement of age [18, 19]. Testosterone and estrogen have been shown to be positively correlated with serum serotonin. The rate of serotonin synthesis in normal males was found to be 52% higher than in normal females. On the other hand, serotonin transporter protein may be reduced in synaptic junctions by the sex hormones and may result in enhancement of synaptic transmission. Thus, the pain perception can be expected to be different between genders and postmenopausal age [19–21]. By advancement of age and consequent decrease in gonadal hormones, serum serotonin regulation by gonadal hormones may be lost and more diverse fluctuation may be seen in stress related conditions. Hence, different levels of sex hormones can be a possible explanation for difference in serotonin levels in different age and gender groups observed in the pre- and postoperative periods of our study. However, further studies including more participants have to be implemented to carefully delineate the observed significant alterations of serum serotonin in different age and gender groups before and after surgery.

In our study, the level of serum serotonin was not significantly changed from the pre- to the postoperative period, in contrast to the level of the pain. Besides, in the postoperative period, the level of serum serotonin was inversely associated with the level of the pain. There is much debate over the association of levels of serum serotonin and chronic low back pain. Similar to ours, an inverse relationship between serum serotonin and pain was reported in healthy individuals and patients performing lumbar exercise for treatment of their low back pain [22, 23]. In an experimental study by Vogel et al., an increment in level of serotonin in a nerve with chronic constriction injury was observed while the level of spinal serotonin decreased [24]. In contrast, some studies showed that the level of spinal serotonin increased or was not changed after spinal nerve injury [25, 26]. Two recent experimental studies have shown that using selective serotonin or serotonin–noradrenaline reuptake inhibitors may be associated with reduction of neuropathic pain related to lumbar disk herniation and inhibition of tumor necrosis factor expression after two or three weeks of treatment suggesting the pronociceptive feature of serotonin in lumbar disk herniation-related pain [27, 28]. On the other hand, in a systematic review by Urquhart et al., in 2008, including nine randomized controlled trials, no significant relief in chronic low back pain was observed in patients who were treated with SSRIs [29]. In contrast, two randomized controlled trials in 2010 suggested that duloxetine as a SSRI associated with improvement of function and pain in patients suffering from chronic low back pain [30, 31].

Chronic low back pain associated with lumbar disk herniation may be related to inflammatory process and mediators such as tumor necrosis factor-alpha and serotonin which are released from mast cells and platelets as a consequence of tissue injury [32]. Serotonin as a neurotransmitter has been proposed to play various roles in pain modulation and signaling mechanisms in both peripheral and central nervous systems. It has been well elucidated that, in peripheral nervous system, serotonin and some mediators of inflammation such as prostaglandins, bradykinin, histamine, potassium ion, and substance P may be responsible for sensitizing the peripheral neurons to inflammation-related pain [33–35]. Nevertheless, in the central nervous system, serotonin may have various effects in stimulating or inhibiting pain signal transmission and its role in nociception in the central nervous system has not been well established yet [36, 37]. The high inconsistency through the various studies may be due to the complex underlying mechanisms of pronociceptive or antinociceptive effects of serotonin in the central nervous system and multiplicity of its receptors. Modulation of tryptophan, precursor of serotonin, has been used as a model for serotonin changes in pain processing [38]. It has been shown that depletion of tryptophan in healthy volunteers diminished morphine induced analgesia or resulted in network disruption similar to disturbance seen in irritable bowel syndrome sufferers with pain [39, 40]. On the other hand, using tryptophan supplementation may be associated with both pain tolerance and mood in healthy subjects [41]. A recent study has indicated an association between reduction of global serotonin and alteration in pain perception, though dissociating these findings from altered mood state [8]. Moreover, it has been reported that patients with chronic tension type headache may have low levels of serum serotonin [42–44]. These data are supported by the fact that using SSRIs may be associated with improvement of chronic pain [45, 46]. Thus, low levels of serotonin may correlate with pain sensitization or perception. However, future studies on the role of serotonin in cognitive and noncognitive characteristics of pain processing and chronic pain is essential to improving individual treatment choice for patients with chronic pain.

5. Conclusions

In summary, preoperative chronic low back pain of our patients reduced in postoperative period; however the level of serum serotonin was not significantly changed. Moreover, a negative medium strength linear relationship between the postoperative serum serotonin and pain was observed in our study.

References

[1] J. K. Freburger, G. M. Holmes, R. P. Agans et al., "The rising prevalence of chronic low back pain," *JAMA Internal Medicine*, vol. 169, no. 3, pp. 251–258, 2009.

[2] J. A. Ricci, W. F. Stewart, E. Chee, C. Leotta, K. Foley, and M. C. Hochberg, "Back pain exacerbations and lost productive time costs in United States workers," *The Spine Journal*, vol. 31, no. 26, pp. 3052–3060, 2006.

[3] Y. Aoki, B. Rydevik, S. Kikuchi, and K. Olmarker, "Local application of disc-related cytokines on spinal nerve roots," *The Spine Journal*, vol. 27, no. 15, pp. 1614–1617, 2002.

[4] S. M. Rothman and B. A. Winkelstein, "Chemical and mechanical nerve root insults induce differential behavioral sensitivity and glial activation that are enhanced in combination," *Brain Research*, vol. 1181, no. 1, pp. 30–43, 2007.

[5] O. Paulsen, B. Laird, N. Aass et al., "The relationship between pro-inflammatory cytokines and pain, appetite and fatigue in patients with advanced cancer," *PLoS ONE*, vol. 12, no. 5, Article ID e0177620, 2017.

[6] H. Obata, "Analgesic mechanisms of antidepressants for neuropathic pain," *International Journal of Molecular Sciences*, vol. 18, no. 11, p. 2483, 2017.

[7] L. Bardin, "The complex role of serotonin and 5-HT receptors in chronic pain," *Behavioural Pharmacology*, vol. 22, no. 5-6, pp. 390–404, 2011.

[8] S. L. Martin, A. Power, Y. Boyle, I. M. Anderson, M. A. Silverdale, and A. K. Jones, "5-HT modulation of pain perception in humans," *Psychopharmacology*, vol. 234, no. 19, pp. 2929–2939, 2017.

[9] C. Sommer, "Serotonin in pain and analgesia: actions in the periphery," *Molecular Neurobiology*, vol. 30, no. 2, pp. 117–125, 2004.

[10] M. Sedighi and A. Haghnegahdar, "Lumbar disk herniation surgery: outcome and predictors," *Global Spine Journal*, vol. 4, no. 4, pp. 233–243, 2014.

[11] K. Fujii, T. Henmi, Y. Kanematsu, T. Mishiro, and T. Sakai, "Surgical treatment of lumbar disc herniation in elderly patients," *The Journal of Bone & Joint Surgery*, vol. 85, no. 8, pp. 1146–1150, 2003.

[12] V. Graver, A. K. Haaland, B. Magnas, and M. Loeb, "Seven-year clinical follow-up after lumbar disc surgery: results and predictors of outcome," *British Journal of Neurosurgery*, vol. 13, no. 2, pp. 178–184, 2009.

[13] W. C. Peul, R. Brand, R. T. W. M. Thomeer, and B. W. Koes, "Influence of gender and other prognostic factors on outcome of sciatica," *PAIN*, vol. 138, no. 1, pp. 180–191, 2008.

[14] F. Strömqvist, M. Ahmad, C. Hildingsson, B. Jönsson, and B. Strömqvist, "Gender differences in lumbar disc herniation surgery," *Acta Orthopaedica*, vol. 79, no. 5, pp. 643–649, 2009.

[15] D. Kerr, W. Zhao, and J. D. Lurie, "What are long-term predictors of outcomes for lumbar disc herniation? A randomized and observational study," *Clinical Orthopaedics and Related Research*, vol. 473, no. 6, pp. 1920–1930, 2015.

[16] C. Behrend, M. Prasarn, E. Coyne, M. Horodyski, J. Wright, and G. R. Rechtine, "Smoking cessation related to improved patient-

reported pain scores following spinal care," *The Journal of Bone & Joint Surgery*, vol. 94, no. 23, pp. 2161–2166, 2012.

[17] A. Sørile, V. Moholdt, K. A. Kvistad et al., "Modic type i changes and recovery of back pain after lumbar microdiscectomy," *European Spine Journal*, vol. 21, no. 11, pp. 2252–2258, 2012.

[18] A. M. Kumar, S. Weiss, J. B. Fernandez, D. Cruess, and C. Eisdorfer, "Peripheral serotonin levels in women: Role of aging and ethnicity," *Gerontology*, vol. 44, no. 4, pp. 211–216, 1998.

[19] S. Nishizawa, C. Benkelfat, S. N. Young et al., "Differences between males and females in rates of serotonin synthesis in human brain," *Proceedings of the National Acadamy of Sciences of the United States of America*, vol. 94, no. 10, pp. 5308–5313, 1997.

[20] H. Jovanovic, L. Kocoska-Maras, A. F. Rådestad et al., "Effects of estrogen and testosterone treatment on serotonin transporter binding in the brain of surgically postmenopausal women - a PET study," *NeuroImage*, vol. 106, pp. 47–54, 2015.

[21] E. Perfalk, S. D. Cunha-Bang, K. K. Holst et al., "Testosterone levels in healthy men correlate negatively with serotonin 4 receptor binding," *Psychoneuroendocrinology*, vol. 81, pp. 22–28, 2017.

[22] G. Pickering, F. Januel, C. Dubray, and A. Eschalier, "Serotonin and experimental pain in healthy young volunteers," *The Clinical Journal of Pain*, vol. 19, no. 4, pp. 276–279, 2003.

[23] O. Sokunbi, P. Watt, and A. Moore, "Changes in plasma concentration of serotonin in response to spinal stabilisation exercises in chronic low back pain patient," *Nigerian Quarterly Journal of Hospital Medicine*, vol. 17, no. 3, 2008.

[24] C. Vogel, R. Mössner, M. Gerlach et al., "Absence of thermal hyperalgesia in serotonin transporter-deficient mice," *The Journal of Neuroscience*, vol. 23, no. 2, pp. 708–715, 2003.

[25] J. A. Lovell, J. C. Novak, S. L. Stuesse, W. L. R. Cruce, and T. Crisp, "Changes in spinal serotonin turnover mediate age-related differences in the behavioral manifestations of peripheral nerve injury," *Pharmacology Biochemistry & Behavior*, vol. 66, no. 4, pp. 873–878, 2000.

[26] O. Satoh and K. Omote, "Roles of monoaminergic, glycinergic and GABAergic inhibitory systems in the spinal cord in rats with peripheral mononeuropathy," *Brain Research*, vol. 728, no. 1, pp. 27–36, 1996.

[27] H. Saito, J. Wakai, M. Sekiguchi, S. Kikuchi, and S. Konno, "The effect of selective serotonin reuptake inhibitor (SSRI) on pain-related behavior in a rat model of neuropathic pain," *European Spine Journal*, vol. 23, no. 11, pp. 2401–2409, 2014.

[28] J. Handa, M. Sekiguchi, O. Krupkova, and S.-I. Konno, "The effect of serotonin–noradrenaline reuptake inhibitor duloxetine on the intervertebral disk-related radiculopathy in rats," *European Spine Journal*, vol. 25, no. 3, pp. 877–887, 2016.

[29] D. M. Urquhart, J. L. Hoving, W. J. Assendelft, M. Roland, and M. W. van Tulder, "Antidepressants for non-specific low back pain," *Cochrane Database of Systematic Reviews*.

[30] M. Mazza, O. Mazza, C. Pazzaglia, L. Padua, and S. Mazza, "Escitalopram 20 mg versus duloxetine 60 mg for the treatment of chronic low back pain," *Expert Opinion on Pharmacotherapy*, vol. 11, no. 7, pp. 1049–1052, 2010.

[31] V. Skljarevski, S. Zhang, D. Desaiah et al., "Duloxetine versus placebo in patients with chronic low back pain: a 12-week, fixed-dose, randomized, double-blind trial," *The Journal of Pain*, vol. 11, no. 12, pp. 1282–1290, 2010.

[32] H. Kobayashi, S.-I. Kikuchi, S.-I. Konno, K. Kato, and M. Sekiguchi, "Interaction of 5-hydroxytryptamine and tumor necrosis factor-α to pain-related behavior by nucleus pulposus applied on the nerve root in rats," *The Spine Journal*, vol. 36, no. 3, pp. 210–218, 2011.

[33] L. Becerra, J. Bishop, G. Barmettler, V. Kainz, R. Burstein, and D. Borsook, "Brain network alterations in the inflammatory soup animal model of migraine," *Brain Research*, vol. 1660, pp. 36–46, 2017.

[34] D. Julius and A. I. Basbaum, "Molecular mechanisms of nociception," *Nature*, vol. 413, no. 6852, pp. 203–210, 2001.

[35] J.-M. Zhang and J. An, "Cytokines, inflammation and pain," *International Anesthesiology Clinics*, vol. 45, no. 2, pp. 27–37, 2007.

[36] F. Bobinski, T. A. A. Ferreira, M. M. Córdova et al., "Role of brainstem serotonin in analgesia produced by low-intensity exercise on neuropathic pain after sciatic nerve injury in mice," *PAIN*, vol. 156, no. 12, pp. 2595–2606, 2015.

[37] D. Yarnitsky, "Role of endogenous pain modulation in chronic pain mechanisms and treatment," *PAIN*, vol. 156, supplement 1, pp. S24–S31, 2015.

[38] H. W. Chase, M. J. Crockett, R. M. Msetfi et al., "5-HT modulation by acute tryptophan depletion of human instrumental contingency judgements," *Psychopharmacology*, vol. 213, no. 2-3, pp. 615–623, 2011.

[39] F. V. Abbott, P. Etienne, K. B. J. Franklin, M. J. Morgan, M. J. Sewitch, and S. N. Young, "Acute tryptophan depletion blocks morphine analgesia in the cold-pressor test in humans," *Psychopharmacology*, vol. 108, no. 1-2, pp. 60–66, 1992.

[40] J. S. Labus, E. A. Mayer, J. Jarcho et al., "Acute tryptophan depletion alters the effective connectivity of emotional arousal circuitry during visceral stimuli in healthy women," *Gut*, vol. 60, no. 9, pp. 1196–1203, 2011.

[41] S. Seltzer, R. Stoch, R. Marcus, and E. Jackson, "Alteration of human pain thresholds by nutritional manipulation and l-tryptophan supplementation," *PAIN*, vol. 13, no. 4, pp. 385–393, 1982.

[42] M. Anthony and J. W. Lance, "Plasma serotonin in patients with chronic tension headaches," *Journal of Neurology, Neurosurgery & Psychiatry*, vol. 52, no. 2, pp. 182–184, 1989.

[43] D. Jonsson, O. Finskas, Y. Fujioka, A. Ståhlberg, and K. Olmarker, "Disc herniation decreases expression of serotonin receptors in the dorsal root ganglion in a tnf-dependent manner - a gene expression analysis in a rat model of disc herniation :.GP47," *Spine Journal Meeting Abstracts*, pp. 132-133, 2014.

[44] Y. C. Lee, N. J. Nassikas, and D. J. Clauw, "The role of the central nervous system in the generation and maintenance of chronic pain in rheumatoid arthritis, osteoarthritis and fibromyalgia," *Arthritis Research & Therapy*, vol. 13, no. 2, article 211, 2011.

[45] M. Khan, S. E. Nishi, S. N. Hassan, M. A. Islam, and S. H. Gan, "Trigeminal neuralgia, glossopharyngeal neuralgia, and myofascial pain dysfunction syndrome: An update," *Pain Research & Management*, vol. 2017, Article ID 7438326, 18 pages, 2017.

[46] P. L. Delgado, "Serotonin noradrenaline reuptake inhibitors: New hope for the treatment of chronic pain," *International Journal of Psychiatry in Clinical Practice*, vol. 10, no. 2, pp. 16–21, 2006.

8

Pain and Stress Response during Intravenous Access in Children with Congenital Adrenal Hyperplasia: Effects of EMLA and Nitrous Oxide Treatment

K. Ekbom[1,2]

[1]*Division of Paediatrics, Department for Clinical Science Intervention and Technology, Karolinska Institute, Karolinska University Hospital, 141 86 Stockholm, Sweden*
[2]*Division of Endocrinology, Diabetes and Metabolism, National Childhood Obesity Centre, Karolinska University Hospital, 141 86 Stockholm, Sweden*

Correspondence should be addressed to K. Ekbom; kerstin.ekbom@sll.se

Academic Editor: Donald A. Simone

Background. Congenital adrenal hyperplasia (CAH) is an endocrine condition that requires regularly blood samples for optimal treatment. The management of CAH in children is complex when intravenous access is one of the most stressful procedures for children. The purpose of this pilot study was to investigate the effects of nitrous oxide inhalation (N2O) in combination with cutaneous application of local anesthetics (EMLA) for improving intravenous access in children with CAH. *Method.* Ten children (7–14 years) were studied. The children received two intravenous procedures: one with EMLA and one with EMLA + N2O. The order of priority was randomized. The outcomes were the children's pain experience (0–10) and an evaluation of satisfaction (1–5) after the procedure. Heart rate, blood pressure, saturation, and analyses of 17-hydroxyprogesterone (17-OHP), norepinephrine, and glucose were analyzed. *Results.* Higher pain scores, heart rate, and glucose levels were reported after EMLA, compared to EMLA + N2O, but 17-OHP levels remained unchanged. The children's satisfaction with the intravenous procedure was more positive for EMLA + N2O. *Conclusions.* EMLA + N2O offers the possibility of improving the intravenous procedure for anxious children with CAH. Although the quality of care was better with N2O treatment, it was not possible to demonstrate that this is a prerequisite for valid 17-OHP measurements.

1. Introduction

Congenital adrenal hyperplasia (CAH) is one of the most prevalent monogenetic autosomal recessive endocrine disorders [1, 2]. Ninety-five percent of all cases are caused by a deficiency in 21-hydroxylase, which results in impaired biosynthesis of cortisol and cortisol deficiency as well as androgen excess with or without aldosterone deficiency. CAH shows a range of severity and is clinically classified into classic forms, the severe form, divided into simple virilizing and salt-wasting forms (33% and 67%, resp.), or nonclassic forms, the mild or late-onset form. Data from newborn infants, screened in 13 countries including Sweden, show an incidence of one in 15,000 livebirths for the classic form of CAH and an incident about one in 1,000 for the nonclassic form [3–5].

Medical treatment for CAH using glucocorticoids needs to be individualized to suppress androgen secretion, yet without total suppression of the hypothalamic-pituitary-adrenal (HPA) axis, which requires high glucocorticoid doses that cause negative side effects [6–10].

The 17-hydroxyprogesterone (17-OHP) levels are used to adjust the hydrocortisone dose and stressful IV access may affect 17-OHP levels, which could be interpreted as a sign of an insufficient glucocorticoid substitution dose.

The management of CAH is complex and adequate monitoring of therapy is important and includes IV access. However, there are other valuable control parameters, such as 17-OHP in saliva or urinary steroids (pregnanetriol), compared to the measurement of serum 17-OHP alone. However, an adequate monitoring includes as well blood samples for analysis of serum androstenedione, indicating if the children have appropriately therapy.

The target of 17-OHP and other hormones vary widely in children depending on the time of day and the interval since the last glucocorticoid dose. A concentration of 17-OHP >40 nmol/L indicates undertreatment [11]. Overtreatment can lead to growth suppression and potentially obesity as well as osteoporosis [7, 8, 10]. Since undertreatment results in an excess of high androgens, close control of medication is necessary [7, 12].

The use of intravenous (IV) access procedures is common in all chronically ill children [13], and IV procedures have been ranked as some of the most unpleasant procedures that children must undergo at a hospital [14]. Stress factors in connection with IV access include both emotional/physical stress and often poor vein selection [15].

Pain relief before venipuncture is an important issue for all anxious children and/or children with poor quality veins. We previously compared the efficiency of the standard procedure using EMLA with EMLA+ inhaled 50% nitrous oxide (N2O) in children with difficulties related to IV access [16]. However, we do not know how anxious children with CAH evaluate the IV procedure using conventional pain relief with EMLA and whether treatment with N2O would be a suitable alternative treatment for these children. Inhalation of nitrous oxide (N2O) is a well-established method and has both pain reduction and sedation effects [17, 18], which may be useful when treating anxious children with CAH.

It is even unclear if procedural pain in connection with IV access affects the analysis of 17-OHP and that connection has not been studied before in children with CAH.

The aim of our study was to compare EMLA with EMLA + N2O in children with CAH reporting anxiety in establishing IV access. We hypothesized that EMLA + N2O would be superior to EMLA reducing pain in children with CAH undergoing IV access and that the pain and anxiety reductions effects of N2O would decrease children's physiological stress markers and adrenal hormone secretion. Children's evaluation of pain, satisfaction with the IV procedure, and children's physiological stress markers were the primary end point. Secondary end point was levels of 17-OHP, norepinephrine, glucose, parents, and nurses satisfaction with the IV procedure.

The study was approved by the Ethical Committee of South Stockholm (Decision 050114).

Trial Registration. Current controlled trial is registered with ISRCTN33779750 (controlled-trials.com) and Karolinska Clinical Trial Registration (KCTR) is registered with CT 20090023.

2. Method

2.1. Design. The study design was a randomized, double-blind, crossover study including 10 children with CAH. The children were randomly allocated to two procedures. One procedure with EMLA and the inhalation of 100% oxygen (EMLA) and one procedure with EMLA and the inhalation of 50% nitrous oxide (EMLA + N2O), Figure 1.

One criterion for inclusion was that children had experienced previous difficulties connected to establishing IV access. The difficulties were defined as either a previous requirement of several attempts before establishing IV access or children rating anticipatory anxiety > 4 using a numeric rating scale (0–10) with 0 = no anxiety and 10 = worst possible anxiety [19, 20].

To be included, children also needed to have the ability to understand and comply with the different treatments, including using a face mask and interpreting the numeric rating scale (0–10) and Likert Scale (1–5) with verbal categorical response options of satisfaction with the IV procedure.

In addition to the double-blind crossover study, 30 children aged 5–18 served as controls. These children underwent blood sampling at the same time points after nitrous oxide sedation.

A research nurse randomized the children and prepared the anesthesia machine. She also set the percentage of nitrous oxide and oxygen according to randomization and concealed the mixing device. A pediatric nurse performed all the IV procedures and when the child had started to breathe into the mask for three minutes, the nurse set up an IV line.

The children, parents, and nurses were unaware of the randomization codes until data entry was completed. The procedure has been described in detail elsewhere [21].

2.1.1. Anesthesia Equipment. Oxygen and nitrous oxide were mixed using the Engstrom 2024® (Engstrom Medical AB Stockholm, Sweden) connected to nitrous oxide and oxygen sources.

2.1.2. Procedure. The children received EMLA® cream (Lidokain Prilokain 25 mg/g Astra Zeneca Södertälje, Sweden) 1 hour before IV access. They were also informed that during one of the procedures N2O treatment would be administered. All children were breathing a gas mixture continuously administered by an anesthesia machine through a mask from 3 minutes before until 3 minutes after the procedure. The anesthesia machine was hidden from the children and investigators by the research nurse. The IV cannulation was performed by an experienced pediatric nurse using a 22 G catheter.

The last dose of hydrocortisone was given in the morning, and no medication doses were adjusted between the 2 IV procedures.

2.2. Data Collection. All procedures were performed and blood samples were collected between the hours of 8:00 and 10:00. Blood samples were taken by venipuncture 5 minutes after venous access. Samples taken for plasma (P-) glucose (mmol/L), serum (S) androstenedione (nmol/L), and P-norepinephrine (NE; nmol/L) were analyzed directly in the Karolinska University Hospital laboratory. Samples obtained for S-17-OHP (nmol/L) were centrifuged immediately and stored at −80°C until they were assayed.

S-Androstenedione was analyzed, to measure if children had appropriately therapy.

30 children aged 5–18 served as controls, treated with EMLA + N2O.

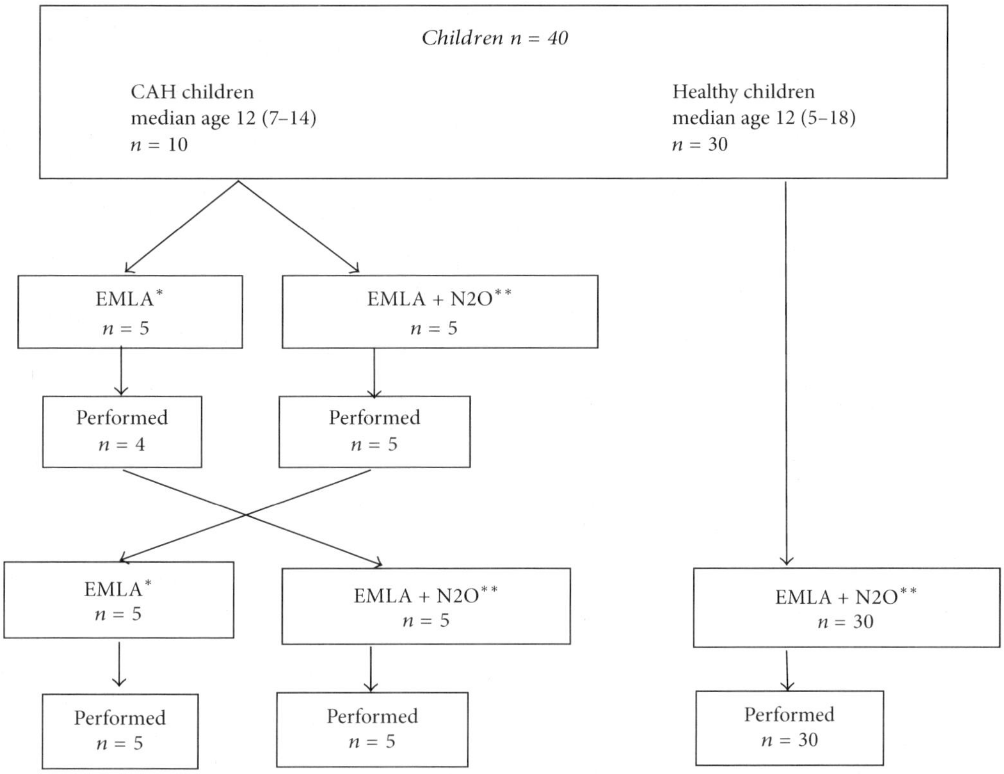

FIGURE 1: Flow diagram of the included children randomly allocated to two procedures, EMLA, and EMLA + N2O. *Inhalation of 100% oxygen. **Inhalation of 50% nitrous oxide.

Fifteen minutes after the IV procedure, the children were asked to rate the pain experience during IV access by using a numeric rating scale (NRS) of 0–10 with zero as no pain and 10 as the worst possible pain [20]. The children, parents, and nurses were also asked to do an evaluation, that is, the satisfaction with the procedure itself on a 5-point Likert Scale (1–5) in which 1 was poor, 2 was fair, 3 was good, 4 was very good, and 5 was excellent [22]. The children performed their evaluations first, and then the parents were asked to evaluate the procedure. The parents were present when the children made their assessments.

Additional variables recorded by the investigator included age, body mass index standard deviation score (BMI SDS) [23], the number of attempts, heart rate, blood pressure (NAIS-Blood Pressure Watch Diagnostic®), and oxygen saturation using pulse oximetry (Date-Ohmeda TUFF SAT®). Hypoxia was defined as a saturation of less than 93%. All side effects were documented in the study protocol.

2.3. Analysis. P-Glucose levels were measured using Modular Analytics P (Roche Diagnostics GmbH, Mannerheim, Germany). S-Androstenedione levels were measured using chromatography and mass spectrometry. P-NE was determined using HPLC (High Pressure Liquid Chromatography) (Dionex Corporation, Sunnyvale, CA, USA). The 17-OHP in serum was measured using a commercially available enzyme immunoassay (ELISA kit, Labor Diagnostic Nord Gmb & Co., KG, Nordhorn, Germany).

2.3.1. Statistical Analysis. All statistical analyses were performed using SPSS for windows version 22 (SPSS, IL, USA).

Descriptive data are presented as median values and ranges. The treatment groups were compared using nonparametric statistics. For treatment comparisons of pain, evaluations, heart rate, blood pressure, saturation, and median values of blood samples of paired data the Wilcoxon test was used. When comparing CAH children with the control group independent t-test was used. Correlations were assessed using Spearman's rank order correlation.

The body mass index standard deviation score was calculated according to the study by Rolland-Cachera et al. [23]. All tests were two-sided, and p values <0.05 were regarded as statistically significant.

3. Results

The demographic characteristics and blood analyzes of the children that were studied are summarized in Table 1.

Three children were classified as nonclassic (NC) CAH, and 7 were classified as classic severe form (2 simple virilizing form and 5 salt-wasting form) [3] and the hydrocortisone doses varied from 7.8 to 17.0 mg/m^2/day, data not shown.

The hydrocortisone doses varied from 7.8 to 17.0 mg/m^2/day. Three children were classified as nonclassic CAH, mean dose of 10,9 mg/m^2/day, and 7 were classified as classic severe form, mean dose 12,2 mg/m^2/day (2 simple virilizing

TABLE 1: Characteristics of CAH children and control children undergoing IV access with EMLA and EMLA + N2O.

(a)

	EMLA	EMLA + N2O	p^*
CAH children		(n = 10)	
Age, year		12 (7–14)	
Gender, male/female		3/7	
BMI SDS		0.38 (0–6.8)	
Attempts, number	1.0 (1–5)	1.0 (1-1)	0.3
Pain, 0–10	4.5 (2–10)	1.5 (1–3)	*0.02*
Children's evaluations 1–5	3.0 (1–5)	5.0 (4-5)	*0.01*
Parent's evaluations, 1–5	3.0 (1–5)	5.0 (4-5)	*0.02*
Nurse's evaluations, 1–5	2.5 (1–5)	5.0 (4-5)	*0.02*
Blood analyses			
17-OHP nmol/L	5.9 (1.7–52.3)	5.3 (2.9–24.2)	0.9
Androstenedione nmol/L	1.9 (0.3–12.0)	1.3 (0.6–11.0)	0.7
Glucose mmol/L	4.5 (4.1–5.6)	4.1 (3.7–5.0)	*0.04*
Norepinephrine nmol/L	1.3 (0.5–2.2)	1.4 (1.3–1.5)	0.6
Heart rate			
Before IV access	87 (67–96)	80 (74–100)	0.8
During IV access	91 (80–115)	81 (72–95)	*0.02*
After IV access	82 (65–104)	82 (67–91)	0.5
Blood pressure			
Before IV access	113/75 (107/67–135/80)	109/70 (85/55–137/80)	0.4
During IV access	114/77 (110/68–122/80)	110/70 (98/60–120/80)	0.05
After IV access	110/75 (106/68–113/75)	103/72 (87/60–115/75)	0.3
Saturation			
Before IV access	98 (97–100)	97 (97–99)	0.9
During IV access	98 (98–100)	98 (97–100)	1.0
After IV access	98 (97–100)	98 (97–100)	1.0

(b)

	EMLA + N2O		p^{**}
Control children		(n = 30)	
Age, year		12 (5–18)	
Gender, male/female		21/9	
BMI SDS		5.0 (−1.2–8.9)	
Pain, 0–10	2.0 (1–10)		0.9
17-OHP nmol/L	2.7 (0.7–7.1)		<0.001
Glucose mmol/L	4.7 (4.1–5.2)		<0.01
Norepinephrine nmol/L	1.5 (0.9–2.7)		0.8

Data are presented as median and range. In the evaluation score, 5 is most satisfactory. *Wilcoxon signed rank test. **Comparing control children with CAH children treated with EMLA + N2O.

forms and 5 salt-wasting forms, mean dose 13,7 and 11,6 mg/m^2/day, resp.).

A higher pain score was reported after EMLA compared to EMLA + N2O (p = 0.02), and the children's evaluations of satisfaction with the IV procedure were more positive for the EMLA + N2O treatment compared to EMLA (p = 0.01). Parents and nurses considered treatment with EMLA + N2O to be significantly better.

The heart rate increased significantly during IV access (p = 0.02) when using EMLA compared with EMLA + N2O as well as a trend of higher blood pressure. No differences were seen in saturation levels before, during, or after the IV access when comparing the different treatments. We found a significant correlation between children's evaluation of pain and number of attempts for a successful IV access (r = 0.6) data not shown.

The level of androstenedione was 1.3 (0.6–11.0), which indicated the children were receiving an appropriate dose.

No differences in levels of 17-OHP and NE after IV access were seen after comparing EMLA and EMLA + N2O, with no differences between children with salt-wasting and simple virilizing forms. However, glucose levels were significantly lower after the EMLA + N2O treatment ($p = 0.04$), as shown in Table 1.

No correlation was found between levels of 17-OHP and children's evaluation of pain.

Levels of 17-OHP were also measured in a control group of 30 healthy children who received IV access through EMLA + N2O. Significant lower glucose levels were seen in CAH children ($p < 0.01$), with no difference in the reported pain score between CAH children and control children.

In the EMLA group, IV access was not achieved in one patient, and the procedure was stopped by the child after the first blood sample. IV access was achieved in all procedures when EMLA + N2O was used. No respiratory adverse events were seen and no other side effects were reported.

4. Discussion

The management of CAH is complex and adequate monitoring of therapy must include IV access. A clinical problem often arises for children, parents, and nurses when IV access has to be done in anxious CAH children who have poor quality veins. The IV procedure has even led discussions about whether the procedural stress affects the blood analysis and subsequent treatment.

In this randomized, double-blind crossover study, self-reported pain and stress markers as well as heart rate, blood pressure, and oxygen saturation were studied after two different procedures associated with IV access were conducted in distressed children with CAH.

Higher self-reported pain and lower satisfaction with the procedures were found after EMLA compared to EMLA + N2O, which was similar to the results of our previous studies [16, 21].

We also measured the evaluations of the IV procedure made by parents and nurses because nurses often take an active role and assist CAH patients and their parents with management of the condition [24]. Overall, the results from children, parents, and nurses showed clearly that they considered the procedure with EMLA to be difficult, which indicated there is a need for a better method for the IV procedure. The studied children's evaluation of pain and satisfaction of IV procedure were similar to results we obtained from evaluations made by obese children on the difficulties of the IV procedure [21].

To involve children, parents, and nurses before and during stressful procedures is necessary, and requests from the family as well as caregivers for good quality of care must be taken into account [25]. Our results clearly showed a possible method for improving IV procedures in anxious children with CAH. Treatment with N2O is easy to perform, and the equipment required includes an anesthetic block, a suction unit, a scavenging system, and a pulse oximeter. Nitrous oxide administration can easily be performed by a single, specially trained nurse if local regulations allow it.

Heart rate and glucose levels were higher when using EMLA, which probably occurred due to a higher stress response. However, number of attempts may be a confounding factor when measuring stress response in anxious children, but the low number of participants in our study does not allow correction for any confounding variables.

No differences in 17-OHP or NE levels were found when comparing the different treatments, which may indicate that clinically relevant 17-OHP levels can be measured despite higher stress markers and pain in connection with IV access. Thus, the values obtained after EMLA varied more than after EMLA + N2O, and it is therefore possible that, for some patients, optimal 17-OHP measurements require good pain relief. The control group of healthy children treated with EMLA + N2O had significantly higher glucose levels compared to CAH children treated with EMLA + N2O. This result coincided with results from a controlled trial that compared CAH adolescents with healthy volunteers to examine their response to high-intensity exercise. The report's authors concluded that patients with classic CAH have an impaired stress-induced capacity, which led to a defective glucose response [26].

Treatment with N2O has a well-known sympathetic effect [27], but no differences in NE levels between EMLA and N2O + EMLA were seen in the children in our study. One explanation for this lack of differences may be that patients with CAH have a reduced capacity to upregulate their sympathetic nervous system [26]. It is also possible that the pain-induced stress that occurred when EMLA was used increased NE secretion to the same levels as seen after N2O inhalation.

A placebo effect may have initiated when the children were informed that during one of the procedures they should be given a treatment which may decrease the pain of venipuncture. We know the placebo effect in children to be high [28], but we considered it unethical not to inform the child about the expected effect of N2O. However, the effects of expectations in children and adolescents, as well as the mediation by parents, need further investigation. Even specific clinical trial-designs for children have been suggested [29].

4.1. Strengths and Limitations of the Study. The principle strength of our study was its randomized, double-blind crossover design.

A weakness was the low number of patients included in the study. The small number was due to, first, CAH being a rare disease and, second, to the inclusion of only anxious children who experienced previous difficulties with IV access.

The children were asked to evaluate the procedure in front of their parents and it is possible that children's evaluation affects the parental evaluation. It is also well-known that parents' values and attitudes influence their children's pain evaluation [30]. Thus, when the study was designed it was considered impossible to separate parents and children after the IV procedure. All evaluations were performed in the same order throughout the study.

The BMI SDS was higher in the control group. However, the pharmacological distribution of N2O is marginally affected of body weight when N2O has a low solubility in blood, leading to rapidly increase of alveolar concentration and a rapidly decrease after the inhalation [31].

We can only speculate how the stress response may have been without any pain relief and whether any difference in 17-OHP levels could have been detected.

As mentioned before, optimizing the hydrocortisone dosage has major clinical importance [3]. Excess glucocorticoids suppress growth [7, 10], and the use of hydrocortisone has also been shown to have a positive correlation with BMI SDS. In other words, children with CAH have a higher risk of obesity [32]. On the other hand, suboptimal glucocorticoid doses may lead to reduced physical and mental capacity [33] as well as a high concentration of sex steroids, which may induce premature epiphyseal closure for the child [10].

Continued care, including frequent blood sampling, is required for children with CAH to prevent long-term adverse consequences from the disease, including metabolic syndrome and osteoporosis [7]. Treatment with N2O offers the possibility of improving the IV access procedure for children with CAH.

5. Conclusion

The management of CAH is complex and adequate monitoring of therapy is important.

Despite higher self-reported pain, heart rate, glucose levels, and lower satisfaction with the IV procedure after EMLA compared to EMLA + N2O, no difference in 17-OHP levels was found in children with CAH. Thus, although the quality of care was better with N2O treatment, it was not possible to demonstrate that this is a prerequisite for valid 17-OHP measurements.

Acknowledgments

The author would like to acknowledge the Swedish Order of Freemasons, the Sallskapet Barnavard Foundation, the Stiftelsen Samariten Foundation, the Crown Princess Lovisa Foundation, and the FAS (the Council for Working Life and Social Research) and finally thank Jan Kowalski, a statistician, for their expert help.

References

[1] D. Merke and M. Kabbani, "Congenital adrenal hyperplasia: Epidemiology, management and practical drug treatment," *Pediatric Drugs*, vol. 3, no. 8, pp. 599–611, 2001.

[2] C. M. Trapp, P. W. Speiser, and S. E. Oberfield, "Congenital adrenal hyperplasia: An update in children," *Current Opinion in Endocrinology, Diabetes and Obesity*, vol. 18, no. 3, pp. 166–170, 2011.

[3] D. P. Merke and S. R. Bornstein, "Congenital adrenal hyperplasia," *The Lancet*, vol. 365, no. 9477, pp. 2125–2136, 2005.

[4] P. W. Speiser, R. Azziz, L. S. Baskin et al., "Congenital adrenal hyperplasia due to steroid 21-hydroxylase deficiency: an Endocrine Society clinical practice guideline," *The Journal of Clinical Endocrinology & Metabolism*, vol. 95, no. 9, pp. 4133–4160, 2010.

[5] H. Falhammar and A. Nordenström, "Nonclassic congenital adrenal hyperplasia due to 21-hydroxylase deficiency: clinical presentation, diagnosis, treatment, and outcome," *Endocrine Journal*, vol. 50, no. 1, pp. 32–50, 2015.

[6] B. L. Linder, N. V. Esteban, A. L. Yergey, J. C. Winterer, D. L. Loriaux, and F. Cassorla, "Cortisol production rate in childhood and adolescence," *Journal of Pediatrics*, vol. 117, no. 6, pp. 892–896, 1990.

[7] E. Marumudi, R. Khadgawat, V. Surana, I. Shabir, A. Joseph, and A. C. Ammini, "Diagnosis and management of classical congenital adrenal hyperplasia," *Steroids*, vol. 78, no. 8, pp. 741–746, 2013.

[8] C. M. Trapp and S. E. Oberfield, "Recommendations for treatment of nonclassic congenital adrenal hyperplasia (NCCAH): an update," *Steroids*, vol. 77, no. 4, pp. 342–346, 2012.

[9] S. F. Witchel, "Non-classic congenital adrenal hyperplasia," *Steroids*, vol. 78, no. 8, pp. 747–750, 2013.

[10] W. Bonfig, S. Bechtold, H. Schmidt, D. Knorr, and H. P. Schwarz, "Reduced final height outcome in congenital adrenal hyperplasia under prednisone treatment: Deceleration of growth velocity during puberty," *The Journal of Clinical Endocrinology & Metabolism*, vol. 92, no. 5, pp. 1635–1639, 2007.

[11] A. Dauber, M. Kellogg, and J. A. Majzoub, "Monitoring of therapy in congenital adrenal hyperplasia," *Clinical Chemistry*, vol. 56, no. 8, pp. 1245–1251, 2010.

[12] H. Falhammar and M. Thorén, "Clinical outcomes in the management of congenital adrenal hyperplasia," *Endocrine Journal*, vol. 41, no. 3, pp. 355–373, 2012.

[13] E. A. Cummings, G. J. Reid, G. A. Finley, P. J. McGrath, and J. A. Ritchie, "Prevalence and source of pain in pediatric inpatients," *Pain*, vol. 68, no. 1, pp. 25–31, 1996.

[14] R. M. Kennedy, J. Luhmann, and W. T. Zempsky, "Clinical implications of unmanaged needle-insertion pain and distress in children," *Pediatrics*, vol. 122, supplement 3, pp. S130–S133, 2008.

[15] G. B. Humphrey, C. M. Boon, G. F. van Linden van den Heuvell, and H. B. van de Wiel, "The occurrence of high levels of acute behavioral distress in children and adolescents undergoing routine venipunctures," *Pediatrics*, vol. 90, no. 1, part 1, pp. 87–91, 1992.

[16] K. Ekbom, J. Jakobsson, and C. Marcus, "Nitrous oxide inhalation is a safe and effective way to facilitate procedures in paediatric outpatient departments," *Archives of Disease in Childhood*, vol. 90, no. 10, pp. 1073–1076, 2005.

[17] S. A. Kanagasundaram, L. J. Lane, B. P. Cavalletto, J. P. Keneally, and M. G. Cooper, "Efficacy and safety of nitrous oxide in alleviating pain and anxiety during painful procedures," *Archives of Disease in Childhood*, vol. 84, no. 6, pp. 492–495, 2001.

[18] D. Annequin, R. Carbajal, P. Chauvin, O. Gall, B. Tourniaire, and I. Murat, "Fixed 50% nitrous oxide oxygen mixture for painful procedures: A French survey.," *Pediatrics*, vol. 105, no. 4, p. E47, 2000.

[19] D. D. Price, F. M. Bush, S. Long, and S. W. Harkins, "A comparison of pain measurement characteristics of mechanical visual analogue and simple numerical rating scales," *Pain*, vol. 56, no. 2, pp. 217–226, 1994.

[20] J. Miró, E. Castarlenas, and A. Huguet, "Evidence for the use of a numerical rating scale to assess the intensity of pediatric pain," *European Journal of Pain*, vol. 13, no. 10, pp. 1089–1095, 2009.

[21] K. Ekbom, S. Kalman, J. Jakobsson, and C. Marcus, "Efficient intravenous access without distress: a double-blind randomized study of midazolam and nitrous oxide in children and adolescents," *Archives of Pediatrics & Adolescent Medicine*, vol. 165, no. 9, pp. 785–791, 2011.

[22] D. A. Lowe, M. C. Monuteaux, S. Ziniel, and A. M. Stack, "Predictors of parent satisfaction in pediatric laceration repair," *Academic Emergency Medicine*, vol. 19, no. 10, pp. 1166–1172, 2012.

[23] M. F. Rolland-Cachera, M. Sempé, M. Guilloud-Bataille, E. Patois, F. Péquignot-Guggenbuhl, and V. Fautrad, "Adiposity indices in children," *The American Journal of Clinical Nutrition*, vol. 36, no. 1, pp. 178–184, 1982.

[24] K. Glatt, D. L. Garzon, and J. Popovic, "Congenital adrenal hyperplasia due to 21-hydroxylase deficiency," *Journal for Specialists in Pediatric Nursing*, vol. 10, no. 3, pp. 104–114, 2005.

[25] I. Coyne and L. Kirwan, "Ascertaining children's wishes and feelings about hospital life," *Journal of Child Health Care*, vol. 16, no. 3, pp. 293–304, 2012.

[26] M. Weise, S. L. Mehlinger, B. Drinkard et al., "Patients with classic congenital adrenal hyperplasia have decreased epinephrine reserve and defective glucose elevation in response to high-intensity exercise," *The Journal of Clinical Endocrinology & Metabolism*, vol. 89, no. 2, pp. 591–597, 2004.

[27] R. D. Sanders, J. Weimann, and M. Maze, "Biologic effects of nitrous oxide: a mechanistic and toxicologic review," *Anesthesiology*, vol. 109, no. 4, pp. 707–722, 2008.

[28] D. R. Hoekman, J. Zeevenhooven, F. S. van Etten-Jamaludin et al., "The placebo response in pediatric abdominal pain-related functional gastrointestinal disorders: a systematic review and meta-analysis," *Journal of Pediatrics*, vol. 182, pp. 155–163.e7, 2017.

[29] K. Weimer, M. D. Gulewitsch, A. A. Schlarb, J. Schwille-Kiuntke, S. Klosterhalfen, and P. Enck, "Placebo effects in children: a review," *Pediatric Research*, vol. 74, no. 1, pp. 96–102, 2013.

[30] P. Kankkunen, A.-M. Pietilä, and K. Vehviläinen-Julkunen, "Families' and children's postoperative pain—literature review," *Journal of Pediatric Nursing*, vol. 19, no. 2, pp. 133–139, 2004.

[31] D. E. Becker and M. Rosenberg, "Nitrous oxide and the inhalation anesthetics," *Anesthesia Progress*, vol. 55, no. 4, pp. 124–132, 2008.

[32] R. P. P. Moreira, S. M. Villares, G. Madureira, B. B. Mendonca, and T. A. S. S. Bachega, "Obesity and familial predisposition are significant determining factors of an adverse metabolic profile in young patients with congenital adrenal hyperplasia," *Hormone Research in Paediatrics*, vol. 80, no. 2, pp. 111–118, 2013.

[33] A. Strandqvist, H. Falhammar, P. Lichtenstein et al., "Suboptimal psychosocial outcomes in patients with congenital adrenal hyperplasia: Epidemiological studies in a nonbiased national cohort in Sweden," *The Journal of Clinical Endocrinology & Metabolism*, vol. 99, no. 4, pp. 1425–1432, 2014.

Morphine Suppository versus Indomethacin Suppository in the Management of Renal Colic: Randomized Clinical Trial

Forough Zamanian,[1] Mohammad Jalili,[2] Maziar Moradi-Lakeh,[3] Maryam Kia,[4] Rokhsareh Aghili,[5] and Seyed Mojtaba Aghili[1]

[1] *Department of Emergency Medicine, Imam Khomeini Hospital, Tehran University of Medical Sciences, Tehran, Iran*
[2] *Emergency Medicine Department, Tehran University of Medical Sciences, Tehran, Iran*
[3] *Department of Community Medicine, Iran University of Medical Sciences, Tehran, Iran*
[4] *Department of Internal Medicine, Dr. Ziaeian Hospital, Tehran University of Medical Sciences, Tehran, Iran*
[5] *Endocrine Research Center, Institute of Endocrinology and Metabolism, Iran University of Medical Sciences, Tehran, Iran*

Correspondence should be addressed to Seyed Mojtaba Aghili; m-aghili@tums.ac.ir

Academic Editor: Giustino Varrassi

Background. Renal colic is a medical emergency due to the rapid onset and devastating nature of its pain. Opioids and nonsteroidal anti-inflammatory drugs (NSAIDs) are both used as first-line choices in its management. *Aim.* This study aimed to compare the efficacy and safety of opioids and NSAIDs in the management of acute renal colic. *Methods.* One hundred and fifty-eight patients were divided into two groups ($n = 79$) and received either 10 mg morphine or 100 mg indomethacin suppositories. The severity of pain was measured using verbal numeric rating scale at baseline and 20, 40, 60, and 90 minutes after the administration of analgesics. Drug side effects as well as patients' vital signs were also recorded. *Results.* The mean decrease in the pain score during the first 20 minutes was significantly higher among those who received morphine suppository. However, no significant difference was observed between the two groups regarding the mean decrease in pain score during the first 40, 60, and 90 minutes after the admission. Prevalence of drug side effects or changes in the vital signs was not significantly different between the two groups. *Conclusions.* Morphine suppositories seem to be more efficient in achieving rapid pain relief comparing to indomethacin.

1. Introduction

Renal colic, as the most common presentation of ureteral calculi, is characterized by a sudden onset and severe sense of pain in the flanks which may radiate to the hypochondrium [1]. This pain is caused by the obstruction and the subsequent increased tension in the urinary tract during the calculi passage and is commonly compared with the delivery pain. Increased pressure of the renal pelvis provokes the secretion of prostaglandins followed by vasodilatation which results in further increase in the intrarenal pressure as a result of diuresis and smooth muscle spasm [2, 3]. Renal colic is generally considered as a serious health problem due to the devastating nature of the pain and its high prevalence in general population which results in a considerable number of lost work days. The annual incidence of renal colic is reported to be around 16 per 10,000 population with a lifetime incidence of 1–20% [4–6]. Interestingly, an increase in the incidence of ureteric calculi and renal colic has been observed during the past decades, most probably due to changes in the life style of the general population [7].

The current standard management of pain during acute renal colic episodes includes administration of opioids as well as nonsteroidal anti-inflammatory drugs (NSAIDs) both alone and in combination with each other. While opioids take advantages of being inexpensive, potent, and titratable, their usage is limited due to the fear of respiratory depression, drug dependency, and potential drug abuse by mimicking renal colic symptoms in order to receive opioids [8]. Morphine suppositories benefit from a sustained and prolonged analgesic effect which requires fewer administrations [9] and could potentially be less favorable for drug abusers who mimic renal colic. In addition, administration of morphine via rectal rout bypasses the need for intravenous catheter placement and can be given to patients in their first encounter in the triage room. Moreover, opioids have no effect on the prostaglandin secretion, as the main cause of pain in renal colic [10]. NSAIDs, on the other hand, directly inhibit the prostaglandin effect and, as a result, are probably more effective than opioids [8, 10]. However, NSAIDs may cause serious side effects, most notably renal impairment and renal failure as well as gastrointestinal bleeding [10]. Moreover, in contrast with opioids, NSAIDs are not titratable and their analgesic benefits take longer to effect [8].

Currently, the choice between opioids and NSAIDs at the clinical setting is highly dependent on clinician's personal preference and experience as well as institutional protocols while there is limited data in order to compare the outcome of these drugs in the management of acute renal colic [11]. Considering the exceedingly busy setting of emergency department and the time needed to achieve intravenous access, the current study was designed to compare the efficacy and adverse effects of the suppository administrated morphine and indomethacin used in the management of renal colic.

2. Methods

The current randomized double-blind clinical trial (IRCT registration ID: 2014050514297N2) was performed between March 2011 and March 2013 in the emergency department of Imam Hospital and Shariati hospital, two tertiary care university affiliated teaching hospitals. The Institutional Review Board has reviewed and approved the process of this study.

Based on the previous studies, a minimum sample size of 79 for each group was desired [12]. This was based on an alpha of 0.05, power of 0.90; and mean (M) and standard deviations (SD) of 24.7 and 9.1 for indomethacin and 27.4 and 9.1 for morphine, using the following formula:

$$N = \frac{\left(Z_{1-\alpha/2} + Z_{\beta}\right)^2 \left(\mathrm{SD}_1^2 + \mathrm{SD}_2^2\right)}{\left(M_1 - M_2\right)^2}. \quad (1)$$

One hundred and fifty-eight patients with a confirmed diagnosis of renal colic who aged between 18 and 75 years were enrolled in this study and were randomly allocated into two groups using permuted-block randomization method ($n = 79$). Based on the patients' clinical presentation, the diagnosis of renal colic was primarily made by triage nurse and was then confirmed by the emergency medicine resident and the attending physician. The process of the study was explained to all participants and they were asked to fill an informed consent before being entered into the study. Patients were ensured that their personal and clinical data would not be revealed under any circumstances and their names were replaced with codes before data entry to ensure data confidentiality. The exclusion criteria were as follows: unwillingness to participate in the study or to receive suppository analgesics, pregnancy, breastfeeding, a history of current or past drug abuse, analgesic intake during up to 4 hours prior to admission, long-term use of NSAIDs, a drug history of hypnotic drugs or phenothiazines, a history of drug hypersensitivity reaction due to morphine or NSAIDs, diarrhea, peritonitis, and a history of chronic diseases including liver disorders, renal disorders, respiratory problems, gastrointestinal problems, and endocrine disorders.

Patients either received 10 mg morphine suppository (group A) or 100 mg indomethacin suppository (group B) for the management of renal colic, respectively. In order to blind the observers as well as patients, morphine and indomethacin suppositories were placed into glass containers labeled as A and B and were administrated for patients by the resident of emergency medicine. Only pharmacy section manager of hospital was aware of the type of suppositories placed into A and B containers. The primary outcome of the study was change in the pain score. The secondary outcome of the study was the safety and tolerability of drugs as measured by hemodynamic changes and adverse effects. Assessment of pain was performed using 11-point numeric rating scale (from 0 for no pain to 10 for most severe pain possible) at the time of admission and 20, 40, 60, and 90 minutes later. Intravenous morphine with a dosage of 5 mg was suggested and administrated for each patient every 20 minutes if the pain remained the same or the patient reported only a minor pain relief. Drug adverse effects including nausea, vomiting, dizziness, and drowsiness as well as patients' vital signs were also assessed every 20 minutes. Demographic data including sex and age, pain score reported by patient at various points, the amount of analgesics needed for pain relief, and the duration of hospital stay was recorded for each patient.

Data analysis was performed using SPSS software package for windows version 21 (IBM, USA). Quantitative variables are expressed as mean ± standard deviation. Repeated measure analysis and chi-squared test were used in order to compare quantitative and qualitative variables between groups, respectively. Effect size (ES) was estimated with a 95% confidence interval (95% CI). P values lower than 0.05 were considered as statistically significant.

3. Results

A total number of 158 cases including 102 (64.6%) male and 56 (35.4%) female cases were enrolled in the current study (Figure 1). The mean age of the study population was 37.4 ± 11.1 years which was not statistically different between groups A and B (37.2 ± 10.6 years versus 37.3 ± 11.5 years, $P = 0.9$, and ES = −0.01 [95% CI = −0.32 to 0.32]). The mean weight of the study population was 73.8 ± 10.4 kilograms which was not statistically different between groups A and B (74.1 ± 8.9 kilograms versus 73.4 ± 11.8 kilograms, $P = 0.9$, and ES = 0.07 [95% CI = −0.25 to 0.38]). Male to female ratio was also similar between groups A and B (1.75 versus 1.88, $P = 0.6$, and ES = 0.74 [95% CI = 0.37 to 1.10]). Table 1 summarizes patients' demographic data.

The mean pain score at the start of measurements was not significantly different between the two groups (8.38 ± 1.08 for group A versus 8.26 ± 1.09 for group B, $P = 0.5$, and ES = 0.1 [95% CI = −0.22 to 0.41]). The mean decrease in the pain score during the first 20 minutes after the admission

TABLE 1: Demographic data of the study population.

	Group A	Group B	Total	P value	EF (95% CI)
Age (year)	37.2 ± 10.6	37.3 ± 11.5	37.4 ± 11.1	0.9	−0.01 (−0.32 to 0.30)
Weight (Kg)	74.1 ± 8.9	73.4 ± 11.8	73.8 ± 10.4	0.9	0.07 (−0.25 to 0.38)
Male/female	1.75	1.88	1.82	0.6	0.74 (0.37 to 1.10)

Group A: patients received morphine suppository.
Group B: patients received indomethacin suppository.
95% CI: 95% confidence interval.
EF: effect size.

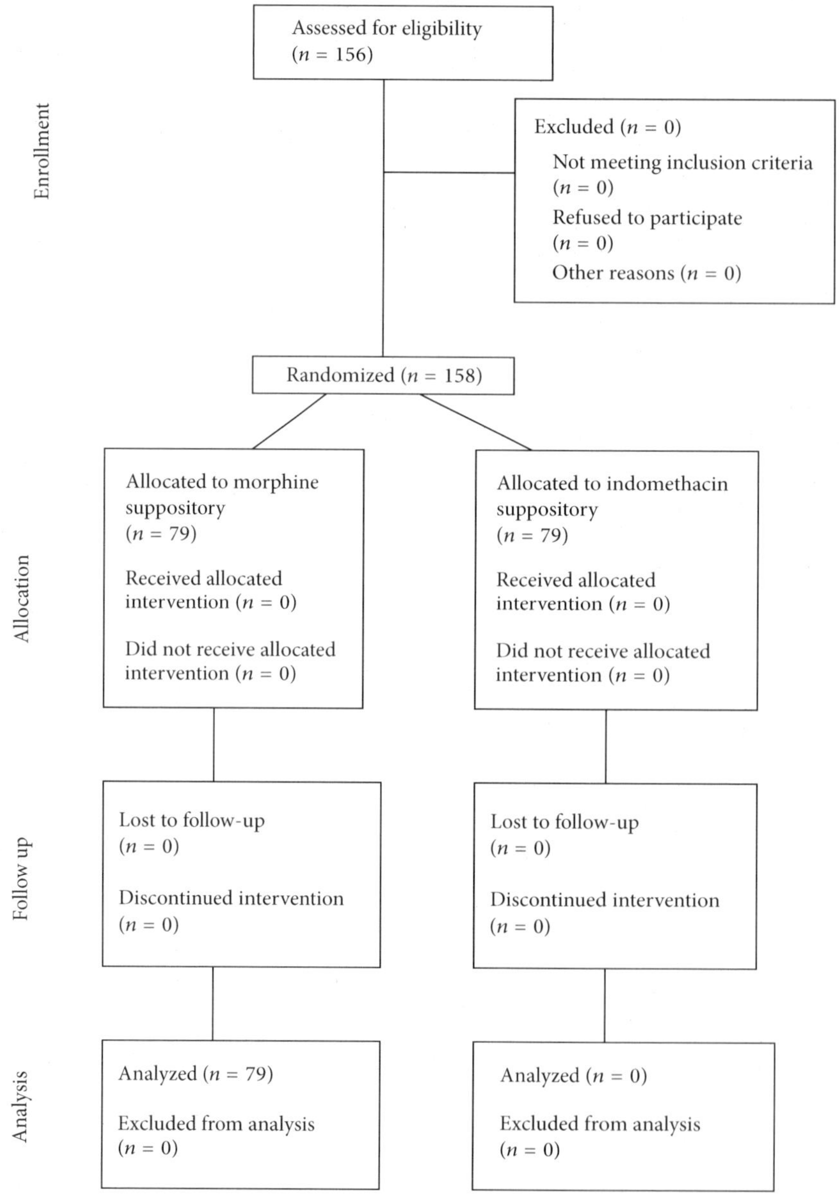

FIGURE 1: CONSORT diagram showing the flow of participants.

was significantly higher among group A cases who received morphine suppository comparing to group B who received indomethacin suppository (5.46 ± 1.34 versus 4.36 ± 1.62, $P < 0.001$, and ES = 0.74 [95% CI = 0.44 to 1.06]). However, no significant difference was observed between the two groups regarding the mean decrease in pain score during the first 40, 60, and 90 minutes after the admission (Table 2). Figure 2 shows the timeline for pain scores in two study groups. The mean change in the systolic and diastolic blood pressure was not also significantly different between the two groups

TABLE 2: The mean decrease in the pain score during the first 20, 40, 60, and 90 minutes after the admission in groups A and B.

Duration	Group	Decrease in the pain score Mean ± SD	P value	EF (95% CI)
0–20 minutes	Group A	5.46 ± 1.34	<0.001*	0.73 (0.40 to 1.05)
	Group B	4.37 ± 1.63		
0–40 minutes	Group A	6.26 ± 1.62	0.3	0.16 (−0.18 to 0.45)
	Group B	6.04 ± 1.59		
0–60 minutes	Group A	6.27 ± 1.79	0.5	0.16 (−0.22 to 0.40)
	Group B	6.11 ± 1.66		
0–90 minutes	Group A	6.28 ± 1.75	0.4	0.13 (−0.18 to 0.44)
	Group B	6.07 ± 1.67		

Group A: patients received morphine suppository.
Group B: patients received indomethacin suppository.
95% CI: 95% confidence interval.
EF: effect size.
SD: standard deviation.
*Statistically significant.

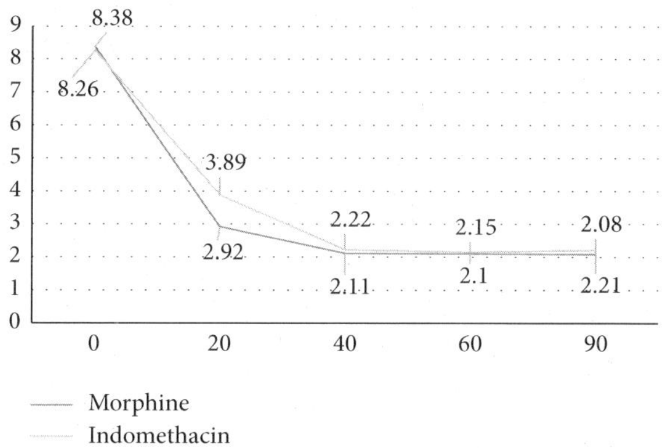

FIGURE 2: Timeline graph of pain scores in the two study groups.

during the first 20, 40, 60, and 90 minutes after the admission (Table 3).

Nausea was reported by 52.7% of patients in group A and by 47.3% of patients in group B which was not significantly different ($P = 0.5$, ES = 0.11 [95% CI = −0.22 to 0.46]). Vomiting was reported by 49% of patients in group A and by 51% of patients in group B which was also not significantly different ($P = 0.7$, ES = −0.04 [95% CI = −0.38 to 0.29]). The prevalence of dizziness was 43.3% in group A and 56.7% in group B which was not significantly different ($P = 0.4$, ES = −0.29 [95% CI = −0.64 to 0.04]). Dryness of the mouth was reported by 48% of patients in group A and by 52% of patients in group B which was also not significantly different ($P = 0.4$, ES = −0.08 [95% CI = −0.43 to 0.25]). Allergic drug reactions were observed in 49.7% of patients in group A and in 50.3% of patients in group B which was also not significantly different ($P = 0.5$, EF = −0.01 [−0.35 to 0.33]). Table 4 compares the adverse effects between the two study groups.

4. Discussion

According to the results of the current study, the mean pain score was not significantly different between renal colic patients who received either morphine or indomethacin suppository. However, those who received morphine experienced a greater relief in pain during the first 20 minutes after the admission. No difference was observed between these two groups regarding the drug side effects including changes in the systolic and diastolic blood pressures.

In one study, Cordell et al. investigated the differences regarding the efficacy in pain relief and probable side effects of intravenous morphine and indomethacin suppositories in patients with renal colic [10]. Their findings showed that those who received intravenous morphine achieved a better pain relief after the first ten minutes but not after 20 and 30 minutes comparing to those who received indomethacin suppository. This is in accordance with the results of this study in which morphine suppository was superior comparing to indomethacin suppository in order to achieve pain relief only during the first 20 minutes after the admission. Moreover, similar to the current study, they found no significant differences regarding the side effects of the two drugs.

Since the analgesic effects of morphine and NSAIDs in renal colic are achieved via different pathways, one may conclude that the combination of these drugs would result in a better pain management or a decrease in the amount of needed morphine as a drug with a high potential for abuse. In a study by Engeler et al. two orally administrated NSAIDs, rofecoxib and diclofenac, were used in combination with morphine in the management of acute pain of renal colic [13]. The mean morphine consumption was not significantly different among patients who received rofecoxib, diclofenac, or placebo in addition to morphine. Moreover, the pain score reported by patients was similar among these three groups. On the contrary, in a study by Safdar et al., renal colic patients who received a combination of intravenous morphine and ketorolac, NSAIDs, achieved a better pain relief with a lesser amount of medication comparing to those who received either of these two drugs alone [14]. In another study by Phillips et al. the efficacy of celecoxib, also an NSAID, in the management of renal colic was evaluated [15]. The authors reported that celecoxib was not efficient in the facilitation

TABLE 3: The mean change in the systolic and diastolic blood pressure among the two groups during the first 20, 40, 60, and 90 minutes after the admission.

Duration	Group	Change in the systolic blood pressure			Change in the diastolic blood pressure		
		Mean ± SD	*P* value	EF (95% CI)	Mean ± SD	*P* value	EF (95% CI)
0–20 minutes	Group A	3.18 ± 3.62	0.1	0.16 (−0.9 to 0.53)	0.65 ± 2.34	0.3	0.15 (−0.16 to 0.46)
	Group B	2.16 ± 5.37			0.13 ± 4.29		
0–40 minutes	Group A	1.43 ± 3.33	0.2	−0.2 (−0.51 to 0.12)	0.71 ± 2.39	0.7	0.05 (−0.26 to 0.36)
	Group B	2.39 ± 5.98			0.52 ± 4.47		
0–60 minutes	Group A	1.79 ± 3.98	0.09	−0.28 (−0.59 to 0.04)	0.97 ± 2.81	0.4	0.12 (0.19 to 0.43)
	Group B	3.19 ± 5.94			0.52 ± 4.38		
0–90 minutes	Group A	1.64 ± 3.5	0.09	−0.29 (0.60 to 0.03)	0.92 ± 3.02	0.7	−0.05 (−0.36 to 0.26)
	Group B	3.03 ± 5.83			1.06 ± 2.39		

Group A: patients received morphine suppository.
Group B: patients received indomethacin suppository.
95% CI: 95% confidence interval.
EF: effect size.
SD: standard deviation.

TABLE 4: Comparison of adverse effects between the two study groups.

	Morphine group	Indomethacin group	*P* value	EF (95% CI)
Nausea	52.7%	47.3%	0.5	0.11 (−0.22 to 0.46)
Vomiting	49%	51%	0.7	−0.04 (−0.38 to 0.29)
Dizziness	43.3%	56.7%	0.4	−0.29 (−0.64 to 0.04)
Mouth dryness	48%	52%	0.4	−0.08 (−0.43 to 0.25)
Allergic reaction	49.7%	50.3%	0.5	−0.01 (−0.35 to 0.33)

95% CI: 95% confidence interval.
EF: effect size.

of the stone passage or decrease in the amount of narcotic administration was evaluated.

Several studies have focused on finding an alternative analgesic for opioids in the management of acute pain of renal colic. Aside from NSAIDs, the efficacy and probable side effects of paracetamol have also been the subject of some investigations. In one study, Bektas et al. compared the intravenous administration of morphine and paracetamol among 146 renal colic patients who visited emergency department [8]. Their findings showed that intravenously administrated morphine and paracetamol were both effective in achieving pain relief comparing to the placebo with no significant difference between the two and both drugs were well tolerated. In another study by Grissa et al. renal colic patients received either intravenous single-dose paracetamol or intramuscular single-dose piroxicam, an NSAID, after being admitted for renal colic at the emergency department [16]. The authors reported a higher rate of pain relief for paracetamol comparing to piroxicam 90 minutes after the administration of these analgesics with minimal side effects for both drugs (80% versus 48%, resp.). Moreover, the superiority in the efficacy of paracetamol comparing to piroxicam began to be apparent 45 minutes after the administration of these drugs.

The current study faces several limitations. First, some of the most serious side effects of analgesics used in this study could not be assessed due to the short period of follow-up. Drug abuse and dependence among those receiving opioids such as morphine and gastrointestinal bleeding among those receiving NSAIDs such as indomethacin are more likely to occur after patient's discharge from the emergency ward. However, it should be noted that the potential for abuse is particular for those who already have a history of drug abuse and should not be generalized to all patients after one admission. Second, it has been previously suggested that nausea and vomiting, which were expected side effects in this study, may affect patient's perception of pain by increasing the level of discomfort [14]. Finally, due to difficulties in obtaining the desired number of patients, we did not include a group receiving both morphine and indomethacin which would help to find out if the combination of these drugs could result in a better pain management and decrease in the amount of opioids administrated.

In conclusion, while the effect of analgesics on patients' vital signs and side effects of both morphine and indomethacin do not differ significantly, morphine suppositories seem to be more efficient in achieving rapid pain relief comparing to their indomethacin counterparts. Hence, morphine remains as a yet irreplaceable analgesic in the acute management of pain among renal colic patients.

Competing Interests

The authors declare no conflict of interests.

Acknowledgments

This study was funded and supported by Tehran University of Medical Sciences (Grant no. 9011307019).

References

[1] J. Edwards, E. P. Sloan, S. Eder, and S. Chan, "Renal colic patient pain management in the emergency department," *Annals of Emergency Medicine*, vol. 44, no. 4, p. S58, 2004.

[2] S. W. Leslie, E. Kim, and F. Talavora, *Nephrolithiasis: Acute Renal Colic*, eMedicine, St. Petersburg, Fla, USA, 2007.

[3] B. K. Welk and J. M. H. Teichman, "Pharmacological management of renal colic in the older patient," *Drugs & Aging*, vol. 24, no. 11, pp. 891–900, 2007.

[4] J. M. H. Teichman, "Acute renal colic from ureteral calculus," *The New England Journal of Medicine*, vol. 350, no. 7, pp. 684–693, 2004.

[5] G. R. Nuss, J. D. Rackley, and D. G. Assimos, "Adjunctive therapy to promote stone passage," *Reviews in Urology*, vol. 7, no. 2, pp. 67–74, 2005.

[6] M. Yakoot, A. Salem, S. Yousef, and S. Helmy, "Clinical efficacy of Spasmofen® suppository in the emergency treatment of renal colic: a randomized, double-blind, double-dummy comparative trial," *Drug Design, Development and Therapy*, vol. 8, pp. 405–410, 2014.

[7] A. Alleemudder, X.-Y. Tai, A. Goyal, and J. Pati, "Raised white cell count in renal colic: is there a role for antibiotics?" *Urology Annals*, vol. 6, no. 2, pp. 127–129, 2014.

[8] F. Bektas, C. Eken, O. Karadeniz, E. Goksu, M. Cubuk, and Y. Cete, "Intravenous paracetamol or morphine for the treatment of renal colic: a randomized, placebo-controlled trial," *Annals of Emergency Medicine*, vol. 54, no. 4, pp. 568–574, 2009.

[9] E. Bruera, R. Fainsinger, K. Spachynski, N. Babul, Z. Harsanyi, and A. C. Darke, "Steady-state pharmacokinetic evaluation of a novel, controlled-release morphine suppository and subcutaneous morphine in cancer pain," *Journal of Clinical Pharmacology*, vol. 35, no. 7, pp. 666–672, 1995.

[10] W. H. Cordell, T. A. Larson, J. E. Lingeman et al., "Indomethacin suppositories versus intravenously titrated morphine for the treatment of ureteral colic," *Annals of Emergency Medicine*, vol. 23, no. 2, pp. 262–269, 1994.

[11] S. E. J. Golzari, H. Soleimanpour, F. Rahmani et al., "Therapeutic approaches for renal colic in the emergency department: a review article," *Anesthesiology and Pain Medicine*, vol. 4, no. 1, Article ID e16222, 2014.

[12] A. Holdgate and T. Pollock, "Systematic review of the relative efficacy of non-steroidal anti-inflammatory drugs and opioids in the treatment of acute renal colic," *British Medical Journal*, vol. 328, no. 7453, p. 1401, 2004.

[13] D. S. Engeler, D. K. Ackermann, J. J. Osterwalder, A. Keel, and H.-P. Schmid, "A double-blind, placebo controlled comparison of the morphine sparing effect of oral rofecoxib and diclofenac for acute renal colic," *The Journal of Urology*, vol. 174, no. 3, pp. 933–936, 2005.

[14] B. Safdar, L. C. Degutis, K. Landry, S. R. Vedere, H. C. Moscovitz, and G. D'Onofrio, "Intravenous morphine plus ketorolac is superior to either drug alone for treatment of acute renal colic," *Annals of Emergency Medicine*, vol. 48, no. 2, pp. 173.e1–181.e1, 2006.

[15] E. Phillips, B. Hinck, R. Pedro et al., "Celecoxib in the management of acute renal colic: a randomized controlled clinical trial," *Urology*, vol. 74, no. 5, pp. 994–999, 2009.

[16] M. H. Grissa, Y.-E. Claessens, W. Bouida et al., "Paracetamol vs piroxicam to relieve pain in renal colic. Results of a randomized controlled trial," *The American Journal of Emergency Medicine*, vol. 29, no. 2, pp. 203–206, 2011.

Central Sensitization and Perceived Indoor Climate among Workers with Chronic Upper-Limb Pain: Cross-Sectional Study

Emil Sundstrup,[1,2] Markus D. Jakobsen,[1,2] Mikkel Brandt,[1,3] Kenneth Jay,[1,2] Roger Persson,[4] and Lars L. Andersen[1,3]

[1] *National Research Centre for the Working Environment, 2100 Copenhagen, Denmark*
[2] *Institute for Sports Science and Clinical Biomechanics, University of Southern Denmark, 5230 Odense, Denmark*
[3] *Physical Activity and Human Performance Group, SMI, Department of Health Science and Technology, Aalborg University, 9220 Aalborg, Denmark*
[4] *Department of Psychology, Lund University, Box 213, 221 00 Lund, Sweden*

Correspondence should be addressed to Emil Sundstrup; esu@nrcwe.dk

Academic Editor: Steve McGaraughty

Monitoring of indoor climate is an essential part of occupational health and safety. While questionnaires are commonly used for surveillance, not all workers may perceive an identical indoor climate similarly. The aim of this study was to evaluate perceived indoor climate among workers with chronic pain compared with pain-free colleagues and to determine the influence of central sensitization on this perception. Eighty-two male slaughterhouse workers, 49 with upper-limb chronic pain and 33 pain-free controls, replied to a questionnaire with 13 items of indoor climate complaints. Pressure pain threshold (PPT) was measured in muscles of the arm, shoulder, and lower leg. Cross-sectional associations were determined using general linear models controlled for age, smoking, and job position. The number of indoor climate complaints was twice as high among workers with chronic pain compared with pain-free controls (1.8 [95% CI: 1.3–2.3] versus 0.9 [0.4–1.5], resp.). PPT of the nonpainful leg muscle was negatively associated with the number of complaints. Workers with chronic pain reported more indoor climate complaints than pain-free controls despite similar actual indoor climate. Previous studies that did not account for musculoskeletal pain in questionnaire assessment of indoor climate may be biased. Central sensitization likely explains the present findings.

1. Introduction

Previous research has documented the importance of a good indoor climate for workers health and safety [1–4]. Effective occupational health and safety programs include workplace assessments, for example, monitoring the indoor climate by asking the workers about complaints such as noise, draught, and temperature. Such analyses can identify physical hazards related to job position or work location and thereby provide key knowledge to preventing work-related health hazards [3]. However, workers with chronic pain may experience the indoor climate differently than pain-free colleagues which could distort conclusions. Thus, to avoid any misinterpretation of workplace health and safety programs and to prevent further worsening of symptoms it is important to identify workers with high prevalence of indoor climate complaints along with the specific bothering factors. Previous studies on indoor climate have mainly focused on symptoms attributed to indoor environment by comparing different workplaces or job positions [3, 5–7]. However, knowledge concerning interindividual variation in indoor climate sensation as a consequence of chronic musculoskeletal pain is lacking.

Chronic musculoskeletal pain is a common problem that affects millions of people worldwide. The consequences of chronic pain are often serious, affecting employee health and wellbeing, and impose a substantial socioeconomic burden due to extensive use of health care services, sickness absence, disability pension, and loss of productivity [8, 9]. Initially pain may emanate from activation of peripheral nociceptors due to tissue damage, but when the perception of pain for some reason (e.g., untreated pain, poor pain treatment, or just too long activation of the pain system) persists beyond the expected time for tissue healing, it has become chronic [10]. Chronic pain is caused by not only physiological pathology but rather a complex interaction between biological, psychological, and social factors [10, 11]. This implies the existence of many workplace risk factors for chronic pain and emphasizes the necessity of an effective and inclusive occupational health and safety system to rehabilitate and prevent aggravation of symptoms. Central sensitization is an important mechanism involved in chronic pain conditions and is defined as "facilitated excitatory synaptic response and depressed inhibition, causing amplified responses to noxious and innocuous inputs" [12, 13]. Thus, central sensitization may not only influence perception of pain, but also amplify other nonpainful stimuli. In line with this, de Klaver and colleagues [14] demonstrated that hyperacusis (intolerance of ordinary sound levels) is common among patients severely affected by complex regional pain syndrome type 1. Hyperacusis has been associated with central nervous system involvement and the authors speculated that hyperacusis may reflect the spreading of central sensitization to auditory circuits in these patients. We have also observed central sensitization in women with frequent neck-shoulder pain and desensitization in response to physical rehabilitation [15]. Also patients with chronic pain conditions such as fibromyalgia and irritable bowel syndrome have been shown more responsive to other stimuli than pain (auditory, visual) suggesting that these individuals have a different interpretation of pain or sensory information that reaches further than to the specific body region where the pain is perceived to be situated [16]. Thus, it could be speculated that central sensitization may spread to sensory processing circuits in workers with chronic pain consequently affecting their perception of specific indoor climate factors.

Slaughtering and meat processing operations involve a high degree of repetitive and forceful upper-limb movements and imply an elevated risk of work-related musculoskeletal disorders [17, 18]. In particular the prevalence of musculoskeletal disorders in the shoulder, arm, and hand is high among slaughterhouse workers, allegedly due to frequently repeated high-force actions and lack of sufficient recovery of these body regions during work [19–23]. Additionally, to comply with the standards on meat processing, ambient temperature is often low increasing the risk of MSD. Previous studies have demonstrated that musculoskeletal complaints, such as shoulder pain and low back pain, are more prevalent when the work is performed in a cold environment compared with work performed in normal temperature and that these symptoms seem to be aggravated as a function of time working in cold conditions [24–26]. Specifically, studies among seafood industry workers have shown that a cold work environment is a risk factor for musculoskeletal symptoms [27] and that workers who often felt cold at work experienced a higher prevalence of musculoskeletal pain compared to workers who never felt cold [6]. The authors concluded that the prevalence of feeling cold at work could be a valuable estimate for exposure in moderate cold exposure situations [6]. In addition to low working temperature, other environmental risk factors for MSD at the slaughterhouse involve draught from compressing machinery or elsewhere as well as noise from the mechanically based production systems. It is, however, unknown whether slaughterhouse workers with chronic pain are more sensitive to these environmental risk factors and to what extent central mechanisms are involved in the perception of these factors.

The aim of this study was to investigate whether workers with chronic pain compared with pain-free colleagues perceive the same indoor climate differently. We hypothesized that workers with chronic pain were more sensitive to the indoor climate (especially cold, draught, noise, and light) and that central sensitization could be involved in this perception.

2. Materials and Methods

2.1. Study Design and Ethics. A cross-sectional study concerning central mechanisms to chronic pain and its relation to perceived indoor climate complaints was conducted among 82 male slaughterhouse workers in Denmark, Europe. The present study was a part of a randomized controlled trial on the effect of strength training or ergonomic counseling on chronic pain [23] and was approved by the Danish National Ethics Committee on Biomedical Research (Ethical Committee of Frederiksberg and Copenhagen, H-3-2010-062) and registered in ClinicalTrials.gov (NCT01716767). All participants were informed about the purpose and content of the project and gave their written informed consent to participate in the study. All experimental conditions conformed to the Declaration of Helsinki.

2.2. Participants. Eighty-two male slaughterhouse workers, 49 with chronic upper-limb pain and 33 pain-free controls, with similar job tasks were recruited from two large scale pig slaughterhouses for the study. Participant characteristics for the two groups are shown in Table 1. The workers were recruited in relation to the before mentioned intervention study [23, 28].

The recruitment process was two-phased and consisted of a brief screening questionnaire followed by a clinical examination and questionnaire. The screening questionnaire was administered to 645 Danish slaughterhouse workers and contained questions on demographics, pain, and diagnosed diseases. Those who were interested in participating and who met the initial inclusion criteria for one of the two groups (chronic pain or pain-free controls, criteria described later) were invited for the clinical examination and questionnaire. Table 1 shows demographics, clinical, and work-related characteristics of the participants in the two groups.

Participants in the chronic pain group were to display (1) pain intensity in the shoulder, elbow/forearm, or hand/wrist of 3 or more on a 0–10 VAS scale during the last 3 months, (2) pain intensity in the shoulder, elbow/forearm, or hand/wrist of 3 or more on a 0–10 VAS scale during the last week, (3) pain that has lasted more than 3 months, (4) frequency of pain of at least 3 days per week during the last week, and (5) statement of at least "*some*" work disability scoring on a five-point scale, "*not at all,*" "*a little,*" "*some,*" and "*much*" to "*very much,*" when asked the question "*During the last 3 months, did you have any difficulty performing your work due to pain*

TABLE 1: Descriptive statistics for the main study variables. Mean (SD).

	Chronic pain ($n = 49$)	Control ($n = 33$)
Demographics		
Age (years)	45 (11)	45 (11)
Height (cm)	179 (7)	178 (7)
Weight (kg)	90 (16)	87 (13)
Body mass index (kg·m^2)	28 (5)	28 (5)
Proportion of smokers (%)	41	25
Clinical		
Shoulder pain intensity in the previous week (0–10)	5.6 (2.3)	0.1 (0.3)
Elbow/forearm pain intensity in the previous week (0–10)	3.9 (2.7)	0.0 (0.2)
Hand/wrist pain intensity in the previous week (0–10)	3.7 (2.9)	0.2 (0.6)
Pain duration >3 months (%)	100	0
PPT tibialis anterior (kPa)	805 (205)	1014 (285)
PPT extensor carpi radialis brevis (kPa)	639 (147)	918 (201)
PPT infraspinatus (kPa)	573 (138)	753 (178)
Hand grip strength (Kg)	39 (14)	51 (10)
Work-related		
Weekly working hours	40 (1)	39 (6)
Duration of slaughterhouse work (years)	17 (10)	16 (13)
DASH work module (0–100)	28 (17)	0 (0)

in the shoulder, arm or hand?" This single-item question was inspired by the work module of the DASH questionnaire [29].

The pain-free controls were a comparison group showing no pain symptoms or work disability. Inclusion criteria for this group were as follows: (1) pain intensity in the shoulder, elbow/forearm, or hand/wrist of 1 or less during the last 3 months, (2) pain intensity in the shoulder, elbow/forearm, or hand/wrist of 1 or less during the last week, and (3) statement of "*not at all*" work disability scoring on a five-point scale, "*not at all*," "*a little*," "*some*," and "*much*" to "*very much*," when asked the question "*During the last 3 months, did you have any difficulty performing your work due to pain in the shoulder, arm or hand?*"

Exclusion criteria for all participants were hypertension (systolic BP > 160, diastolic BP > 100), a medical history of cardiovascular diseases, symptoms of carpal tunnel syndrome, recent traumatic injury of the neck, shoulder, arm, or hand regions, or pregnancy.

2.3. Experimental Procedure. After the initial screening questionnaire, eligible participants were asked to present at the slaughterhouse for a questionnaire and clinical examination. In the questionnaire, participants were to rate the prevalence of indoor environmental complaints by the MM-indoor climate questionnaire [30, 31]. The MM-questionnaire contained questions on 13 different indoor environmental factors, and the participant had to rate whether the single factor is a bothering workplace-factor by stating "yes, often," "yes, sometimes," or "no, never." Only the alternative "yes, often" (meaning every week) was used as a positive outcome in the analyses. The 13 indoor environmental factors were draught, room temperature too high, varying room temperature, room temperature too low, stuffy "bad" air, dry air, unpleasant odour, static electricity, passive smoking, noise, lighting problems, reflections, and dust and dirt. Additionally, participants were asked about year of birth, height and weight, seniority, and primary job function. Primary job function was further trichotomized into "meat cutters," "meat packers," and "slaughterer." Smoking habits were identified by the question "do you smoke?"—"yes" or "no." Further, work disability was rated by the work module of the Disability of the Arm, Shoulder and Hand (DASH) questionnaire [23, 29].

The clinical examination of participants included pressure algometry using an electronic pressure algometer (Somedic Productions AB, Sollentuna, Sweden, Europe). The examiner was blinded to group allocation and measured pressure pain threshold (PPT) of the painful muscles (infraspinatus and extensor carpi radialis brevis) and a nonpainful reference muscle (tibialis anterior). The contact area of the circular probe was 1 cm^2 and pressure was applied perpendicular to the skin at the mid-belly of the 3 muscles at a rate of 30 kPa·s-1 [15]. The participant was not aware of the reading of PPT on the display and was instructed to push the patient operated switch on a pinch handle mounted on the algometer when the sensation of "pressure" changed to "pain". PPT was measured 3 times at the infraspinatus, extensor carpi radialis brevis, and tibialis anterior with 1.5 min between each measurement alternating between the 3 muscles [15]. PPT for each muscle was subsequently expressed as the average value of the 3 measurements. Previous studies have shown satisfactory to good test-retest reliability of PPT [32, 33].

2.4. Statistical Analysis. Pearson chi-square tests were performed to investigate between-group differences in indoor climate complaints for each of the 13 environmental factors by the use of the frequency procedure of SAS version 9.3.

Using general linear models (PROC GLM of SAS version 9.3) we estimated the relationships between indoor climate complaints, PPT, and chronic pain in two sets of analyses. The first set of analyses included average number of indoor climate complaints as a dependent variable and job position (meat cutter, meat packer, and slaughterer) and smoking habits (yes, no) as independent classification variables. In model 1, the relationship between indoor climate complaints and chronic pain was investigated by including group allocation (chronic pain, pain-free controls) as an independent classification variable. In model 2, the relationship between indoor climate complaints and central sensitization was investigated by adding tibialis anterior PPT (very low, low, moderate, and high) as an independent classification variable. Both models were adjusted for age.

The second set of analyses included PPT as a dependent variable and job position and smoking habits as independent classification variables. The analyses were adjusted for age. In model 3, we investigated the association between central sensitization and chronic pain by including PPT of tibialis anterior (pain-free muscle) as the dependent variable. In models 4 and 5, the relationship between peripheral sensitization and chronic pain was estimated by adding extensor carpi radialis brevis and infraspinatus (painful muscles) as dependent variables, respectively.

Results are given as least square means and 95% confidence intervals. An alpha level of less than 0.05 was accepted as statistically significant.

3. Results

Table 1 shows descriptive statistics for the main study variables. No difference existed in job position between participants in the two groups.

Table 2 summarizes specific indoor climate complaints for workers with chronic pain and the pain-free controls. A significantly greater proportion of workers with chronic pain reported higher prevalence of ("often") draught ($p < 0.001$) and noise ($p < 0.05$) during work compared with the healthy controls (Table 2). There were no differences between the two groups for the remainder of the indoor climate factors.

Table 3 summarizes the relationship between average indoor climate complaints and chronic pain (model 1) and PPT of tibialis anterior (model 2). Model 1 explained 9% of the variance observed for average indoor complaints and shows that slaughterhouse workers with chronic pain reported twice as many indoor climate complaints as pain-free controls (95% CI 1.8 versus 0.9, $p = 0.0163$) corresponding to a between-group difference of 0.9 complaints (95% CI 0.2 to 1.5). Model 2 explained 14% of the variance observed for average indoor complaints and indicates a significant negative association between tibialis PPT and indoor climate complaints ($p = 0.019$). However, only "very low" PPT scores were associated with more complaints. Compared with "low to high" PPT workers, workers with "very low" tibialis PPT reported a twofold increase in indoor complaints (2.4 versus 1.2). We found no significant influence of job function, age, or smoking habits on indoor climate complaints for both models.

TABLE 2: Prevalence of indoor climate complaints among slaughterhouse workers with chronic pain and pain-free controls.

	Chronic pain (n = 49) Prevalence (%)	Control (n = 33) Prevalence (%)
Draught	40*	6
Room temperature too high	2	3
Varying room temperature	4	3
Room temperature too low	24	15
Stuffy "bad" air	0	3
Dry air	6	6
Unpleasant odour	9	3
Static electricity	0	3
Passive smoking	4	0
Noise	58*	33
Lightning problems	6	0
Reflections	6	6
Dust and dirt	9	9
Average complaints (mean; 95% CI)	1.8 (1.3–2.3)*	0.9 (0.4–1.5)

*Significantly different from the pain-free control group ($p < 0.05$).

Table 4 summarizes the relationship between PPT of different muscles and chronic pain. PPT for both tibialis anterior and extensor carpi radialis brevis and infraspinatus were significantly lower in workers with chronic pain compared with pain-free controls (Figure 1). A significant association was observed for chronic pain and PPT of tibialis anterior, extensor carpi radialis brevis, and infraspinatus. The model explained 20%, 31%, and 23% of the variance observed for tibialis anterior PPT (model 3), extensor carpi radialis PPT (model 4), and infraspinatus PPT (model 5), respectively. We found no significant influence of job function, age, or smoking habits on PPT of any of the muscles tested.

4. Discussion

Workers with chronic pain reported twice as many indoor climate complaints as pain-free controls despite similar actual indoor climate. The number of complaints was associated with PPT of the nonpainful tibialis anterior suggesting a spreading of central sensitization to sensory processing circuits and thereby an amplification of external stimuli.

Workers with chronic pain displayed increased sensitivity to pressure, evidenced by lower PPT, in the painful muscles of the arm and shoulder compared with pain-free controls. This hyperalgesia may partly be explained by local cellular muscle mechanisms. However, in any chronic pain condition there is a fine tuned interplay of peripheral and central factors that

Table 3: The relationship between average indoor climate complaints (dependent variable) and chronic pain (model 1) and pressure pain threshold (PPT) of tibialis anterior (model 2). We found no significant influence of job function, age, or smoking habits on indoor climate complaints for both models.

	Dependent variable: number of indoor climate symptoms					
	Model 1			Model 2		
	LS mean	95% CI	p value (F-value)	LS mean	95% CI	p value (F-value)
Status			0.0163* (6.05)			
Chronic pain	1.8	1.3–2.3				
Pain-free	0.9	0.4–1.5				
Job position			0.5567 (0.59)			0.9613 (0.04)
Meat cutter	1.3	0.9–1.7		1.4	1.0–1.8	
Meat packer	1.1	0.4–1.7		1.4	0.7–2.0	
Slaughterer	1.6	0.7–2.7		1.5	0.5–2.6	
Smoking			0.9275 (0.01)			0.6404 (0.22)
Yes	1.3	0.7–2.0		1.5	0.9–2.2	
No	1.4	0.9–1.8		1.4	0.9–1.8	
PPT tibialis anterior						0.0190* (3.54)
Very low				2.4	1.6–3.1	
Low				0.9	0.1–1.7	
Moderate				1.2	0.5–1.9	
High				1.3	0.7–2.0	

*Significantly associated to average indoor climate complaints ($p < 0.05$).

Table 4: The relationship between pressure pain threshold (PPT) of the different muscles and chronic pain. We found no significant influence of job function, age, or smoking habits on PPT for either of the muscles.

	Dependent variable: PPT								
	Model 3 Tibialis anterior			Model 4 Extensor carpi radialis brevis			Model 5 Infraspinatus		
	LS mean	95% CI	p value (F-value)	LS mean	95% CI	p value (F-value)	LS mean	95% CI	p value (F-value)
Status			0.0023* (9.99)			<0.0001* (26.42)			0.0006* (13.03)
Chronic pain	805	701–910		639	554–725		573	494–652	
Pain-free	1015	900–1130		918	824–1013		753	666–839	
Job position			0.1021 (2.35)			0.1500 (1.95)			0.7458 (0.29)
Meat cutter	806	721–891		763	694–833		635	571–699	
Meat packer	877	751–1003		694	591–797		655	561–750	
Slaughterer	1047	841–1253		879	710–1048		698	543–854	
Smoking			0.0593 (3.67)			0.1830 (1.81)			0.0980 (2.81)
Yes	977	847–1107		817	711–924		707	609–805	
No	843	751–934		740	665–815		618	550–687	

*Statistically significant association between the PPT of respective muscle and status (chronic pain versus pain-free control) ($p < 0.05$).

can mutually influence and reinforce each other [16]. In line with this, we observed lower PPT in the nonpainful tibialis anterior among the workers with chronic pain reflecting a certain degree of general sensitization and thus the involvement of a central mechanism in the perception of upper-limb chronic pain. Generalized hypersensitivity, evidenced by enhanced nociceptive sensitivity and reduced pressure pain threshold, has also been reported in patients with chronic pain conditions such as fibromyalgia, trapezius myalgia, and chronic low back pain [15, 34, 35]. The proposed mechanisms of central sensitization involve an enhancement in the function of neurons and circuits in nociceptive pathways caused by increases in membrane excitability and synaptic efficacy as well as reduced inhibition [36].

The neural changes that lead to central sensitization may not only influence the perception of chronic pain, but also amplify other nonpainful stimuli [13, 36]. Hence, patients with chronic pain conditions have been shown more sensitive to other stimuli than pain, such as visual and auditory sensations [16]. This shows that these patients have a fundamental problem with pain or sensory processing rather than an abnormality confined to the specific body region where the pain is perceived to be situated [16]. In the present study, workers with chronic pain reported twice as many

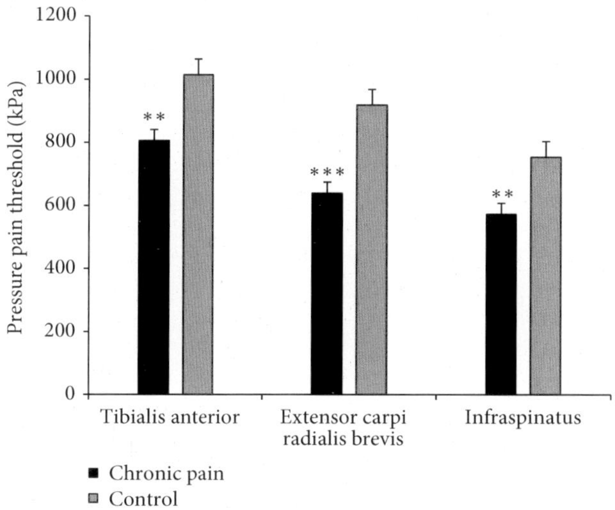

FIGURE 1: Average pressure pain threshold (PPT) of nonpainful (tibialis anterior) and painful (extensor carpi radialis brevis and infraspinatus) muscles among slaughterhouse workers with chronic pain and pain-free controls. $**$, $***$ denotes difference from the pain-free control group ($p < 0.01$; $p < 0.0001$, resp.).

indoor climate complaints as healthy controls despite similar environmental working conditions. This higher complaint rate was additionally associated with lower PPT in the tibialis anterior suggesting that central sensitization may amplify normal innocuous factors to make them intolerable to workers with chronic upper-limb pain. Of the 13 single indoor climate factors of the indoor climate questionnaire, the chronic pain group reported significantly higher prevalence of bothering from draught and noise. Possibly this reflects a spreading of central sensitization to sensory processing circuits involved in noise and draught perception in workers with chronic pain. The existence of a biological amplification of sensory stimuli to chronic pain has support from functional imaging studies in patients with fibromyalgia that shows hyperactivity in the insula which plays a critical role in sensory integration and emotional processing of sensation [16, 37, 38]. Additionally, de Klaver and colleagues [14] demonstrated that hyperacusis (intolerance of ordinary sound levels) is common among patients severely affected by complex regional pain syndrome type 1. Hyperacusis has been associated with central nervous system involvement and the authors speculated that hyperacusis may reflect the spreading of central sensitization to auditory circuits in these patients.

To foster a safe and healthy work environment, occupational health and safety programs have strong focus on primary prevention of workplace hazards along with monitoring of workers symptoms and perception of the work environment. Altogether, these analyses can indicate the best mode of prevention and rehabilitate work-related illness and discomfort. Environmental hazards in the slaughterhouse involve, among others, low ambient temperatures, draught from compressing machinery or elsewhere, and noise from the mechanically based production systems. In the present study, the prevalence of complaints from draught and noise was higher among workers with chronic pain compared with pain-free controls, whereas no difference was observed for low temperature or light complaints. In contrast, Bang et al. [6] reported a large interindividual variation in cold sensation among seafood industrial workers in Norway and found that workers who often felt cold reported increased prevalence of musculoskeletal pain. However, no physiological measures were obtained to propose a mechanistic explanation and the authors speculated that the interindividual variation in cold sensation was due to variations in activity levels, clothing, and cold adaptation. Spreading of central sensitization to sensory circuits as a function of chronic pain could possibly explain the increased sensitivity to draught and noise as a function of chronic pain in the present study. However, from this perspective one would perhaps expect more complaints in relation to lighting and temperature. Surprisingly, however, central sensitization did not seem to influence the processing of cold or light sensation among the workers with chronic pain.

The observed existence of an interindividual variation in indoor climate sensation among workers with and without chronic pain suggests that conclusions of occupational health and safety programs that assess the indoor environment with self-reports may be distorted. Additionally, we found that persons with very low PPT, regardless of chronic pain, likewise experienced the indoor climate more bothering than subjects with higher PPT. Occupational physicians monitoring workers' symptoms and their perception of the work environment should take into account musculoskeletal pain and pressure soreness of employees in the evaluation of environmental workplace hazards. Additionally, future studies on indoor climate perception should be adjusted for musculoskeletal pain or pressure threshold.

5. Strength and Limitations

Our study has both strengths and limitations. Combining direct measures of pressure pain threshold with subjective reporting on indoor climate among workers with chronic pain is a strength. To our knowledge this is the first study to focus on the interindividual variance in indoor climate complaints as a function of chronic disease and additionally to offer a mechanistic explanation for this variance. A limitation is that we did not collect any objective data of the specific indoor climate factors such as draught and noise to support the workers perception of the indoor work environment. Because this part of the study was exploratory in nature, that is, assessing several indoor climate complaints, there is a chance of random findings. However, the p value of <0.001 for "draught" shows that even correcting conservatively for type I errors, for example, by Bonferroni correction, would not change the overall results. Furthermore, the complaints that reached significance are in agreement with those expected in the hypothesis. Unfortunately we did not have brain imaging to support the spreading of central sensitization to sensory processing circuits. However it would be optimal if future studies on chronic disease and climate perception could include brain imaging techniques to investigate whether hyperactivity exists in the areas of the brain involved in sensory processing. Even though the nociceptive responses to different types of painful stimuli largely converge, using only the tibialis anterior as reference could be a limitation. Finally, the cross-sectional design of the present study makes it impossible to conclude any causal relationship between the number of indoor climate complaints and central sensitization, and the generalizability of the results is limited to workers with heavy manual job tasks. Thus studying the longitudinal effect of climate complaints and pain with an additional focus on development of central sensitization would be of interest. It would also be relevant to investigate whether changes in pain over time follow changes in the perception of indoor climate among workers remaining in the same workplace with the same actual indoor climate.

6. Conclusion

Workers with chronic pain reported more indoor climate complaints than pain-free controls despite similar actual indoor climate. Previous studies that did not account for musculoskeletal pain in questionnaire assessment of indoor climate may be biased. Central sensitization likely explains the present findings.

Acknowledgments

This study was supported by a grant from the Danish Parliament (Satspuljen 2012; Nye Veje, Grant no. § 17.21.02.60) and a grant from the Danish Working Environment Research Fund (Grant no. 48-2010-03).

References

[1] J. F. Brundage, R. M. Scott, W. M. Lednar, D. W. Smith, and R. N. Miller, "Building-associated risk of febrile acute respiratory diseases in Army trainees," *Journal of the American Medical Association*, vol. 259, no. 14, pp. 2108–2112, 1988.

[2] W. J. Fisk and A. H. Rosenfeld, "Estimates of improved productivity and health from better indoor environments," *Indoor Air*, vol. 7, no. 3, pp. 158–172, 1997.

[3] N. Magnavita, "Work-related symptoms in indoor environments: a puzzling problem for the occupational physician," *International Archives of Occupational and Environmental Health*, vol. 88, no. 2, pp. 185–196, 2015.

[4] M. J. Mendell, W. J. Fisk, K. Kreiss et al., "Improving the health of workers in indoor environments: priority research needs for a National Occupational Research Agenda," *American Journal of Public Health*, vol. 92, no. 9, pp. 1430–1440, 2002.

[5] J. Pejtersen, L. Allermann, T. S. Kristensen, and O. M. Poulsen, "Indoor climate, psychosocial work environment and symptoms in open-plan offices," *Indoor Air*, vol. 16, no. 5, pp. 392–401, 2006.

[6] B. E. Bang, L. Aasmoe, L. Aardal et al., "Feeling cold at work increases the risk of symptoms from muscles, skin, and airways in seafood industry workers," *American Journal of Industrial Medicine*, vol. 47, no. 1, pp. 65–71, 2005.

[7] C. A. Redlich, J. Sparer, and M. R. Cullen, "Sick-building syndrome," *The Lancet*, vol. 349, no. 9057, pp. 1013–1016, 1997.

[8] E. K. Hansson and T. H. Hansson, "The costs for persons sick-listed more than one month because of low back or neck problems. A two-year prospective study of Swedish patients," *European Spine Journal*, vol. 14, no. 4, pp. 337–345, 2005.

[9] L. L. Andersen, O. S. Mortensen, J. V. Hansen, and H. Burr, "A prospective cohort study on severe pain as a risk factor for long-term sickness absence in blue- and white-collar workers," *Occupational and Environmental Medicine*, vol. 68, no. 8, pp. 590–592, 2011.

[10] D. C. Turk, H. D. Wilson, and A. Cahana, "Treatment of chronic non-cancer pain," *The Lancet*, vol. 377, no. 9784, pp. 2226–2235, 2011.

[11] R. J. Gatchel, Y. B. Peng, M. L. Peters, P. N. Fuchs, and D. C. Turk, "The biopsychosocial approach to chronic pain: scientific advances and future directions," *Psychological Bulletin*, vol. 133, no. 4, pp. 581–624, 2007.

[12] C. J. Woolf, "Central sensitization: implications for the diagnosis and treatment of pain," *Pain*, vol. 152, no. 3, upplement, pp. S2–S15, 2011.

[13] C. J. Woolf and M. W. Salter, "Neuronal plasticity: increasing the gain in pain," *Science*, vol. 288, no. 5472, pp. 1765–1768, 2000.

[14] M. J. M. de Klaver, M. A. van Rijn, J. Marinus, W. Soede, J. A. P. M. de Laat, and J. J. van Hilten, "Hyperacusis in patients with complex regional pain syndrome related dystonia," *Journal of Neurology, Neurosurgery and Psychiatry*, vol. 78, no. 12, pp. 1310–1313, 2007.

[15] L. L. Andersen, C. H. Andersen, E. Sundstrup, M. D. Jakobsen, O. S. Mortensen, and M. K. Zebis, "Central adaptation of pain perception in response to rehabilitation of musculoskeletal pain: randomized controlled trial," *Pain Physician*, vol. 15, no. 5, pp. 385–394, 2012.

[16] K. Phillips and D. J. Clauw, "Central pain mechanisms in chronic pain states—maybe it is all in their head," *Best Practice and Research: Clinical Rheumatology*, vol. 25, no. 2, pp. 141–154, 2011.

[17] M. Magnusson, R. Örtengren, G. B. J. Andersson, I. Petersén, and B. Sabel, "An ergonomic study of work methods and physical disorders among professional butchers," *Applied Ergonomics*, vol. 18, no. 1, pp. 43–50, 1987.

[18] L. Punnett and D. H. Wegman, "Work-related musculoskeletal disorders: the epidemiologic evidence and the debate," *Journal of Electromyography and Kinesiology*, vol. 14, no. 1, pp. 13–23, 2004.

[19] B. P. Bernard, *Musculoskeletal Disorders and Workplace Factors: A Critical Review of Epidemiologic Evidence for Work-Related Musculoskeletal Disorders of the Neck, Upper Extremity, and Low Back*, US Department of Health and Human Servises, Public Health Service, Center for Disease Control and Prevention, National Institute for Occupational Safety and Health, Washington, DC, USA, 1997.

[20] D. A. W. M. Van Der Windt, E. Thomas, D. P. Pope et al., "Occupational risk factors for shoulder pain: a systematic review," *Occupational and Environmental Medicine*, vol. 57, no. 7, pp. 433–442, 2000.

[21] E. Viikari Juntura, "Neck and upper limb disorders among slaughterhouse workers. An epidemiologic and clinical study," *Scandinavian Journal of Work, Environment and Health*, vol. 9, no. 3, pp. 283–290, 1983.

[22] E. Sundstrup, M. D. Jakobsen, K. Jay, M. Brandt, and L. L. Andersen, "High intensity physical exercise and pain in the neck

and upper limb among slaughterhouse workers: cross-sectional study," *BioMed Research International*, vol. 2014, Article ID 218546, 5 pages, 2014.

[23] E. Sundstrup, M. D. Jakobsen, C. H. Andersen et al., "Effect of two contrasting interventions on upper limb chronic pain and disability: a randomized controlled trial," *Pain Physician*, vol. 17, no. 2, pp. 145–154, 2014.

[24] F. Chen, T. Li, H. Huang, and I. Holmér, "A field study of cold effects among cold store workers in China," *Arctic Medical Research*, vol. 50, supplement 6, pp. 99–103, 1991.

[25] I. Niedhammer, M.-F. Landre, A. Leclerc et al., "Shoulder disorders related to work organization and other occupational factors among supermarket cashiers," *International Journal of Occupational and Environmental Health*, vol. 4, no. 3, pp. 168–178, 1998.

[26] T. Pienimäki, "Cold exposure and musculoskeletal disorders and diseases. A review.," *International Journal of Circumpolar Health*, vol. 61, no. 2, pp. 173–182, 2002.

[27] L. Aasmoe, B. Bang, C. Egeness, and M.-L. Løchen, "Musculoskeletal symptoms among seafood production workers in North Norway," *Occupational Medicine*, vol. 58, no. 1, pp. 64–70, 2008.

[28] E. Sundstrup, M. D. Jakobsen, M. Brandt et al., "Workplace strength training prevents deterioration of work ability among workers with chronic pain and work disability: a randomized controlled trial," *Scandinavian Journal of Work, Environment and Health*, vol. 40, no. 3, pp. 244–251, 2014.

[29] D. E. Beaton, J. N. Katz, A. H. Fossel, J. G. Wright, V. Tarasuk, and C. Bombardier, "Measuring the whole or the parts? Validity, reliability, and responsiveness of the disabilities of the arm, shoulder and hand outcome measure in different regions of the upper extremity," *Journal of Hand Therapy*, vol. 14, no. 2, pp. 128–146, 2001.

[30] K. Andersson, G. Stridh, I. Fagerlund, W. Aslaksen, and S. Rudblad, "Comparison of the perveived indoor climate and symptoms reported by students and personnel in 16 senior high schools in Sweden," in *Proceedings of the 9th International Conference on Indoor Air Quality and Climate: Indoor Air*, vol. 3, pp. 399–403, Monterey, Calif, USA, June-July 2002.

[31] K. Reijula and C. Sundman-Digert, "Assessment of indoor air problems at work with a questionnaire," *Occupational and Environmental Medicine*, vol. 61, no. 1, pp. 33–38, 2004.

[32] A. L. Persson, C. Brogårdh, and B. H. Sjölund, "Tender or not tender: test-retest repeatability of pressure pain thresholds in the trapezius and deltoid muscle of healthy women," *Journal of Rehabilitation Medicine*, vol. 36, no. 1, pp. 17–27, 2004.

[33] J. Ylinen, M. Nykänen, H. Kautiainen, and A. Häkkinen, "Evaluation of repeatability of pressure algometry on the neck muscles for clinical use," *Manual Therapy*, vol. 12, no. 2, pp. 192–197, 2007.

[34] S. O'Neill, C. Manniche, T. Graven-Nielsen, and L. Arendt-Nielsen, "Generalized deep-tissue hyperalgesia in patients with chronic low-back pain," *European Journal of Pain*, vol. 11, no. 4, pp. 415–420, 2007.

[35] F. Petzke, D. J. Clauw, K. Ambrose, A. Khine, and R. H. Gracely, "Increased pain sensitivity in fibromyalgia: effects of stimulus type and mode of presentation," *Pain*, vol. 105, no. 3, pp. 403–413, 2003.

[36] A. Latremoliere and C. J. Woolf, "Central sensitization: a generator of pain hypersensitivity by central neural plasticity," *Journal of Pain*, vol. 10, no. 9, pp. 895–926, 2009.

[37] A. D. Craig, "Pain mechanisms: labeled lines versus convergence in central processing," *Annual Review of Neuroscience*, vol. 26, pp. 1–30, 2003.

[38] I. Tracey, "Neuroimaging of pain mechanisms," *Current Opinion in Supportive and Palliative care*, vol. 1, no. 2, pp. 109–116, 2007.

11

The Association between Patient-Reported Pain and Doctors' Language Proficiency in Clinical Practice

Marianne Mustajoki,[1] Tom Forsén,[2] and Timo Kauppila[2]

[1] *Department of General Practice and Primary Health Care, University of Helsinki, Kiskontie 23 B, 00280 Helsinki, Finland*
[2] *Department of General Practice and Primary Health Care, University of Helsinki, PB 20 (Tukholmankatu 8 B), 00014 Helsinki, Finland*

Correspondence should be addressed to Marianne Mustajoki; marianne.mustajoki@duodecim.fi

Academic Editor: Anna Maria Aloisi

Patients' limited literacy and language fluency of different kinds cause them problems in navigating the medical interview. However, it is not known how physicians' native language skills affect the reported intensity of pain among Finnish emergency patients. Data were collected with two consecutive questionnaires in 16 healthcare centres and outpatient departments along the Finnish coast. Swedish and Finnish speaking 18–65-year-old emergency patients were eligible for this study. Our patients were predominantly Finnish speakers. Patient-rated poor language skills in Finnish among the physicians in ED setting increased statistically significantly pain reported by the Finnish speaking patients and their dissatisfaction with the health service. These patients were also less motivated to adhere to the instructions given by their physician. Patients speaking various languages reported less degree of pain. Foreign physicians' poor language proficiency in Finnish was expected to explain only some of the patients' pain experience. Physicians' good native language skills may help to reduce pain experience. Despite concordant language communication, other unknown barriers in the interaction might reduce the magnitude of pain reported.

1. Introduction

Healthcare is ideally delivered in language concordance which means that both the patient and the physician speak the same preferred language. Mutual language and understanding are critical in generating good functional relationships between health staff and patients. Language barriers cause communication difficulties which may hamper the treatment of a disease [1]. Patients with difficulties to express themselves in a nonnative language are less adherent to health instructions and report significantly decreased patient satisfaction [2–5]. Furthermore, communication problems with the patients affect also the physicians and impede their decision making and adequate medical treatment. On the other hand, limited literacy and insufficient language fluency cause the patients problems in navigating the medical interview. Diagnosing, for example, acute chest pain patients in emergency departments (ED) may be hampered because of language barriers [6]. In line with this, language barriers have been associated with a higher rate of resource utilization for the diagnostic process and increased ED visit times [7]. Yet common cultural and lingual conditions do not necessarily prevent the patients and physicians from miscommunication, thus compromising mutual understanding. Patients' limited comprehension of their disease can also undermine effective communication and distract physicians from investigating symptoms. The patients and physicians might have different explanations for diseases which are reflected in the clinical information gained in the medical interview. Patients suffering from chronic diseases may also be exposed to cognitive problems affecting their ability to express reliably vital symptoms such as pain [8, 9].

Measuring the pain intensity in a clinical situation is challenging and as a rule healthcare personnel underestimate the severity of pain [10, 11]. In line with this, a paired survey demonstrated that socially discordant physician-patient interaction resulted in the physicians' overestimation of patients' confidence and trust but underestimation of their pain. The physicians' inability to effectively communicate with their patients may lead to frustration, which in turn leads to the patients' increasing concern of not being heard [12]. On the other hand, the physicians' ability to assess pain severity has been reported not to differ for Hispanic and non-Hispanic white patients in an ED in the USA, suggesting that there may be other explanations for observed differences in analgesic practice than ethnicity-based misinterpretation of the patients' pain intensity [13]. However, the physicians' language skills might affect the estimation of pain, resulting in poorer diagnostic confidence and increased need of ancillary tests [14]. Foreign physicians are not automatically able to fluently communicate in the patients' native language. The amount of mainly native Russian and Estonian speaking physicians has increased during recent years in Finland and they are likely to be overrepresented in EDs. A majority of them report very good communication skills in Finnish, but no data are available about their proficiency in Finland's second national language Swedish [15]. Thus this study about patients' experience concerning the physicians' communication skills in an ED setting and the effects on estimation of pain severity is a relevant issue in Finland.

By tradition Finland is an ethnically broadly homologous but bilingual country where patients have the right to get health service either in Finnish or in Swedish. The great amount of language contacts had exposed the minority of Swedish speakers to increasing Finnicization ("language transition") [16]. This linguistic instability typical for Finland means that the linguistic exchange in public services generally proceeds in Finnish and not in Swedish. Thus we have good opportunities to study how exclusively linguistic factors impact on the communication in EDs. As the Swedish speaking minority in Finland lives along the south and southwest coasts intermingled with the Finnish speaking majority this exceptional setting is ideal for testing the importance of linguistic factors in pain measuring. More important for the present study is that, unlike the conditions for minorities in general, these two language groups studied here—the Swedish speakers or Finnish speakers Finns—are quite similar in most aspects, including socioeconomic status, education, religion, and access to health services [17, 18]. According to this we were able to specifically study how the patients' and physicians' language skills affect the intensity of patient-reported pain.

2. Materials and Methods

Our study was approved by the Ethics Committee of the Hospital District of Helsinki and Uusimaa (Reference number 5/13/03/00/2008). Data were collected in 2008-2009 in 15 healthcare centres and outpatient departments along the south coast and in one healthcare centre in South Ostrobothnia. Only Swedish and Finnish speaking 18–65-year-old emergency patients were eligible for this study. Patients with major mental disturbances as well as life threatening symptoms were excluded by the personnel.

Everyone visiting healthcare in Finland is registered electronically. The personal data in the registration for population are automatically transferred into everyone's electronic case record. These data contain also information about the patients' native language. The arriving emergency patient was informed by a receptionist or a nurse about the possibility to voluntarily participate in the study. Interested and applicable patients were provided with language concordant information about the study and an agreement-form plus a questionnaire. All corresponding data-collection material was also accessible on a table in the waiting-room for entering patients in order to facilitate participation by oneself. The patients completed the questionnaire before the physician's appointment and were advised to drop the sealed questionnaire into a locked box in the waiting-room. The questionnaire included 43 closed questions, of which 15 were standardised questions about socioeconomic and health conditions used in periodical population surveys in Finland; 23 questions about native and nonnative language proficiency, the relatives' native language, language spoken at home and stated in registration for population, Finnish or Swedish schooling, and preferred communication language with the general practitioner (GP); and 5 questions about the frequency and quality of health centre visits and the reason for the visit.

Two weeks after the emergency visit, the patients who agreed to a follow-up were sent a second questionnaire including detailed filling instructions by mail. The language in the second questionnaire was specified according to the patient-reported native language during the visit. This structured questionnaire included 30 closed questions about the GP's language proficiency in the patient's native language and patient-preferred communication language, the patient's feeling of confidence and satisfaction on a 1–5 graded scale, pain experience on standardized VAS scale, frequency of laboratory tests and X-rays during the visit, medication prescriptions, pain medication, written and verbal instructions in the patient-preferred language, and length of sick leave. To quantify the language discordance between the patients and the GPs, the patients were asked to assess the GP's language proficiency in Finnish or Swedish according to a numerical, well-established Finnish school grade of 4–10. The patients' numeric ratings of the GP's language proficiency in the patient-preferred language were pooled into good, average, and poor by means of a data reduction technique for statistical analysis [19]. A measure of the patients' language proficiency was obtained by asking them to assess their ability to communicate in their second nonnative language.

Data were statistically analysed with SPSS system. Correlations between variables were calculated using linear regression. Statistical significance was set at $p < 0.05$. Adjustment was used for age, income, education, and gender.

3. Results

875 patients in total filled in the first questionnaire during their emergency visit on the healthcare centres. 53% of them ($n = 466$), predominantly Finnish speaking female patients, replied to the second questionnaire. All respondents did not

TABLE 1: Characteristics of the respondents.

	Finnish speakers (n = 383)	Swedish speakers (n = 79)
Gender		
M/F (n)	80/303	25/54
M/F (%)	21/79	32/68
Age, yrs (mean), M/F	46.0/43.0	56.0/49.8
Annual income (%)		
0–20 000	44.1	54.2
20 001–30 000	32.7	30.6
>30 000	23.1	15.3
Education, yrs (mean), M/F	13.4/14.2	12.2/13.2
BMI (mean kg/m^2), M/F	28.0/25.9	2.6/26.6

reply on every question in the questionnaire. Tables include only individuals with available data.

The characteristics of the respondents reveal that the Swedish speaking respondents were on average ten years older than the Finnish speaking respondents (Table 1).

The statistical analyses were performed according to the patient-preferred language stated in the questionnaire by the respondents. The Swedish speaking patients were less likely to estimate the GP's language proficiency in their native language since they generally communicated in Finnish. 55% of the patients reported that the GP's native language was Finnish, 10% Swedish, and 35% another language rather than Finnish or Swedish.

Comparison between Swedish speakers (n = 24) and Finnish speakers (n = 407) revealed that the Swedish speakers were significantly less confident about the GP's professional qualification ($p < 0.001$) and the care quality ($p < 0.001$) during the visit. They also reported significantly less motivation to adhere to the GP's instructions ($p < 0.001$) (Table 2). The Swedish speakers reported less pain when they were treated by a Swedish speaking GP than did the Finnish speakers although the difference did not reach the level of significance (Table 3).

The Finnish speakers reported significantly less unspecified pain when the GP's language proficiency in Finnish was good. On the contrary, the GP's poor language skills in Finnish increased significantly the degree of patient-reported pain in all diseases, except in musculoskeletal diseases ($p < 0.01$) (Table 4). The patients with good proficiency in a second nonnative language reported less unspecified pain compared to patients who knew only one language (Table 5). One-third of all patients were prescribed analgesics, but the small sample size made analysis of the significance between language groups impossible.

The GP's language proficiency in patients' native language, in both Finnish and Swedish, influenced the patients' experiences of the emergency visit. Deficient language competence among the GPs tended to increase both Finnish speakers' and Swedish speakers' dissatisfaction with the emergency visit and their insecurity, uncertainty, and fear during the visit. Furthermore, those patients were significantly less motivated to adhere to the instructions ($p < 0.001$) given by the GP (Table 6). One-third of the patients had undergone laboratory tests and 12% an X-ray during the visit.

4. Discussion

Our results suggest that the patients report a lower level of pain if they have estimated the GP's language skills highly in the patient-preferred language. This result is in line with previous findings among Spanish speaking cancer patients in the USA [20]. We also found that the patients' ability to speak an additional nonnative language was associated with a lower degree of reported pain. Patients with good nonnative language proficiency seemed to have generally advantageous communication conditions. These findings were independent of the GP's patient-rated language proficiency.

Patients' higher level of self-efficacy for pain communication has been reported to be associated with significantly lower levels of pain, physical and psychological disability, and pain catastrophizing and with lower levels of partner negative affect [21]. In the light of these findings, our results regarding the reasons for more intensive patient-reported pain are not surprising, although all pain decreasing factors are not known. Our results can, however, also indicate that the patients' estimation of the GP's language skills mirrors a plausible social discordance between the patients and GPs. We suppose, furthermore, that the patients' impression of the GP's personality is likely to influence patients' estimation of the GP's language proficiency.

The perception of the interaction and different ethnicity between the patient and the GP tends to affect the GP's perception of patients' pain [22]. Unfortunately, we did not collect any data about the GPs' nationalities from the healthcare centres, and so we do not know how many patients visited a nonnative (e.g., Swedish or Finnish is not the mother tongue) GP. From the patients' spontaneous remarks in the questionnaires we could, however, conclude that some foreign GPs were on duty during the study time indicating that lingual and cultural disparities might cause some patients' communication problems including uncertainty and fear. This topic would be exceptionally difficult to study with minorities in several other communities. However, the equal socioeconomic conditions among the broadly homologous but bilingual population living along the south coast and in South Ostrobothnia region provide an ideal test group for our study [16–18].

Our study revealed that, despite concordant language communication, other barriers had impact on reported pain intensity. As noted, low literate patients have less capability to spontaneously relate their symptoms in a structured and precise way. Our respondents had between 13.0 and 14.5 years of education and thus low literacy seems unlikely to cause any major problems in the medical interview. The GPs' preference to use difficult words, mainly Latin, when explaining the origin of disease might, however, also cause the patients uncertainty about the severity of their symptoms.

Greater depth of patient-physician relationship in primary care has been suggested to increase the GPs' detection of patients' emotional distress [23]. Altogether 41% of our

TABLE 2: Correlations between the GP's patient-reported language proficiency (1 = poor, 2 = average, and 3 = good) and the patients' experience of the visit (scale 1–5*).

	Mean ± SD (*n*)**	Total	*p* value
Very secure	2.8 ± 0.5 (155)		
Secure	2.6 ± 0.6 (172)		
Neither secure nor insecure	2.4 ± 0.7 (81)	2.6 ± 0.6 (432)	<0.001
Insecure	2.4 ± 0.7 (21)		
Very insecure	1.5 ± 1.0 (4)		
Very fearless	2.6 ± 0.6 (259)		
Fearless	2.5 ± 0.6 (87)		
Neither afraid nor fearless	2.5 ± 0.7 (45)	2.6 ± 0.6 (420)	0.02
Afraid	2.3 ± 0.8 (16)		
Very afraid	2.6 ± 0.8 (14)		
Great confidence in the GP's skills	2.8 ± 0.5 (122)		
Confidence	2.7 ± 0.5 (176)		
Neither confident nor uncertain	2.4 ± 0.7 (92)	2.6 ± 0.6 (433)	<0.001
Uncertain	2.7 ± 0.7 (30)		
Weak confidence	1.7 ± 0.9 (13)		
Very satisfied with the service	2.8 ± 0.5 (151)		
Satisfied	2.6 ± 0.6 (135)		
Neither satisfied nor dissatisfied	2.5 ± 0.7 (88)	2.6 ± 0.6 (435)	<0.001
Dissatisfied	2.4 ± 0.8 (38)		
Very dissatisfied	2.1 ± 0.8 (23)		
Very motivated to follow the GP's instructions	2.7 ± 0.5 (242)		
Motivated	2.5 ± 0.7 (129)		
Neither motivated nor unmotivated	2.5 ± 0.7 (43)	2.6 ± 0.6 (434)	<0.001
Unmotivated	2.4 ± 0.8 (14)		
Very unmotivated	1.8 ± 1.0 (6)		

*1–5 graded scale: 1 = the most negative experience, 5 = the most positive experience.
**Adjusted for age, gender, income, education, and native language.

TABLE 3: Correlations between the GP's patient-reported proficiency in Swedish and Finnish* and the patients' experience of pain**.

	Poor	Average	Good	*p* value
The GP's language proficiency in				
Swedish % (*n*)	76.9 (13)	19.0 (12)	60.3 (38)	
Finnish % (*n*)	5.1 (19)	26.1 (98)	68.8 (258)	
Both Swedish and Finnish % (*n*)	7.3 (32)	24.8 (109)	67.6 (296)	
The patients' pain experience mean ± SD (*n*)				
GP's proficiency in Swedish	3.7 ± 2.43 (12)	2.7 ± 2.0 (11)	2.8 ± 1.9 (33)	Ns
GP's proficiency in Finnish	4.4 ± 1.7 (18)	3.7 ± 1.9 (91)	3.3 ± 2.1 (252)	0.005
Proficiency in Swedish and Finnish	4.1 ± 2.0 (30)	3.7 ± 1.9 (103)	3.3 ± 2.1 (285)	0.007

*Language proficiency scale: 1 = poor, 2 = average, and 3 = good.
**Adjusted for age, gender, income, education, and native language.

respondents reported having earlier visited an assigned GP. One emergency patient out of five had the ED visit made to a previously assigned Finnish speaking GP. Our study, however, could not demonstrate less patient-reported pain among those patients who met their assigned GP during their emergency visit.

Although pain is an important symptom in most diseases, the emergency situation might prevent especially stressed patients from being active in the medical interview. Our findings can also indicate that increased patient-reported pain reflects GPs' emphasising laboratory tests or X-rays instead of asking the patients what is wrong with them. Compared to Finnish data from 1998 our study could not demonstrate the GPs compensating poor communication by a need of more tests to narrow the diagnosis [24].

The patients reported more pain when the GP's language proficiency was poor in all other reasons for the visit other than musculoskeletal diseases. Obesity (body mass index,

TABLE 4: Correlations between the GP's patient-reported language proficiency* in Swedish and Finnish and pain experience (pain scale VAS 0–10) related to the reason for emergency visit**.

	Pain experience, mean ± SD (n) when the GP's language proficiency was as follows			p value
	Poor	Average	Good	
Reason for visit				
Musculoskeletal problems	5.1 ± 1.5 (6)	4.7 ± 1.0 (27)	4.3 ± 1.8 (77)	0.2
Other health problems	3.8 ± 2.0 (23)	3.3 ± 2.0 (75)	2.9 ± 2.1 (202)	0.01
All problems	4.1 ± 2.0 (30)	3.6 ± 1.9 (102)	3.3 ± 2.1 (285)	0.007

*Language proficiency scale: 1 = poor, 2 = average, and 3 = good.
**Adjusted for age, gender, income, education, and native language.

TABLE 5: Correlation between the patient's pain experience and their language proficiency in a nonnative language*.

	VAS pain scale 0–10	Mean ± SD (n)	p value
The patients' nonnative language proficiency, 1–4 graded scale (1 = none/poor, 4 = fluent)	None or very poor proficiency	3.6 ± 1.9 (78)	
	Speaking satisfactory well	3.5 ± 2.0 (132)	
	Speaking well	3.2 ± 2.1 (121)	
	Fluent proficiency	3.0 ± 2.0 (66)	
	Total	3.4 ± 2.0 (396)	0.02

*Adjusted for age, gender, income, education, and native language.

TABLE 6: Correlations between the patients' native language and their experience during the visit (1–5 graded scale*).

	Swedish speakers Mean ± SD (n)**	Finnish speakers Mean ± SD (n)**	p value
Sense of security/insecurity	4.23 ± 0.9 (77)	4.0 ± 0.9 (379)	0.99
Trust/fear	1.5 ± 1.0 (71)	1.7 ± 1.0 (372)	0.7
Confidence in/uncertainty of the GP's skills	3.8 ± 1.0 (76)	3.8 ± 1.0 (381)	0.1
Motivated/unmotivated to follow the GP's instructions	4.2 ± 1.0 (76)	4.5 ± 0.9 (381)	0.005
Satisfied/dissatisfied with the service	3.9 ± 1.4 (77)	3.8 ± 1.2 (382)	0.27

*1–5 graded scale: 1 = the most negative experience, 5 = the most positive experience.
**Adjusted for age, gender, income, and education.

BMI, > 30 kg/m^2) has been noted to increase the patient-reported pain compared to normal-weight and underweight patients [25]. Our respondents reported average BMI < 30 kg/m^2 indicating that obesity was not the exclusive explanation for pain. Furthermore, pain is the most prominent symptom in musculoskeletal diseases and therefore is likely to be noted by the GP in the medical interview, but we assume that urological, gynaecological, obstetrical, and abdominal symptoms including pain might embarrass many patients minimizing their information especially if the communication with the GPs is poor. Unquoted and unexplained pain can increase the patients' worries for the situation which in turn intensify the symptoms. Being disbelieved by healthcare providers or reassured that nothing is physically wrong has also been noted to worsen symptoms [26]. Many symptoms are, furthermore, difficult for patients to identify and explain without GPs' verbal navigation. Any significant differences in GPs' prescription of analgesics and the patient-preferred language were not possible to demonstrate in this study as the Swedish speaking patients were few. However, based on earlier minority studies, we assume that a larger sample size could reveal putative significance. By paying more attention to the GPs' language education, language barriers are possible to reduce in healthcare service.

5. Conclusions

The GPs' deficient native language proficiency affects negatively patients' experience of the emergency visit which might affect also pain communication. Our study could thus verify that although language concordant communication is a prerequisite for mutual understanding, pain revealing requires additionally good language skills.

Previous studies have consistently confirmed that language minority patients are in general at risk for communication problems in healthcare mainly caused by their unfavourable socioeconomic conditions as well as cultural and lingual disparities. We could, however, demonstrate that language discordance alone in a sociocultural homogenous population is sufficient to increase both minority and majority patients' insecurity and fear and can also intensify patient-reported pain.

Study Limitations and Strengths

The strengths of this study were that the respondents represented typical acutely ill native patients making out-of-hour visits to healthcare centres in Finland. The coastal region of Finland is an ethnically and culturally relatively homogenous but bilingual part of the country providing exceptionally favourable opportunities to study how linguistic factors impact pain measuring in EDs.

A considerable proportion of our Swedish speaking minority patients reported impediments during the medical interview performed in a nonpreferred language. Our sample was, however, too small to reach the level of significance due to minority patients' reported pain. Further studies are required to reveal how often pain other than that caused by musculoskeletal diseases remains unobserved by the GPs.

Acknowledgments

This study was supported by Svenska Kulturfonden, Nursing Association in Finland, and Vasa Central Hospital (EVO Government subsidy).

References

[1] R. N. J. Cioffi, "Communicating with culturally and linguistically diverse patients in an acute care setting: nurses' experiences," *International Journal of Nursing Studies*, vol. 40, no. 3, pp. 299–306, 2003.

[2] J. C. M. Van Wieringen, J. A. M. Harmsen, and M. A. Bruijnzeels, "Intercultural communication in general practice," *European Journal of Public Health*, vol. 12, no. 1, pp. 63–68, 2002.

[3] M. Mustajoki and K. Saranto, "The influence of language barriers on patient care," *Journal of Nursing Science*, vol. 21, pp. 109–119, 2009.

[4] J. A. M. Harmsen, R. M. D. Bernsen, M. A. Bruijnzeels, and L. Meeuwesen, "Patients' evaluation of quality of care in general practice: what are the cultural and linguistic barriers?" *Patient Education and Counseling*, vol. 72, no. 1, pp. 155–162, 2008.

[5] Q. Ngo-Metzger, D. H. Sorkin, R. S. Phillips et al., "Providing high-quality care for limited english proficient patients: the importance of language concordance and interpreter use," *Journal of General Internal Medicine*, vol. 22, supplement 2, pp. 324–330, 2007.

[6] S. A. Farmer, D. L. Roter, and I. J. Higginson, "Chest pain: communication of symptoms and history in a London emergency department," *Patient Education and Counseling*, vol. 63, no. 1-2, pp. 138–144, 2006.

[7] L. C. Hampers, S. Cha, D. J. Gutglass, H. J. Binns, and S. E. Krug, "Language barriers and resource utilization in a pediatric emergency department," *Pediatrics*, vol. 103, no. 6, pp. 1253–1256, 1999.

[8] P. K. Elias, M. F. Elias, R. B. D'Agostino et al., "NIDDM and blood pressure as risk factors for poor cognitive performance: the Framingham study," *Diabetes Care*, vol. 20, no. 9, pp. 1388–1395, 1997.

[9] A. Pesonen, T. Kauppila, P. Tarkkila, A. Sutela, L. Niinistö, and P. H. Rosenberg, "Evaluation of easily applicable pain measurement tools for the assessment of pain in demented patients," *Acta Anaesthesiologica Scandinavica*, vol. 53, no. 5, pp. 657–664, 2009.

[10] K. Puntillo, M. Neighbor, N. O'Neil, and R. Nixon, "Accuracy of emergency nurses in assessment of patient's pain," *Pain Management Nursing*, vol. 4, no. 4, pp. 171–175, 2003.

[11] N. Davoudi, P. Afsharzadeh, S. Mohammadalizadeh, and A. A. Haghdoost, "A comparison of patients' and nurses' assessments of pain intensity in patients with coronary artery disease," *International Journal of Nursing Practice*, vol. 14, no. 5, pp. 347–356, 2008.

[12] J. J. Coran, T. Koropeckyj-Cox, and C. L. Arnold, "Are physicians and patients in agreement? Exploring dyadic concordance," *Health Education and Behavior*, vol. 40, no. 5, pp. 603–611, 2013.

[13] K. H. Todd, T. Lee, and J. R. Hoffman, "The effect of ethnicity on physician estimates of pain severity in patients with isolated extremity trauma," *The Journal of the American Medical Association*, vol. 271, no. 12, pp. 925–928, 1994.

[14] G. Garra, H. Albino, H. Chapman, A. J. Singer, and H. C. Thode Jr., "The impact of communication barriers on diagnostic confidence and ancillary testing in the emergency department," *Journal of Emergency Medicine*, vol. 38, no. 5, pp. 681–685, 2010.

[15] The Finnish Medical Association, "Data about foreign physicians in Finland," 2010.

[16] K. D. McRae, *Conflict and Compromise in Multilingual Societies. Volume 3, Finland*, Wilfrid Laurier University Press, Waterloo, Canada, 1997.

[17] M. T. Hyyppä and J. Mäki, "Individual-level relationships between social capital and self-rated health in a bilingual community," *Preventive Medicine*, vol. 32, no. 2, pp. 148–155, 2001.

[18] M. T. Hyyppä and J. Mäki, "Why do Swedish-speaking Finns have longer active life? An area for social capital research," *Health Promotion International*, vol. 16, no. 1, pp. 55–64, 2001.

[19] J. Metsämuuronen, *Tutkimuksen Tekemisen Perusteet Ihmistieteissä*, International Methelp, Helsinki, Finland, 2003.

[20] C. E. Mosher, K. N. Duhamel, J. Egert, and M. Y. Smith, "Self-efficacy for coping with cancer in a multiethnic sample of breast cancer patients: associations with barriers to pain management and distress," *Clinical Journal of Pain*, vol. 26, no. 3, pp. 227–234, 2010.

[21] L. S. Porter, F. J. Keefe, C. Wellington, and A. de Williams, "Pain communication in the context of osteoarthritis: patient and partner self-efficacy for pain communication and holding back from discussion of pain and arthritis-related concerns," *Clinical Journal of Pain*, vol. 24, no. 8, pp. 662–668, 2008.

[22] J. Miner, M. H. Biros, A. Trainor, D. Hubbard, and M. Beltram, "Patient and physician perceptions as risk factors for oligoanalgesia: a prospective observational study of the relief of pain in the emergency department," *Academic Emergency Medicine*, vol. 13, no. 2, pp. 140–146, 2006.

[23] M. Ridd, G. Lewis, T. J. Peters, and C. Salisbury, "Detection of patient psychological distress and longitudinal patient-doctor relationships: a cross-sectional study," *The British Journal of General Practice*, vol. 62, no. 596, pp. 132–133, 2012.

[24] A. Aromaa, A. Linnala, T. Maljanen, and K. Mattila, *Private Practitioners As Family Doctors. A Report from the Social*

12

Incidence and Health Related Quality of Life of Opioid-Induced Constipation in Chronic Noncancer Pain Patients: A Prospective Multicentre Cohort Study

Dalila R. Veiga,[1] **Liliane Mendonça**,[2] **Rute Sampaio**,[3,4,5,6]
José C. Lopes,[2,3,4,6,7] **and Luís F. Azevedo**[8]

[1] *Anesthesiology Department, Chronic Pain Center, Centro Hospitalar Universitário do Porto, Largo do Prof. Abel Salazar, 4099-001 Porto, Portugal*
[2] *Centro Nacional de Observação em Dor, OBSERVDOR, Alameda Prof. Hernâni Monteiro, 4200-319 Porto, Portugal*
[3] *Departamento de Biomedicina, Unidade de Biologia Experimental, Faculdade de Medicina da Universidade do Porto, Portugal*
[4] *i3S, Instituto de Investigação e Inovação em Saúde, Universidade do Porto, Portugal*
[5] *Instituto de Biologia Molecular e Celular (IBMC), Universidade do Porto, Portugal*
[6] *Alameda Prof. Hernâni Monteiro, 4200-319 Porto, Portugal*
[7] *Instituto de Biologia Molecular e Celular (IBMC), Universidade do Porto, Portugal Faculty of Medicine University of Porto, Department of Biomedicine, Porto, Portugal*
[8] *Center for Health Technology and Services Research (CINTESIS); Faculdade de Medicina da Universidade do Porto, Departamento de Medicina da Comunidade Informação e Decisão em Saúde (MEDCIDS); Faculdade de Medicina da Universidade do Porto, Alameda Prof. Hernâni Monteiro, 4200-319 Porto, Portugal*

Correspondence should be addressed to Dalila R. Veiga; dalilaveiga@gmail.com

Academic Editor: Giustino Varrassi

Background. High rates of opioid use for chronic noncancer pain (CNCP) have been reported worldwide, despite its association with adverse events, inappropriate use, and limited analgesic effect. Opioid-induced constipation (OIC) is the most prevalent and disabling adverse effect associated with opioid therapy. Our aim was to assess the incidence, health related quality of life (HRQOL), and disability in OIC patients. *Methods.* A prospective cohort study was performed, with 6 months of follow-up, of adult CNCP patients consecutively admitted in 4 multidisciplinary pain clinics (MPC). Demographic and clinical data have been collected. Brief Pain Inventory (BPI) and Short version of Treatment Outcomes in Pain Survey (S-TOPS) were used to measure functional outcomes and HRQOL. OIC was assessed using Bowel Function Index (BFI). *Results.* 694 patients were recruited. OIC prevalence at baseline was 25.8%. At 6 months, OIC incidence was 24.8%. Female gender (OR = 1.65, $p = 0.039$), opioid therapy (OR 1.65, $p = 0.026$), and interference pain score on BPI (OR 1.10, $p = 0.009$) were identified as OIC independent predictors. OIC patients presented higher disability and pain interference and severity scores. OIC patients reported less satisfaction with outcome ($p = 0.038$). *Discussion.* Constipation is a common adverse event among opioid users with major functional and quality of life impairment. These findings emphasise the need of OIC adequate assessment and management.

1. Introduction

Chronic pain is a major public healthcare problem worldwide [1]. It has an estimated prevalence of 20% in the European population and is an important cause of quality of life impairment and substantial burden in healthcare systems [2–4]. Opioids may be a safe and reliable therapeutic option for moderate or severe chronic pain treatment, but their adequate prescription requires suitable patients' selection, clinicians' training, and patients' education. Indeed, opioid use in chronic noncancer pain (CNCP) treatment is recommended in several guidelines [5–7], and high prescription rates were observed in several countries of Europe and the United States in the last decade [8–10], although there has been a decreasing trend in prescription rates since 2011 [10, 11].

Opioid use is associated with adverse effects development such as gastrointestinal disorders, neuroendocrine dysfunction, osteoporosis, immunosuppression, cognitive disorders, drowsiness, respiratory depression, physical dependence, hyperalgesia, and addiction [12–16]. Therefore, opioid prescription requires adequate and regular clinical supervision in order to monitor their efficacy and safety.

Gastrointestinal disorders, including constipation, nausea, vomiting, abdominal cramping, and bloating, are often associated with opioid use and represent an important cause of opioid withdrawal [17]. Opioid-induced constipation, a type of secondary constipation [18], is the most prevalent and disabling adverse effect associated with chronic opioid therapy. There is no consensual definition in the literature for OIC [19]. According to Gaertner et al., OIC is defined as a "change from baseline in bowel habits and change in defecation patterns after initiating opioid therapy, which is characterized by any of the following: reduced frequency of spontaneous bowel movements (BM), development or worsening of straining to pass BMs, a sense of incomplete rectal evacuation, and harder stool consistency" [20]. One useful and reliable tool in clinical setting for OIC diagnosis is the Bowel Function Index (BFI), a self-reported patient questionnaire, with 3 variables: ease of defecation, feeling of incomplete evacuation, and personal judgment of constipation [21–23].

OIC prevalence is estimated to be as high as 40-64% in CNCP patients on opioid therapy. Moreover, OIC is the most common secondary cause of constipation to which patients do not become tolerant [24]. This prevalence may vary according to the type and dose of opioid prescribed, route of administration, and treatment duration. Morphine seems to be the opioid with the highest associated risk of OIC, while transdermal preparations of Buprenorphine and Fentanyl are associated with lower risk [25]. However, the prevalence may also vary due to differences in clinical supervision on OIC development and prophylactic laxative therapy prescription, as well as variability in patient's perception of their constipation symptoms [19, 26–28].

In clinical practice, it is important to keep a high index of suspicion concerning OIC since many patients do not feel comfortable to discuss this problem with their doctor [29].

According to the literature, the economic impact of OIC among long-term opioid users is significant [30]. Therefore, effective therapies on OIC are needed in order to reduce OIC related costs and improve patient's quality of life [30, 31]. Moreover, CNCP patients have a high prevalence of associated depression, occurring in up to 50% of these patients [32], and depression is also a prevalent condition associated with functional constipation. Because OIC has a similar clinical presentation as functional constipation, it is important for clinicians to be aware of functional constipation prevalence in this specific population when considering opioid therapy prescription. Adequate prophylactic measures and a high index of suspicion may contribute to a higher success on OIC symptoms management [17, 32, 33].

The primary aim of this study was to assess and estimate the incidence of OIC, health related quality of life and disability in CNCP patients followed in Chronic Pain Clinics. Secondary aims include assessment of pain clinical characteristics, analgesic prescription, laxative therapy, and interference in activities of daily living among OIC patients.

2. Methods

2.1. Study Design. A prospective cohort study with 6 months of follow-up was performed in 4 multidisciplinary pain clinics (MPC). This study was conducted in accordance with the Guideline for Good Clinical Practice of the International Conference on Harmonization and the ethical principles of the Declaration of Helsinki. The approvals from the National Committee for Data Protection and from local Ethical Committees were obtained. All patients were informed of the study details and signed an informed consent.

2.2. Patient Selection. Participants were recruited during their first appointment in one of the MPC and were included if they provided consent to participate, were 18 years or older, and presented CNCP ≥ 3 months.

Patients with psychiatric or cognitive disorders that could interfere with data collection, those physically or psychologically unable to communicate, and those unable to speak Portuguese were excluded.

2.3. Data Collection. Data was collected in a face to face interview with a trained interviewer at patient's first consultation in the MPC and through consultation of hospital records. Patient follow-up contacts were made by telephone by trained interviewers at 1 week and 3 and 6 months. During this period, data collection was complemented with consultation and analysis of hospital records.

A structured questionnaire was used to collect the following patients' data: demographic characteristics, clinical and pain characteristics, follow-up, pharmacological treatment prescribed, daily activities pain interference, health related quality of life (HRQOL), and clinical outcomes. The following translated, culturally adapted, and validated instruments for Portuguese population were used: Bowel Function Index (BFI) questionnaire [22, 35]; Brief Pain Inventory [BPI] [36, 37], and Short version of the Treatment Outcomes in Pain Survey (S-TOPS) [38, 39].

The BFI self-report questionnaire consists of three questions about constipation symptoms in the last 7 days: ease of defecation, feeling of incomplete evacuation, and personal judgment of constipation. Each item is scored from 0 to 100 by the patient according to the last 7 days. The BFI score is calculated as the mean of the three items scores [21, 23]. The cut-off definition BFI score for OIC is 28.8 points [34]. In cases were constipation was present at baseline, OIC was considered in patients under opioid therapy that presented a clinically significant change ≥ 12 points in BFI score, according to the criteria defined by Rentz et al. (Rentz,

2009 #2) or an increase in the dosage of previously used laxatives.

The BPI questionnaire is a self-report questionnaire measuring both the intensity of pain (sensory dimension) and interference of pain in the patient's life (reactive dimension). Each item is rated in a scale from 0 to 10. Pain severity and interference scores are calculated by the mean of the answers on each dimension of the questionnaire [35, 37, 40].

The S-TOPS questionnaire was used to assess changes in OIC related quality of life (QOL) from baseline to 6 months. S-TOPS is composed by 7 validated independent subscales with a total of 29 items: (1) Pain Symptom; (2) Physical Disability-Lower Body; (3) Physical Disability-Upper Body; (4) Family/Social Disability; (5) Role Emotional Disability; (6) Patient Satisfaction with Care; and (7) Patient Satisfaction with Outcomes. Each subscale score from S-TOPS is expressed from 0 ("no pain/disability") to 100 ("maximum pain/disability"). The satisfaction with care and satisfaction with outcomes subscales are inverted, with 0 representing "no satisfaction" and 100 representing "maximum satisfaction". The mean of the answers in each subscale was calculated [41].

Pain aetiology classification was conducted according to IASP Taskforce on Pain Classification for ICD-11 [42].

2.4. Outcome Assessment. The primary outcome assessment of our study was OIC incidence at 6 months, as previously defined, and OIC related QOL change from baseline to 6 months concerning physical disability, family and social disability, role emotional disability, and patient satisfaction with outcomes. Secondary outcomes included change from baseline in the following: pain severity and pain interference scales of the BPI, opioid consumption, laxative prescription, and general health status perception.

2.5. Statistical Analysis. We described our population considering OIC prevalence at baseline and pain clinical characterization. The primary analysis was stratified on OIC incidence at 6 months of follow-up. Descriptive statistics of patient characteristics and clinical variables are presented as frequencies with percentages (%), median with interquartile range or mean with standard deviation [43] when appropriate. Nonparametric and parametric tests were performed for comparisons between numerical variables according their distribution and chi-squared test for categorical variables.

A p-value ≤ 0.05 was considered significant for all tests.

Multivariate logistic regression analysis was performed. Univariate predictors of outcome with a p-value <0.10 were selected for multivariate logistic regression analysis with stepwise backward elimination. The dependent variable was OIC and possible predictors were used as independent variables. We have evaluated goodness of fit of the logistic regression model using the Hosmer-Lemeshow test and receiver operating characteristic (ROC) curve to evaluate its predictive and discriminative power.

Statistical analysis was performed using the Statistical Package for the Social Sciences version 24.0 (SPSS, USA).

3. Results

3.1. Prevalence and Incidence of OIC. 694 patients with CNCP diagnosis were recruited. The general characteristics of the cohort are described in Table 1.

OIC prevalence at baseline was 25.8% (n = 174; BFI median 18.9 ± 30.9). At their first consultation, OIC patients were mostly >75 years old (n = 29, 33.0%), female (n = 131, 75.3%), with a low level of education (1-4 years; n = 94, 54.3%), and with a median BMI of 26.3 ± 3.8. 63.2% of OIC patients (n = 110) were prescribed with weak opioids and 36.8% (n = 54) with strong opioids. Most OIC patients were not prescribed with laxative therapy (n = 162; 93.1%) before their first consultation at MPC. At six-month follow-up, OIC was persistent in 51.7% (n = 90) of patients having OIC at baseline and resolved in 48.3% (n = 84) of them. There were no significant differences among these two subgroups except concerning prescription of laxative therapy in persistent OIC patients ($p < 0.001$) (Table 2).

At 6 months, OIC prevalence was 32.0% (n = 216), and OIC incidence was 24.8% (n = 126; BFI mean 18.8 ± 28.5). OIC patients at 6 months were mostly 40-65 years old (n = 60, 35.9%), female (n = 134, 80.2%), with low levels of education (1-4 years; n = 94, 56.3%), and with a median BMI of 26.9 ± 5.1. There was a significant association among OIC development and opioid prescription (p = 0.034), but there were no significant differences among strong and weak opioids prescriptions in these patients. Patients with OIC had a higher prescription rate of laxative therapy ($p < 0.001$).

Although other adverse drug reactions [44] associated with opioids were not our primary focus, we obtained data regarding other ADR, at 6 months, for 145 patients. Among those, the most frequently reported ADRs associated with opioids, besides OIC, were nausea and vomiting (27%), rash (11%), somnolence/sleepiness (10%), dizziness (10%), and pruritus (9%).

3.2. Clinical Characteristics, Severity, and Interference of Pain in OIC Patients. Pain characteristics are described in Table 4.

Compared to non-OIC patients, OIC patients had longer pain duration and presented more often pain at cervical region, lumbar region, upper limbs, and lower limbs, both at baseline and at 6 months of follow-up. More frequent pain aetiologies were chronic musculoskeletal pain and chronic neuropathic pain. However, these were not statistically different from non-OIC patients except for pain location at cervical region (baseline and 6 months) and upper limb (baseline). There were no significant differences in pain severity and interference scores at baseline among OIC and non-OIC patients (Figure 1). However, at baseline OIC patients reported statistically significant higher interference pain scores in general activity, mood, walking ability, normal work, relations with other people, sleep, and enjoyment of life ($p < 0.05$).

At 6-month follow-up, OIC patients presented significant higher pain severity scores (5.5 P25-P75 4.0-7.0 versus 5.0 P25-P75 3.2-6.5, p = 0.021) and higher pain interference scores (5.9 P25-P75 4.0-7.3 versus 4.9 P25-P75 2.1-7.0, $p < 0.001$) in all domains (Figure 2).

TABLE 1: General characteristics of CNCP patients at baseline.

Variable		No Constipation	Constipation
Total	674 (100%)	500 (74.2%)	174 (25.8%)
Age, years			
18-45	151	110 (22.0%)	41 (23.6%)
45-60	214	162 (32.4%)	52 (29.9%)
60-75	221	169 (33.8%)	52 (29.9%)
>75	88	59 (11.8%)	29 (16.7%)
Gender			
Female	488	357 (71.4%)	131 (75.3%)
Male	186	143 (28.6%)	43 (24.7%)
BMI	27.0 (±5.20)	27.1 (±5.20)	26.5 (±5.20)
Education level			
No education	19	12 (2.4%)	7 (4.0%)
1-4 years (basic 1st cycle)	340	246 (49.2%)	94 (54.3%)
5-9 years (basic 2nd and 3rd cycles)	163	127 (25.4%)	36 (20.8%)
10-12 years (secondary)	78	60 (12.0%)	18 (10.4%)
More than 12 years(higher)	73	55 (11.0%)	18 (10.4%)
Opioid therapy	402	228 (56.7%)	174 (43.2%)
Analgesic prescription			
Non-opioid	213	163 (32.6%)	50 (28.7%)
Weak opioid	339	229 (45.8%)	110 (63.2%)
Strong opioid	126	62 (12.4%)	64 (36.8%)
Laxatives use	24	12 (15.8%)	12 (30.8%)
Current depressive disorder on treatment	139	97 (20.8%)	42 (25.8%)

OIC: opioid-induced constipation; BMI: body mass index; data are presented as n (%) except BMI which is presented as mean ± standard deviation. Proportions are calculated as column proportions.

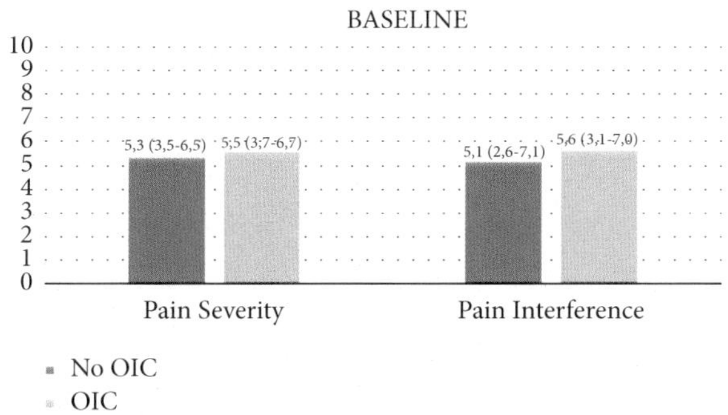

FIGURE 1: Brief Pain Inventory questionnaire at baseline. Data are presented as median (interquartile range). P values are derived from T test (pain severity) and Mann-Whitney U test (pain interference),

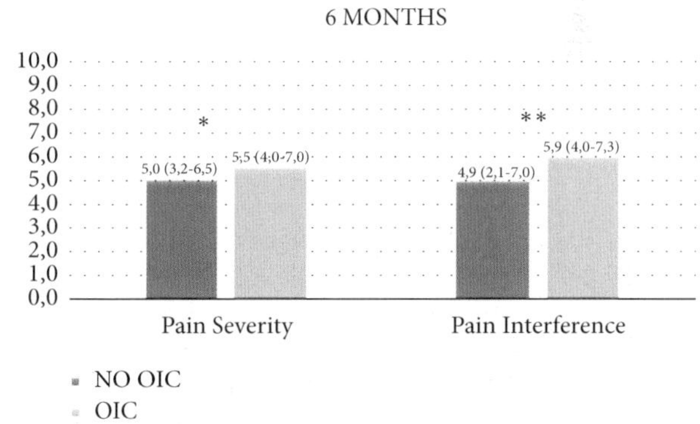

FIGURE 2: Brief Pain Inventory at 6 months. Data are presented as median (interquartile range). P values are derived from T test (Pain severity) and Mann-Whitney U test (Pain interference). $^{*}p < 0.05$, $^{**}p < 0.001$.

3.3. Outcomes Assessment of OIC and Related Quality of Life (QoL). At baseline, OIC patients reported significantly higher disability in physical lower function (59.8 ± 30.9 versus 53.9 ± 32.5, $p = 0.028$), physical upper function (34.0 ± 24.0 versus 26.7 ± 21.5, $p < 0.001$), and family/social disability (41.6 ± 24.9 versus 35.5 ± 24.7, $p < 0.001$) (Figure 3), and 32.9% ($n = 222$) considered that their health was poor.

At 6 months, OIC patients reported significantly higher disability in all subscales of S-TOPS questionnaire except physical upper function: pain severity (62.3 ± 20.9 versus 55.8 ± 25.2, $p = 0.011$), physical lower function (57.5 ± 31.1 versus 52.8 ± 33.7, $p = 0.026$), family/social disability (36.2 ± 27.5 versus 28.8 ± 26.8, $p = 0.005$), and role emotional disability (45.4 ± 34.5 versus 53.9 ± 32.5, $p = 0.028$). OIC patients reported significantly less satisfaction with outcomes than non-OIC patients (54.5 ± 22.0 versus 56.0 ± 26.1, $p = 0.038$) (Figure 4). At 6 months of follow-up, 38.0% ($n = 256$) of OIC patients considered that their health was poor.

Table 2: Follow-up at 6 months of patients with OIC at baseline.

6 Months Follow-up of OIC patients at baseline			
Variable	Previous OIC (OIC absent at 6 months)	Current OIC (OIC still present at 6 months)	*P* value
Total	84 (48.3%)	90 (51.7%)	
Age, years			0.349[a]
18-45	23 (27.4%)	18 (20.0%)	
45-60	27 (32.1%)	25 (27.8%)	
60-75	20 (16.7%)	32 (35.6%)	
>75	14 (48.3%)	15 (16.7%)	
Gender			
Female	60 (71.4%)	71 (78.9%)	0.293[a]
Male	24 (28.6%)	19 (21.1%)	
BMI	27.15	26.49	0.178[b]
Mean [34];	(±5.20)	(±5.20)	
Education level			**0.047**[a]
No education	4 (4.8%)	3 (3.3%)	
1-4 years (basic 1st cycle)	40 (48.2%)	54 (60.0%)	
5-9 years (basic 2nd and 3rd cycles)	15 (18.1%)	21 (23.3%)	
10-12 years (secondary)	12 (14.5%)	6 (6.7%)	
More than 12 years(higher)	12 (14.5%)	6 (6.7%)	
Opioid therapy			0.409[a]
Weak opioid	43 (51.2%)	50 (55.6%)	
Strong opioid	41 (48.8%)	40 (44.4%)	
Laxatives use	0 (0%)	19 (100%)	**<0.001**[a]
Current depressive disorder on treatment	20 (24.4%)	14 (27.2%)	0.686

OIC: opioid-induced constipation; BMI: body mass index. Data are presented as *n* (%) except BMI which is presented as mean ± standard deviation. Proportions are calculated as column proportions. *P* values are derived from (a) x2 comparisons; (b) *T* test.

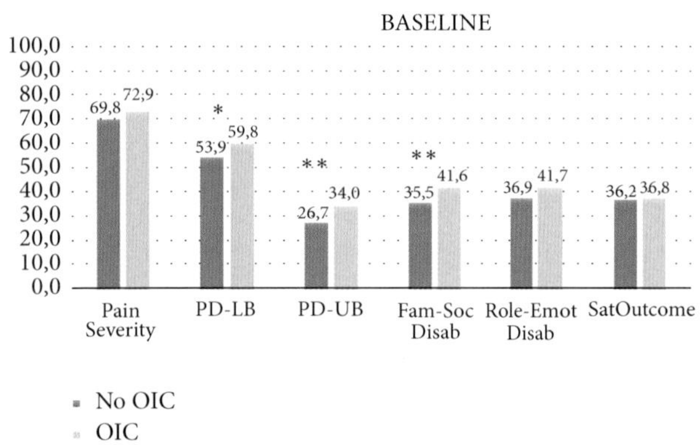

Figure 3: Short-Treatment Outcomes in Pain Survey (S-TOPS) questionnaire at baseline. OIC: opioid-induced constipation; PD-LB: physical Disability lower body; PD-LB: physical disability upper body; FAM-SOC DISAB: family and social disability; ROLE-EMOT DISAB: role emotional disability; SATOUTCOME: satisfaction with outcomes. Data are presented as median of each subscale. *P* values are derived from Mann-Whitney U test comparisons. $^{*}p < 0.05$, $^{**}p < 0,001$.

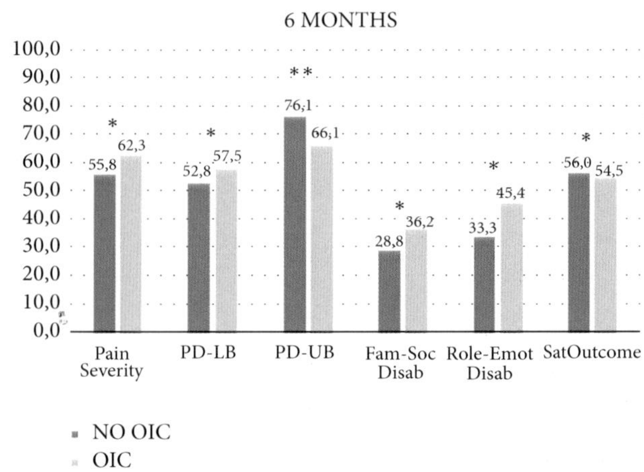

Figure 4: Short-Treatment Outcomes in Pain Survey (S-TOPS) questionnaire at 6 months. OIC: opioid-induced constipation; PD-LB: physical disability lower body; PD-LB: physical disability upper body; FAM-SOC DISAB: family social disability; ROLE-EMOT DISAB: role emotional disability; SATOUTCOME: satisfaction with outcomes. Data are presented as median of each subscale. *P* values are derived from Mann-Whitney U test comparisons. $^{*}p < 0.05$, $^{**}p < 0.001$.

TABLE 3: OIC incidence at 6 months.

	OIC Incidence at 6 months of follow-up		
Variable	**No Constipation**	**Constipation**	*P* value
Age, years			0.171[a]
18-45	123 (24.3%)	28 (16.8%)	
45-60	154 (30.4%)	60 (35.9%)	
60-75	167 (32.9%)	54 (32.3%)	
>75	63 (12.4%)	25 (15.0%)	
Gender			
Female	354 (69.8%)	134 (80.2%)	**0.009**[a]
Male	153 (30.2%)	33 (19.8%)	
BMI	27.33 (5.50)	26.87 (5.10)	0.357[b]
Education level			0.562[a]
No education	15 (3.0%)	4 (2.4%)	
1-4 years (basic 1st cycle)	246 (48.6%)	94 (56.3%)	
5-9 years (basic 2nd and 3rd cycles)	127 (25.1%)	36 (21.6%)	
10-12 years (secondary)	61 (12.1%)	17 (10.2%)	
More than 12 years (higher)	57 (11.3%)	16 (9.6%)	
Opioid therapy			**0.034**[a]
Yes	338 (72.8%)	126 (75.4%)	
No	169 (80.5%)	41 (24.6%)	
Analgesic Therapy			0.087[a]
Non-opioid	168 (80.4%)	41 (24.6%)	
Weak opioid	233 (71.9%)	91 (54.5%)	
Strong opioid	104 (74.8%)	35 (21.0%)	
Laxatives use	2 (100%)	51 (100%)	**<0.001**[a]
Depressive disorder	102 (21.4%)	37 (24.0%)	0.504[a]

OIC: opioid-induced constipation; BMI: body mass index. Data are presented as n (%) except BMI which is presented as mean ± standard deviation. Proportions are calculated as column proportions. *P* values are derived from (a) x2; (b) *T* test comparisons.

3.4. Predictors of OIC at 6 Months. Tables 3 and 4 and Figure 2 present factors associated with OIC incidence development at 6 months. Gender ($p = 0.009$), opioid use ($p = 0.034$), BPI severity score ($p = 0.021$), and BPI interference score ($p < 0.001$) are significantly associated with OIC. Taking into account the available literature [28, 40, 41], we decided to include depressive disorders diagnosis in our multivariate regression analysis model.

Table 5 describes independent predictors of OIC at 6 months identified in a multivariate logistic regression analysis with stepwise backward elimination. In our multivariate model, opioid therapy (OR 1.65, $p = 0.026$), female gender (OR 1.65, $p = 0.039$), and higher interference pain score (OR 1.10, $p = 0.009$) are independent predictors of higher risk of OIC at 6 months. Our model had a good predictive power (Hosmer and Lemeshow test: $p = 0.107$) and a moderate discriminative power (AUC 0,678, $p < 0.001$).

4. Discussion

Opioid-induced constipation is a prevalent and debilitating condition with a significantly high impact in patient's quality of life and well-being. OIC has an estimated prevalence of 15-90 % in chronic noncancer pain patients. Our estimated prevalence of 25.8% at baseline and 32.0% at 6-month follow-up is in accordance with previous data [19, 27]. Indeed, in the last decades there has been an increment of opioid prescription for chronic noncancer pain management that may explain high OIC prevalence among this specific population [6, 15, 45]. Long-term exposure, high opioid doses and absence of laxative therapy are some of the conditions associated with OIC development [17, 27].

Chronic noncancer pain is more prevalent in female gender and with increasing age [6]. Therefore, a similar demographic data in the OIC population was expected [46, 47].

In our study, at 6 months OIC patients reported higher pain severity score ($p = 0.021$) and higher pain interference score ($p < 0.001$). These results are in accordance with the statistically significant association with opioid prescription in these patients ($p = 0.034$). Indeed, it is expected that patients with more severe pain are more often prescribed with opioids and for longer periods, and, therefore, present a higher risk of OIC development. Several studies have reported the association of OIC with the burden of opioid prescription in CNCP in the last decades [1, 48, 49].

OIC is the most prevalent adverse effect associated with opioid use and has severe impact on patient's quality of life

Table 4: Pain characteristics.

Pain Characteristics		Baseline				6 Months		
		Total	**No constipation**	**Constipation**	**P value**	**No Constipation**	**Constipation**	**P value**
Pain duration	Pain duration in years	4.0 (2.0-12.0)	4.0 (2.0-13.0)	5.0 (2.0-10.5)	0.207[c]	4.0 (2.0-12.0)	4.7 (2.0-14.0)	0.782[b]
Pain location	Head	67 (65.0%)	67 (65.0%)	36 (35.0%)	**0.021**[a]	69 (67.0%)	34 (33.0%)	0.931[a]
	Face	26 (61.9%)	26 (61.9%)	16 (38.1%)	0.060[a]	28 (66.7%)	14 (33.3%)	0.921[a]
	Cervical region	172 (68.5%)	172 (68.5%)	79 (31.5%)	**0.010**[a]	156 (62.2%)	95 (37.8%)	**0.028**[a]
	Dorsal region	41 (64.1%)	41 (64.1%)	23 (35.9%)	0.052[a]	46 (71.9%)	18 (28.1%)	0.485[a]
	Lumbar region	292 (73.7%)	292 (73.7%)	104 (26.3%)	0.324[a]	265 (66.9%)	131 (33.1%)	0.803[a]
	Abdominal region	21 (73.8%)	21 (73.8%)	11 (26.2%)	0.954[a]	28 (66.7%)	14 (33.3%)	0.921[a]
	Upper Limb	240 (70.4%)	240 (70.4%)	101 (29.6%)	**0.022**[a]	226 (66.3%)	115 (31.5%)	0.566[a]
	Lower Limb	314 (72.5%)	314 (72.5%)	119 (27.5%)	0.185[a]	294 (67.9%)	139 (33.6%)	0.732[a]
Pain aetiology	Chronic primary pain	50 (7.4%)	32 (64.0%)	18 (36.0%)	0.087[a]	18 (43.9%)	23 (56.1%)	**0.008**[a]
	Chronic postsurgical and posttraumatic pain	92 (13.6%)	66 (71,7%)	26 (28.3%)	0.564[a]	47 (62.7%)	28 (37.3%)	0.813[a]
	Chronic neuropathic pain	170 (25.2%)	128 (75.3%)	42 (24.7%)	0.702[a]	99 (67.8%)	47 (32.2%)	0.926[a]
	Chronic headache and orofacial pain	15 (2.2%)	6 (40.0%)	9 (60.0%)	**0.002**[a]	7 (58.3%)	5 (41.7%)	0.581[a]
	Chronic visceral pain	26 (3.9%)	15 (57.7%)	11 (42.3%)	0.050[a]	14 (63.6%)	8 (36.4%)	0.833[a]
	Chronic musculoskeletal pain	254 (37.7%)	183 (72%)	71 (28.0%)	0.324[a]	249 (69.9%)	107 (30.1%)	0.310[a]

Data are presented as *n* (%) except pain duration which is presented as median (interquartile range). Proportions are calculated as row proportions. *P* values are derived from (a) x^2 comparisons; (b) *T* test; (c) Mann-Whitney *U* test.

and ability to perform daily life activities and work [27, 50]. OIC results from opioid action on mu-opioid receptors in the gastrointestinal tract that induces delayed gastric emptying, decreased bowel movements, increased intestinal fluids absorption, and increased anal sphincter tone [17]. However, opioids may present different effects depending on their location in the gastrointestinal tract. For instance, there is tolerance development for mu-opioid receptor actions for all gastrointestinal tract except for colon [51]. Therefore, while other gastrointestinal disorders tend to disappear in long-term opioid exposure, constipation is a persistent and debilitating side effect that must be appropriately treated [51, 52]. Moreover, OIC is such a distressing adverse event that, as a consequence, some patients prefer to reduce or discontinue their opioid therapy and be in pain rather than experiencing severe constipation.

OIC symptoms management is challenging and often with unsatisfactory response to the available therapeutics. OIC treatment encompasses either nonpharmacological approaches (dietary fibre, fluid intake, and physical activity) or nonspecific pharmacological approaches with laxatives use (stimulants, softeners, bulk forming, and enemas) and prokinetics. However, even with these therapeutic measures many patients do not have significant OIC symptoms relief. LoCasale et al. reported in a prospective longitudinal study of 489 OIC noncancer pain patients, a high rate (48%) of inadequate OIC relief despite adequate laxative therapy prescribed [24]. Nowadays, new specific pharmacological treatments with formulations containing peripherally acting opioid antagonists such as methylnaltrexone bromide and oxycodone/naloxone are available and may allow more efficacy in OIC management without analgesia impairment [26, 27, 53, 54]. However, in spite of the available recommendations, early prescription of prophylactic measures such as dietary fibre, fluid intake, physical activity, and laxative use are not routine when starting an opioid prescription [24, 27, 53]. In our study, the prescription rate of laxative therapy at baseline was only of 6.9% ($n = 12$) in spite of a prevalence of opioid use of 59.6% ($n = 402$) and an OIC prevalence of 25.8% ($n = 174$). At 6 months of follow-up, our prescription rate of laxative therapy in patients with persistent OIC was still low ($n = 19$, 16.7%). These results may reflect the lack of awareness of healthcare professionals about the real impact of OIC on patient's quality of life and well-being. More efforts should be made to promote physician's education on OIC and increase safe and responsible opioid use.

At six-month follow-up, OIC patients reported significantly higher disability in all subscales of S-TOPS questionnaire except physical upper function, which is consistent with previous studies [20, 27]. Indeed, OIC has a severe and

TABLE 5: Predictors of OIC at 6 months.

	Crude OR (95%CI)	Adjusted OR (95%CI)
Gender	**p = 0.010**	**p = 0.039**
Female	1.76 (1.15-2.69)	1.65 (1.03-2.67)
Male	1	1
Current depressive disorders	*P* = 0.50	-
	1.16 (0.76-1.78)	
Opioid therapy	**p = 0.036**	**p = 0.026**
Yes	1.53 (1.03-2.28)	1.65 (1.06-2.56)
No	1	1
Severity Scale	*P* = 0.058	-
	1.06 (1.00-1.13)	
Interference Scale	**p = 0.001**	**p = 0.009**
	1.13 (1.06-1.21)	1.10 (1.02-1.19)

95% CI, 95% confidence interval; OR, odds ratio. Predictors of opioid induced constipation defined by simple and multiple logistic regression; crude and adjusted ORs for categories of demographic variables, opioid therapy, and pain characteristics variables. Adjusted ORs were calculated using multivariate logistic regression models. Multivariate model included adjustment all variables with crude association measures with P values < 0.1 in the univariate analysis. P values for the omnibus tests evaluating the significance of each predictor variable.

debilitating repercussion in the patients' quality of life and impairs their ability to perform daily life activities. In our sample, OIC patients reported significantly less satisfaction with outcomes than non-OIC patients ($p = 0.034$). LoCasale et al. reported in another prospective observational study of six-month follow-up that OIC patients despite adequate laxative therapy prescription presented persistent constipation and a small improvement in their quality of life and ability to perform daily life activities [55]. This may lead patients to reduce their opioid analgesic doses or even to opioid withdrawal, which can compromise their CNCP management. Another additional problem is related to patients' long-term exposure to opioid therapy and, therefore, to persistent OIC symptoms and associated morbidity with significant economic and societal costs [30, 31, 50, 56].

We have identified as independent predictors of incident OIC at six-month follow-up, female gender, higher interference pain score on BPI, and opioid therapy. The latter finding was expected since opioid therapy is the major risk factor for constipation development in CNCP patients. Moreover, this risk increases with higher doses and longer exposure times and varies with the type of opioid prescribed and route of administration [19, 25, 27]. On the other hand, patients with higher interference pain scores are those at increased risk of being prescribed with opioids and in higher doses in order to control their pain. Therefore, it was also expected that patients with higher severity pain scores were also associated with higher risk of OIC development at 6 months. However, we have not found this association, which may be explained by a more significant difference of interference than severity pain scores among OIC and non-OIC patients. Taking into account the higher prevalence of CNCP in female gender and with increasing age, it is reasonable to expect that OIC also presents a similar demographic characterization [25, 46]. To the best of our knowledge, there has been only one publication concerning OIC predictors' identification in a sample of 2324 Italian patients on chronic pain treatment [57]. According to the results of this study, opioid use, female gender, and increasing age are risk factors for OIC development. In cancer pain patients the risk of OIC development seems to be higher when higher opioid doses are needed.

Our study has several strengths. It was an observational prospective study with 6-month follow-up period regarding OIC incidence, its predictive factors, functional outcomes, and quality of life assessment based in the seven subscales of the S-TOPS questionnaire following IMMPACT recommendations [58]. We provided a detailed assessment based on standardized and validated questionnaires. We believe that our cohort is representative of the CNCP population taking into account the fact that we included data from 4 different MPC. This study also presents some limitations. As a prospective observational study, it may present selection bias from losses of follow-up. To overcome this, we have developed retention strategies since eligible patients have consented and those who have continued for all duration of the study in order to reduce our follow-up losses.

5. Conclusions

Opioid use is associated with the potential risk of adverse effects development. OIC is the most prevalent side effect and may negatively impact patients' adherence to their analgesic prescription. It is important to promote clinician's awareness on OIC since it is still a grossly underrecognized and undertreated condition. A high index of suspicion in high risk populations such as CNCP patients, utilization of adequate diagnostic tools, and routine implementation of prophylactic therapies such as laxatives prescription are key measures to improve OIC management and reduce its associated disability and costs.

Abbreviations

BFI:	Bowel Function Index
BPI:	Brief Pain Inventory
CNCP:	Chronic noncancer pain
CI:	Confidence interval
IASP:	International Association for the Study of Pain
ICD:	International Classification of Diseases
IMMPACT:	Initiative on Methods, Measurement, and Pain Assessment in Clinical Trials
MCPC:	Multidisciplinary Chronic Pain Clinics
OIC:	Opioid-induced constipation
P25:	25th percentile
P75:	75th percentile

SD: Standard deviation
S-TOPS: Shortened Treatment Outcomes in Pain Survey.

Disclosure

This manuscript has been presented as a poster at Meeting with Science and Technology in Portugal-Lisbon 2017.

Acknowledgments

This work was supported by intramural funds from the Chair on Pain Medicine of the Faculty of Medicine, University of Porto, and by projects "Porto Neurosciences and Neurologic Disease Research Initiative at i3S" (NORTE-01-0145-FEDER-000008) and "NanoSTIMA" (NORTE-01-0145-FEDER-000016), which are financed by the North Portugal Regional Operational Programme (NORTE 2020), under the Portugal 2020 Partnership Agreement, and through the European Regional Development Fund (ERDF).

References

[1] D. S. Goldberg and S. J. McGee, "Pain as a global public health priority," *BMC Public Health*, vol. 11, no. 1, article 770, 2011.

[2] H. Breivik, E. Eisenberg, and T. O'Brien, "The individual and societal burden of chronic pain in Europe: the case for strategic prioritisation and action to improve knowledge and availability of appropriate care," *BMC Public Health*, vol. 13, no. 1, article 1229, 2013.

[3] L. F. Azevedo, A. Costa-Pereira, L. Mendonça, C. C. Dias, and J. M. Castro-Lopes, "The economic impact of chronic pain: a nationwide population-based cost-of-illness study in Portugal," *European Journal of Health Economics*, vol. 17, no. 1, pp. 87–98, 2016.

[4] L. F. Azevedo, A. Costa-Pereira, L. Mendonça, C. C. Dias, and J. M. Castro-Lopes, "Chronic pain and health services utilization: Is there overuse of diagnostic tests and inequalities in nonpharmacologic treatment methods utilization?" *Medical Care*, vol. 51, no. 10, pp. 859–869, 2013.

[5] C. R. Chapman, D. L. Lipschitz, M. S. Angst et al., "Opioid pharmacotherapy for chronic non-cancer pain in the United States: A research guideline for developing an evidence-base," *The Journal of Pain*, vol. 11, no. 9, pp. 807–829, 2010.

[6] T. O'Brien, L. L. Christrup, A. M. Drewes et al., "European Pain Federation position paper on appropriate opioid use in chronic pain management," *European Journal of Pain*, vol. 21, no. 1, pp. 3–19, 2017.

[7] R. Chou, G. J. Fanciullo, P. G. Fine et al., "Clinical guidelines for the use of chronic opioid therapy in chronic noncancer pain," *The Journal of Pain*, vol. 10, no. 2, pp. 113.e22–130.e22, 2009.

[8] CDC guidelines for Prescribing Opioids for Chronic Pain—United States, 2016.

[9] J. van Amsterdam and W. van den Brink, "The misuse of prescription opioids: A threat for Europe?" *Current Drug Abuse Reviews*, vol. 8, no. 1, pp. 3–14, 2015.

[10] W. Häuser, S. Schug, and A. D. Furlan, "The opioid epidemic and national guidelines for opioid therapy for chronic noncancer pain," *PAIN Reports*, vol. 2, no. 3, p. e599, 2017.

[11] E. J. Pezalla, D. Rosen, J. G. Erensen, J. D. Haddox, and T. J. Mayne, "Secular trends in opioid prescribing in the USA," *Journal of Pain Research*, vol. 10, pp. 383–387, 2017.

[12] M. Noble, S. J. Tregear, J. R. Treadwell, and K. Schoelles, "Long-Term Opioid Therapy for Chronic Noncancer Pain: A Systematic Review and Meta-Analysis of Efficacy and Safety," *Journal of Pain and Symptom Management*, vol. 35, no. 2, pp. 214–228, 2008.

[13] S. Raghavan, A. D. Harvey, and S. R. Humble, "New opioid side effects and implications for long-term therapy," *Trends in Anaesthesia and Critical Care*, vol. 1, no. 1, pp. 18–21, 2011.

[14] R. Duarte and J. Raphael, "The pros and cons of long-term Opioid therapy," *Journal of Pain and Palliative Care Pharmacotherapy*, vol. 28, no. 3, pp. 308–310, 2014.

[15] H. Blake, P. Leighton, G. van der Walt, and A. Ravenscroft, "Prescribing opioid analgesics for chronic non-malignant pain in general practice—a survey of attitudes and practice," *British Journal of Pain*, vol. 9, no. 4, pp. 225–232, 2015.

[16] J. C. Ballantyne, "Opioid Therapy in Chronic Pain," *Physical Medicine and Rehabilitation Clinics of North America*, vol. 26, no. 2, pp. 201–218, 2015.

[17] A. D. Nelson and M. Camilleri, "Opioid-induced constipation: advances and clinical guidance," *Therapeutic Advances in Chronic Disease*, vol. 7, no. 2, pp. 121–134, 2016.

[18] C. Hsieh, "Treatment of constipation in older adults," *American Family Physician*, vol. 72, no. 11, pp. 2277–2284, 2005.

[19] S. J. Panchal, P. Müller-Schwefe, and J. I. Wurzelmann, "Opioid-induced bowel dysfunction: prevalence, pathophysiology and burden," *International Journal of Clinical Practice*, vol. 61, no. 7, pp. 1181–1187, 2007.

[20] J. Gaertner, W. Siemens, M. Camilleri et al., "Definitions and outcome measures of clinical trials regarding opioid-induced constipation: A systematic review," *Journal of Clinical Gastroenterology*, vol. 49, no. 1, pp. 9–16, 2015.

[21] L. Abramowitz, N. Béziaud, C. Caussé, B. Chuberre, F. A. Allaert, and S. Perrot, "Further validation of the psychometric properties of the Bowel Function Index for evaluating opioid-induced constipation (OIC)," *Journal of Medical Economics*, vol. 16, no. 12, pp. 1434–1441, 2013.

[22] M. Dueñas, L. Mendonça, R. Sampaio et al., "Reliability and validity of the Bowel Function Index for evaluating opioid-induced constipation: translation, cultural adaptation and validation of the Portuguese version (BFI-P)," *Current Medical Research and Opinion*, vol. 33, no. 3, pp. 563–572, 2017.

[23] M. A. Ueberall, S. Müller-Lissner, C. Buschmann-Kramm, and B. Bosse, "The bowel function index for evaluating constipation in pain patients: Definition of a reference range for a non- constipated population of pain patients," *Journal of International Medical Research*, vol. 39, no. 1, pp. 41–50, 2011.

[24] R. J. LoCasale, C. Datto, M. K. Margolis, and K. S. Coyne, "Satisfaction with Therapy Among Patients with Chronic Noncancer Pain with Opioid-Induced Constipation," *Journal of managed care & specialty pharmacy*, vol. 22, no. 3, pp. 246–253, 2016.

[25] S. Müller-Lissner, G. Bassotti, B. Coffin et al., "Opioid-induced constipation and bowel dysfunction: A clinical guideline," *Pain Medicine*, vol. 18, no. 10, pp. 1837–1863, 2017.

[26] W. Siemens, J. Gaertner, and G. Becker, "Advances in pharmacotherapy for opioid-induced constipation - A systematic

review," *Expert Opinion on Pharmacotherapy*, vol. 16, no. 4, pp. 515–532, 2015.

[27] L. Kumar, C. Barker, and A. Emmanuel, "Opioid-Induced Constipation: Pathophysiology, Clinical Consequences, and Management," *Gastroenterology Research and Practice*, vol. 2014, Article ID 141737, 6 pages, 2014.

[28] H. Y. Chang and A. J. Lembo, "Opioid-induced bowel dysfunction," *Current Treatment Options in Gastroenterology*, vol. 11, no. 1, pp. 11–18, 2008.

[29] R. J. LoCasale, C. Datto, H. Wilson, K. Yeomans, and K. S. Coyne, "The Burden of Opioid-Induced Constipation: Discordance Between Patient and Health Care Provider Reports," *Journal of managed care & specialty pharmacy*, vol. 22, no. 3, pp. 236–245, 2016.

[30] B. Alemayehu, K. Coyne, and F. King, "Self Reported Health Care Resource Use and Indirect Economic Burden of Opioid Induced Constipation (Oic)," *Value in Health*, vol. 17, no. 7, p. A541, 2014.

[31] Y. Wan, S. Corman, X. Gao, S. Liu, H. Patel, and R. Mody, "Economic burden of opioid-induced constipation among long-term Opioid users with non cancer pain," *American Health and Drug Benefits*, vol. 8, no. 2, pp. 93–101, 2015.

[32] R. L. Barkin, S. J. Barkin, G. A. Irving, and A. Gordon, "Management of chronic noncancer pain in depressed patients," *Postgraduate Medical Journal*, vol. 123, no. 5, pp. 143–154, 2011.

[33] S. T. Hosseinzadeh, S. Poorsaadati, B. Radkani, and M. Forootan, "Psychological disorders in patients with chronic constipation," *Gastroenterology and Hepatology from Bed to Bench*, vol. 4, no. 3, pp. 159–163, 2011.

[34] S. H. Ahmedzai, F. Nauck, G. Bar-Sela, B. Bosse, P. Leyendecker, and M. Hopp, "A randomized, double-blind, active-controlled, double-dummy, parallel-group study to determine the safety and efficacy of oxycodone/naloxone prolonged-release tablets in patients with moderate/severe, chronic cancer pain," *Palliative Medicine*, vol. 26, no. 1, pp. 50–60, 2012.

[35] L. F. Azevedo, A. C. Pereira, C. Dias, and J. Romão, "Translation, cultural adaptation and multicentric validation study of chronic pain screening and impact assessment instruments," *DOR*, pp. 6–56, 2007.

[36] L. Furler, "Validity and reliability of the pain questionnaire "Brief Pain Inventory". A literature research," *Pflegezeitschrift*, vol. 66, no. 9, pp. 546–550, 2013.

[37] S. Keller, C. M. Bann, S. L. Dodd, J. Schein, T. R. Mendoza, and C. S. Cleeland, "Validity of the brief pain inventory for use in documenting the outcomes of patients with noncancer pain," *The Clinical Journal of Pain*, vol. 20, no. 5, pp. 309–318, 2004.

[38] R. H. Dworkin, D. C. Turk, J. T. Farrar et al., "Core outcome measures for chronic pain clinical trials: IMMPACT recommendations," *PAIN*, vol. 113, no. 1-2, pp. 9–19, 2005.

[39] S. M. Mulla, A. Maqbool, L. Sivananthan et al., "Reporting of IMMPACT-recommended core outcome domains among trials assessing opioids for chronic non-cancer pain," *PAIN*, vol. 156, no. 9, pp. 1615–1619, 2015.

[40] G. Tan, M. P. Jensen, J. I. Thornby, and B. F. Shanti, "Validation of the brief pain inventory for chronic nonmalignant pain," *The Journal of Pain*, vol. 5, no. 2, pp. 133–137, 2004.

[41] S. Haroutiunian, G. Donaldson, J. Yu, and A. G. Lipman, "Development and validation of shortened, restructured Treatment Outcomes in Pain Survey instrument (the S-TOPS) for assessment of individual pain patients' health-related quality of life," *PAIN*, vol. 153, no. 8, pp. 1593–1601, 2012.

[42] R.-D. Treede, W. Rief, A. Barke et al., "A classification of chronic pain for ICD-11," *PAIN*, vol. 156, no. 6, pp. 1003–1007, 2015.

[43] M. Ortiz-Catalan, R. A. Guðmundsdóttir, M. B. Kristoffersen et al., "Phantom motor execution facilitated by machine learning and augmented reality as treatment for phantom limb pain: a single group, clinical trial in patients with chronic intractable phantom limb pain," *The Lancet*, vol. 388, no. 10062, pp. 2885–2894, 2016.

[44] J. P. Headrick, S. Pepe, and J. N. Peart, "Non-analgesic effects of opioids: Cardiovascular effects of opioids and their receptor systems," *Current Pharmaceutical Design*, vol. 18, no. 37, pp. 6090–6100, 2012.

[45] J. C. Ballantyne, "Opioid controls: Regulate to educate," *Pain Medicine*, vol. 11, no. 4, pp. 480-481, 2010.

[46] C. I. Campbell, C. Weisner, L. LeResche et al., "Age and gender trends in long-term opioid analgesic use for noncancer pain," *American Journal of Public Health*, vol. 100, no. 12, pp. 2541–2547, 2010.

[47] Y. S. Almakadma and K. Simpson, "Opioid therapy in non-cancer chronic pain patients: Trends and efficacy in different types of pain, patients age and gender," *Saudi Journal of Anaesthesia*, vol. 7, no. 3, pp. 291–295, 2013.

[48] D. Boudreau, M. Von Korff, C. M. Rutter et al., "Trends in long-term opioid therapy for chronic non-cancer pain," *Pharmacoepidemiology and Drug Safety*, vol. 18, no. 12, pp. 1166–1175, 2009.

[49] R. Foy, B. Leaman, C. McCrorie et al., "Prescribed opioids in primary care: Cross-sectional and longitudinal analyses of influence of patient and practice characteristics," *BMJ Open*, vol. 6, no. 5, Article ID e010276, 2016.

[50] K. S. Coyne, M. K. Margolis, K. Yeomans et al., "Opioid-Induced Constipation Among Patients with Chronic Noncancer Pain in the United States, Canada, Germany, and the United Kingdom: Laxative Use, Response, and Symptom Burden Over Time," *Pain Medicine*, vol. 16, no. 8, pp. 1551–1565, 2015.

[51] H. I. Akbarali, A. Inkisar, and W. L. Dewey, "Site and mechanism of morphine tolerance in the gastrointestinal tract," *Neurogastroenterology & Motility*, vol. 26, no. 10, pp. 1361–1367, 2014.

[52] G. W. Pasternak, "Molecular biology of opioid analgesia," *Journal of Pain and Symptom Management*, vol. 29, no. 5, pp. S2–S9, 2005.

[53] P. Holzer, "New approaches to the treatment of opioid-induced constipation," *European Review for Medical and Pharmacological Sciences*, pp. 119–127, 2008.

[54] F. M. Reichle and P. F. Conzen, "Methylnaltrexone, a new peripheral μ-receptor antagonist for the prevention and treatment of opioid-induced extracerebral side effects," *Current Opinion in Infectious Diseases*, vol. 9, no. 1, pp. 90–100, 2008.

[55] R. J. Locasale, C. J. Datto, M. K. Margolis, J. Tack, and K. S. Coyne, "The impact of opioid-induced constipation among chronic pain patients with sufficient laxative use," *International Journal of Clinical Practice*, vol. 69, no. 12, pp. 1448–1456, 2015.

[56] S. M. Holliday, C. Hayes, A. J. Dunlop et al., "Does brief chronic pain management education change opioid prescribing rates? A pragmatic trial in Australian early-career general practitioners," *PAIN*, vol. 158, no. 2, pp. 278–288, 2017.

[57] G. Rosti, A. Gatti, A. Costantini, A. F. Sabato, and F. Zucco, "Opioid-related bowel dysfunction: Prevalence and identification of predictive factors in a large sample of Italian patients on chronic treatment," *European Review for Medical and Pharmacological Sciences*, vol. 14, no. 12, pp. 1045–1050, 2010.

13

Factors Associated with Opioid use in a Cohort of Patients Presenting for Surgery

Jennifer M. Hah,[1] Yasamin Sharifzadeh,[2] Bing M. Wang,[2] Matthew J. Gillespie,[2] Stuart B. Goodman,[3] Sean C. Mackey,[1] and Ian R. Carroll[1]

[1] *Division of Pain Medicine, Department of Anesthesiology, Perioperative, and Pain Medicine, Stanford University, Palo Alto, CA, USA*
[2] *Stanford Systems Neuroscience and Pain Lab (SNAPL), Stanford University, Palo Alto, CA, USA*
[3] *Department of Orthopaedic Surgery, Stanford University, Palo Alto, CA, USA*

Correspondence should be addressed to Jennifer M. Hah; jhah@stanford.edu

Academic Editor: Anna Maria Aloisi

Objectives. Patients taking opioids prior to surgery experience prolonged postoperative opioid use, worse clinical outcomes, increased pain, and more postoperative complications. We aimed to compare preoperative opioid users to their opioid naïve counterparts to identify differences in baseline characteristics. *Methods.* 107 patients presenting for thoracotomy, total knee replacement, total hip replacement, radical mastectomy, and lumpectomy were investigated in a cross-sectional study to characterize the associations between measures of pain, substance use, abuse, addiction, sleep, and psychological measures (depressive symptoms, Posttraumatic Stress Disorder symptoms, somatic fear and anxiety, and fear of pain) with opioid use. *Results.* Every 9-point increase in the Screener and Opioid Assessment for Patients with Pain-Revised (SOAPP-R) score was associated with 2.37 (95% CI 1.29–4.32) increased odds of preoperative opioid use ($p = 0.0005$). The SOAPP-R score was also associated with 3.02 (95% CI 1.36–6.70) increased odds of illicit preoperative opioid use ($p = 0.007$). Also, every 4-point increase in baseline pain at the future surgical site was associated with 2.85 (95% CI 1.12–7.27) increased odds of legitimate preoperative opioid use ($p = 0.03$). *Discussion.* Patients presenting with preoperative opioid use have higher SOAPP-R scores potentially indicating an increased risk for opioid misuse after surgery. In addition, legitimate preoperative opioid use is associated with preexisting pain.

1. Introduction

Previous research has reported prolonged postoperative opioid use in patients already taking opioids prior to surgery [1–3]. A small retrospective study of patients undergoing orthopedic surgery for trauma reported that positive toxicology results at the time of injury predicted an extended duration of postoperative prescription opioid use [1]. Similarly, 30% of women taking preoperative opioids were taking them 6 months after gynecologic surgery compared to 2.2% of women not taking preoperative opioids [2]. These findings extend to patients with preoperative chronic opioid use. 77% of chronic opioid users undergoing bariatric surgery continued to use opioids in the year after surgery [4]. Likewise, a higher proportion of chronic opioid users compared to nonusers continued to take opioids 58 months after total hip arthroplasty [5]. Furthermore, compared to their opioid naïve counterparts, preoperative prescription opioid users have worse functional outcomes [3], worse clinical outcomes [5, 6], increased hospital length of stay [5, 6], increased pain severity after surgery [7] even in the context of increased opioid requirements [8], increased specialist referrals for pain management [6], more dissatisfaction with the surgical outcome [7], and a higher prevalence of postsurgical complications [6]. Particularly notable is the increased mortality associated with preoperative chronic opioid use. A history of chronic opioid use in patients with end-stage renal disease was associated with 1.6- to 2-fold increased risk of death after kidney transplantation [9].

Mechanisms for reduced opioid cessation after surgery in patients taking preoperative opioids are unclear. Research suggests a decreased resolution of postoperative allodynia

[10]. In mice, morphine leads to enhanced nociceptive sensitivity and significant sensitization for several days after incision which may be due to excess cytokine production [11]. Also, patients receiving methadone maintenance display mood stabilization at peak concentrations and increased mood disturbance at trough concentrations implying that opioids may directly affect mood states [12–17]. In the future, more patients will be presenting to surgery on opioids. Research indicates that postoperative pain management in these patients will be challenging [18–21].

We conducted an analysis of the data from a previously reported [22, 23] prospective, observational study of opioid cessation after 5 discrete surgical procedures (thoracotomy, total hip replacement, total knee replacement, mastectomy, and lumpectomy). Of 20 variables, only preoperative elevated depressive symptoms, self-perceived susceptibility to addiction, and legitimate preoperative opioid use were independent predictors of delayed opioid cessation after surgery [22].

The aim of this cross-sectional cohort study was to further compare this at-risk population of patients taking opioids prior to surgery to their opioid naïve counterparts. In addition, this study also compared patients taking legitimate, prescribed or illicit, nonprescribed opioids prior to surgery to opioid naïve patients in order to further characterize the distinction between patients with medical and nonmedical use of opioids prior to surgery.

2. Materials and Methods

Subjects were recruited between January 2007 and April 2009. Exclusion criteria were any mental incapacity or language barrier precluding completion of assessments. The Stanford University IRB approved the entire protocol, and all participants provided written informed consent.

2.1. Measures of Pain and Opioid Use. Prior to surgery, the Brief Pain Inventory (BPI) [24] was administered twice to capture pain limited to the future surgical site, as well as pain elsewhere on the body. Preoperative opioid use was categorized as "legitimate preoperative opioid use" (subjects reported taking opioids directly prescribed to them for pain), "illicit preoperative opioid use" (subjects reported taking opioids not directly prescribed to them), or "any preoperative opioid use" (all subjects from either of the two previous categories).

2.2. Measures of Substance Use, Abuse, and Addiction. The Screener and Opioid Assessment for Patients with Pain-Revised (SOAPP-R) was administered to assess the risk of opioid misuse [25]. The self-perceived susceptibility to addiction measure was administered as a response to the question "How likely do you think it is that you will develop an addiction problem from pain medication you take after surgery?" Subjects chose from 4 responses: (1) "not at all"; (2) "unlikely"; (3) "somewhat likely"; or (4) "very likely." The Addiction Severity Index Drug and Alcohol Use section was used to assess lifetime and previous 30-day use of illicit substances and alcohol [26, 27].

2.3. Sleep. The Pittsburgh Sleep Quality Index (PSQI) is a self-rated questionnaire assessing sleep disturbances over the past month [28]. 19 items are administered to generate 7 subscores of subjective sleep quality, sleep latency, sleep duration, habitual sleep efficiency, sleep disturbances, use of sleeping medication, and daytime dysfunction. A global PSQI score was calculated as the sum of these subscores [28].

2.4. Psychological Measures. The Beck Depression Inventory-II (BDI-II) [29], Primary Care Posttraumatic Stress Disorder Screen [30], Anxiety-Sensitivity Index [31], and Fear of Pain Questionnaire [32] were administered to assess depressive symptoms, PTSD symptoms, somatic fear and anxiety, and fear of pain, respectively. All baseline questionnaires were assessed between 1 and 2 weeks prior to surgery.

2.5. Statistical Analyses. SAS version 9.3 (SAS Institute, Inc., Cary, NC) was used for all analyses. A t-test was used to compare all numerical variables, and Chi-square or Fisher's exact test was used to compare all categorical variables. Any preoperative opioid use was analyzed as a distinct dependent variable in the primary logistic regression analyses. As sub-analyses, legitimate and illicit preoperative opioid use were then analyzed as distinct dependent variables using separate logistic regression analyses. For each of the subanalyses, those patients reporting both legitimate and illicit preoperative opioid use were excluded in order to directly compare each opioid-using subgroup to their opioid naïve counterparts. SAS PROC LOGISTIC was used for logistic regression, calculation of odds ratios, and model building. The linearity assumption of all significant predictors was met by plotting a linear relationship of the independent variable to the log odds.

Given the paucity of data regarding preoperative characteristics associated with legitimate or illicit preoperative opioid use, we were unable to construct a multivariate model of preselected variables a priori. Instead, all variables found to be significant in univariate analysis were considered for inclusion in the multivariate model. Subsequent multivariate model selection was accomplished by comparing the results of automated stepwise, backward, and forward variable-selection algorithms in order to account for potential errors in model building, sensitivity of the results to the specific model building algorithm, and order effects and to determine optimal model fit.

3. Results

Table 1 shows patient characteristics comparing preoperative opioid users to their opioid naïve counterparts. One hundred seven of 134 patients approached for inclusion agreed to participate in the study and provided data on preoperative opioid use. Table 2 shows patient characteristics comparing illicit and legitimate preoperative opioid users. Of the entire cohort, 8 patients reported both legitimate and illicit preoperative opioid use.

3.1. Factors Associated with Preoperative Opioid Use. As shown in Table 1, preoperative opioid users had elevated

TABLE 1: Patient characteristics.

	No preoperative opioid use	Any preoperative opioid use	p value
Preoperative characteristic (SD)[a]			
Patients (n)	80	27	
Age (y)	58 (13)	56 (14)	0.48
Male gender (n)	28% (22)	37% (10)	0.35
Baseline pain other than surgical site (0–10)	2.04 (2.45)	3.78 (2.58)	0.002
Baseline pain at surgical site (0–10)	1.58 (2.42)	3.44 (3.03)	0.002
Self-Perceived Risk of Addiction	1.27 (0.55)	1.44 (0.58)	0.15
History of Addiction Treatment (n)	4% (3)	4% (1)	1
SOAPP-R score	11.91 (5.74)	19.26 (12.57)	0.006
Used tobacco regularly (lifetime) (n)	23% (18)	41% (11)	0.07
Beck Depression Inventory-II score	7.75 (6.11)	14.65 (12.49)	0.01
Anxiety Sensitivity Index Score	14.54 (10.55)	19.48 (15.81)	0.14
Fear of Pain Score	70.12 (22.53)	74.19 (21.92)	0.42
Primary Care PTSD Screen Score	0.49 (1.04)	0.88 (1.45)	0.21
PSQI Total Score	6.96 (3.69)	9.92 (4.67)	0.002
Surgery type (n)			0.02
Thoracotomy	28% (22)	19% (5)	
Total knee replacement	14% (11)	30% (8)	
Total hip replacement	19% (15)	37% (10)	
Radical mastectomy	26% (21)	15% (4)	
Lumpectomy	14% (11)	0% (0)	

SOAPP-R, Screener and Opioid Assessment for Patients with Pain-Revised; PTSD, Posttraumatic Stress Disorder; PSQI, Pittsburgh Sleep Quality Index.
[a]Values are presented as means and SD except where noted otherwise.

TABLE 2: Patient characteristics amongst opioid use subgroups[a].

	Illicit preoperative opioid use	Legitimate preoperative opioid use
Preoperative characteristic (SD)[b]		
Patients (n)	14	21
Age (y)	52 (17)	57 (12)
Male gender (n)	43% (6)	43% (9)
Baseline pain other than surgical site (0–10)	3.79 (2.58)	3.76 (2.81)
Baseline pain at surgical site (0–10)	3.36 (3.43)	3.62 (2.64)
Self-Perceived Risk of Addiction	1.57 (0.65)	1.43 (0.60)
History of Addiction Treatment (n)	7% (1)	5% (1)
SOAPP-R score	23.00 (16.03)	18.43 (11.74)
Used tobacco regularly (lifetime) (n)	57% (8)	38% (8)
Beck Depression Inventory-II score	19.92 (15.28)	13.35 (9.98)
Anxiety Sensitivity Index Score	22.71 (18.31)	18.52 (14.17)
Fear of Pain Score	74.29 (25.88)	72.10 (22.11)
Primary Care PTSD Screen Score	1.15 (1.57)	0.85 (1.46)
PSQI Total Score	9.58 (4.08)	10.55 (4.56)
Surgery type (n)		
Thoracotomy	21% (3)	19% (4)
Total knee replacement	29% (4)	29% (6)
Total hip replacement	29% (4)	48% (10)
Radical mastectomy	21% (3)	5% (1)
Lumpectomy	0% (0)	0% (0)

SOAPP-R, Screener and Opioid Assessment for Patients with Pain-Revised; PTSD, Posttraumatic Stress Disorder; PSQI, Pittsburgh Sleep Quality Index.
[a]Eight patients reported both illicit and legitimate preoperative opioid use.
[b]Values are presented as means and SD except where noted otherwise.

Table 3: Univariate analysis of preoperative variables associated with any preoperative opioid use.

	OR (95% CI)	p value
Beck Depression Inventory-II score	1.08 (1.02–1.15)	0.001
SOAPP-R score	1.10 (1.03–1.18)	0.005
PSQI Total Score	1.14 (1.01–1.28)	0.04
Primary Care PTSD Screen Score	1.48 (0.99–2.20)	0.06
Used tobacco regularly (lifetime)	2.40 (0.90–6.38)	0.08
Self-Perceived Risk of Addiction	1.91 (0.87–4.16)	0.11
Baseline pain other than surgical site (0–10)	1.16 (0.95–1.41)	0.15
Anxiety Sensitivity Index Score	1.03 (0.99–1.06)	0.19
Age (y)	0.98 (0.94–1.01)	0.21
Baseline pain at surgical site (0–10)	1.14 (0.92–1.42)	0.24
Fear of Pain Score	1.01 (0.99–1.03)	0.37
Male gender	0.86 (0.31–2.37)	0.77
History of Addiction Treatment	1.04 (0.10–11.39)	0.97

SOAPP-R, Screener and Opioid Assessment for Patients with Pain-Revised; PTSD, Posttraumatic Stress Disorder; PSQI, Pittsburgh Sleep Quality Index.

levels of baseline pain at sites other than their surgical site, elevated SOAPP-R scores, elevated depressive symptoms, and worse sleep. Of note, global PSQI scores >5 are associated with poor sleep quality which would apply to both the preoperative opioid users and the opioid naïve group [28]. Of the entire patient cohort, 65 patients (61%) had a global PSQI score >5. Specifically, 56% (n = 45) of the preoperative opioid naïve patients and 74% (n = 20) of the preoperative opioid users reported poor sleep quality.

Table 3 shows the results of univariate logistic regression of preoperative variables associated with preoperative opioid use. Of all the variables, only the BDI-II score, SOAPP-R score, and global PSQI score were significantly associated with preoperative opioid use. Table 4 shows the final multivariate logistic regression model reflecting the adjusted OR for SOAPP-R score. Every 9-point increase in the SOAPP-R score (interquartile range in this cohort) is associated with 2.37 (95% CI 1.29–4.32) increased odds of presenting with preoperative opioid use (p = 0.0005). Previous research has reported a cutoff score of 18 or higher to identify patients at high risk for aberrant medication-related behavior [33]. Using these criteria, 21 patients (20%) of the entire cohort had a positive SOAPP-R score. Specifically, 16% (n = 13) of the preoperative opioid naïve patients and 30% (n = 8) of the preoperative opioid users reported positive SOAPP-R scores.

Table 4: Multivariate analysis of preoperative variables associated with any preoperative opioid use.

	Adjusted OR (95% CI)	p value
SOAPP-R Score	2.37 (1.29–4.32)	0.0005

Adjusted OR represents every 9-point increase in the SOAPP-R (Screener and Opioid Assessment for Patients with Pain-Revised) score, which is the interquartile range.

Table 5: Univariate analysis of preoperative variables associated with legitimate preoperative opioid use.

	OR (95% CI)	p value
PSQI Total Score	1.20 (1.04–1.39)	0.01
Baseline pain at surgical site (0–10)	1.33 (1.07–1.65)	0.01
Baseline pain other than surgical site (0–10)	1.28 (1.03–1.59)	0.03

PSQI, Pittsburgh Sleep Quality Index.

3.2. Factors Associated with Legitimate Preoperative Opioid Use. Table 5 shows the results of univariate logistic regression of preoperative variables associated with legitimate preoperative opioid use. Of all the variables, only the global PSQI score, baseline pain at the future surgical site, and baseline pain elsewhere over the body were significant. Table 6 shows the final multivariate logistic regression model reflecting the adjusted OR for baseline pain at the future surgical site. Every 4-point increase in baseline pain at the surgical site (interquartile range in this cohort) is associated with 2.85 (95% CI 1.12–7.27) increased odds of presenting with legitimate preoperative opioid use (p = 0.03). Also, the global PSQI score was a confounder of the relationship between baseline pain and legitimate opioid use. In the final model, every 7-point increase in the global PSQI score (interquartile range in this cohort) is associated with 2.82 (95% CI 0.98–8.12) increased odds of presenting with legitimate preoperative opioid use.

3.3. Factors Associated with Illicit Preoperative Opioid Use. Table 7 shows the results of univariate logistic regression of preoperative variables associated with illicit preoperative opioid use stratified by surgery type. Of all the variables, BDI-II score and SOAPP-R score were significantly associated with illicit preoperative opioid use. Table 8 shows the final multivariate logistic regression model reflecting the adjusted OR for SOAPP-R score. Every 9-point increase in the SOAPP-R score (interquartile range in this cohort) is associated with

Table 6: Multivariate analysis of preoperative variables associated with legitimate preoperative opioid use.

	Adjusted OR (95% CI)	p value
Baseline pain at surgical site (0–10)	2.85 (1.12–7.27)	0.03
PSQI Total Score	2.82 (0.98–8.12)	0.06

Adjusted OR represents every 4-point increase in the baseline pain score and every 7-point increase in the global PSQI (Pittsburgh Sleep Quality Index) score, which is the interquartile range.

Table 7: Univariate analysis of preoperative variables associated with illicit preoperative opioid use.

	OR (95% CI)	p value
SOAPP-R score	1.13 (1.04–1.24)	0.007
Beck Depression Inventory-II score	1.11 (1.02–1.20)	0.02

SOAPP-R, Screener and Opioid Assessment for Patients with Pain-Revised.

Table 8: Multivariate analysis of preoperative variables associated with illicit preoperative opioid use.

	Adjusted OR (95% CI)	p value
SOAPP-R score	3.02 (1.36–6.70)	0.007

Adjusted OR represents every 9-point increase in the SOAPP-R (Screener and Opioid Assessment for Patients with Pain-Revised) score, which is the interquartile range.

3.02 (95% CI 1.36–6.70) increased odds of presenting with illicit preoperative opioid use ($p = 0.007$).

4. Discussion

The main purpose of this study was to identify preoperative factors associated with preoperative opioid use. Of all the preoperative variables examined, only an elevated SOAPP-R score was significantly associated with preoperative opioid use in the final multivariate model. In addition, legitimate and illicit preoperative opioid users were compared to opioid naïve patients as subanalyses. Of all the preoperative variables, baseline pain at the future surgical site was associated with legitimate opioid use, and poor sleep was a confounder of this association. As those patients taking prescribed opioids for pain were classified as legitimate opioid users, we would expect to see an association between elevated levels of pain and legitimate opioid use. Also, an elevated SOAPP-R score was associated with illicit preoperative opioid use. Thus, elevated SOAPP-R scores in illicit preoperative opioid users are potentially driving the association in the entire opioid-using cohort. An important note is that the original study from which this data was drawn was not powered for the present analyses [22]. As the global PSQI score and BDI-II score were both significantly associated with any preoperative opioid use in univariate analyses, it is possible that these associations may be just as important as the SOAPP-R in relation to preoperative opioid use. These findings should be considered in future studies.

The SOAPP-R is a self-reported measure of the risk potential for aberrant medication behavior amongst people with chronic pain [34]. The SOAPP-R has been validated as a screening tool in this population and intended for administration to patients being considered for long-term opioid therapy [34]. Amongst a cross-validation sample for the SOAPP-R, 33.5% of patients had a score of 18 or higher, which was reported as a cutoff score with 80% sensitivity and 52% specificity in identifying patients at risk for aberrant drug-related behavior. In other words, at this cutoff score, the SOAPP-R has a higher chance of identifying false-positives due to this lower specificity. Nonetheless, the SOAPP-R has demonstrated superiority over other self-report measures including the Pain Medication Questionnaire and Opioid Risk Tool to predict discharge from opioid treatment and the presence of aberrant drug-related behavior [35].

Use of the SOAPP-R in the preoperative setting has never been previously reported. Of interest, 30% of the preoperative opioid users and only 16% of the preoperative opioid naïve patients had a positive SOAPP-R score. Furthermore, 24% of legitimate opioid users and 43% of illicit opioid users had a positive SOAPP-R score. These findings are concerning in the context of research showing prolonged postoperative opioid use in patients taking opioids prior to surgery [2–5, 7, 22]. Although this study did not distinguish whether or not patients were already receiving chronic opioid therapy, our results suggest that the positive SOAPP-R score may indicate a potential for aberrant medication behaviors and opioid misuse in the postoperative setting with prolonged opioid use. This is especially likely, as elevated SOAPP-R scores were associated with preoperative self-reported illicit opioid use. In a cohort of chronic pain patients continuing opioid therapy for 12 weeks, a SOAPP-R score greater than or equal to 18 was predictive of a Current Opioid Misuse Measure (COMM) greater than or equal to 9 [36]. The COMM asks patients to describe how they are currently using their medication to identify current opioid misuse. A score of 9 or higher on the COMM has 94% sensitivity and 73% specificity to identify opioid misuse amongst patients with persistent pain [37]. In our present study, we cannot make any assumptions whether or not elevated SOAPP-R scores precede initiation of either legitimate or illicit opioid use. However, the SOAPP-R may be a valuable screening tool in the perioperative setting to identify patients taking preoperative opioids, who are at risk for opioid misuse. Future research should focus on whether elevated preoperative SOAPP-R scores are predictive of elevated postoperative COMM scores.

The global PSQI score was positive (>5) in 61% of our entire patient cohort indicating pervasive poor self-reported sleep quality. While 56% of opioid naïve patients had a positive score, the global PSQI score was positive in 74% of all preoperative opioid users, 81% of legitimate opioid users, and 71% of illicit opioid users, respectively. In addition, the global PSQI score was a confounder of the relationship between baseline pain at the future surgical site and preoperative legitimate opioid use. Although research has established an association between chronic pain and sleep disorders [38], much of the literature examining the effects of chronic opioid therapy on sleep involves patients receiving opioid replacement therapy. Methadone maintenance patients have a high prevalence of sleep disturbances as measured through elevated PSQI scores [39], worse daytime function, and increased subjective daytime somnolence. Less attention has focused on patients with chronic pain, who are also using prescription opioids. In a cross-sectional study of VA patients in a single VA medical center, patients with chronic pain prescribed opioids were more likely to have a sleep apnea diagnosis, as well as an elevated PSQI global score. Opioid dose was also a significant predictor of impaired sleep latency and global PSQI score. In our study, patients reporting legitimate opioid use may have had more consistent opioid exposure resulting in a higher proportion of elevated PSQI scores. In patients with chronic pain receiving chronic opioid therapy, opioid dose is associated with unrefreshing sleep and worse sleep maintenance. Also, use of long-acting opioids is associated with increased napping [40]. In the perioperative setting, screening for poor sleep quality amongst prescription opioid users may be particularly important given the increased and prolonged opioid requirements in the postoperative period through recovery. As a dose-dependent relationship between opioid use, central sleep apneas, and ataxic breathing exists, patients reporting elevated global PSQI scores may be at increased risk for respiratory depression [41]. Research is needed to examine the association between preoperative elevated global PSQI scores and objective measures of impaired sleep in the postoperative setting.

Although depressive symptoms were not associated with preoperative opioid use in any of the final multivariate models, our study found that elevated depressive symptoms were associated with any preoperative opioid use and illicit opioid use in univariate analyses. Previous research has demonstrated an association between nonmedical prescription opioid use with panic, depressive, and social phobic/agoraphobic symptoms [42]. Of note, 57% of the preoperative illicit opioid users in our study also reported legitimate opioid use. In a cohort of primary care patients with chronic pain, Posttraumatic Stress Disorder was a factor associated with prescription drug use disorder [43]. Although we are unable to make assumptions regarding the chronicity of opioid use in our surgical cohort, an association exists between long-term prescription opioid use, affective disorders, and substance abuse. Increased rates of substance abuse and depression exist in long-term prescription opioid users compared to nonusers with chronic pain, and pain intensity does not predict treatment with opioids versus nonopioid analgesics [44]. Other research shows that depression and anxiety contribute to substance use disorders amongst long-term opioid users [45]. As more than half of the illicit opioid users in our cohort were also receiving legitimately prescribed opioids, it is possible that elevated depressive symptoms may have led to nonmedical prescription opioid use.

Similarly, psychological comorbidities are common amongst patients with prescribed opioids for chronic noncancer pain. For example, patients with chronic pain who have psychological comorbidity and higher pain severity ratings are more likely to present on opioids to a tertiary pain clinic [46]. Likewise, veterans with prescribed high doses of opioids (greater than or equal to 180 morphine equivalents daily for 90 days) are more likely to have the highest rates of medical, psychiatric, and substance use disorders (major depressive disorder, Posttraumatic Stress Disorder, anxiety disorders, sleep disorders, or a substance use disorder) [47]. Higher opioid doses are associated with higher levels of patient-reported opioid-related psychosocial problems (loss of interest in activities, trouble concentrating, feeling slowed down and sluggish, feeling depressed or anxious, interference with activities, and decreased alertness), opioid control concerns (being worried about opioid dependence, wanting to stop or cut down use of opioids, and reporting that family or friends think the patient may be addicted to opioids), and depressive symptoms and are more likely to be clinically depressing [48].

Although our study did not capture the chronicity or quantity of preoperative opioid use in our surgical cohort, our previously reported findings demonstrated that an elevated preoperative BDI-II score is an independent predictor of delayed opioid cessation after surgery [22]. Therefore, preoperative assessment of depressive symptoms may have two important benefits: (1) to identify patients who may be using illicit opioids and (2) to identify patients at risk for prolonged opioid use after surgery. Furthermore, testosterone deficiency is a less commonly discussed adverse effect of prescription opioid use. Particularly, testosterone serves a function in endogenous opioid activity through facilitation of opioid receptor binding, activation of dopamine and norepinephrine activity, and maintenance of blood-brain barrier transport [49]. Clinically, decreased testosterone can result in impaired pain control, depression, anxiety, weight gain, decreased muscle mass, reduced quality of life, osteoporosis, fatigue, sleep disturbances, irregular menses, reduced libido, erectile dysfunction, and hot flashes [49, 50]. This opioid-induced androgen deficiency may play a key role in precipitating pain sensitivity and mood disturbances. Future work to preoperatively diagnose opioid-induced hypogonadism and to correlate this endocrinopathy to preoperative mood disturbances and increased pain sensitivity may pinpoint an underlying mechanism for our findings, as well as an important future intervention target.

5. Conclusions

Opioid users presenting for surgery have elevated SOAPP-R scores relative to their opioid naïve counterparts. As preoperative opioid users are exposed to surgical injury and escalated and prolonged opioid use in the postoperative period, these elevated SOAPP-R scores may also indicate the potential for opioid misuse. Notably, a high proportion of the entire surgical cohort reported poor sleep quality through elevated global PSQI scores. Future research is needed to further examine objective measures of impaired sleep in the postoperative period.

Acknowledgments

Dr. Hah was supported by K23 Grant 1K23DA035302 from the National Institute on Drug Abuse. Dr. Mackey was supported by NIH K24DA029262 and the Chris Redlich Pain Research Fund. Dr. Carroll gratefully acknowledges funding from the Foundation for Anesthesia Education and Research (FAER) in the form of a mentored research training grant. Subsequent funding was provided by K23 Grant 1K23DA025152 from the National Institute on Drug Abuse.

References

[1] G. M. Massey, H. N. Dodds, C. S. Roberts, T. J. Servoss, and R. D. Blondell, "Toxicology screening in orthopedic trauma patients predicting duration of prescription opioid use," *Journal of Addictive Diseases*, vol. 24, no. 4, pp. 31–41, 2005.

[2] E. G. VanDenKerkhof, W. M. Hopman, D. H. Goldstein et al., "Impact of perioperative pain intensity, pain qualities, and opioid use on chronic pain after surgery: a prospective cohort study," *Regional Anesthesia and Pain Medicine*, vol. 37, no. 1, pp. 19–27, 2012.

[3] J. T. R. Lawrence, N. London, H. H. Bohlman, and K. R. Chin, "Preoperative narcotic use as a predictor of clinical outcome: results following anterior cervical arthrodesis," *Spine*, vol. 33, no. 19, pp. 2074–2078, 2008.

[4] M. A. Raebel, S. R. Newcomer, L. M. Reifler et al., "Chronic use of opioid medications before and after bariatric surgery," *The Journal of the American Medical Association*, vol. 310, no. 13, pp. 1369–1376, 2013.

[5] R. Pivec, K. Issa, Q. Naziri, B. H. Kapadia, P. M. Bonutti, and M. A. Mont, "Opioid use prior to total hip arthroplasty leads to worse clinical outcomes," *International Orthopaedics*, vol. 38, no. 6, pp. 1159–1165, 2014.

[6] M. G. Zywiel, D. A. Stroh, S. Y. Lee, P. M. Bonutti, and M. A. Mont, "Chronic opioid use prior to total knee arthroplasty," *The Journal of Bone & Joint Surgery—American Volume*, vol. 93, no. 21, pp. 1988–1993, 2011.

[7] P. D. Franklin, J. A. Karbassi, W. Li, W. Yang, and D. C. Ayers, "Reduction in narcotic use after primary total knee arthroplasty and association with patient pain relief and satisfaction," *Journal of Arthroplasty*, vol. 25, no. 6, pp. 12–16, 2010.

[8] S. E. Rapp, L. B. Ready, and M. L. Nessly, "Acute pain management in patients with prior opioid consumption: a case-controlled retrospective review," *Pain*, vol. 61, no. 2, pp. 195–201, 1995.

[9] F. Barrantes, F. L. Luan, M. Kommareddi et al., "A history of chronic opioid usage prior to kidney transplantation may be associated with increased mortality risk," *Kidney International*, vol. 84, no. 2, pp. 390–396, 2013.

[10] R. J. Horvath, R. P. Landry, E. A. Romero-Sandoval, and J. A. DeLeo, "Morphine tolerance attenuates the resolution of postoperative pain and enhances spinal microglial p38 and extracellular receptor kinase phosphorylation," *Neuroscience*, vol. 169, no. 2, pp. 843–854, 2010.

[11] D. Liang, X. Shi, Y. Qiao, M. S. Angst, D. C. Yeomans, and J. Clark, "Chronic morphine administration enhances nociceptive sensitivity and local cytokine production after incision," *Molecular Pain*, vol. 4, article 7, 2008.

[12] K. R. Dyer, J. M. White, D. J. R. Foster, F. Bochner, A. Menelaou, and A. A. Somogyi, "The relationship between mood state and plasma methadone concentration in maintenance patients," *Journal of Clinical Psychopharmacology*, vol. 21, no. 1, pp. 78–84, 2001.

[13] I. I. Galynker, D. Eisenberg, J. A. Matochik et al., "Cerebral metabolism and mood in remitted opiate dependence," *Drug and Alcohol Dependence*, vol. 90, no. 2-3, pp. 166–174, 2007.

[14] S. M. Savvas, A. A. Somogyi, and J. M. White, "The effect of methadone on emotional reactivity," *Addiction*, vol. 107, no. 2, pp. 388–392, 2012.

[15] D. Filliol, S. Ghozland, J. Chluba et al., "Mice deficient for δ- and μ-opioid receptors exhibit opposing alterations of emotional responses," *Nature Genetics*, vol. 25, no. 2, pp. 195–200, 2000.

[16] T. R. Kosten, C. Morgan, and T. A. Kosten, "Depressive symptoms during buprenorphine treatment of opioid abusers," *Journal of Substance Abuse Treatment*, vol. 7, no. 1, pp. 51–54, 1990.

[17] M. O. Rojas-Corrales, E. Berrocoso, J. Gibert-Rahola, and J. A. Micó, "Antidepressant-like effects of tramadol and other central analgesics with activity on monoamines reuptake, in helpless rats," *Life Sciences*, vol. 72, no. 2, pp. 143–152, 2002.

[18] M. Doverty, A. A. Somogyi, J. M. White et al., "Methadone maintenance patients are cross-tolerant to the antinociceptive effects of morphine," *Pain*, vol. 93, no. 2, pp. 155–163, 2001.

[19] P. Athanasos, C. S. Smith, J. M. White, A. A. Somogyi, F. Bochner, and W. Ling, "Methadone maintenance patients are cross-tolerant to the antinociceptive effects of very high plasma morphine concentrations," *Pain*, vol. 120, no. 3, pp. 267–275, 2006.

[20] A. E. Patanwala, D. L. Jarzyna, M. D. Miller, and B. L. Erstad, "Comparison of opioid requirements and analgesic response in opioid-tolerant versus opioid-naïve patients after total knee arthroplasty," *Pharmacotherapy*, vol. 28, no. 12, pp. 1453–1460, 2008.

[21] S. L. Ingram, T. A. Macey, E. N. Fossum, and M. M. Morgan, "Tolerance to repeated morphine administration is associated with increased potency of opioid agonists," *Neuropsychopharmacology*, vol. 33, no. 10, pp. 2494–2504, 2008.

[22] I. Carroll, P. Barelka, C. K. M. Wang et al., "A pilot cohort study of the determinants of longitudinal opioid use after surgery," *Anesthesia & Analgesia*, vol. 115, no. 3, pp. 694–702, 2012.

[23] J. M. Hah, S. Mackey, P. L. Barelka et al., "Self-loathing aspects of depression reduce postoperative opioid cessation rate," *Pain Medicine*, vol. 15, no. 6, pp. 954–964, 2014.

[24] C. S. Cleeland and K. M. Ryan, "Pain assessment: global use of the Brief Pain Inventory," *Annals of the Academy of Medicine Singapore*, vol. 23, no. 2, pp. 129–138, 1994.

[25] S. F. Butler, S. H. Budman, K. Fernandez, and R. N. Jamison, "Validation of a screener and opioid assessment measure for patients with chronic pain," *Pain*, vol. 112, no. 1-2, pp. 65–75, 2004.

[26] A. T. McLellan, L. Luborsky, G. E. Woody, and C. P. O'Brien, "An improved diagnostic evaluation instrument for substance abuse patients. The Addiction Severity Index," *The Journal of Nervous and Mental Disease*, vol. 168, no. 1, pp. 26–33, 1980.

[27] K. Mäkelä, "Studies of the reliability and validity of the Addiction Severity Index," *Addiction*, vol. 99, no. 4, pp. 398–410, 2004.

[28] D. J. Buysse, C. F. Reynolds III, T. H. Monk, S. R. Berman, and D. J. Kupfer, "The Pittsburgh sleep quality index: a new instrument for psychiatric practice and research," *Psychiatry Research*, vol. 28, no. 2, pp. 193–213, 1989.

[29] A. T. Beck, C. H. Ward, M. Mendelson, J. Mock, and J. Erbaugh, "An inventory for measuring depression," *Archives of General Psychiatry*, vol. 4, pp. 561–571, 1961.

[30] R. Kimerling, P. Ouimette, A. Prins et al., "Brief report: utility of a short screening scale for DSM-IV PTSD in primary care," *Journal of General Internal Medicine*, vol. 21, no. 1, pp. 65–67, 2006.

[31] S. Reiss, R. A. Peterson, D. M. Gursky, and R. J. McNally, "Anxiety sensitivity, anxiety frequency and the prediction of fearfulness," *Behaviour Research and Therapy*, vol. 24, no. 1, pp. 1–8, 1986.

[32] D. W. McNeil and A. J. Rainwater III, "Development of the fear of pain questionnaire—III," *Journal of Behavioral Medicine*, vol. 21, no. 4, pp. 389–410, 1998.

[33] S. F. Butler, K. Fernandez, C. Benoit, S. H. Budman, and R. N. Jamison, "Validation of the revised Screener and Opioid Assessment for Patients with Pain (SOAPP-R)," *The Journal of Pain*, vol. 9, no. 4, pp. 360–372, 2008.

[34] S. F. Butler, S. H. Budman, K. C. Fernandez, G. J. Fanciullo, and R. N. Jamison, "Cross-validation of a screener to predict opioid misuse in chronic pain patients (SOAPP-R)," *Journal of Addiction Medicine*, vol. 3, no. 2, pp. 66–73, 2009.

[35] T. Jones, T. Moore, J. L. Levy et al., "A comparison of various risk screening methods in predicting discharge from opioid treatment," *Clinical Journal of Pain*, vol. 28, no. 2, pp. 93–100, 2012.

[36] S. D. Passik, A. Narayana, and R. Yang, "Aberrant drug-related behavior observed during a 12-week open-label extension period of a study involving patients taking chronic opioid therapy for persistent pain and fentanyl buccal tablet or traditional short-acting opioid for breakthrough pain," *Pain Medicine*, vol. 15, no. 8, pp. 1365–1372, 2014.

[37] S. F. Butler, S. H. Budman, K. C. Fernandez et al., "Development and validation of the current opioid misuse measure," *Pain*, vol. 130, no. 1-2, pp. 144–156, 2007.

[38] D. A. Fishbain, B. Cole, J. E. Lewis, and J. Gao, "What is the evidence for chronic pain being etiologically associated with the DSM-IV category of sleep disorder due to a general medical condition? A structured evidence-based review," *Pain Medicine*, vol. 11, no. 2, pp. 158–179, 2010.

[39] M. D. Stein, D. S. Herman, S. Bishop et al., "Sleep disturbances among methadone maintained patients," *Journal of Substance Abuse Treatment*, vol. 26, no. 3, pp. 175–180, 2004.

[40] A. Zgierska, R. T. Brown, M. Zuelsdorff, D. Brown, Z. Zhang, and M. F. Fleming, "Sleep and daytime sleepiness problems among patients with chronic noncancerous pain receiving long-term opioid therapy: a cross-sectional study," *Journal of Opioid Management*, vol. 3, no. 6, pp. 317–327, 2007.

[41] J. M. Walker, R. J. Farney, S. M. Rhondeau et al., "Chronic opioid use is a risk factor for the development of central sleep apnea and ataxic breathing," *Journal of Clinical Sleep Medicine*, vol. 3, no. 5, pp. 455–461, 2007.

[42] W. C. Becker, L. E. Sullivan, J. M. Tetrault, R. A. Desai, and D. A. Fiellin, "Non-medical use, abuse and dependence on prescription opioids among U.S. adults: psychiatric, medical and substance use correlates," *Drug and Alcohol Dependence*, vol. 94, no. 1–3, pp. 38–47, 2008.

[43] J. M. Liebschutz, R. Saitz, R. D. Weiss et al., "Clinical factors associated with prescription drug use disorder in urban primary care patients with chronic pain," *Journal of Pain*, vol. 11, no. 11, pp. 1047–1055, 2010.

[44] J. Breckenridge and J. D. Clark, "Patient characteristics associated with opioid versus nonsteroidal anti-inflammatory drug management of chronic low back pain," *Journal of Pain*, vol. 4, no. 6, pp. 344–350, 2003.

[45] M. J. Edlund, M. Sullivan, D. Steffick, K. M. Harris, and K. B. Wells, "Do users of regularly prescribed opioids have higher rates of substance use problems than nonusers?" *Pain Medicine*, vol. 8, no. 8, pp. 647–656, 2007.

[46] A. Mailis-Gagnon, S. F. Lakha, T. O. A. Louffat et al., "Chronic noncancer pain: characteristics of patients prescribed opioids by community physicians and referred to a tertiary pain clinic," *Canadian Family Physician*, vol. 57, no. 3, pp. e97–e105, 2011.

[47] B. J. Morasco, J. P. Duckart, T. P. Carr, R. A. Deyo, and S. K. Dobscha, "Clinical characteristics of veterans prescribed high doses of opioid medications for chronic non-cancer pain," *Pain*, vol. 151, no. 3, pp. 625–632, 2010.

[48] J. O. Merrill, M. Von Korff, C. J. Banta-Green et al., "Prescribed opioid difficulties, depression and opioid dose among chronic opioid therapy patients," *General Hospital Psychiatry*, vol. 34, no. 6, pp. 581–587, 2012.

[49] J. A. Gudin, A. Laitman, and S. Nalamachu, "Opioid related endocrinopathy," *Pain Medicine*, vol. 16, supplement 1, pp. S9–S15, 2015.

[50] C. De Maddalena, M. Bellini, M. Berra, M. C. Meriggiola, and A. M. Aloisi, "Opioid-induced hypogonadism: why and how to treat it," *Pain Physician*, vol. 15, no. 3, supplement, pp. ES111–ES118, 2012.

14

Comparison of Dry Needling versus Orthopedic Manual Therapy in Patients with Myofascial Chronic Neck Pain

Irene Campa-Moran,[1] Etelvina Rey-Gudin,[1] Josué Fernández-Carnero,[2,3,4] Alba Paris-Alemany,[1,3,4,5] Alfonso Gil-Martinez,[1,3,4,5] Sergio Lerma Lara,[1,4,6] Almudena Prieto-Baquero,[7] José Luis Alonso-Perez,[7] and Roy La Touche[1,3,4,5]

[1] *Faculty of Health Science, Department of Physiotherapy, The Center for Advanced Studies University La Salle, Faculty of Health Science, The Autonomous University of Madrid, Aravaca, Madrid, Spain*
[2] *Department of Physical Therapy, Occupational Therapy, Rehabilitation and Physical Medicine, King Juan Carlos University, Alcorcón, Madrid, Spain*
[3] *Hospital La Paz Institute for Health Research, IdiPAZ, Madrid, Spain*
[4] *Motion in Brains Research Group, The Center for Advanced Studies University La Salle, The Autonomous University of Madrid, Spain*
[5] *Institute of Neuroscience and Craniofacial Pain (INDCRAN), Madrid, Spain*
[6] *Movement Analysis Laboratory, University Hospital Niño Jesus, Madrid, Spain*
[7] *Department of Physiotherapy, European University of Madrid, Villaviciosa de Odón, Madrid, Spain*

Correspondence should be addressed to Roy La Touche; roylatouche@yahoo.es

Academic Editor: Giustino Varrassi

Objective. The aim of this study was to compare the efficacy of three interventions for the treatment of myofascial chronic neck pain. *Methods.* Thirty-six patients were randomly assigned to one of three intervention groups: orthopedic manual therapy (OMT), dry needling and stretching (DN-S), and soft tissue techniques (STT). All groups received two treatment sessions with a 48 h time interval. Outcome measures included neck pain intensity measured using a visual analogue scale, cervical range of motion (ROM), pressure pain threshold for measuring mechanical hyperalgesia, and two self-reported questionnaires (neck disability index and pain catastrophizing scale). *Results.* The ANOVA revealed significant differences for the group × time interaction for neck disability, neck pain intensity, and pain catastrophizing. The DN-S and OMT groups reduced neck disability. Only the OMT group showed decreases in mechanical hyperalgesia and pain catastrophizing. The cervical ROM increased in OMT (i.e., flexion, side-bending, and rotation) and DN-S (i.e., side-bending and rotation) groups. *Conclusions.* The three interventions are all effective in reducing pain intensity. Reduction in mechanical hyperalgesia and pain catastrophizing was only observed in the OMT group. Cervical ROM improved in the DN-S and OMT groups and also neck disability being only clinically relevant for OMT group.

1. Introduction

Neck pain is one of the most frequent pain conditions; the prevalence of neck pain in the general population has been estimated between 10% and 15%, being more common in females than in males [1]. In a recent study, the prevalence of neck pain in the adult Spanish population has been estimated at 19.5% [2].

There have been many studies to determine the causes of neck pain, but there remains a lack of knowledge about the etiology of this condition. Myofascial pain (MP) is a common variety of such pain, usually caused by myofascial trigger points (MTrPs) [3]. The MTrPs in the neck muscles have been associated with a possible source of referred facial and cranial pain [3].

Myofascial trigger points (MTrPs) in the muscles of the neck and shoulder often coexist with neck pain conditions and can contribute to the symptoms [4]. Therefore, there is increasing evidence that MTrPs often play a role in the symptoms of patients with neck pain [5]. The muscle most often affected with the presence of MTrPs in the neck region is the trapezius muscle [6, 7], specifically the upper fibers, and this is the most hyperalgesic muscle of the neck and shoulder [8].

Active MTrPs are defined as hyperirritable spots within a taut band in skeletal muscles that are painful on compression and when stimulated (by digital compression or dry needling) can evoke a characteristic pattern of referred pain and related autonomic phenomena [3]. These findings are supported by other outcomes such as altered EMG activity, which has also been associated with chronic neck pain [9, 10]. In other recent studies, an altered motor control strategy of the trapezius muscle during isometric shoulder exercise has been reported [11].

Other major locations responsible for neck pain in patients are the articular zygapophysial joints (facet joints) [12]. Some studies have determined the prevalence of painful zygapophysial joints in patients with neck pain by blocking the medial branch of the spinal dorsal horn, with very positive results for the reduction of pain [12].

The majority of patients with chronic neck pain are treated in primary care by either medical intervention or physiotherapy [13]. Manual therapy, such as manipulation and mobilization, is frequently used for the treatment for neck pain and has great support in Cochrane reviews [14]. The preferred techniques for the treatment of articular origin pain are the manipulation or mobilization of the affected segments; the handling achieves a more immediate effect in reducing the pain, whereas the mobilization effect acts in the medium-to-long term [15, 16]. It has been shown that the mobilization has an effect on pain perception in patients with neck pain [17, 18]. Neurophysiologic effects have been demonstrated after mobilization techniques have been applied over the cervical spine [18]. However, a recent systematic review [14] reported that there is a lack of evidence to allow definitive conclusions about which groups of patients will benefit the most from what type of manual therapy technique (manipulation or mobilization) applied.

Many forms of treatment, such as ischemic compression [19, 20] and dry needling [21–24], have shown positive effects of reduction of pain intensity when they are applied at the MTrPs in the trapezius muscle of patients with neck pain. Furthermore, in a systematic review, it was concluded that the effect of injection therapies is likely to be due to the physical prick of the needle rather than to the type of substance injected [25].

Experts recommend that a multimodal approach must be investigated in patients with neck pain [26], because the clinical patterns of patients often do not respond to a single intervention, but they do with a multimodal approach. This is because, in real cases, patients with neck pain may present several disorders, and the symptoms of the patients therefore do not automatically respond to a single treatment.

In our investigation, a randomized clinical trial was designed to respond to three objectives: (1) to compare the efficacy of orthopedic manual therapy (OMT), dry needling, stretching (DN-S), and soft tissue techniques (STT) for the treatment of MTrP in patients with myofascial chronic neck pain, (2) to compare the treatment effects over disability and catastrophizing in patients with neck pain, and finally (3) to evaluate the likely neurophysiological effects produced by these techniques in the neck.

2. Materials and Methods

2.1. Research Design. A randomized, single-blind study design was used. An independent "blind" assessor made the measurements and registered the data. Patients were randomly allocated to one of three different intervention groups (DN-S group, STT group, and OMT group) performed by a computer-generated random-sequence table created before the start of the study with GraphPad software (GraphPad Software, Inc., CA 92037, USA).

2.2. Participants. Participants were recruited from the Public Valleagudo Primary Health Care Center in Coslada, Madrid, Spain. Patients with cervical pain of muscular origin were referred and screened for possible eligibility criteria. In this research we defined cervical pain as mechanical pain in the cervical muscles, which can be provoked both by maintained postures and by movements. Patients were selected if they met all of the following criteria: (a) bilateral pain involving the upper trapezius and elevator muscle of the scapula; (b) a duration of pain of at least 3 months; (c) a pain intensity corresponding to at least 20 mm on a 100 mm visual analogue scale (VAS); (d) neck pain with symptoms provoked by either neck postures or neck movement; (e) pain localized at least in the cervical and occipital regions but not in the orofacial region; (f) neck disability index (NDI) [27, 28] greater than or equal to 15 points; (g) restricted cervical range of movements (flexion, extension, rotation, and side-bending); (h) presence of bilateral MTrPs in upper trapezius and levator scapulae muscles. MTrPs were diagnosed according to the following criteria [29]: (1) presence of a palpable taut band in skeletal muscle, (2) presence of a hypersensitive tender spot within this taut band, and (3) reproduction of referred pain in response to MTrP compression. In order to meet the criteria to participate in the study, patients had to pass an initial physical examination performed by a single investigator to rule out the presence of nerve root compression. (i) Patients were between 18 and 75 years of age.

Patients were excluded if they presented any signs, symptoms, or history of the following diseases: (a) orofacial pain and temporomandibular disorders according to the Research Diagnostic Criteria of Temporomandibular Disorders (RDC/TMD); (b) a history of traumatic injuries (e.g., contusion, fracture, and whiplash injury); (c) systemic diseases such as fibromyalgia, systemic erythematous lupus, and psoriatic arthritis; (d) neurologic disorders (e.g., trigeminal neuralgia or occipital neuralgia); (e) concomitant medical diagnosis of any primary headache (tension type or migraine); (f) unilateral neck pain; (g) cervical spine surgery; (h) clinical diagnosis of cervical radiculopathy or myelopathy; (i) needle phobia; (j) history of previous physical therapy intervention for the cervical region.

Each participant received a thorough explanation about the content and purpose of the treatment before signing an informed consent form relative to the procedures. All of the procedures used in this study were planned under the ethical norms of the Helsinki Declaration and were approved by the local ethics committee.

2.3. Demographic and Clinical Data. Each of the eligible patients had to complete a basic questionnaire to determine if they met the criteria for inclusion or exclusion. This questionnaire included demographic data (gender, age, height, and weight), a body chart where patients had to mark the location of their pain, and several questions about their characteristics of their pain; for example, when did it start? How does it worsen or alleviate? What kind of pain is it?

2.4. Self-Report Questionnaires. The following questionnaires have been used to asses psychological and disability variables: the Spanish version of the Pain Catastrophizing Scale (PCS) [30, 31] was used to measure the catastrophic level associated with pain and the Spanish version of the NDI [27, 28] to measure perceived neck disability in order to quantify the psychophysical state of the patients. All patients included in the research had to complete all these questionnaires before the first intervention and a week after the last intervention (follow-up period).

2.4.1. Pain Catastrophizing. The PCS instructions ask participants to reflect on past painful experiences and to indicate the degree to which they experienced each of 13 thoughts or feelings (items) when experiencing pain. Items are scored on a 5-point scale with the end points "0" (not at all) and "4" (all the time). The PCS yields a total score ranging from 0 to 52. Three subscale scores can be obtained assessing rumination, magnification, and helplessness. The Spanish version of the PCS has been used in this research. It also showed appropriate internal consistency (Cronbach alpha = 0.79) and test-retest reliability (intraclass correlation coefficient = 0.84) [31].

2.4.2. Neck Disability Index (NDI). It consists of 10 items assessing different functional activities and uses a 6-point Likert scale ranging from 0 (no disability) to 5 (complete disability). The overall score (out of 100) is obtained by adding the score for each item and multiplying by 2. A higher score indicates greater pain and disability. The validated Spanish version was used in this study [27]. The minimum detectable change is 5 points out of 50, and it is recommended that 7 points is the minimum clinically important difference [32].

2.5. Outcome Measures. Outcome measures included neck pain intensity measured with VAS, the cervical range motion (ROM), and the pressure pain threshold (PPT) for measuring the mechanical hyperalgesia. Measurements were performed before the first treatment session (baseline), after the first session (post 1), after the second session (post 2), and one week after the last measurement (follow-up period).

2.5.1. Visual Analogue Scale (VAS). A VAS was used to measure pain intensity before and after each treatment. The VAS comprises a 100 mm horizontal line from 0 mm representing "no pain" to 100 mm representing "pain as bad as you can imagine". The patient placed a mark on the line at the point that they felt represented their intensity at the time, which was quantified by the assessor in mm. This scale has proven its reliability and validity for the measurement of pain intensity [33].

2.5.2. Pressure Pain Threshold (PPT). PPT is defined as the minimum amount of pressure needed to provoke a pain sensation [34]. We used a digital algometer (Model FDX 10, Wagner Instruments, Greenwich, CT, USA) that consists of a rubber head (1 cm^2) attached to a pressure gauge which measures in kg, with thresholds expressed in kg/cm^2. The protocol was a sequence of three measurements, with an interval of 30 seconds between each. The average of the three outcomes was calculated in order to obtain only one value for all the measured points in each of the assessments. This algometric method has a high reliability (ICC = 0.91, IC of 95%: 0.82–0.97) for PPT measurement. PPT were assessed at one point in the C5 zygapophysial joint and upper trapezius, all of them bilaterally. The device was applied perpendicular to the skin. The patients were asked to raise their hand at the moment the pressure started to change to a pain sensation, at which point the assessor stopped applying pressure. This sequence was performed three times. Anatomic references for the algometric measurements were C5 zygapophysial joint: 2 cm lateral to the spinous process of C6; trapezius muscle: 2.5 cm above the superior medial angle of the scapula.

2.5.3. Cervical Range of Motion (CROM). Cervical ROM was measured with a cervical goniometer called a CROM. This device has three inclinometers, one at each plane of movement. A plastic glasses-like support houses two of the inclinometers which allows the measurement of flexion, extension, and side-bending of the neck. Adding another part of the device with the third inclinometer and the magnets around the neck allows rotations to be measured. The subjects were instructed to sit upright, relax their shoulders, and rest their hands on their thighs, with hips and knees flexed at 90°. Different verbal commands were given to the subjects to perform the neck movements properly. For flexion, "bring your chin downwards and then tilt your head forwards as far as possible"; for extension, "bring your chin up and then tilt your head backward as far as possible"; for side-bending, "bring your ear toward your shoulder as far as possible, maintaining your face to the front and not moving your shoulder"; for rotations, "turn your head to the side without moving your shoulders". All movements had to be done without pain. In some of the subjects the movement had to be hand-guided to achieve a proper movement. This procedure has demonstrated its reliability in patients with neck pain [35].

2.6. Procedure. Once the subjects went through the final assessment and were included in the research, a randomization into three groups was performed. The DN-S group received dry needling and stretching; the STT group received soft tissue techniques treatment focused on the muscle; the

OMT group received an OMT focused in joints and nerves. All groups received two treatment sessions, with a 48 h interval between them.

2.6.1. DN-S Group. DN-S group received two treatments of bilateral dry needling on levator scapulae and upper trapezius muscles and a passive stretching technique. We chose those muscles because they are more affected in patients with neck pain [36]. The needling technique applied was performed according to the method of Hong et al. The needles used were 0.26 × 25 mm. The technique began with palpation of the active MTrP localizing the more sensitive taught band of the muscle. The needle was inserted in the direction of the taught band and perpendicular to the skin and was directed to the muscle MTrP until a first local twitch response was provoked. Then, the needle was inserted and withdrawn; the local twitch response was perceived by the therapist as a transient and involuntary contraction of the taut band. The needle insertions were repeated to achieve at least three local twitch responses. Then, the needle was withdrawn. The needling procedure at each MTrP lasted about 2 minutes. Once the needle was withdrawn, firm compression was exerted on the insertion site for 40 seconds to avoid excessive bleeding.

Following the needling procedure, a passive stretching to the levator scapulae and trapezius muscles was applied bilaterally for 20 seconds to each muscle.

2.6.2. STT Group. These patients received a bilateral OMT treatment based on the ischemic compression technique over both the levator scapulae and upper trapezius muscles, but also a dynamic soft tissue mobilization (DSTM) was applied on the upper trapezius for four minutes. For the ischemic compression technique, the physiotherapist (PT) applied gradually increasing pressure to the MTrP until the patient felt the sensation of pressure changed into pain; at that time the pressure was maintained until the discomfort eased, at which moment the pressure was increased until discomfort was again perceived by the patient. This process was repeated for 90 s while the patient was lying prone. This technique has been used in previous studies [19, 20].

The DSTM are a group of techniques used to treat the muscle, a direct stimulus over a specific region of the muscle (pressure, gliding pressure, etc.) added to stretching of the muscle or a mobilization of the closest joint or both together.

For group 2, a DSTM over the trapezius muscle was used. The patient was in lateral decubitus; the PT positioned one hand over the acromion and the other hand at the distal part of the upper trapezius. The technique consisted of performing a circular movement of the scapular belt while a slow gliding pressure was applied over the trapezius muscle in the direction to the occipital bone while the muscle was in a relaxed position. When the shoulder was depressed and therefore the muscle was stretched, nothing was performed over the muscle but the stretching itself. The technique was applied bilaterally for two minutes.

2.6.3. OMT Group. OMT group received an OMT protocol with a neural/joint approach, with three techniques: (1) anterior-posterior upper cervical mobilization (APUCM) with wedge (four min); (2) the cervical lateral glide mobilization technique at C4 and C5 (two min each side); and (3) neural thoracic mobilization with wedge (four min):

(1) APUCM: with the patient lying supine with a neutral position of the cervical spine, the wedge was positioned under the C2 spinous process. The PT held the occipital region of the patient with both hands to stabilize and maintain the position of the upper cervical structures, while with the anterior part of his shoulder applying a posteriorly directed force on the frontal region of the patient (anterior to posterior force). The mobilization was applied at a slow rate of one oscillation per two seconds (0.5 Hz) controlled with a digital metronome MA-30 (Korg Inc., Japan). The total time of mobilization was four minutes, applied for two intervals of two minutes each, with 30 seconds rest in between. This technique has been used in previous studies [37].

(2) Cervical lateral glide mobilization technique: with the patient in a supine position, the PT cradled the head and neck of the patient and, including the levels to be treated (C4-C5), performed a lateral translatory movement while minimizing gross cervical side flexion or rotation [38, 39], spending two min at each point and side and a total of eight min. This technique has been used in previous studies [38–40].

(3) Neural thoracic mobilization: patient was lying supine, with both knees in flexion and one leg crossed over the other, maintaining the knees together. A wedge is placed under the patient's back, with the upper side at T4-T5 level. The PT holds the head with the forearm in a craniocervical flexion and submaximal cervical flexion; the hand is placed under the spine at the mobilization level, to ensure the vertebrae are mobilizing. A towel is placed over the sternum of the patient and the other hand of the PT is placed over the towel to exert an anterior-posterior pressure. This is a dynamic technique; the patient is asked to extend the crossed leg without losing the knee-knee contact, and when the patient again flexed the knee, the PT applied the pressure over the sternum.

2.7. Statistical Analysis. Data were analyzed using the SPSS software package, version 19 (SPSS, Chicago, IL). Normal distribution was confirmed with the Shapiro-Wilk test ($P > 0.05$) for NDI, PCS, and VAS variables, so parametric statistics were used. Means and standard deviations were calculated for each variable. The baseline and demographic data at pretreatment were compared among groups using a one-way analysis of variance (ANOVA). A 2-way repeated measures ANOVA was performed to evaluate the effect in all the variables, with intervention (DN-S group 1, STT group 2, and OMT group 3) and time (before treatment, immediately after the first session, after the second session, and one week

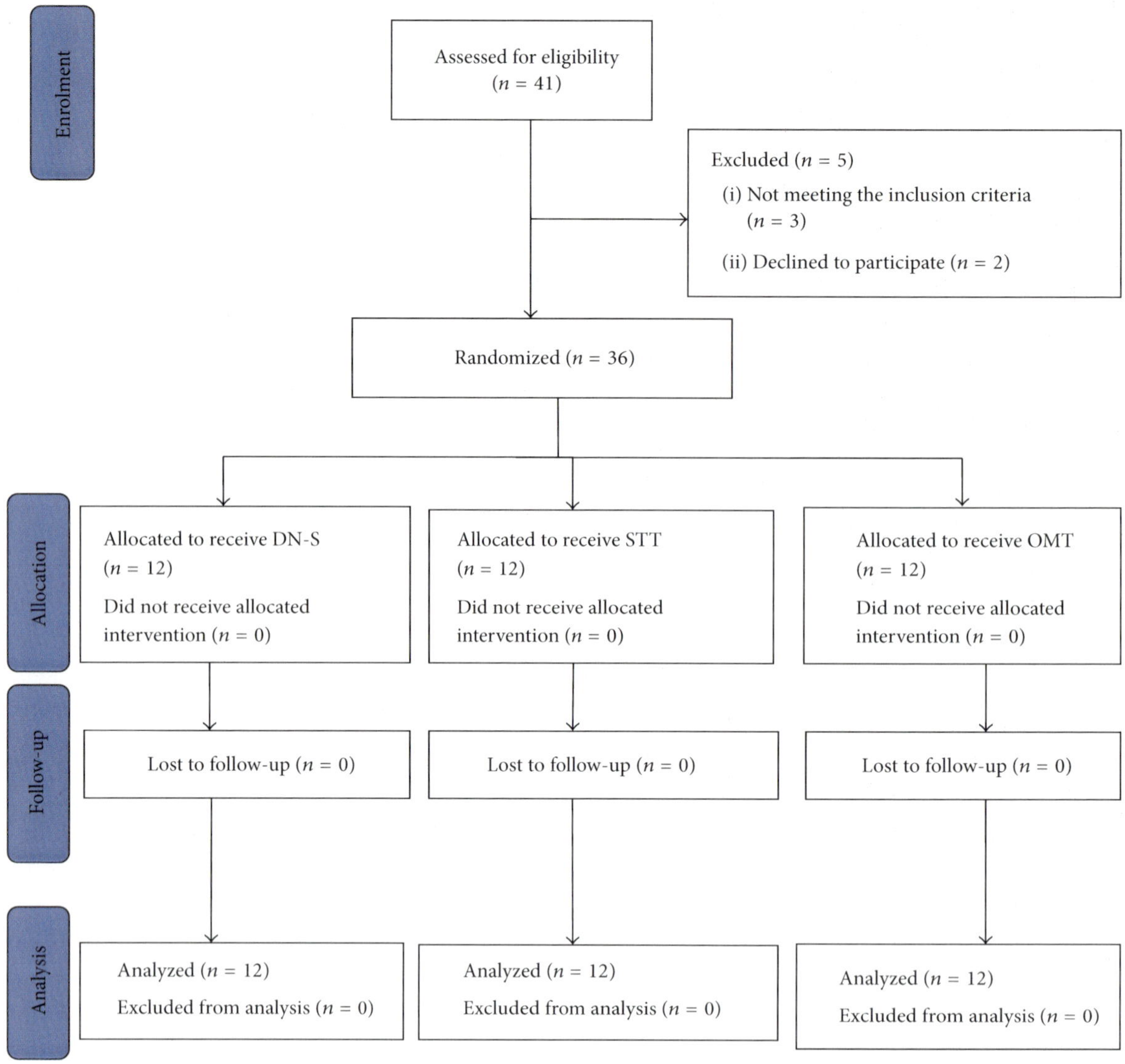

FIGURE 1: Flow fiagram.

after treatment) as factors. Tests of within-patients *post hoc* simple effects (i.e., changes in time for all variables for each group separately) were performed with Bonferroni corrections. Partial eta-squared (η_p^2) was calculated as a measure of effect size (strength of association) for each main effect and interaction in the ANOVAs, with 0.01–0.059 representing a small effect, 0.06–0.139 a medium effect, and > 0.14 a large effect [41].

The PPTs and CROM variables did not meet the normal distribution test, so nonparametric statistics were used. Descriptive statistics were used to summarize the data, including means and SDs, medians, and interquartile ranges (IQR) for continuous data. The Kruskal-Wallis test was used for the analysis and was used to compare data among the three groups to baseline data. The Friedman test was used to analyze the change from the intragroup results, and the Wilcoxon signed rank test was used for *post hoc* intragroup comparisons. In all statistical comparisons, $P < 0.05$ was used as the criterion for statistical significance.

3. Results

Thirty-six patients (7 males and 29 females) with chronic mechanical neck pain, aged 18 to 73 years (mean 49.5 ± 13.05 years; mean height 160 ± 7 cm; mean weight 66 ± 13 kg), were included in this study and assigned to one of three groups (Figure 1). No significant differences were found between groups for age ($F = 1.19$, $P = 0.31$), height ($F = 0.6$, $P = 0.55$), weight ($F = 2.72$, $P = 0.08$), and NDI ($F = 0.19$, $P = 0.82$), and pain duration ($F = 2.1$, $P = 0.13$). However, significant differences between groups appeared for pain intensity ($F = 3.38$, $P = 0.04$). Demographic and clinical data for each group are detailed in Table 1. There were no subject drop-outs during the different phases of the study, and

Table 1: Demographic and clinical data of three groups at the beginning of the study.

	DN-S group $N = 12$	STT group $N = 12$	OMT group $N = 12$	P value
Gender (male/female)	3/9	2/10	2/10	0.83
Age (years)	53.9 ± 12.7 (45.8 to 62)	45.8 ± 15.4 (36 to 55.6)	48.7 ± 10.2 (42.2 to 55.2)	0.31
Height (cm)	159.1 ± 7.4 (154.4 to 163.9)	160.8 ± 8.2 (154.4 to 163.9)	162.5 ± 6.9 (158.1 to 167)	0.52
Weight (kg)	71.1 ± 8.3 (65.8 to 76.4)	69.5 ± 17.3 (58.5 to 80.5)	60.1 ± 9.8 (53.8 to 66.4)	0.08
PCS	19.25 ± 6.48 (15.13 to 23.36)	17.50 ± 4.58 (14.58 to 20.41)	18.33 ± 4.27 (15.61 to 21.04)	0.71
NDI (points)	17.5 ± 5.5 (14 to 21.1)	17.5 ± 4.5 (14.6 to 20.3)	18.9 ± 3.4 (16.7 to 21)	0.69
Pain duration (months)	10.0 ± 2.9 (8.2 to 11.9)	11.8 ± 4.4 (9 to 14.6)	14.0 ± 3.6 (11.7 to 15.4)	0.12
Pain intensity (VAS)	33.8 ± 11.7 (26.3 to 41.3)	50.2 ± 17.6 (39 to 61.4)	42.1 ± 16.2 (31.8 to 52.5)	0.04*

Values are expressed as mean ± standard deviation (95% confidence interval). *$P < 0.05$.

Table 2: Comparison of changes in PSC and NDI over time for each treatment group.

Measure	Groups	Baseline mean (SD)	Follow-up mean (95% CI)	Follow-up versus baseline	
				Mean difference (95% CI)	P value
PSC	DN-S	19.2 ± 6.4	18.2 (15.3 to 21.1)	−1.0 (−3.6 to 1.6)	0.45
	STT	17.5 ± 4.5	16.4 (13.4 to 19.3)	−1.1 (−3.7 to 1.5)	0.41
	OMT	18.3 ± 4.2	13.1 (10.1 to 16.0)	−5.2 (−8.0 to −2.6)	0.001*
NDI	DN-S	18.0 ± 5.4	12.2 (8.6 to 15.6)	−5.8 (−9.1 to−2.5)	0.001*
	STT	17.4 ± 4.8	15.2 (11.6 to 18.7)	−2.2 (−5.5 to 1.0)	0.17
	OMT	18.5 ± 3.2	10.0 (6.5 to 13.5)	−8.6 (−11.8 to −5.2)	0.001*

PSC = pain catastrophizing scale, NDI = neck disability index, DN-S = dry needling + stretching, STT = soft tissue techniques, OMT = orthopedic manual therapy, and 95% CI = 95% confidence interval. *$P < 0.001$.

no adverse effects were registered after the application of the three treatments. None of the subjects started drug therapy during the lifetime of the study.

3.1. Self-Report Psychological Questionnaires: Catastrophizing and Neck Disability Outcomes. The ANOVA revealed significant differences for time factor ($F = 35.29$, $P < 0.000$; $\eta_p^2 = 0.51$) and for group × time interaction ($F = 3.84$, $P = 0.032$; $\eta_p^2 = 0.19$) for neck disability. Statistical descriptive data and *post hoc* results are represented in Table 2. For catastrophizing, differences were found for time factor ($F = 10.45$, $P = 0.003$; $\eta_p^2 = 0.24$) and for group × time interaction ($F = 3.44$, $P = 0.04$; $\eta_p^2 = 0.17$).

The *post hoc* analysis showed significant differences in the comparison between pretreatment and follow-up period ($P < 0.001$) for neck disability for groups 2 and 3. Descriptive data and *post hoc* results are shown in Table 2.

The *post hoc* analysis showed significant differences in the comparison between pretreatment and follow-up period ($P < 0.001$) for pain catastrophizing for group 3. Descriptive data and *post hoc* results are shown in Table 2.

3.2. Visual Analogue Scale. The ANOVA revealed that significant differences are present for time factor ($F = 25.8$, $P < 0.001$; $\eta_p^2 = 0.44$) and group × time interaction ($F = 5.0$, $P < 0.001$; $\eta_p^2 = 0.23$) regarding pain intensity. The *post hoc* analysis found significant differences between pretreatment, post 1, post 2, and follow-up data ($P < 0.05$) for pain intensity in group 2 and group 3 (Table 3). However, regarding group 1, differences were found in the comparisons of pretreatment with the follow-up period ($P = 0.001$), post 1 with follow-up period ($P < 0.001$), and post 2 with follow-up period ($P < 0.001$).

3.3. Pressure Pain Thresholds in the Cervical Region. In the Kruskal-Wallis test, differences were found for PPT in C5-C6 in post 1, post 2, and follow-up at two weeks ($P < 0.05$) and for PPT in trapezius muscle in the baseline, post 1, and follow-up at two weeks ($P < 0.05$). The Wilcoxon test showed significant differences for PPT in C5-C6 and PPT over trapezius outcomes when the baseline data were compared with post 1, post 2, and follow-up at two weeks for group OMT, but not for the groups DN-S and STT. The Friedman test showed that, in the group OMT, the PPT over C5-C6 and trapezius variables were found to be statistically significant ($P < 0.01$), but not for groups DN-S and STT. Comparisons between groups 1 and 3 at follow-up and between groups 2 and 3 in post 1, post 2, and the follow-up period for PPT over C5-C6 and between groups 1 and 2 at follow-up and between groups 2 and 3 in post 1, post 2, and follow-up period for PPT over trapezius were examined using the Mann-Whitney U test. The results for PPT are presented in Table 4.

3.4. Active Cervical Range of Motion Assessment. In the Kruskal-Wallis test, differences were found for flexion and

TABLE 3: Comparison of changes in VAS over time for each treatment group.

Measure	Groups	Baseline mean ± SD	Post 1 mean (95% CI)	Post 2 mean (95% CI)	Follow-up mean (95% CI)	Follow-up versus baseline Mean difference (95% CI)[b]	Follow-up versus baseline P value	Post 1 versus baseline Mean difference (95% CI)[b]	Post 1 versus baseline P value	Post 2 versus baseline Mean difference (95% CI)[b]	Post 2 versus baseline P value
VAS	DN-S	33.8 ± 11.7	39.7 (28.4 to 51.0)	36.0 (24.0 to 48.0)	13.3 (3.9 to 22.7)	20.5 (7.0 to 33.9)	0.001*	−5.9 (−5.9 to 17.7)	1.0	−2.1 (−14.1 to 18.4)	1.0
	STT	50.2 ± 17.7	38.2 (26.0 to 49.4)	30.1 (18.0 to 42.1)	34.3 (24.9 to 43.7)	15.9 (2.4 to 15.0)	0.001*	−12.0 (−23.9 to −0.2)	0.04*	−20.1 (−36.4 to −3.8)	0.01*
	OMT	42.1 ± 16.3	29.8 (18.5 to 41.1)	23.0 (10.8 to 35.0)	9.4 (0.03 to 18.8)	32.7 (19.3 to 46.2)	0.001*	−12.3 (−24.2 to −0.4)	0.03*	−19.2 (−35.5 to −3.0)	0.01*

VAS = visual analog scale, DN-S = dry needling + stretching, STT = soft tissue techniques, OMT = orthopedic manual therapy, and 95% CI = 95% confidence interval. * $P < 0.05$.
[b]Mean diff = difference among groups for the least squares mean (adjusted for baseline and missing data).

TABLE 4: Nonparametric tests of outcome data of pressure pain thresholds.

Variable	Groups	Median (interquartile range) Pressure pain thresholds (PPT) Baseline	Post 1	Post 2	Follow-up	Friedman ANOVA	Wilcoxon (a) Base versus post 1 (b) Base versus post 2 (c) Base versus follow-up
C5-C6	DN-S	2.34 (1.16–3.29)	2.42 (1.26–3.39)	2.88 (1.28–3.65)	2.09 (1.45–3.63)	0.545	(a) 0.721 (b) 0.182 (c) 0.695
	STT	2.19 (1.31–3.08)	1.74 (0.88–2.14)	1.57 (1.21–2.55)	2.25 (1.64–2.45)	0.058	(a) 0.239 (b) 0.480 (c) 0.638
	OMT	1.94 (1.44–2.19)	3.05 (2.16–4.37)	3.60 (2.59–3.74)	3.11 (2.81–3.92)	0.001	(a) 0.006 (b) 0.003 (c) 0.002
	K-W	0.612	0.008	0.019	0.011		
	Mann-Whitney *U* test						
	DN-S versus STT	0.729	0.073	0.166	0.908		
	DN-S versus OMT	0.354	0.224	0.325	0.043		
	STT versus OMT	0.487	0.002	0.003	0.002		
Trapezius	DN-S	3.13 (1.42–4.45)	3.20 (1.80–4.09)	3.52 (1.30–4.31)	2.85 (1.50–5.23)	0.682	(a) 0.937 (b) 0.638 (c) 0.239
	STT	2.19 (1.72–3.03)	1.84 (0.94–2.51)	1.78 (1.33–2.83)	2.49 (1.64–3.50)	0.117	(a) 0.530 (b) 0.814 (c) 0.583
	OMT	3.15 (1.62–3.24)	3.24 (2.95–4.28)	3.65 (3.21–3.68)	4.06 (3.75–4.38)	0.001	(a) 0.005 (b) 0.003 (c) 0.005
	K-W	0.453	0.008	0.072	0.012		
	Mann-Whitney *U* test						
	DN-S versus STT	0.355	0.050	0.326	0.488		
	DN-S versus OMT	0.524	0.297	0.885	0.057		
	STT versus OMT	0.247	0.002	0.005	0.003		

DN-S = dry needling + stretching, STT = soft tissue techniques, and OMT = orthopedic manual therapy.
K-W = Kruskal-Wallis test.

for extension in the follow-up at two weeks ($P < 0.05$). The Wilcoxon test showed significant differences for flexion outcomes when the baseline data were compared with follow-up at two weeks for group 1 and when the baseline data were compared with post 1, post 2, and follow-up at two weeks for group 3, but not for group 2 ($P < 0.05$). Significant differences were observed for side-bending outcomes when the baseline data were compared with post 2 and follow-up at 2 weeks for group 1 and when the baseline data were compared with post 2 for group 2, but not for group 3 ($P < 0.05$), and for rotation outcomes when the baseline data were compared with post 2 for group 1 and when the baseline data were compared with post 2 and with follow-up for group 3, but not for group 2 ($P < 0.05$). The Friedman test showed that, in group 3, the flexion was found to be statistically significant ($P < 0.01$), but not for groups 1 and 2, and, in groups 1 and 3, the side-bending and rotation were found to be statistically significant ($P < 0.01$), but not for group 2. In comparisons between groups 1 and 3 at post 2 and follow-up and between groups 2 and 3 in follow-up period for flexion, between groups 1 and 3 at post 2 and follow-up and between groups 2 and 3 in follow-up period for extension, and between groups 1 and 3 at post 2 for rotation, using the Mann-Whitney *U* test, the results for CROM are presented in Tables 5 and 6.

4. Discussion

In the present study all groups experienced a statistically significant improvement in neck pain intensity 1 week after intervention in patients with myofascial chronic neck pain. However, only the OMT and DN-S had an immediate effect reducing neck pain intensity after the first and second sessions. In addition, only the OMT group had a short term hypoalgesic effect for reducing the catastrophizing level and for increasing of CROM for flexion and extension, but not the DN-S and STT groups. The DN-S and OMT groups showed a short term effect reducing neck disability, but not the STT group. There were no differences in side-bending and rotation movements between groups, but the DN-S and OMT had an increase of range of motion higher than the STT group.

4.1. Neck Pain Intensity. The effects of pain reduction produced by the three groups were at their strongest two weeks

Table 5: Nonparametric tests of outcome data of cervical ROM (flexion and extension).

Variable	Groups	Median (interquartile range) Range of motion (ROM) in grades Baseline	Post 1	Post 2	Follow-up	Friedman ANOVA	Wilcoxon (a) Base versus post 1 (b) Base versus post 2 (c) Base versus follow-up
Flexion	DN-S	38.7 (35.6–40)	40 (30.2–49.37)	41.2 (37–46.9)	45 (40–49.4)	0.085	(a) 0.448 (b) 0.079 (c) 0.009
	STT	40.0 (30.6–49.4)	46.2 (35–58.1)	50 (32.2–56.9)	40.5 (32.5–50)	0.692	(a) 0.325 (b) 0.108 (c) 0.674
	OMT	40.0 (31.5–47.5)	45.7 (35–55)	50 (50–55)	52.5 (47.5–60)	0.017	(a) 0.031 (b) 0.007 (c) 0.008
	K-W	0.804	0.626	0.070	0.036		
	Mann-Whitney *U* test						
	DN-S versus STT	0.557	0.467	0.338	0.622		
	DN-S versus OMT	0.883	0.369	0.009	0.014		
	STT versus OMT	0.597	0.816	0.517	0.046		
Extension	DN-S	46.25 (33.7–51)	50.7 (40–59.4)	50 (40.2–59.7)	50 (41.7–60)	0.193	(a) 0.169 (b) 0.154 (c) 0.054
	STT	42.5 (27.5–60)	41.2 (30.6–50)	45 (40–58.7)	50 (45.6–50.7)	0.633	(a) 0.580 (b) 0.635 (c) 0.422
	OMT	48.75 (40–70)	50 (40–75)	62.5 (50–65)	60 (57.5–63.7)	0.846	(a) 0.526 (b) 0.477 (c) 0.074
	K-W	0.491	0.332	0.080	0.005		
	Mann-Whitney *U* test						
	DN-S versus STT	0.794	0.210	0.839	0.726		
	DN-S versus OMT	0.257	0.816	0.044	0.022		
	STT versus OMT	0.381	0.195	0.062	0.001		

DN-S = dry needling + stretching, STT = soft tissue techniques, and OMT = orthopedic manual therapy.
K-W = Kruskal-Wallis test.

after treatment (mean difference −20.5 mm, −15.9 mm, and −32.7 mm for DN-S, STT, and OMT, resp.) indicating that the changes are clinically relevant, since the magnitude of change of clinically important difference is established in 8.5 mm [42]. The pain reduction represents a change of 39.3% for the DN-S group, 68.3% for the STT group, and 89% for the OMT group. Changes of 30% or more are considered to be clinically meaningful improvements in spinal pain conditions [43]. The DN-S group started at a lower level of pain intensity than the others; this is why even though the mean difference at follow-up is greater than in the STT group, the percentage of pain reduction is the lowest of the three groups. The group of DN-S had more pain after the first session, although 15 days later the OMT and DN-S showed no differences. This could be because the local twist response is necessary to obtain positive effects producing pain and elicit referred pain. For that reason, patients in the DN-S group could have had more pain at the beginning of the treatment [44, 45].

Ay et al. did not find differences when comparing two groups (2 mL lidocaine 1% versus dry needling) for cervical spine pain on pain intensity at 4 and 12 weeks after the treatment [21]. Other studies showed similar results on pain intensity when they compared the effect 1 week, 4 weeks, and 12 weeks after one session of three different injections (dry needling versus lidocaine 0.5% versus botulinum toxin 10–20 U) in patients with myofascial pain syndrome and headache [46]. Previous studies treating patients with MTrPs in the neck region have reported pain relief after several sessions (between 5 and 6 sessions) of ischemic compression [47–49]. These outcomes agree with our study because we obtained similar differences (15.9 mm) in the STT group. However in a study in which ischemic compression was applied after a single session of lidocaine injection over MTrPs in patients with neck pain, the intensity improved to 42 mm one week after treatment [50], but that could be because drug injection was carried out.

4.2. Outcomes Related to Catastrophizing. In current study we have found that patients who received OMT have more improvement of catastrophizing than DN-S and soft tissue therapy. These are valuable findings because a previous study has reported that catastrophizing and disability are an important predictor of poor outcome in patients with neck pain treated by physical therapy [51]. In a prospective

TABLE 6: Nonparametric tests of outcome data of cervical ROM (side-bending and rotation).

Variable	Groups	Median (interquartile range) Range of motion (ROM) Baseline	Post 1	Post 2	Follow-up	Friedman ANOVA	Wilcoxon (a) Base versus post 1 (b) Base versus post 2 (c) Base versus follow-up
Side-bending	DN-S	66.2 (50–71.9)	62.2 (60–75.6)	70 (62.9–78.7)	70 (63.7–78.7)	0.005	(a) 0.858 (b) 0.028 (c) 0.014
	STT	75 (61.2–81.9)	72 (68.1–77.5)	80.5 (70–95.6)	70.5 (68.9–80.6)	0.062	(a) 0.724 (b) 0.008 (c) 0.637
	OMT	80.2 (60.1–80.5)	70 (70–72.5)	80.5 (70–86)	80 (70–95)	0.019	(a) 0.345 (b) 0.454 (c) 0.062
	K-W	0.318	0.238	0.270	0.182		
	Mann-Whitney *U* test						
	1 versus 2	0.154	0.098	0.104	0.663		
	1 versus 3	0.257	0.268	0.324	0.092		
	2 versus 3	0.543	0.597	0.602	0.154		
Rotation	DN-S	105 (88.1–116.9)	107.7 (92.5–122.5)	110.2 (89.9–129.4)	117.5 (96.2–131.9)	0.043	(a) 0.420 (b) 0.033 (c) 0.059
	STT	110 (102.5–123)	113.7 (106.2–120)	120 (110–129.6)	100 (87.5–120)	0.290	(a) 0.919 (b) 0.054 (c) 0.455
	OMT	110 (110–116.9)	120 (106.2–120)	129.5 (124–139.4)	120.7 (99.5–133.7)	0.000	(a) 0.279 (b) 0.002 (c) 0.033
	K-W						
	Mann-Whitney *U* test	0.586	0.605	0.092	0.191		
	1 versus 2	0.295	0.418	0.325	0.236		
	1 versus 3	0.598	0.447	0.040	0.664		
	2 versus 3	0.653	0.514	0.164	0.068		

DN-S = dry needling + stretching, STT = soft tissue techniques, and OMT = orthopedic manual therapy.
K-W = Kruskal-Wallis test.

cohort study, it was found that more complaints and catastrophizing showed an interaction with the success of the treatment, decreasing the OR for every point increase on the catastrophizing scale. Patients with higher catastrophizing levels were more likely to achieve treatment success with manual therapy but not with physiotherapy [52]. We obtained markedly reduced PCS values in the OMT group. However, this result should be treated with caution because we obtained a mean difference of 4.8, which is not clinically significant, as it should be at least a change of 9.1 points [53].

4.3. Disability. The neck disability improved significantly in the DN-S and OMT groups but not in the STT group. It has been suggested that the minimum clinically important difference required for NDI is 7 points [32, 54], although others have found higher values (10.2) for their patient population [55]. In our study, the DN-S group showed difference of 5.9 points, but the OMT group showed a higher score at 8.5 points. Nevertheless, soft tissue manual therapy group did not show statistical changes in disability. However, our results are in contrast to a recent study [50] which has reported that when ischemic compression is applied, but after lidocaine injection, it produces a statically significant decrease of disability after one week when compared with lidocaine injection only after a single intervention; the range of change was clinically relevant reaching 9.5 points of difference after treatment. According to the results obtained for the self-reported variables and pain intensity, the articular-neural approach would have a greater influence over the disability and catastrophizing of the patient than the other approaches.

4.4. Pressure Pain Threshold. Mechanical hypoalgesia was found over the C5-C6 level and trapezius muscle in the OMT group at post 1, post 2, and 1 week later, but not for the other two groups. The PPT results showed the minimal detectable change [56] which is defined between 0.45 Kg/cm^2 and 1.13 kg/cm^2, with 1.45 Kg/cm^2 for C5-C6 and 1.63 Kg/cm^2 for trapezius muscle. The OMT group increase was 76.7% for C5-C6 level and 63.9% for the trapezius muscle. These findings are higher than those noted in previous studies which were found to be between 22.55% [18] and 40%–56% [57]. These differences could be because in our study we designed a protocol with different techniques in manual therapy, and the others have only carried out one single technique. This indicates that hyperalgesia is decreased with the articular-neural approach (OMT) and no significant difference was observed with the other therapies. A specific and specialized physical therapy must be applied to obtain the best results in this kind of patient.

This indicates that cervical pain is decreased with the articular-neural approach and no significant difference is observed with the other therapies. Although in other studies, where the patients were instructed in self-treatment using ischemic compression for 5 days, they reported a change of 1.2 kg/cm^2, that value is considered clinically significant but is in contrast to our study for group 2. That difference could be explained because it related to different doses of treatment. In another study [49], where ischemic compression was applied, an increase of PPT of 0.79 kg/cm^2 was found, similar to our outcomes in the STT group. Nevertheless our results are in contrast to those of Kim et al. [50] who reported a statically significant increase of PPT after lidocaine injection (3 kg/cm^2) and ischemic compression versus lidocaine injection only (0.67 kg/cm^2) one week after [50].

In a recent study which compared one session of dry needling versus 10 sessions of physical therapy (superficial heat, TENS 25 min, ultrasound 5 min, and trapezius stretching), there were no statistically significant differences between the groups either one week or one month after in the pressure pain threshold [58]. Nevertheless, the pressure pain threshold of myofascial trigger point hyperalgesia improved in the OMT group. Our outcomes agree with previous studies of the group, where the patients improved on the PPT after eight sessions of IC [59]. However another study showed that PPTs in a group treated with IC were significantly greater than in an ultrasound and control group [48].

The exact mechanism by which manual therapy and dry needling modulate nociceptive information remains unknown. However, many algogenic substances and neuropeptides have been found where MTrPs occur, producing peripheral sensitization [60, 61], and neuroplastic changes in the dorsal horn soon appear when a MTrPS is developed [62]. A few studies have also found enhanced activity of brain areas of pain process when MTrPs are stimulated [63], suggesting that a central and peripheral sensitization is induced. The likely mechanism of OTM for pain relief is mean central nociceptive process. On the one hand, studies have demonstrated that manual therapy could activate inhibitory descending pain system and produce hypoalgesic effects, suggesting a mechanism mediated by the periaqueductal gray via serotoninergic and noradrenergic activation [64–67]. On the other hand, decreased temporal summation following NM is applied suggesting that the dorsal horn of the spinal cord could be involved in hypoalgesic effects in healthy patients [68, 69]. It has been suggested that facet and myofascial trigger point nociceptors could be connected in the spinal cord. Therefore if facet joint pain is eliminated, then the pain of myofascial trigger point can be relieved [16, 70, 71] but not vice versa (to our knowledge there has not been any study where the cervical facet joint pain can be controlled with a trigger point injection).

4.5. Cervical Range of Motion. There were statistically significant differences between groups in CROM for flexion and extension the OMT group being the one that increased more than the others at posttreatments (mean difference of 13° for flexion and 8.8° for extension). The range gained exceeded the minimal detectable change, which is established at 6.5° for flexion and 5.1° for extension [35].

This outcome agrees with other studies which compared efficacy of local anesthetic injection versus dry needling on the trapezius muscle; all groups improved at CROM in patients with myofascial pain syndrome at 4 weeks and 12 weeks after a single intervention [21].

A previous study where cervical facet joint injection was used in patients with cervical myofascial pain showed that patients who received facet injection improved in CROM and experienced reduced pain intensity during 1 year of follow-up. Other previous studies have found similar effects on myofascial pain syndrome when injection into muscles of the cervical region was carried out [71, 72]. Another study found that patients with myofascial trigger points in the cervical region improved after high velocity and low amplitude were applied to cervical spine [16].

In relation to the STT group, few studies have demonstrated an increase in ROM after a single or several sessions of ischemic compression [49, 73, 74]. Cagnie et al. [59] reported that the patients treated with IC resulted in a significant improvement in flexion, extension, and side-bending immediately after eight sessions.

However, the results of this study support the results of the OMT group because joint mobilization techniques improve the pain in patients with myofascial pain syndrome [70].

In observational studies it has been reported that active MTrPs are more common in patients with cervical root compression than in healthy controls (51.2% of the patients with cervical radiculopathy). These findings suggest to us that neural pain could be involved in the MTrPs, and for this reason in our study the patients who received neural mobilization techniques can show an improvement of the outcomes. The muscle which is most frequently involved with active MTrPS was the levator scapula and the muscle more frequently involved with latent MTrPS was the upper trapezius; both muscles have been treated in the dry needling group [75].

One possible explanation of the effects of the OMT on cervical joints is that cervical facet joints are innervated by the medial branch of the posterior rami of the cervical root. When the facet joint is in disorder, the facet nociceptors transmit input to the spinal cord, and in the spinal cord other neurons can be involved; this is the underlying mechanism to explain the referred muscle pain.

4.6. Limitations. There are several limitations that must be taken into account in this current study. The data obtained at this research are preliminary outcomes and they are useful to calculate the sample size for future research. In order to extrapolate accurate and representative results of a future clinical trial on patients with myofascial chronic neck pain, the sample size should be of 108 patients. The necessary sample size was estimated using G*Power 3.1.7 for Windows (G*Power©, University of Dusseldorf, Germany) [76]. The sample size calculation was considered as a power calculation to detect between-group differences in the neck disability outcome measures. To obtain 95% statistical power (1-β error probability) with an α error level probability of 0.05, we used repeated-measured analysis of variance (ANOVA), within-between interaction, and an effect size of 0.19 to consider three groups and three measurements, generating a sample size of 30 patients per group (total simple size of 90 patients). Allowing a drop-out rate of 20% and aiming to increase the statistical power of the results, the simple size should be increased to at least 18 patients more, with a total simple size of 108 patients.

We did not include a placebo and a control group, so we are not able to know the influence of others factors like the natural evolution of the neck pain or any nonspecific effects of the treatment. However, it has been reported in the literature that manual therapy treatment is superior to a control group [14, 77] and DN is superior to a placebo, decreasing the pain in myofascial pain patients in the upper quadrant [78]. Only two sessions were applied to patients, and in clinical practice more sessions are provided; thus more sessions should be included in future studies. We only collected data for a short follow-up of 1 week; perhaps a longer follow-up time could change the course of evolution. In spite of attempts to assess the changes of catastrophizing, many other psychological variables may be assessed such as depression, anxiety, or kinesiophobia because these are involved in chronic neck pain. Only two muscles were treated in DN-S and STT groups, but myofascial trigger points of other muscles are involved with symptoms in patients with chronic neck pain. Future studies should continue to evaluate the effectiveness of various therapies in patients suffering myofascial chronic neck pain with long-term follow-up periods, including placebo and a control group. Data of the neck pain intensity should be taken with caution because the study started with a significant difference between groups at the VAS baseline outcomes.

5. Conclusions

The results showed that all groups experienced an improvement in neck pain intensity in the follow-up period. However, only OMT and SST had an immediate effect on reducing neck pain intensity after the first session and second session. The OMT techniques decreased mechanical hyperalgesia and pain catastrophizing and increased the cervical ROM in patients with cervical myofascial pain syndrome. In addition, the DN-S and OMT approaches showed a short term effect reducing neck disability, but only the reduction of disability in the OMT group can be considered clinically relevant.

References

[1] J. A. J. Borghouts, B. W. Koes, H. Vondeling, and L. M. Bouter, "Cost-of-illness of neck pain in The Netherlands in 1996," *Pain*, vol. 80, no. 3, pp. 629–636, 1999.

[2] C. Fernández-de-las-Peñas, V. Hernández-Barrera, C. Alonso-Blanco et al., "Prevalence of neck and low back pain in community-dwelling adults in Spain: a population-based national study," *Spine*, vol. 36, no. 3, pp. E213–E219, 2011.

[3] D. G. Simons and J. S. L. Travell, *Myofascial Pain and Dysfunction: The Trigger Point Manual*, vol. 1, Lippincott Williams & Wilkins, Baltimore, Md, USA, 1999.

[4] S. Muñoz-Muñoz, M. T. Muñoz-García, F. Alburquerque-Sendín, M. Arroyo-Morales, and C. Fernández-De-Las-Peñas, "Myofascial trigger points, pain, disability, and sleep quality in individuals with mechanical neck pain," *Journal of Manipulative and Physiological Therapeutics*, vol. 35, no. 8, pp. 608–613, 2012.

[5] C. Fernández-de-las-Peñas, C. Alonso-Blanco, and J. C. Miangolarra, "Myofascial trigger points in subjects presenting with mechanical neck pain: a blinded, controlled study," *Manual Therapy*, vol. 12, no. 1, pp. 29–33, 2007.

[6] V. M. Sciotti, V. L. Mittak, L. DiMarco et al., "Clinical precision of myofascial trigger point location in the trapezius muscle," *Pain*, vol. 93, no. 3, pp. 259–266, 2001.

[7] A. L. Meleger and L. S. Krivickas, "Neck and back pain: musculoskeletal disorders," *Neurologic Clinics*, vol. 25, no. 2, pp. 419–438, 2007.

[8] A. A. Fischer, "Pressure algometry over normal muscles. Standard values, validity and reproducibility of pressure threshold," *Pain*, vol. 30, no. 1, pp. 115–126, 1987.

[9] D. L. Falla, G. A. Jull, and P. W. Hodges, "Patients with neck pain demonstrate reduced electromyographic activity of the deep cervical flexor muscles during performance of the craniocervical flexion test," *Spine*, vol. 29, no. 19, pp. 2108–2114, 2004.

[10] D. Falla, G. Jull, and P. W. Hodges, "Feedforward activity of the cervical flexor muscles during voluntary arm movements is delayed in chronic neck pain," *Experimental Brain Research*, vol. 157, no. 1, pp. 43–48, 2004.

[11] E. Zakharova-Luneva, G. Jull, V. Johnston, and S. O'Leary, "Altered trapezius muscle behavior in individuals with neck pain and clinical signs of scapular dysfunction," *Journal of Manipulative and Physiological Therapeutics*, vol. 35, no. 5, pp. 346–353, 2012.

[12] G. Cooper, B. Bailey, and N. Bogduk, "Cervical zygapophysial joint pain maps," *Pain Medicine*, vol. 8, no. 4, pp. 344–353, 2007.

[13] C. J. Vos, A. P. Verhagen, J. Passchier, and B. W. Koes, "Management of acute neck pain in general practice: a prospective study," *British Journal of General Practice*, vol. 57, no. 534, pp. 23–28, 2007.

[14] A. Gross, J. Miller, J. D'Sylva et al., "Manipulation or mobilisation for neck pain: a cochrane review," *Manual Therapy*, vol. 15, no. 4, pp. 315–333, 2010.

[15] J. D. Cassidy, A. A. Lopes, and K. Yong-Hing, "The immediate effect of manipulation versus mobilization on pain and range of motion in the cervical spine: a randomized controlled trial," *Journal of Manipulative and Physiological Therapeutics*, vol. 15, no. 9, pp. 570–575, 1992.

[16] R. Martínez-Segura, C. Fernández-de-las-Peñas, M. Ruiz-Sáez, C. López-Jiménez, and C. Rodríguez-Blanco, "Immediate effects on neck pain and active range of motion after a single

cervical high-velocity low-amplitude manipulation in subjects presenting with mechanical neck pain: a randomized controlled trial," *Journal of Manipulative and Physiological Therapeutics*, vol. 29, no. 7, pp. 511–517, 2006.

[17] A. Schmid, F. Brunner, A. Wright, and L. M. Bachmann, "Paradigm shift in manual therapy? Evidence for a central nervous system component in the response to passive cervical joint mobilisation," *Manual Therapy*, vol. 13, no. 5, pp. 387–396, 2008.

[18] M. Sterling, G. Jull, and A. Wright, "Cervical mobilisation: concurrent effects on pain, sympathetic nervous system activity and motor activity," *Manual Therapy*, vol. 6, no. 2, pp. 72–81, 2001.

[19] F. J. Montañez-Aguilera, N. Valtueña-Gimeno, D. Pecos-Martín, R. Arnau-Masanet, C. Barrios-Pitarque, and F. Bosch-Morell, "Changes in a patient with neck pain after application of ischemic compression as a trigger point therapy," *Journal of Back and Musculoskeletal Rehabilitation*, vol. 23, no. 2, pp. 101–104, 2010.

[20] F. J. M. Aguilera, D. P. Martín, R. A. Masanet, A. C. Botella, L. B. Soler, and F. B. Morell, "Immediate effect of ultrasound and ischemic compression techniques for the treatment of trapezius latent myofascial trigger points in healthy subjects: a randomized controlle," *Journal of Manipulative and Physiological Therapeutics*, vol. 32, no. 7, pp. 515–520, 2009.

[21] S. Ay, D. Evcik, and B. S. Tur, "Comparison of injection methods in myofascial pain syndrome: a randomized controlled trial," *Clinical Rheumatology*, vol. 29, no. 1, pp. 19–23, 2010.

[22] A. Kamanli, A. Kaya, O. Ardicoglu, S. Ozgocmen, F. O. Zengin, and Y. Bayik, "Comparison of lidocaine injection, botulinum toxin injection, and dry needling to trigger points in myofascial pain syndrome," *Rheumatology International*, vol. 25, no. 8, pp. 604–611, 2005.

[23] P. Peloso, A. Gross, T. Haines, K. Trinh, C. H. Goldsmith, and S. Burnie, "Medicinal and injection therapies for mechanical neck disorders," *Cochrane Database of Systematic Reviews*, no. 3, Article ID CD000319, 2007.

[24] A. Venâncio Rde, F. G. PJ. Alencar, and C. Zamperini, "Different substances and dry-needling injections in patients with myofascial pain and headaches," *Cranio*, vol. 26, no. 2, pp. 96–103, 2008.

[25] T. M. Cummings and A. R. White, "Needling therapies in the management of myofascial trigger point pain: a systematic review," *Archives of Physical Medicine and Rehabilitation*, vol. 82, pp. 986–992, 2001.

[26] G. Jull and A. Moore, "Systematic reviews assessing multimodal treatments," *Manual Therapy*, vol. 15, no. 4, pp. 303–304, 2010.

[27] J. A. Andrade Ortega, A. D. Delgado Martínez, and R. Almécija Ruiz, "Validation of the Spanish version of the neck disability index," *Spine*, vol. 35, no. 4, pp. E114–E118, 2010.

[28] H. Vernon and S. Mior, "The neck disability index: a study of reliability and validity," *Journal of Manipulative and Physiological Therapeutics*, vol. 14, no. 7, pp. 409–415, 1991.

[29] D. Simons, J. Travell, and L. Simons, *Myofascial Pain and Dysfunction: The Trigger Point Manual*, vol. 1, Lippincott Williams & Wilkins, Baltimore, Md, USA, 2nd edition, 1999.

[30] M. J. L. Sullivan, S. R. Bishop, and J. Pivik, "The pain catastrophizing scale: development and validation," *Psychological Assessment*, vol. 7, no. 4, pp. 524–532, 1995.

[31] J. García Campayo, B. Rodero, M. Alda, N. Sobradiel, J. Montero, and S. Moreno, "Validation of the Spanish version of the Pain Catastrophizing Scale in fibromyalgia," *Medicina Clinica*, vol. 131, no. 13, pp. 487–492, 2008.

[32] J. C. MacDermid, D. M. Walton, S. Avery et al., "Measurement properties of the neck disability index: a systematic review," *Journal of Orthopaedic & Sports Physical Therapy*, vol. 39, no. 5, pp. 400–417, 2009.

[33] P. E. Bijur, W. Silver, and E. J. Gallagher, "Reliability of the visual analog scale for measurement of acute pain," *Academic Emergency Medicine*, vol. 8, no. 12, pp. 1153–1157, 2001.

[34] P. Svensson, L. Arendt-Nielsen, H. Nielsen, and J. K. Larsen, "Effect of chronic and experimental jaw muscle pain on pain-pressure thresholds and stimulus-response curves," *Journal of Orofacial Pain*, vol. 9, no. 4, pp. 347–356, 1995.

[35] I. Audette, J.-P. Dumas, J. N. Côté, and S. J. De Serres, "Validity and between-day reliability of the cervical range of motion (CROM) device," *Journal of Orthopaedic and Sports Physical Therapy*, vol. 40, no. 5, pp. 318–323, 2010.

[36] D. G. Simons, "Review of enigmatic MTrPs as a common cause of enigmatic musculoskeletal pain and dysfunction," *Journal of Electromyography and Kinesiology*, vol. 14, no. 1, pp. 95–107, 2004.

[37] R. La Touche, A. París-Alemany, J. S. Mannheimer et al., "Does mobilization of the upper cervical spine affect pain sensitivity and autonomic nervous system function in patients with cervico-craniofacial pain?: a randomized-controlled trial," *The Clinical Journal of Pain*, vol. 29, no. 3, pp. 205–215, 2013.

[38] M. W. Coppieters, K. H. Stappaerts, L. L. Wouters, and K. Janssens, "The immediate effects of a cervical lateral glide treatment technique in patients with neurogenic cervicobrachial pain," *Journal of Orthopaedic and Sports Physical Therapy*, vol. 33, no. 7, pp. 369–378, 2003.

[39] B. Vicenzino, R. Neal, D. Collins, and A. Wright, "The displacement, velocity and frequency profile of the frontal plane motion produced by the cervical lateral glide treatment technique," *Clinical Biomechanics*, vol. 14, no. 8, pp. 515–521, 1999.

[40] I. M. Cowell and D. R. Phillips, "Effectiveness of manipulative physiotherapy for the treatment of a neurogenic cervicobrachial pain syndrome: a single case study—experimental design," *Manual Therapy*, vol. 7, no. 1, pp. 31–38, 2002.

[41] J. Cohen, "Eta-squared and partial eta-squared in fixed factor anova designs," *Educational and Psychological Measurement*, vol. 33, no. 1, pp. 107–112, 1973.

[42] R. Emshoff, S. Bertram, and I. Emshoff, "Clinically important difference thresholds of the visual analog scale: a conceptual model for identifying meaningful intraindividual changes for pain intensity," *Pain*, vol. 152, no. 10, pp. 2277–2282, 2011.

[43] R. W. J. G. Ostelo, R. A. Deyo, P. Stratford et al., "Interpreting change scores for pain and functional status in low back pain: towards international consensus regarding minimal important change," *Spine*, vol. 33, no. 1, pp. 90–94, 2008.

[44] C.-Z. Hong, T.-S. Kuan, J.-T. Chen, and S.-M. Chen, "Referred pain elicited by palpation and by needling of myofascial trigger points: a comparison," *Archives of Physical Medicine and Rehabilitation*, vol. 78, no. 9, pp. 957–960, 1997.

[45] C.-Z. Hong, "Lidocaine injection versus dry needling to myofascial trigger point. The importance of the local twitch response," *American Journal of Physical Medicine & Rehabilitation*, vol. 73, no. 4, pp. 256–263, 1994.

[46] R. A. De Venancio, F. G. P. Alencar, and C. Zamperini, "Botulinum toxin, lidocaine, and dry-needling injections in patients with myofascial pain and headaches," *Cranio*, vol. 27, no. 1, pp. 46–53, 2009.

[47] W. P. Hanten, S. L. Olson, N. L. Butts, and A. L. Nowicki, "Effectiveness of a home program of ischemic pressure followed

by sustained stretch for treatment of myofascial trigger points," *Physical Therapy*, vol. 80, no. 10, pp. 997–1003, 2000.

[48] J. Sarrafzadeh, A. Ahmadi, and M. Yassin, "The effects of pressure release, phonophoresis of hydrocortisone, and ultrasound on upper trapezius latent myofascial trigger point," *Archives of Physical Medicine and Rehabilitation*, vol. 93, no. 1, pp. 72–77, 2012.

[49] C.-R. Hou, L.-C. Tsai, K.-F. Cheng, K.-C. Chung, and C.-Z. Hong, "Immediate effects of various physical therapeutic modalities on cervical myofascial pain and trigger-point sensitivity," *Archives of Physical Medicine and Rehabilitation*, vol. 83, no. 10, pp. 1406–1414, 2002.

[50] S. A. Kim, K. Y. Oh, W. H. Choi, and I. K. Kim, "Ischemic compression after trigger point injection affect the treatment of myofascial trigger points," *Annals of Rehabilitation Medicine*, vol. 37, no. 4, pp. 541–546, 2013.

[51] J. C. Hill, M. Lewis, J. Sim, E. M. Hay, and K. Dziedzic, "Predictors of poor outcome in patients with neck pain treated by physical therapy," *Clinical Journal of Pain*, vol. 23, no. 8, pp. 683–690, 2007.

[52] A. P. Verhagen, C. H. Karels, J. M. Schellingerhout, S. P. Willemsen, B. W. Koes, and S. M. A. Bierma-Zeinstra, "Pain severity and catastrophising modify treatment success in neck pain patients in primary care," *Manual Therapy*, vol. 15, no. 3, pp. 267–272, 2010.

[53] S. Z. George, C. Valencia, and J. M. Beneciuk, "A psychometric investigation of fear-avoidance model measures in patients with chronic low back pain," *Journal of Orthopaedic and Sports Physical Therapy*, vol. 40, no. 4, pp. 197–205, 2010.

[54] B. A. Young, M. J. Walker, J. B. Strunce, R. E. Boyles, J. M. Whitman, and J. D. Childs, "Responsiveness of the neck disability index in patients with mechanical neck disorders," *Spine Journal*, vol. 9, no. 10, pp. 802–808, 2009.

[55] J. A. Cleland, J. D. Childs, and J. M. Whitman, "Psychometric properties of the neck disability index and numeric pain rating scale in patients with mechanical neck pain," *Archives of Physical Medicine and Rehabilitation*, vol. 89, no. 1, pp. 69–74, 2008.

[56] D. M. Walton, J. C. Macdermid, W. Nielson, R. Teasell, M. Chiasson, and L. Brown, "Reliability, standard error, and minimum detectable change of clinical pressure pain threshold testing in people with and without acute neck pain," *Journal of Orthopaedic & Sports Physical Therapy*, vol. 41, no. 9, pp. 644–650, 2011.

[57] H. T. Vernon, P. Aker, S. Burns, S. Viljakaanen, and L. Short, "Pressure pain threshold evaluation of the effect of spinal manipulation in the treatment of chronic neck pain: a pilot study," *Journal of Manipulative and Physiological Therapeutics*, vol. 13, no. 1, pp. 13–16, 1990.

[58] S. M. Rayegani, M. Bayat, M. H. Bahrami, S. A. Raeissadat, and E. Kargozar, "Comparison of dry needling and physiotherapy in treatment of myofascial pain syndrome," *Clinical Rheumatology*, vol. 33, no. 6, pp. 859–864, 2014.

[59] B. Cagnie, V. Dewitte, I. Coppieters, J. Van Oosterwijck, A. Cools, and L. Danneels, "Effect of ischemic compression on trigger points in the neck and shoulder muscles in office workers: a cohort study," *Journal of Manipulative and Physiological Therapeutics*, vol. 36, no. 8, pp. 482–489, 2013.

[60] J. P. Shah, T. M. Phillips, J. V. Danoff, and L. H. Gerber, "An in vivo microanalytical technique for measuring the local biochemical milieu of human skeletal muscle," *Journal of Applied Physiology*, vol. 99, no. 5, pp. 1977–1984, 2005.

[61] J. P. Shah, J. V. Danoff, M. J. Desai et al., "Biochemicals associated with pain and inflammation are elevated in sites near to and remote from active myofascial trigger points," *Archives of Physical Medicine and Rehabilitation*, vol. 89, no. 1, pp. 16–23, 2008.

[62] T.-S. Kuan, C.-Z. Hong, J.-T. Chen, S. M. Chen, and C. H. Chien, "The spinal cord connections of the myofascial trigger spots," *European Journal of Pain*, vol. 11, no. 6, pp. 624–634, 2007.

[63] D. M. Niddam, R.-C. Chan, S.-H. Lee, T.-C. Yeh, and J.-C. Hsieh, "Central representation of hyperalgesia from myofascial trigger point," *NeuroImage*, vol. 39, no. 3, pp. 1299–1306, 2008.

[64] D. A. Skyba, R. Radhakrishnan, J. J. Rohlwing, A. Wright, and K. A. Sluka, "Joint manipulation reduces hyperalgesia by activation of monoamine receptors but not opioid or GABA receptors in the spinal cord," *Pain*, vol. 106, no. 1-2, pp. 159–168, 2003.

[65] A. Paungmali, S. O'Leary, T. Souvlis, and B. Vicenzino, "Naloxone fails to antagonize initial hypoalgesic effect of a manual therapy treatment for lateral epicondylalgia," *Journal of Manipulative and Physiological Therapeutics*, vol. 27, no. 3, pp. 180–185, 2004.

[66] B. Vicenzino, D. Collins, H. Benson, and A. Wright, "An investigation of the interrelationship between manipulative therapy-induced hypoalgesia and sympathoexcitation," *Journal of Manipulative and Physiological Therapeutics*, vol. 21, no. 7, pp. 448–453, 1998.

[67] A. Paungmali, B. Vicenzino, and M. Smith, "Hypoalgesia induced by elbow manipulation in lateral epicondylalgia does not exhibit tolerance," *Journal of Pain*, vol. 4, no. 8, pp. 448–454, 2003.

[68] J. M. Beneciuk, M. D. Bishop, and S. Z. George, "Effects of upper extremity neural mobilization on thermal pain sensitivity: a sham-controlled study in asymptomatic participants," *Journal of Orthopaedic and Sports Physical Therapy*, vol. 39, no. 6, pp. 428–438, 2009.

[69] J. E. Bialosky, M. D. Bishop, D. D. Price, M. E. Robinson, K. R. Vincent, and S. Z. George, "A randomized sham-controlled trial of a neurodynamic technique in the treatment of carpal tunnel syndrome," *Journal of Orthopaedic and Sports Physical Therapy*, vol. 39, no. 10, pp. 709–723, 2009.

[70] S.-C. Park and K.-H. Kim, "Effect of adding cervical facet joint injections in a multimodal treatment program for long-standing cervical myofascial pain syndrome with referral pain patterns of cervical facet joint syndrome," *Journal of Anesthesia*, vol. 26, no. 5, pp. 738–745, 2012.

[71] C.-T. Tsai, L.-F. Hsieh, T.-S. Kuan, M.-J. Kao, and C.-Z. Hong, "Injection in the cervical facet joint for shoulder pain with myofascial trigger points in the upper trapezius muscle," *Orthopedics*, vol. 32, no. 8, 2009.

[72] K.-H. Kim, S.-H. Choi, T.-K. Kim, S.-W. Shin, C.-H. Kim, and J.-I. Kim, "Cervical facet joint injections in the neck and shoulder pain," *Journal of Korean Medical Science*, vol. 20, no. 4, pp. 659–662, 2005.

[73] Y.-C. Lin, C.-H. Lai, W.-H. Chang, J.-C. Lin, and S.-W. Chou, "Immediate effects of ischemic compression on neck function in patients with cervicogenic cephalic syndrome," *Journal of Manipulative and Physiological Therapeutics*, vol. 35, no. 4, pp. 301–307, 2012.

[74] A. V. Nagrale, P. Glynn, A. Joshi, and G. Ramteke, "The efficacy of an integrated neuromuscular inhibition technique on upper trapezius trigger points in subjects with non-specific neck pain: a randomized controlled trial," *Journal of Manual and Manipulative Therapy*, vol. 18, no. 1, pp. 37–43, 2010.

[75] H. Sari, U. Akarirmak, and M. Uludag, "Active myofascial trigger points might be more frequent in patients with cervical radiculopathy," *European Journal of Physical and Rehabilitation Medicine*, vol. 48, no. 2, pp. 237–244, 2012.

[76] F. Faul, E. Erdfelder, A.-G. Lang, and A. Buchner, "G* Power 3: a flexible statistical power analysis program for the social, behavioral, and biomedical sciences," *Behavior Research Methods*, vol. 39, no. 2, pp. 175–191, 2007.

[77] J. Miller, A. Gross, J. D'Sylva et al., "Manual therapy and exercise for neck pain: a systematic review," *Manual Therapy*, vol. 15, no. 4, pp. 334–354, 2010.

[78] D. M. Kietrys, K. M. Palombaro, E. Azzaretto et al., "Effectiveness of dry needling for upper-quarter myofascial pain: a systematic review and meta-analysis," *Journal of Orthopaedic and Sports Physical Therapy*, vol. 43, no. 9, pp. 620–634, 2013.

15

Factors Related to Postoperative Pain Trajectories following Total Knee Arthroplasty: A Longitudinal Study of Patients Admitted to a Russian Orthopaedic Clinic

Nikolai Kornilov,[1] Maren Falch Lindberg,[2,3] Caryl Gay,[4,5] Alexander Saraev,[1] Taras Kuliaba,[6] Leiv Arne Rosseland,[7,8] Konstantin Muniz,[1] and Anners Lerdal[3,5]

[1]*Department of Knee Surgery N 17, Russian Research Institute of Traumatology and Orthopaedics n.a. R.R. Vreden, Saint Petersburg 195427, Russia*
[2]*Department of Surgery, Lovisenberg Diakonale Hospital, 0440 Oslo, Norway*
[3]*Department of Nursing Science, Institute of Health and Society, Faculty of Medicine, University of Oslo, 0318 Oslo, Norway*
[4]*Department of Family Health Care Nursing, University of California, San Francisco, CA 94143-0606, USA*
[5]*Department of Research and Development, Lovisenberg Diakonale Hospital, 0440 Oslo, Norway*
[6]*Department of Knee Surgery N 10, Russian Research Institute of Traumatology and Orthopaedics n.a. R.R. Vreden, Saint Petersburg 195427, Russia*
[7]*Department of Research and Development, Division of Emergencies and Critical Care, Oslo University Hospital, 0424 Oslo, Norway*
[8]*Institute of Clinical Medicine, University of Oslo, 0316 Oslo, Norway*

Correspondence should be addressed to Nikolai Kornilov; drkornilov@hotmail.com

Academic Editor: Giustino Varrassi

This study explores sociodemographic, clinical, and surgical factors in relation to pain trajectories during the first 3 days following total knee arthroplasty (TKA). 100 patients (mean age 63.5 ± 7.8 years and 93% female) consecutively admitted for uncomplicated primary TKA were prospectively included. Postoperative pain was assessed using pain diaries. Measures of preoperative pain, symptoms, daily functioning, quality of life, comorbidities, knee function, perioperative characteristics, and physical/biochemical parameters were also evaluated. All pain ratings decreased in the three days following surgery ($p < .001$) as well as the reported number of daily hours in moderate/severe pain ($p < .001$). Women reported more pain than men ($p = .009$). Pain trajectories did not differ by education, employment, cohabitation, or any patient clinical and biochemical characteristics but were significantly related to preoperative anxiety ($p = .029$). Patients reporting moderate/severe pain prior to surgery also reported more hours in moderate/severe pain on days 0–3 postoperatively ($p = .029$). Patients with surgeries longer than 90 min reported more hours of moderate/severe pain compared with patients who had shorter surgeries ($p = .008$), and similar results were observed for ratings of pain with activity ($p = .012$). In this sample, only female gender, higher levels of preoperative pain and anxiety, and longer surgical duration were associated with increased pain after TKA.

1. Introduction

Total knee arthroplasty (TKA) is known to be a very painful orthopedic procedure [1]. Despite the fact that individual surgical technique and corresponding amount of tissue damage are usually similar from case to case in uncomplicated primary TKA, the level of postoperative pain varies widely among patients [2]. About half of patients experience moderate or severe pain in the first days after surgery, and this pain may become even worse once rehabilitation is started [3, 4]. Effective pain control is therefore important for optimizing the rehabilitation process in order to achieve patient satisfaction with a good functional outcome as well as reduce hospitalization length and costs [5].

Surgeons try to reduce the tissue damage by shortening the length of skin, capsule, and extensor apparatus incisions, modifying the type of arthrotomy (e.g., quadriceps-sparing, minimidvastus, or subvastus approaches), reducing the amount of unnecessary soft-tissue releases, or optimizing tourniquet pressure and time [6]. In addition, various multimodal analgesic options have been developed and their different combinations are currently used in clinical practice [7, 8]: paracetamol, nonsteroidal anti-inflammatory drugs (NSAIDs), opioids, ketamine [9], alpha-2 adrenergic agonists [10], corticosteroids [11], gabapentinoids, local infiltration analgesia (LIA), prolonged epidural anesthesia, continuous or single-shot peripheral nerve blocks, and cryotherapy.

All of these options have established advantages and disadvantages both from clinical and economical points of view [12, 13], but consensus on what protocols are most beneficial among different patient subgroups is still lacking [14]. Despite the fact that modern multimodal approaches to analgesia have decreased the prevalence of persistent postsurgical pain after TKA, further improvement is necessary.

There is growing attention to cognitive and emotional patient characteristics that together with other multiple factors like age, gender, ethnicity, level of preoperative pain, and length of waiting time before the surgery may influence the amount of acute and chronic postoperative pain after knee replacement [15–17]. Negative psychological conditions like anxiety, depression, sleep disturbance, pain catastrophising, hypervigilance, and perceived injustice were found to be very important [18–22].

Thus, the aim of this study was to explore sociodemographic, clinical, and surgical factors in relation to pain trajectories during the first 3 postoperative days following total knee arthroplasty (TKA).

2. Materials and Methods

2.1. Patients and Study Procedures. This study is the first report from a prospective longitudinal study of pain, symptoms, and health-related quality of life in 100 consecutive Caucasian patients receiving total knee arthroplasty. The study was conducted at the Russian Research Institute of Traumatology and Orthopedics n.a. R.R. Vreden (Vreden's Institute) in St. Petersburg, Russia. The study was approved by the local Ethics Committee at Vreden's Institute. Informed written consent was obtained from all patients.

Patients admitted to Vreden's Institute for TKA were recruited for the study between April and September 2014. Patients were included if they were ≥18 years of age; were able to read, write, and understand Russian; and were scheduled for unilateral primary TKA. Patients were excluded if they underwent unicompartmental or revision surgery, had prior TKA on the contralateral knee, or had primary TKA complicated by one of the following conditions: extensive bone defects requiring substitution by graft or metal, collateral ligament insufficiency, frontal deformities over 30 degrees, hyperextension >15 degrees, fibrous or bony knee ankylosis, femur or tibia extra-articular deformities in more than one plane and over 10 degrees, extensor mechanism deficit, or hip fusion.

Patients received written information about the study on the day of admission. Patients were admitted to the hospital between 1 and 7 days prior to surgery depending on comorbidities. Patients who met the inclusion criteria were invited to participate by the senior surgeons (NK and TK) on the day of admission. After obtaining written informed consent, patients completed a questionnaire that assessed demographic characteristics, preoperative symptoms, and psychological factors. Preoperative pain was assessed the day before surgery, and acute postoperative pain was assessed using a 4-day pain diary, which was completed every evening starting on the day of surgery (Day 0) until postoperative Day 3. The completed questionnaires and the pain diary were collected by the junior surgeons (AS and KM).

2.2. Surgical, Anesthesiological, and Pain Management Procedures. The surgery, anesthesia, and postoperative pain management procedures were standardized. All patients received the primary cemented unconstrained posterior cruciate retaining or substituting implants for the TKA. A tourniquet was used during surgery in a minority of cases (21%). To avoid potential harm to the arterial or vein wall, tourniquet was not used in patients with comorbidities, such as varicose vein disease, atherosclerosis of peripheral arteries, diabetes, and other factors associated with increased risk of venous thromboembolism. Because the application of tourniquet within recommended pressure range is ineffective for patients with excessive subcutaneous fat in the middle of the thigh, tourniquet was also not used for obese patients. The low rate of tourniquet use was due to these contraindications. The less-invasive medial parapatellar approach was utilized in all patients without eversion or resurfacing of patella [23]. Drains were placed and removed on postoperative Day 1.

Neuraxial block with bupivacaine and sedation were used for anesthesia for all patients. Spinal anesthesia has been the method of choice for TKA patients in Vreden's Institute for the last two decades because it is safe, well tolerated by patients with comorbidities, and not only clinically effective, but cost-effective as well. In one patient, an incomplete effect of the spinal anesthesia was noticed, so general anesthesia was used as an adjunct because the patient refused a peripheral nerve blockade. Although prolonged epidural anesthesia was previously widely utilized in TKA patients during surgery and even for a few days after it, it is now rarely used at our institution for several reasons. First, the achieved block is more variable in strength and the failure rate of the technique may reach 28% [24]. Second, some patients experience muscle weakness that postpones early ambulation. Third, hypotension and urinary retention are additional concerns. The last but probably most important reason is that the use of direct anticoagulants in the postoperative period makes all our patients ineligible for this technique.

For postoperative pain management, all patients received an intramuscular (IM) injection of ketoprofen 100 mg 3 times per day until discharge from the clinic. If this did not provide adequate pain relief on the first day, the second line drug was a single IM injection of opiate trimeperidine (Promedol) (0.01 mg). On the second and third days, the second line drugs were tramadol (100 mg IM twice per day) or Zaldiar (1 pill every 6 hours). This has been the standard pain management at our institution for many years. All patients received a single intravenous injection of Dexamed (Dexamethasone) (8 mg) just before incision.

Mobilization and physical therapy were standardized. After surgery, patients spent several hours in the recovery room supervised by an anesthesiologist. Patients were then returned to the ward and remained in bed until the next morning when physical therapy was initiated. Beginning on postoperative Day 1, a physiotherapist mobilized the patients out of bed, assisted them with exercises, and helped them ambulate on crutches with partial weight bearing on the operated leg. During the following days, patients received daily physical therapy, which included ambulation as tolerated, and performed flexion and extension of the knee exercises two to three times daily. Most patients were discharged on postoperative Day 7.

2.3. Clinical and Perioperative Characteristics. Data on brand of implant, American Society of Anesthesiologists (ASA) physical status classification [25], length of surgery, tourniquet use, infections (i.e., deep prosthetic, wound), as well as comorbidities, preoperative blood pressure, hemoglobin, C-reactive protein, and creatinine levels were obtained from medical records. Data on anesthesia regimen and postoperative pain medications were obtained from patients' medical records.

2.4. Preoperative Pain

The Brief Pain Inventory (BPI). Patients' level of preoperative pain and its impact on function were assessed using the BPI [26]. The BPI consists of four items that measure pain intensity on a 0 to 10 numeric rating scale (NRS); one item that measures pain relief; a body map to assess pain locations; and seven items that measure interference with function. The Russian version of the BPI has well-established psychometric validity and reliability [27]. For this analysis, the level of average pain reported preoperatively was used to categorize those with moderate or severe pain (NRS ≥ 4) or severe pain (NRS ≥ 7).

2.5. Acute Postoperative Pain

Pain Diary. Patients rated their acute postoperative pain every evening starting on the day of surgery and continuing through Day 3. Six different aspects of pain were rated (i.e., worst, average, least, with activity, at rest, and duration), but this analysis emphasizes pain with activity and pain duration given their potential to impact physical rehabilitation [28]. Patients rated their pain using a 0 (no pain) to 10 (worst imaginable pain) NRS and estimated their pain duration as the number of hours in the prior 24 hours with moderate to severe pain (i.e., rated on the NRS as 4 or higher).

2.6. Symptom Measures. Several measures were used to assess patients' other symptoms. The 14-item Hospital Anxiety and Depression Scale (HADS) [29] was used to evaluate anxiety and depression in the past week; a score above 8 on either the anxiety or depression subscale is clinically significant. The Pittsburgh Sleep Quality Index was used to assess sleep disturbance in the past month, and scores above 5 are considered indicative of poor sleep. The 7-item Fatigue Severity Scale (FSS-7) [30] was used to evaluate fatigue interference during the past week. Total scores can range from 1 to 7 with higher scores indicating higher levels of interference. The FSS-7 has good psychometric properties among adults with a variety of medical conditions. For this study, the FSS was translated into Russian and its Cronbach's alpha was 0.93.

2.7. Functional Ability and Quality of Life Measures. The Knee Society Score (KSS) [31] and Function Score were used to assess the level of knee function. The Knee Score is based on 9 items, of which 3 assess patient-reported pain and 6 involve physiotherapist assessments of range of motion, stability, and alignment. The Function Score consists of 5 items assessing the patient's ability to walk (i.e., maximum distance and up and down stairs) and rise from a chair, as well as their use of support devices (i.e., cane, crutches, and walker). Both scores range 0–100, with higher scores indicating better knee function.

The Lawton Instrumental Activities of Daily Living (IADL) Scale [32] was used to assess patients' abilities to perform everyday tasks. The scale consists of 8 items assessing domains such as shopping, housekeeping, transportation, and finances. Mean substitution was used for up to two items the patient did not consider applicable to them, typically because someone else in the household managed that task. Total scores were considered missing when more than 2 items were not answered or were not considered applicable. Scores range 0–8, with higher scores indicating greater independence with activities of daily living.

The EQ-5D-3L [33] was used to assess patients' quality of life. The scale consists of 5 items assessing the following 5 domains: mobility, self-care, usual activities, pain/discomfort, and anxiety/depression. Each item is rated on a 3-point scale: no problems, some problems, extreme problems. In addition, a visual analogue scale (VAS) is used to assess the patient's self-rated health on a 0–100 scale, where 0 indicates "worst imaginable health state" and 100 indicates "best imaginable health state" [34]. Only the EQ VAS was used in this analysis, and scores of 80 and higher were considered indicative of good health-related quality of life.

2.8. Statistical Analyses. Descriptive statistics and frequency distributions were performed on the preoperative demographic and clinical sample characteristics. Independent sample t-tests and chi-squared tests were used to compare groups on continuous and categorical variables, respectively. Fisher's Exact Test was used instead of the chi-square test when expected cell frequencies were below 5. Repeated measures analysis of variance was used to evaluate the within-subjects effect of time evaluated at 4 points (i.e., Days 0–3) and various between-subjects effects (i.e., sociodemographic, clinical, and surgical factors). Table 1 presents a list of the proposed predictors that was developed based on a review of the literature on perioperative pain intensity in patients undergoing TKA [35–39]. For continuous measures without established cut-points, a median split was used to compare the pain trajectories of patients scoring relatively high and low. All analyses were conducted using SPSS version 22 (IBM, Armonk, NY). A p value of <.05 indicated statistical significance.

3. Results

3.1. Sample Characteristics. Of the 241 knee arthroplasty patients evaluated for inclusion in the study, 14 were not eligible because they had had prior knee replacement, 12 were transferred to other departments due to the necessity of other surgeries prior to the TKA, 23 were discharged prior to surgery due to severe comorbidities, and 92 declined to participate. The remaining 100 patients were enrolled in the study and are included in the analysis. Demographic, clinical, and surgical characteristics are summarized in Table 1. The sample was mostly female (93%) and had a mean age of 63.5 (±7.8) years.

3.2. Pain Trajectories. As shown in Table 2 and Figure 1, all pain ratings decreased in the three days following knee surgery (all main effects for time, $p < .001$). Similarly, the reported number of hours per day in moderate/severe pain (i.e., NRS ≥ 4) decreased over time ($p < .001$). Given the similar trajectories for the different pain ratings, subsequent analyses focus only on pain with activity as a measure of pain intensity and hours in moderate to severe pain as a measure of pain duration or burden.

3.3. Pain by Sociodemographic Characteristics. Women reported more pain than men across Days 0–3 (average pain ratings of 5.5 (SD 1.62) for women versus 3.8 (SD 1.34) for men, $p = .009$), but with only 7 men in the sample, this may not be a robust finding. Age had modest negative correlations (range of −0.20 to −0.25) with pain ratings on Days 1 and 2 but was not correlated with pain ratings on Day 0 or Day 3. Pain trajectories did not differ by education, employment, or cohabitation status.

3.4. Pain by Clinical Characteristics. Pain trajectories from the day of surgery through the first three postoperative days were largely unrelated to patient clinical characteristics. Pain ratings over time did not differ based on the patient's preoperative Knee Society Score, Function Score, their level of independence with activities of daily living, or their health-related quality of life. In addition, pain ratings did not differ based on patient ratings of preoperative sleep quality (PSQI), fatigue (FSS-7), or depression (HADS). However, pain ratings over time were significantly related to preoperative anxiety, with the patients who reported higher anxiety reporting more pain with activity, but only on the day of surgery, not on the subsequent three postoperative days (interaction of time and anxiety $p = .034$). As shown in Figure 2, anxious patients also reported more hours in moderate/severe pain, particularly on the day of surgery and first postoperative day (main effect for anxiety $p = .029$; interaction between anxiety and time, $p = .046$). Not surprisingly, patients who reported moderate to severe average pain *prior to surgery* also reported more hours in moderate to severe pain on Days 0–3 *postoperatively* ($p = .029$). However, preoperative average pain rating was unrelated to ratings of pain with activity on postoperative Days 0–3.

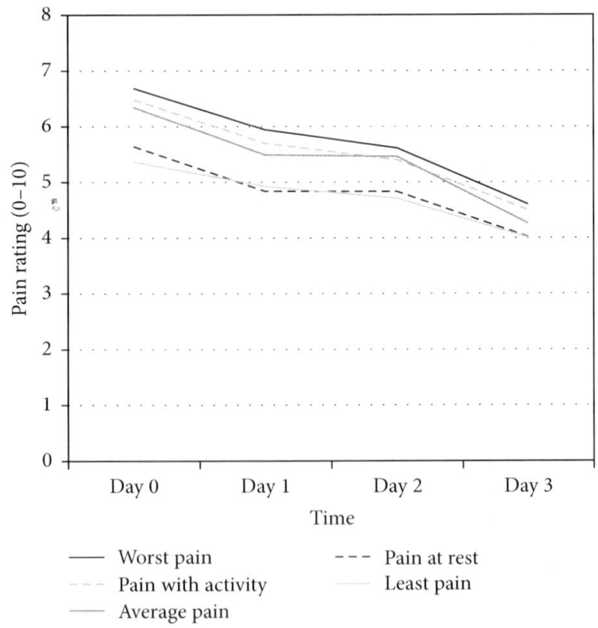

FIGURE 1: Pain severity ratings from day of knee replacement surgery (Day 0) through the third postoperative day. The five types of pain ratings all decreased in a similar pattern across the first three days after surgery (all main effects for time had $p < .001$). Hours in moderate to severe pain (NRS ≥ 4) are not included in the figure but showed a similar decreasing trend over time ($p < .001$).

3.5. Pain Management. All patients received spinal anesthesia and sedation, except one who received total intravenous anesthesia (TIVA). Excluding the one patient with TIVA did not alter any of the results. Medications administered to patients to manage postsurgical pain are summarized in Table 3. There was little variation in the medications administered on Days 1–3, and analysis of medication regimen on the day of surgery (Day 0) indicated no relationship to pain ratings. Dose information was not available for this analysis.

3.6. Pain by Surgical Characteristics

3.6.1. Surgery Duration. The mean surgery duration was 95.6 (SD 23.6) minutes, with a median of 90 minutes. A comparison of shorter (<90 minutes) and longer (>90 minutes) surgeries indicated that longer surgeries were associated with higher postoperative pain ratings. As shown in Figure 3, patients with longer surgeries reported consistently more hours per day of moderate/severe pain (NRS ≥ 4) compared with patients who had shorter surgeries ($p = .008$). Similar results were observed for ratings of pain with activity ($p = .012$).

Table 1: Sample Characteristics and their Relationship to Pain on Postoperative Days 0 to 3.

	Mean (SD)	% (n)	Relationships to pain severity in activity ($p < .10$)	Relationships to hours in moderate to severe pain ($p < .10$)
Demographic characteristics				
Age in years, (range 47–81)	63.5 (7.8)		None (using cutpoint of 65)	None (using cutpoint of 65)
Sex				
Male		7% (7)	Main effect for sex, $p = .052$ (more pain for females)	Interaction of sex and time, **p = .032** (more hours of pain for females)
Female		93% (93)		
Living situation				
Lives alone		18% (18)		
Lives with spouse		58% (58)	None	None
Lives with other(s)		24% (24)		
Education				
Less than high school		45% (45)	None	None
Completed high school		55% (55)		
Employment status				
Paid work or self-employed		24% (24)	None	None
No paid work or retired		76% (76)		
Preoperative clinical characteristics				
EQ VAS health-related quality of life (0–100 scale)	55.6 (15.6)		Main effect for EQ VAS, $p = .061$ (healthier patients reported slightly more pain)	None
<80		88% (88)		
Fatigue Severity Scale (1–7 scale)	3.17 (1.66)			
≥5		14% (14)	None (using cutpoint of either 4 or 5)	None (using cutpoint of either 4 or 5)
≥4		28% (28)		
Pittsburgh Sleep Quality Index	8.35 (3.50)		None (using cutpoint of 5)	None (using cutpoint of 5)
>5		73% (73)		
HADS Depression Subscale	6.12 (4.03)			
0–8 (none)		70% (70)		
9-10 (mild)		17% (17)	None	None
>10 (moderate/severe)		13% (13)		
HADS Anxiety Subscale	7.34 (4.18)			
0–8 (none)		61% (61)	Interaction of anxiety and time, **p = .034** (anxious patients reported more pain on day 0, but not after	Main effect of anxiety, **p = .029**; interaction of anxiety and time, **p = .046** (anxious patients had more hours of pain, particularly on days 0 and 1)
9-10 (mild)		20% (20)		
>10 (moderate/severe)		19% (19)		
BPI Average preoperative pain rating (0–10 scale)	4.76 (2.54)			Main effect for pre-operative pain ≥4, **p = .029** (patients with more pre-op pain reported more hours of post-op pain)
≥4 (moderate or severe pain)		67% (67)	None (using cutpoint of either 4 or 7)	
≥7 (severe pain)		24% (24)		
IADL (0–8 scale) ($n = 95$)[a]	6.43 (1.10)		None (median split at 6)	None (median split at 6)
KSS Knee Score (0–100 scale)	33.5 (20.3)		None (median split at 30)	None (median split at 30)
KSS Function score (0–100 scale)	45.2 (17.1)		None (median split at 44)	None (median split at 44)

Table 1: Continued.

	Mean (SD)	% (n)	Relationships to pain severity in activity ($p < .10$)	Relationships to hours in moderate to severe pain ($p < .10$)
Surgery characteristics				
Anesthesia				
Spinal/sedation		99% (99)	Not analyzed	Not analyzed
TIVA		1% (1)		
Surgery duration in minutes (range 50–210)	95.6 (23.6)		Main effect for surgery duration, **p = .012** (more pain for surgeries >90 minutes)	Main effect for surgery duration, **p = .008** (more hours of pain for surgeries >90 mins)
Implant type			None	Main effect for implant, $p = .060$ (common implants [first 2] had slightly less hours of pain than uncommon implants [last 3])
Sigma (DePuy Johnson & Johnson)		43% (43)		
AGC (Zimmer Biomet)		34% (34)		
LCS (DePuy Johnson & Johnson)		14% (14)		
Scorpio NRG (Stryker)		5% (5)		
NexGen (Zimmer Biomet)		4% (4)		
Tourniquet use		21% (21)	None	None
Bleeding (ml)	341.7 (183.2)		None	Main effect for bleeding, $p = .085$ (slightly more hours of pain for bleeding > 300 ml)
Hemoglobin (g/L)				
Females ($n = 93$)				
Pre-operative (% (n) < 120)	128.6 (12.0)	26% (24)	Main effect for preop Hgb, $p = .086$ (slightly more pain among patients with preop Hgb ≥ 120). When only women are included, **p = .039**. No effects for postop Hgb, but the numbers with normal postop Hgb were small.	Main effect for preop Hgb, $p = .071$ (slightly more hours of pain among patients with higher preop Hgb ≥ 120). When only women are included, **p = .045**. No effects for postop Hgb, but the numbers with normal postop Hgb were small.
Day 0 at 20:00 (% (n) < 120)	106.9 (11.7)	89% (83)		
Day 4 (% (n) < 120)	99.0 (13.4)	92% (86)		
Males ($n = 7$)				
Pre-operative (% (n) < 120)	139.1 (12.3)	0% (0)		
Day 0 at 20:00 (% (n) < 120)	110.1 (11.9)	71% (5)		
Day 4 (% (n) < 120)	106.4 (14.4)	86% (6)		
C-reactive protein, preoperative (mg/L)	4.07 (5.40)		None (split at 5)	None (split at 5)
≥5		24% (24)		
Creatinine, preoperative (mcmol/L)				
Female ($n = 93$) (% (n) < 44)	63.9 (16.5)	5% (5)	None (split at 44)	None (split at 44)
Males ($n = 7$) (% (n) < 44)	79.8 (15.7)	0% (0)		
Length of hospital stay in days				
Pre-operative	7.2 (4.1)		None (median split at 16)	None (median split at 16)
Post-operative	9.2 (2.4)			
Total	16.4 (4.3)			

Note. Relationships to pain were determined by including each variable as a between-subjects factor in a repeated measures analysis of pain in activity and hours in moderate/severe pain. Variables with gender differences were evaluated both with and without men.

[a]Five patients were missing IADL total score because they answered "does not apply" to more than 2 of the IADL items.

TABLE 2: Pain ratings on Days 0–3 after knee replacement surgery.

	Mean pain rating (SD)			
	Day 0	Day 1	Day 2	Day 3
Average pain	6.35 (2.35)	5.49 (2.11)	5.46 (2.20)	4.26 (1.86)
Least pain	5.37 (2.44)	4.93 (2.24)	4.71 (2.36)	4.01 (2.24)
Worst pain	6.69 (2.46)	5.94 (2.40)	5.61 (2.29)	4.60 (1.98)
Pain at rest	5.64 (2.20)	4.84 (2.20)	4.83 (2.09)	4.02 (2.14)
Pain with activity	6.49 (2.41)	5.70 (2.41)	5.40 (2.35)	4.50 (2.16)
Hours > NRS4	8.99 (6.69)	7.46 (5.22)	7.02 (4.75)	6.31 (4.54)

Effects of change over time, all $p < .001$.

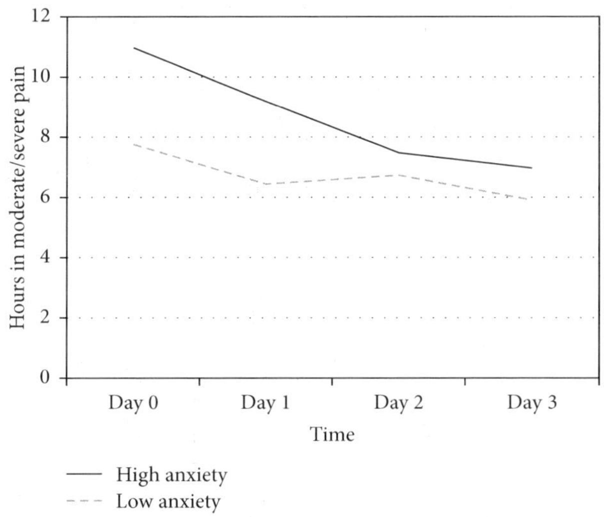

FIGURE 2: Hours of moderate to severe pain over time by preoperative anxiety. Patients with more preoperative anxiety (HADS anxiety score >8) reported more hours per day in moderate to severe pain compared with patients who had less anxiety (HADS score ≤8; main effect for anxiety, $p = .029$; interaction with time, $p = .046$).

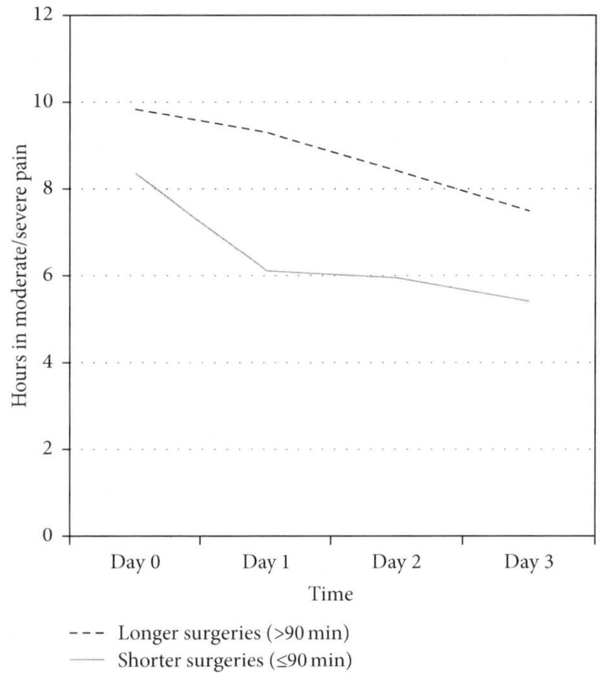

FIGURE 3: Hours in moderate/severe postoperative pain by duration of surgery. Longer knee replacement surgeries were associated with consistently more hours in moderate/severe postoperative pain (NRS ≥ 4) compared with shorter surgeries ($p = .008$). Similar difference was observed for ratings of pain with activity in relation to surgery duration ($p = .012$).

3.6.2. Implant Type. Five different types of knee replacement implants were used in this study, with varying frequencies of use. The Scorpio NRG (Stryker, Kalamazoo, MI, USA) and NexGen (Zimmer Biomet, Warsaw, IN, USA) were only used 4 or 5 times each and were grouped with the LCS DePuy (Johnson & Johnson, Warsaw, IN, USA) for the purpose of analysis. The Sigma DePuy (Johnson & Johnson, Warsaw, IN, USA) and AGC (Zimmer Biomet, Warsaw, IN, USA) were the most commonly used implants and were utilized in 77% of the surgeries in this study. Although the difference did not reach statistical significance ($p = .060$), the less commonly used implants (i.e., LCS, Scorpio NRG, and NexGen) were associated with slightly more hours in moderate/severe pain on Days 0–3 than the more commonly used implants (i.e., the Sigma and AGC) (Figure 4). The implants did not differ with respect to postoperative pain with activity.

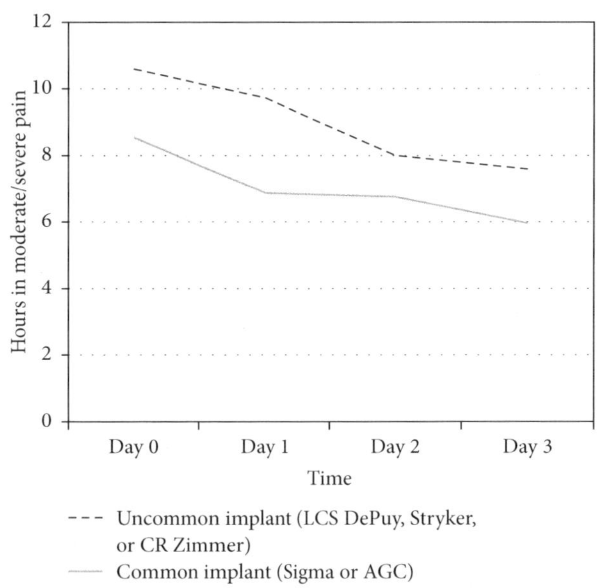

FIGURE 4: Hours of moderate to severe pain by implant type. The more commonly used implants were associated with slightly fewer hours per day in moderate to severe postoperative pain than the less commonly used implants, although the difference did not reach statistical significance ($p = .060$).

3.7. Factors Related to Surgery Duration. As shown in Tables 4 and 5, several factors were related to longer surgery duration, particularly implant type, amount of bleeding, preoperative

TABLE 3: Pain management 0–96 hours after knee replacement surgery.

	0–24 hours	24–48 hours	48–72 hours	72–96 hours
Trimeperidine (Promedol) (Moscow, Russia), %	30%	—	1%	—
Ketoprofen (ketoprofen) (Stavropol, Russia), %	81%	98%	98%	97%
Tramadol (tramadol) (Novokuznetsk, Russia), %	56%	7%	—	—
Paracetamol and tramadol (Zaldiar) (Aachen, Germany), %	3%	7%	5%	5%

Note. Each percentage refers to the proportion of patients who received the listed medication during the indicated time period.

TABLE 4: Descriptive surgical and clinical characteristics by duration of surgery.

Characteristic	Surgery duration		Statistics
	≤90 minutes	>90 minutes	
Implant type, % (n)			All 5, Fisher's exact **p < .001**
Sigma	47.4% (27)	37.2% (16)	Sigma versus AGC versus others
AGC	43.9% (25)	20.9% (9)	$\chi^2(2) = 16.0$, **p < .001**
Other implants:	21.7% (5)	78.3% (18)	Common versus uncommon
LCS	35.7% (5)	64.3% (9)	$\chi^2(1) = 15.2$, **p < .001**
Scorpio NRG	0% (0)	100% (5)	
NexGen	0% (0)	100% (4)	
Tourniquet use, % (n)	24.6% (14)	16.3% (7)	$\chi^2(1) = 1.01$, $p = .314$
Bleeding, mL, mean (SD)	297 (142)	401 (215)	$t(98) = 2.93$, **p = .004**
Hemoglobin, mL			
Preoperative, mean (SD)	126.9 (11.4)	132.6 (12.9)	$t(98) = 2.34$, **p = .022**
Day 0 at 20:00, mean (SD)	106.3 (11.9)	108.1 (11.4)	$t(98) = 0.78$, $p = .437$
Day 4, mean (SD)	100.6 (13.7)	98.2 (13.3)	$t(98) = 0.88$, $p = .379$
Creatinine, Day 0	63.2 (13.3)	67.3 (20.5)	$t(98) = 1.20$, $p = .231$
C-reactive Protein, Day 0	4.23 (4.68)	3.86 (6.29)	$t(98) = 0.33$, $p = .742$
Days in hospital, mean (SD)			
Preoperative	6.7 (4.4)	8.0 (3.6)	$t(98) = 1.53$, $p = .128$
Postoperative	8.9 (2.0)	9.5 (2.9)	$t(98) = 1.15$, $p = .255$
Total	15.6 (4.1)	17.4 (4.4)	$t(98) = 2.14$, **p = .035**

Note. Surgery duration did not differ by patient age or sex. Common implants were Sigma and AGC, and uncommon implants were LCS, Scorpio NRG, and NexGen.

TABLE 5: Descriptive characteristics of surgery duration (minutes), tourniquet use, and postsurgical hemoglobin for five different types of knee replacement implants.

	n	Surgery duration[a] Mean (SD)	Tourniquet use[b] % (n)	Bleeding, mL Mean (SD)	Hemoglobin, g/L[c]		Postoperative length of stay Mean (SD)
					Day 0, 20:00 Mean (SD)	Day 4 Mean (SD)	
Sigma	43	93.6 (20.0)	11.6% (5)	381 (172)	107.9 (11.7)	101.4 (15.0)	9.60 (2.89)
AGC	34	87.8 (20.6)	26.5% (9)	291 (165)	108.4 (10.9)	101.0 (12.1)	8.74 (1.68)
Other implants:	23	110.7 (27.7)	30.4% (7)	343 (215)	103.7 (12.5)	93.8 (11.5)	8.91 (2.21)
LCS	*14*	*105.4 (21.1)*	*50.0% (7)*	*318 (192)*	*100.4 (9.2)*	*91.1 (11.5)*	*8.29 (2.16)*
Scorpio NRG	*5*	*104.0 (5.5)*	*0%*	*470 (311)*	*110.0 (4.9)*	*99.4 (8.5)*	*10.80 (1.64)*
NexGen	*4*	*137.5 (49.9)*[a]	*0%*	*275 (126)*	*107.0 (24.8)*	*96.5 (14.2)*	*8.75 (2.06)*

Note. Italicized text represents the 3 types of implants grouped together as "other implants." Implant types did not differ with respect to bleeding, length of postoperative hospital stay, creatinine values (not shown), or CRP values (not shown).

[a]Surgery duration differed significantly by implant type ($p < .001$). In post hoc testing, the Sigma ($p = .014$) and AGC ($p = .001$) implants had significantly shorter surgery durations than the other three implants. One patient with a NexGen implant had a surgery duration of 210 minutes; a sensitivity analysis excluding this patient yielded similar omnibus results ($p = .004$), and the remaining NexGen implants still had a mean surgery duration of 113.3 (SD 15.3) minutes.

[b]Tourniquet was used with the LCS more often than with the other implants ($p = .009$).

[c]On the night of the surgery, hemoglobin values did not differ by implant type. However, on postoperative Day 4, the more common implants (Sigma and AGC) were associated with higher hemoglobin values than the other implants ($p = .020$).

hemoglobin value, and days in hospital. The more commonly used implants (i.e., Sigma and AGC) were associated with shorter surgery durations compared to the less commonly used implants (i.e., LCS, Scorpio NRG, and NexGen). One of the patients who received the NexGen implant had a surgery duration of 210 minutes, but a sensitivity analysis excluding this patient ($p = .004$) and the nonparametric Kruskal-Wallis test ($p < .001$) confirmed robust differences in surgery duration by implant type. Longer surgeries were also associated with more bleeding, but surgery duration was unrelated to tourniquet use. Longer surgeries were also associated with lower preoperative hemoglobin values, but surgery duration was unrelated to postoperative hemoglobin values. Surgery duration was also unrelated to creatinine and CRP values. Although surgeries longer than 90 minutes were not significantly associated with longer preoperative or postoperative stays in hospital, they were associated with longer hospital stays overall (i.e., combining pre- and postoperative days in hospital).

4. Discussion

A primary finding of this study was that the pain management protocol implemented at our institution was providing insufficient pain relief for some patients. Patients reported mean levels of pain in the moderate to severe range (NRS ≥ 4) on the day of surgery and first three postoperative days. Patients also reported a mean of 9 hours per day in moderate to severe pain. As a result of these findings, new modalities, such as local infiltration analgesia during surgery and intravenous Perfalgan (paracetamol) (Agen, France), were recently added to the protocol. In addition, single-injection femoral nerve blocks are now also used more widely. The levels of pain reported by the patients in this study may have also impacted the study results. The factors evaluated may have somewhat subtle effects that might be more evident among patients with greater pain relief. Thus, due to the possibility of ceiling effects, negative findings should be interpreted with caution. Nonetheless, our study identified several factors as predictors of heightened pain experience, even in this more limited pain management context.

Our study evaluated a variety of different psychological and clinical preoperative patient characteristics and found that only female gender and higher levels of preoperative anxiety and pain were associated with higher levels of pain reported in the early postoperative period after TKA. Anxiety is a recognized risk factor for persistent postsurgical pain [19]. Roth et al. [39] have found that high catastrophisation is predictive of greater postoperative pain, specifically pain at Day 2 and later following TKA. Ip et al. [40] mentioned both presurgical anxiety and psychological distress as predictive factors of postoperative pain intensity. Pinto et al. [41] suggested that pain catastrophising may act as a mediator in the relationship between preoperative anxiety and acute postsurgical pain. Preoperative anxiety is an important pain predictor not only for the first days after surgery but also at 6 weeks [42] and 6 months [43] and has even been linked to residual long-term pain after TKA [16, 44].

Numerous publications indicate that patients who are depressed preoperatively have worse results after TKA surgery in terms of pain, functionality, and satisfaction [17, 45, 46]. In our cohort of patients, we did not find any association between depression and pain trajectories. This is consistent with a recent study by Riddle et al. [47] in which they found no association between preoperative depressive symptom severity and postoperative pain. Furthermore, preoperative and postoperative depressive symptoms in patients before and after TKA did not appreciably change over a 6-year perioperative period. Pérez-Prieto et al. [48] also showed that although depressed patients have worse outcomes after TKA surgery, they also tend to start with worse pain and function levels preoperatively and the degree of improvement is the same as that for nondepressed patients. They conclude that it is equally worthwhile for depressed patients to undergo TKA surgery as is the case for nondepressed patients because to some extent the surgery may also cure the depression.

Other reported predictors for increased postoperative pain include female gender, younger age, increased BMI, increased severity of preoperative pain at the surgical site, preoperative use of opioids, general anesthesia, preoperative use of anticonvulsants, and preoperative use of antidepressants [36]. Among our cohort of patients, we observed similar associations with gender and preoperative pain but found no association with age and could not evaluate the remaining factors. Women reported more pain than men ($p = .009$), but the male subgroup consisted of only 7 patients, which reflects the typical gender distribution among primary TKA patients in our institution in recent years [49]. Patients who had a moderate to severe level of preoperative pain also reported more hours of moderate to severe pain during the first 3 postoperative days, ($p = .029$), although preoperative pain was unrelated to postoperative pain in activity. Neuropathic pain was not addressed in the current study, but Lavand'homme et al. [35] found that, during the first week after TKA, a subgroup of patients whose pain had a neuropathic component reported worse maximal pain and pain associated with mobilization, while no differences were demonstrated in trajectories of pain at rest.

The second finding of the study was that, among intraoperative variables, surgeries longer than 90 minutes were associated with more postoperative pain in activity, as well as more hours of moderate to severe pain. This finding is consistent with those of Niki et al. [50] that reduction of the duration of the surgical procedure as well as minimization of tissue damage and decrease of tourniquet time may also play a role in postoperative recovery [50]. Unexpectedly, surgery time was related to the brand name of the implant. The most commonly used among this cohort of patient implants, Sigma and AGC (77% of all cases), were associated with shorter surgery duration and correspondingly less postoperative pain than the other less commonly used brands. The implant choice was performed randomly the day before surgery, depending upon availability of instrument sets, taking into consideration that the indications for using the primary TKA implants do not differ between the manufacturers. All surgeons involved in the study have vast experience in knee arthroplasty with over 500 implantations per year in total.

All of the less commonly used implants in the study were familiar to the surgeons for several years, so it is unlikely that this finding is explained by a learning curve with these instrumentation systems. While this finding may be due to the fact that the more commonly a specific instrument is used, the faster the surgery is performed, it could also reflect the relative ease of implementation for the different systems.

This study has several strengths and limitations that need to be considered. A strength of the study is that Vreden's Institute used a standard protocol for patient care, thereby limiting the number of potential variables that may have influenced the results. In addition, the study evaluated a fairly comprehensive set of factors, including demographics, psychological well-being, knee function, physiological parameters, and intrasurgical factors, as well as an array of pain measures, including a 4-day pain diary. However, the sample size was small and likely underpowered for the number of factors being evaluated, and the sample was relatively homogeneous, particularly with respect to gender. Although the sample's gender distribution is representative of the patient population admitted for TKA at Vreden's Institute, applying the study findings to male patients should be done with caution, given the small number of men included in the study and the observed gender differences in pain. The surgeries were performed by several different surgeons, which may have added some individuality in soft-tissue handling. Nevertheless, all were trained by senior surgeon (NK) to do the surgery methodically and in a manner corresponding to the principles of less invasive surgery, such as dissecting as little tissue as possible, minimizing the length of incision during approach, avoiding excessive tension by retractors, utilizing the principle of mobile window during all steps of TKA, avoiding eversion of the patella or full subluxation of the tibial plateau anteriorly, and keeping soft-tissue releases minimal but sufficient for correction of both alignment and contracture, as well as gap balancing. Finally, although the pain management protocol was standardized, with little variation in dosing, this study did not include an extensive evaluation of the patients' pain management, which seemed to provide inadequate pain relief for some patients. Future research is needed to evaluate the complex relationships between the timing and dosing of pain management medication and postoperative pain trajectories.

5. Conclusions

Postoperative pain levels were generally high in this sample of TKA patients. Of the numerous previously reported medical and psychological comorbidities associated with pain following TKA, only gender, anxiety, and a higher level of preoperative pain were associated with increased postoperative pain after TKA in our cohort of patients. Among the surgical factors examined, surgery duration, which varied by the brand of implant, was associated with postoperative pain trajectories. Better understanding of which TKA patients are at greatest risk for postoperative pain will allow health care providers to individualize both preventive and protective analgesic peri- and postoperative treatments [35, 51].

References

[1] H. J. Gerbershagen, S. Aduckathil, A. J. M. van Wijck, L. M. Peelen, C. J. Kalkman, and W. Meissner, "Pain intensity on the first day after surgery: a prospective cohort study comparing 179 surgical procedures," *Anesthesiology*, vol. 118, no. 4, pp. 934–944, 2013.

[2] I. Grosu, P. Lavand'homme, and E. Thienpont, "Pain after knee arthroplasty: an unresolved issue," *Knee Surgery, Sports Traumatology, Arthroscopy*, vol. 22, no. 8, pp. 1744–1758, 2014.

[3] M. Sommer, J. M. de Rijke, M. van Kleef et al., "The prevalence of postoperative pain in a sample of 1490 surgical inpatients," *European Journal of Anaesthesiology*, vol. 25, no. 4, pp. 267–274, 2008.

[4] S. Srikandarajah and I. Gilron, "Systematic review of movement-evoked pain versus pain at rest in postsurgical clinical trials and meta-analyses: a fundamental distinction requiring standardized measurement," *Pain*, vol. 152, no. 8, pp. 1734–1739, 2011.

[5] S. S. Liu and C. L. Wu, "The effect of analgesic technique on postoperative patient-reported outcomes including analgesia: a systematic review," *Anesthesia and Analgesia*, vol. 105, no. 3, pp. 789–808, 2007.

[6] C. Li, Y. Zeng, B. Shen et al., "A meta-analysis of minimally invasive and conventional medial parapatella approaches for primary total knee arthroplasty," *Knee Surgery, Sports Traumatology, Arthroscopy*, vol. 23, no. 7, pp. 1971–1985, 2015.

[7] E.-Y. Chan, M. Fransen, S. Sathappan, N. H. L. Chua, Y.-H. Chan, and N. Chua, "Comparing the analgesia effects of single-injection and continuous femoral nerve blocks with patient controlled analgesia after total knee arthroplasty," *Journal of Arthroplasty*, vol. 28, no. 4, pp. 608–613, 2013.

[8] C. B. Chang and W.-S. Cho, "Pain management protocols, peri-operative pain and patient satisfaction after total knee replacement: a multicentre study," *The Journal of Bone & Joint Surgery—British Volume*, vol. 94, no. 11, pp. 1511–1516, 2012.

[9] F. Adam, M. Chauvin, B. Du Manoir, M. Langlois, D. I. Sessler, and D. Fletcher, "Small-dose ketamine infusion improves postoperative analgesia and rehabilitation after total knee arthroplasty," *Anesthesia and Analgesia*, vol. 100, no. 2, pp. 475–480, 2005.

[10] G. Blaudszun, C. Lysakowski, N. Elia, and M. R. Tramèr, "Effect of perioperative systemic $\alpha 2$ agonists on postoperative morphine consumption and pain intensity: systematic review and meta-analysis of randomized controlled trials," *Anesthesiology*, vol. 116, no. 6, pp. 1312–1322, 2012.

[11] T. H. Lunn, B. B. Kristensen, L. Ø. Andersen et al., "Effect of high-dose preoperative methylprednisolone on pain and recovery after total knee arthroplasty: a randomized, placebo-controlled trial," *British Journal of Anaesthesia*, vol. 106, no. 2, pp. 230–238, 2011.

[12] M. Bauer, L. Wang, O. K. Onibonoje et al., "Continuous femoral nerve blocks: decreasing local anesthetic concentration to minimize quadriceps femoris weakness," *Anesthesiology*, vol. 116, no. 3, pp. 665–672, 2012.

[13] R. L. Johnson, S. L. Kopp, J. R. Hebl, P. J. Erwin, and C. B. Mantilla, "Falls and major orthopaedic surgery with peripheral

nerve blockade: a systematic review and meta-analysis," *British Journal of Anaesthesia*, vol. 110, no. 4, pp. 518–528, 2013.

[14] J. E. Paul, M. Nantha-Aree, N. Buckley et al., "Gabapentin does not improve multimodal analgesia outcomes for total knee arthroplasty: a randomized controlled trial," *Canadian Journal of Anesthesia*, vol. 60, no. 5, pp. 423–431, 2013.

[15] P. A. E. Puolakka, M. G. F. Rorarius, M. Roviola, T. J. S. Puolakka, K. Nordhausen, and L. Lindgren, "Persistent pain following knee arthroplasty," *European Journal of Anaesthesiology*, vol. 27, no. 5, pp. 455–460, 2010.

[16] M. M. Vissers, J. B. Bussmann, J. A. N. Verhaar, J. J. V. Busschbach, S. M. A. Bierma-Zeinstra, and M. Reijman, "Psychological factors affecting the outcome of total hip and knee arthroplasty: a systematic review," *Seminars in Arthritis and Rheumatism*, vol. 41, no. 4, pp. 576–588, 2012.

[17] J. A. Singh and D. G. Lewallen, "Medical and psychological comorbidity predicts poor pain outcomes after total knee arthroplasty," *Rheumatology*, vol. 52, no. 5, pp. 916–923, 2013.

[18] J. Blackburn, A. Qureshi, R. Amirfeyz, and G. Bannister, "Does preoperative anxiety and depression predict satisfaction after total knee replacement?" *Knee*, vol. 19, no. 5, pp. 522–524, 2012.

[19] P. R. Pinto, T. McIntyre, R. Ferrero, A. Almeida, and V. Araújo-Soares, "Risk factors for moderate and severe persistent pain in patients undergoing total knee and hip arthroplasty: a prospective predictive study," *PLoS ONE*, vol. 8, no. 9, Article ID e73917, 2013.

[20] E. Yakobov, W. Scott, W. Stanish, M. Dunbar, G. Richardson, and M. Sullivan, "The role of perceived injustice in the prediction of pain and function after total knee arthroplasty," *Pain*, vol. 155, no. 10, pp. 2040–2046, 2014.

[21] D. C. Ayers, P. D. Franklin, and D. C. Ring, "The role of emotional health in functional outcomes after orthopaedic surgery: extending the biopsychosocial model to orthopaedics: AOA critical issues," *The Journal of Bone & Joint Surgery—American Volume*, vol. 95, no. 21, article e165, 2013.

[22] H. Kehlet, T. S. Jensen, and C. J. Woolf, "Persistent postsurgical pain: risk factors and prevention," *The Lancet*, vol. 367, no. 9522, pp. 1618–1625, 2006.

[23] G. R. Scuderi and A. J. Tria, *Minimally Invasive Surgery in Orthopedics: Knee Handbook*, Springer, New York, NY, USA, 2012.

[24] J. Hermanides, M. W. Hollmann, M. F. Stevens, and P. Lirk, "Failed epidural: causes and management," *British Journal of Anaesthesia*, vol. 109, no. 2, pp. 144–154, 2012.

[25] W. D. Owens, J. A. Felts, and E. L. Spitznagel Jr., "ASA physical status classifications: a study of consistency of ratings," *Anesthesiology*, vol. 49, no. 4, pp. 239–243, 1978.

[26] C. S. Cleeland, "Measurement and prevalence of pain in cancer," *Seminars in Oncology Nursing*, vol. 1, no. 2, pp. 87–92, 1985.

[27] S. A. Kalyadina, T. I. Ionova, M. O. Ivanova et al., "Russian brief pain inventory: validation and application in cancer pain," *Journal of Pain and Symptom Management*, vol. 35, no. 1, pp. 95–102, 2008.

[28] H. Breivik, P. C. Borchgrevink, S. M. Allen et al., "Assessment of pain," *British Journal of Anaesthesia*, vol. 101, no. 1, pp. 17–24, 2008.

[29] A. S. Zigmond and R. P. Snaith, "The hospital anxiety and depression scale," *Acta Psychiatrica Scandinavica*, vol. 67, no. 6, pp. 361–370, 1983.

[30] A. Lerdal, A. K. Wahl, T. Rustøen, B. R. Hanestad, and T. Moum, "Fatigue in the general population: a translation and test of the psychometric properties of the Norwegian version of the fatigue severity scale," *Scandinavian Journal of Public Health*, vol. 33, no. 2, pp. 123–130, 2005.

[31] J. N. Insall, "Total knee arthroplasty in rheumatoid arthritis," *Ryumachi*, vol. 33, no. 6, p. 472, 1993.

[32] M. P. Lawton and E. M. Brody, "Assessment of older people: self-maintaining and instrumental activities of daily living," *Gerontologist*, vol. 9, no. 3, pp. 179–186, 1969.

[33] R. Brooks and F. De Charro, "EuroQol: the current state of play," *Health Policy*, vol. 37, no. 1, pp. 53–72, 1996.

[34] P. M. Fayers and D. Machin, *Quality of Life: The Assessment, Analysis, and Interpretation of Patient-Reported Outcomes*, Wiley, Chichester, UK, 2nd edition, 2007.

[35] P. M. Lavand'homme, I. Grosu, M.-N. France, and E. Thienpont, "Pain trajectories identify patients at risk of persistent pain after knee arthroplasty: an observational study," *Clinical Orthopaedics and Related Research*, vol. 472, no. 5, pp. 1409–1415, 2014.

[36] S. S. Liu, A. Buvanendran, J. P. Rathmell et al., "Predictors for moderate to severe acute postoperative pain after total hip and knee replacement," *International Orthopaedics*, vol. 36, no. 11, pp. 2261–2267, 2012.

[37] P. R. Pinto, T. McIntyre, R. Ferrero, A. Almeida, and V. Araújo-Soares, "Predictors of acute postsurgical pain and anxiety following primary total hip and knee arthroplasty," *Journal of Pain*, vol. 14, no. 5, pp. 502–515, 2013.

[38] B. A. Rakel, N. P. Blodgett, M. B. Zimmerman et al., "Predictors of postoperative movement and resting pain following total knee replacement," *Pain*, vol. 153, no. 11, pp. 2192–2203, 2012.

[39] M. L. Roth, D. A. Tripp, M. H. Harrison, M. Sullivan, and P. Carson, "Demographic and psychosocial predictors of acute perioperative pain for total knee arthroplasty," *Pain Research & Management*, vol. 12, no. 3, pp. 185–194, 2007.

[40] H. Y. V. Ip, A. Abrishami, P. W. H. Peng, J. Wong, and F. Chung, "Predictors of postoperative pain and analgesic consumption: a qualitative systematic review," *Anesthesiology*, vol. 111, no. 3, pp. 657–677, 2009.

[41] P. R. Pinto, T. McIntyre, A. Almeida, and V. Araújo-Soares, "The mediating role of pain catastrophizing in the relationship between presurgical anxiety and acute postsurgical pain after hysterectomy," *Pain*, vol. 153, no. 1, pp. 218–226, 2012.

[42] M. Sullivan, M. Tanzer, W. Stanish et al., "Psychological determinants of problematic outcomes following Total Knee Arthroplasty," *Pain*, vol. 143, no. 1-2, pp. 123–129, 2009.

[43] D. L. Riddle, J. B. Wade, W. A. Jiranek, and X. Kong, "Preoperative pain catastrophizing predicts pain outcome after knee arthroplasty," *Clinical Orthopaedics and Related Research*, vol. 468, no. 3, pp. 798–806, 2010.

[44] M. P. Bonnin, L. Basiglini, and H. A. P. Archbold, "What are the factors of residual pain after uncomplicated TKA?" *Knee Surgery, Sports Traumatology, Arthroscopy*, vol. 19, no. 9, pp. 1411–1417, 2011.

[45] M. T. Hirschmann, E. Testa, F. Amsler, and N. F. Friederich, "The unhappy total knee arthroplasty (TKA) patient: higher WOMAC and lower KSS in depressed patients prior and after TKA," *Knee Surgery, Sports Traumatology, Arthroscopy*, vol. 21, no. 10, pp. 2405–2411, 2013.

[46] T. Duivenvoorden, M. M. Vissers, J. A. N. Verhaar et al., "Anxiety and depressive symptoms before and after total hip and knee arthroplasty: a prospective multicentre study," *Osteoarthritis and Cartilage*, vol. 21, no. 12, pp. 1834–1840, 2013.

[47] D. L. Riddle, R. A. Perera, W. T. Nay, and L. Dumenci, "What is the relationship between depressive symptoms and pain during functional tasks in persons undergoing TKA? A 6-year perioperative cohort study," *Clinical Orthopaedics and Related Research*, vol. 473, no. 11, pp. 3527–3534, 2015.

[48] D. Pérez-Prieto, S. Gil-González, X. Pelfort, J. Leal-Blanquet, L. Puig-Verdié, and P. Hinarejos, "Influence of depression on total knee arthroplasty outcomes," *Journal of Arthroplasty*, vol. 29, no. 1, pp. 44–47, 2014.

[49] N. N. Kornilov, T. A. Kulyaba, A. S. Fil, and Y. V. Muravyeva, "Data of knee arthroplasty register of Vreden Russian Research Institute of Traumatology and Orthopedics for period 2011–2013," *Travmatologiya i ortopediya Rossii*, vol. 1, pp. 136–151, 2015.

[50] Y. Niki, T. Mochizuki, S. Momohara, S. Saito, Y. Toyama, and H. Matsumoto, "Is minimally invasive surgery in total knee arthroplasty really minimally invasive surgery?" *Journal of Arthroplasty*, vol. 24, no. 4, pp. 499–504, 2009.

[51] D. Yarnitsky, "Conditioned pain modulation (the diffuse noxious inhibitory control-like effect): its relevance for acute and chronic pain states," *Current Opinion in Anaesthesiology*, vol. 23, no. 5, pp. 611–615, 2010.

16

Using Picture and Text Schedules to Inform Children: Effects on Distress and Pain during Needle-Related Procedures in Nitrous Oxide Sedation

Merja Vantaa Benjaminsson,[1] Gunilla Thunberg,[2] and Stefan Nilsson[3,4]

[1] *Södra Älvsborg Hospital, 504 55 Borås, Sweden*
[2] *DART-Center for AAC and AT, The Queen Silvia Children's Hospital, Sahlgrenska University Hospital, 411 04 Gothenburg, Sweden*
[3] *Faculty of Caring Science, Work Life and Social Welfare, University of Borås, 501 90 Borås, Sweden*
[4] *Institute of Health and Care Sciences, University of Gothenburg, 405 30 Gothenburg, Sweden*

Correspondence should be addressed to Stefan Nilsson; stefan.nilsson.4@gu.se

Academic Editor: Anna Maria Aloisi

During hospital visits, children often undergo examinations and treatments that may involve an experience of pain and distress that is also connected to the staff's treatment. The United Nation's Convention on the Rights of Persons with Disability advocates the use of Universal Design. One way of implementing this idea within paediatric nursing is to increase the use of pictorial supports, and the few studies that have been published show promising results. The aim of this study was to do a comparison between two groups of children in regard to the pre- and postconditions of implementing an intervention including staff instruction and the use of pictorial support. The support consisted of a visual schedule with pictures and text, used both preparatory to and during the hospital visit. One hundred children aged 5–15 (50 children during the preinterventional data collection and 50 children postinterventionally) reported pain intensity and distress during needle-related procedures in nitrous oxide sedation. The results showed that the intervention had a positive effect in significantly lowering the level of preprocedural distress. The results showed that the pain intensity was also lowered however not reaching statistical significance. This confirms other positive research results on the use of visual supports within paediatric care, a topic that has to be further studied.

1. Introduction

The United Nation's (UN) Convention on the Rights of the Child states that all children should be provided with information that is adequate according to their cognitive, physical, and social development, including the right to get information that is important for health and well-being [1]. Article 12 of the UN's Convention on the Rights of the Child stresses that health care professionals "*shall assure the child who is capable of forming his or her own views the right to express those views freely in all matters affecting the child*" [1]. Because of this, it is important to find ways of giving information and providing strategies that are suitable for a child and his/her family. However, a systematic review found that few paediatric clinical practice guidelines for acute procedural pain were clear, concise, and specific or given in an easy-to-follow format; that is, most guidelines for children were in need of improvement [2]. Earlier research has also identified a lack of strategies in nursing literature about how to facilitate communication between the nurse and the child [3].

Communicative rights are reinforced in the UN's Convention on the Rights of Persons with Disability (CRPD), a document that stresses a child's right to accessibility and that health care staff must take all measures to ensure that persons with disabilities have access to information on equal conditions as others have [4]. The use of Universal Design is also put forth (Articles 2, 3, and 21 [4]). When it comes to information and communication, this means that augmentative and alternative communication (AAC) forms should be used to make health care accessible to as many individuals as possible [4]. Hitherto, parents of children with communicative disabilities have experienced a lack of access to information when their children visit the hospital [5, 6]. This stresses the need for adequate access to communication tools, as well as access to individual health information [5]. To achieve this goal, it is necessary to give nurses education about how to use these communication tools [5, 6]. There is a need for educating nurses in using simple, functional, and generic augmentative communication strategies [5]. However, there is a lack of strategies in the literature and a need for research into effects [5]. This lack of knowledge might cause unnecessary suffering for a child [3]. The few studies that have been published point to good results [7, 8].

During hospital visits, children often undergo examinations and treatments that may involve an experience of pain and distress. Procedural pain, which often means a pain induced by a stick, is mediated primarily through nociceptive A-delta fibres [9]. Pain from A-delta fibres is treated effectively using local anaesthetics, such as a Eutectic Mixture of Local Anaesthetics (EMLA) (lidocaine 25 mg/g and prilocaine 25 mg/g) [10]. When a procedure is expected to give children moderate pain and distress, local anaesthetics may be insufficient as the only drug in pain management. This is especially true if a child also worries about how he or she will manage the situation. In these cases, it is effective to add a drug that is both analgesic and sedative. Accordingly, 50% nitrous oxide and 50% oxygen in combination with EMLA are often effective to reduce the pain caused by injections [11]. Acetaminophen and cyclooxygenase (cox) inhibitors (ibuprofen, diclofenac, and ketorolac) may relieve the pain that can be traced to the inflammation that may occur afterwards, but the evidence for this is low [12].

As stated above, a child's right to be provided with adequate information and to express himself/herself is important also in needle-related procedures. When nurses lack the ability to explain what is going to happen, this decreases the possibility of calming a child. At times, this situation may make it necessary to overpower and restrain a child during a procedure [13]. Sometimes, a needle-related procedure even has to be cancelled, which generates extra costs for the organization and decreases the child's will to come back voluntarily to the hospital.

The project KomHIT—communication in care settings using communicative support and IT—has the overall purpose of improving the communicative rights of children during paediatric or dental care situations according to the CRPD, focusing on the use of AAC as Universal Design (Articles 2, 3, and 21 [4]). The hypothesis is that when care staff have better knowledge about communication and routinely use AAC in information and communication processes to meet the rights of children with a communicative disability, the communication situation and quality of care are increased for all children. Furthermore, not only are the numbers of individuals who have communicative problems during care situations limited to children with a disability and their parents but they also include a large proportion of the population [14]. For example, young children, being at early linguistic levels, and their parents have problems, as have immigrant families that are not acquainted with the often complicated language used by medical staff and/or medical culture [14]. KomHIT, therefore, tries to implement AAC strategies, mainly in the form of pictorial supports, to be used generally and routinely to all children within paediatric care. The first studies within this project have shown promising results [15].

Table 1: Demographic data.

	Preinterventional (numbers)	Postinterventional (numbers)
Participants	50	50
Planned visits	39	32
Acute visits	11	18
Girls	24	24
Boys	26	26
Age (years)	9.64	9.12
Lumbar puncture	14	19
Joint injection	10	4
Pin removal	17	19
Others	9	8

2. Aim

The aim of this study was to evaluate the KomHIT-intervention using education to the staff and pictorial supports as Universal Design for communication and information implemented at a paediatric unit. More specifically, the purpose was to investigate whether instruction to the staff and the use of a visual schedule, provided before and during the hospital visit, decreased distress and pain intensity in children who underwent needle-related procedures in nitrous oxide sedation.

3. Methods

3.1. Study Design. A nonrandomised clinical trial was conducted [16] in which data were consecutively collected from groups of participants.

3.2. Participants. One hundred children participated: 50 children during the preinterventional data collection (26 boys and 24 girls; mean 9.64 years) and 50 children after the intervention was implemented (26 boys and 24 girls; mean 9.12 years) (Table 1).

Universal Design was used also in regard to the inclusion of participants. This means that all children were invited; that is, no child was excluded due to disability. According to the medical records, five children in the preinterventional group and eight children in the postinterventional group had a communicative disability. In the preinterventional group, three boys and one girl had Attention Deficit Hyperactivity Disorder (ADHD), and one girl had intellectual disability. In the postinterventional group, five boys had ADHD, one girl had intellectual disability, and two boys had specific language

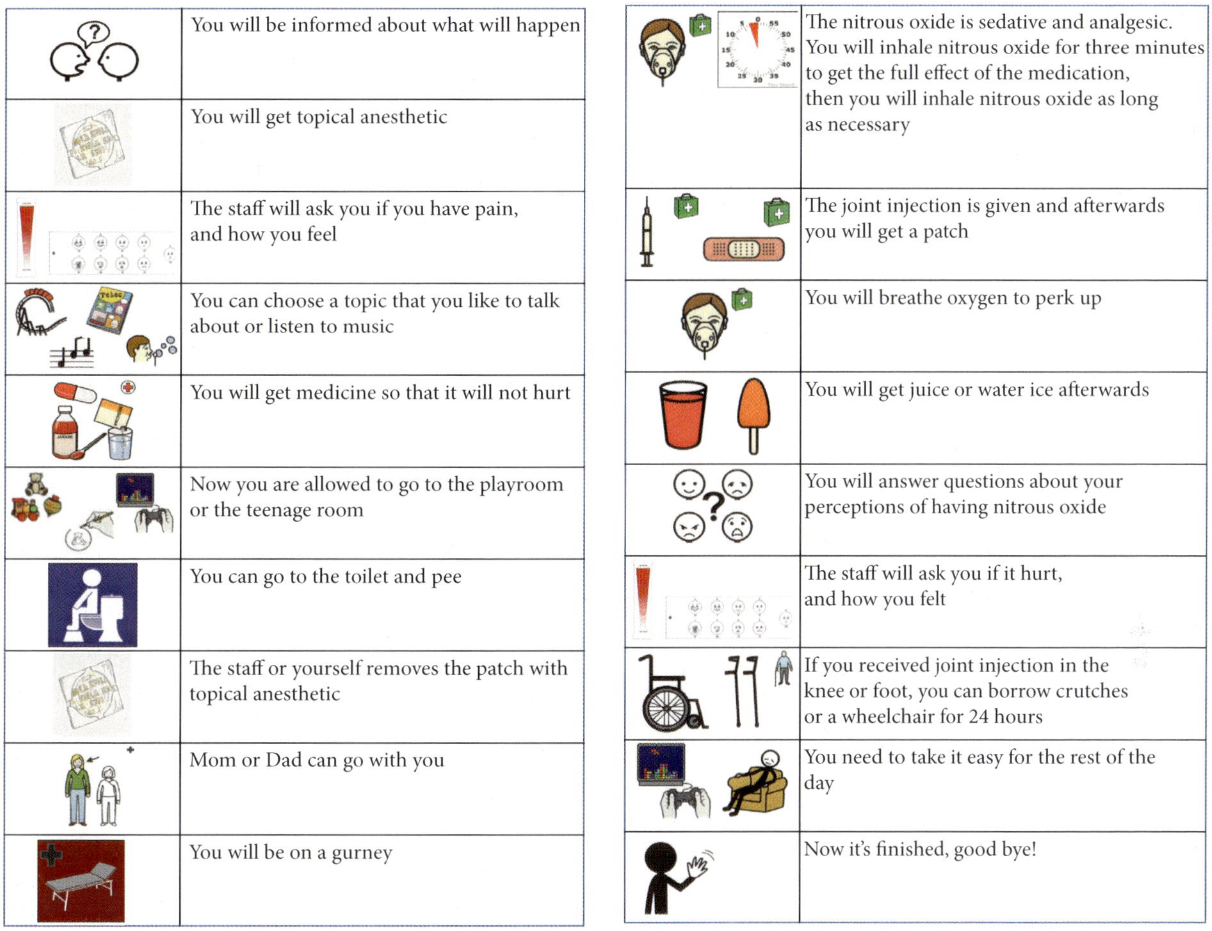

Figure 1: A visual schedule.

impairment. No statistical calculation was conducted due to the low number of participants with a communicative disability.

3.3. Instruments

3.3.1. Distress. The Facial Affective Scale (FAS) is a self-reported scale with nine faces that assesses a child's distress, ranging from 0.04 (happiest feeling possible) to 0.97 (saddest feeling possible) [17]. Distress was reported on three occasions, that is, before, during, and after each needle-related procedure.

3.3.2. Pain Intensity. The Coloured Analogue Scale (CAS) is a self-reported scale that assesses a child's pain intensity, ranging from zero (no pain) to ten (worst possible pain). This scale is designed to provide gradations in colour, area, and length, reflecting different values of pain intensity [17]. Pain intensity was reported on three occasions, that is, before, during, and after each needle-related procedure.

3.4. Intervention. All children underwent a needle-related procedure in nitrous oxide (50% nitrous oxide/50% oxygen) sedation (Table 1). Needle-related procedures are often defined as injections, venepunctures, sutures, and lumbar punctures [18]. In this study, the concept of needle-related procedures also included pin-drawing, which is associated with similar pain and distress as other needle-related procedures [19]. No changes were conducted in the guidelines that were used for the pain management. Based on the guidelines, the children got acetaminophen, cox inhibitors (ibuprofen, diclofenac), and EMLA.

The intervention included a (a) preparatory phase and a (b) procedural phase. During the preparatory phase (a), a visual schedule was sent home by post to the family, depicting and in short text explaining the different steps of a nitrous oxide process (Figure 1). If the procedure was performed acutely, the family received the same visual schedule about two hours before the procedure. In both cases, the parents were instructed to go through the material with the child. The procedural phase (b) included the use of the same visual schedule during the nitrous oxide process at the hospital ward. The staff supplied each child with a schedule and pointed to the pictures when verbally informing the family of everything that was going to happen. The family used the information throughout the procedure. This meant that the child had control over how many steps were finished and how many steps were left to undergo. If something had to be

Table 2: The differences of distress and pain intensity between preinterventional and postinterventional groups.

	Preinterventional mean (range, SD)	Postinterventional mean (range, SD)	p value
FAS (0.04–0.97) before	0.52 (0.04–0.97, 0.27)	0.41 (0.04–0.85, 0.28)	0.04*
FAS during	0.32 (0.04–0.97, 0.28)	0.33 (0.04–0.85, 0.28)	0.85
FAS after	0.25 (0.04–0.85, 0.24)	0.19 (0.04–0.85, 0.20)	0.16
CAS (0–10) before	1.19 (0–8, 2.17)	0.62 (0–6, 1.39)	0.12
CAS during	1.67 (0–9, 2.52)	1.74 (0–8, 2.28)	0.88
CAS after	0.90 (0–9, 1.96)	0.42 (0–5, 1.08)	0.13

*$p < 0.05$.

changed, the visual schedule also could be used as a resource for understanding.

3.5. Data Collection. Data were collected preinterventionally between May and November 2013. Children were invited consecutively until 50 children had agreed to participate in this study. The intervention was introduced after the completion of this first data collection. After the preinterventional phase, the nurses were given education, totalling two hours, including both a theoretical background and practical training. The theory covered knowledge about communicative rights, the idea of Universal Design, communicative disabilities, and augmentative communication strategies. The practical training included the use of the pictorial supports within role-plays. When the intervention had been implemented, a second data collection with another 50 participants was conducted. The data were collected between November 2013 and July 2014.

3.6. Data Analysis. The statistics were calculated using IBM SPSS Statistics for Windows, version 22. Statistical significance was considered if $p < 0.05$. Primary outcome was the FAS, and a power calculation showed that each group needed to be at least 33 participants. The hypothesis was that the FAS should decrease from the mean score of 0.68 to 0.54, and the standard deviation was assumed to be 0.20. This assumption was based on the use of the FAS in an earlier study [20]. The CAS and the FAS have been validated in earlier studies using parametric statistics [17], which led to the selection of parametric statistics in this study.

3.7. Ethical Considerations. The study was carried out according to the rules and recommendations of the regional ethics committee. This means that the benefits of the study were considered greater than the risks. The children underwent this procedure, whether or not they decided to participate in the study, meaning that the situation was not arranged due to this study. Written information was provided to the parents and was supplemented with verbal information to the children. The voluntary nature of the study, as well as the right to withdraw from the study at any time without any explanation or consequence, was highlighted. If the children agreed to participate, the parents were asked for written consent.

4. Results

4.1. Distress. It was seen that the children were distressed before the procedure (Table 2) but that the children that were provided with the visual schedule reported significantly lower levels on the Facial Affective Scale (FAS) (mean 0.41) compared to the case with the preinterventional group (mean 0.52). The FAS scores during and after the procedure were low in both groups (mean $\leq$ 0.33). The children with a communicative disability (in both groups) reported a mean value of 0.60/0.44 before the procedure, 0.48/0.23 during the procedure, and 0.24/0.16 after the procedure on the FAS.

4.2. Pain Intensity. The level of self-reported pain intensity (CAS) before, during, and after the procedures turned out to be low in all children (mean $\leq$ 1.74). There were no differences between the two groups reaching statistical significance before, during, or after the procedure. However, the trend was that the CAS scores were lower in the intervention group both before (mean 0.62 compared to 1.19) and after (mean 0.42 compared to 0.90) the procedure (Table 2). The children with a communicative disability (in both groups) reported a mean value of 2.40/0.69 before the procedure, 2.40/1.38 during the procedure, and 0.40/0.81 after the procedure on the CAS.

5. Discussion

The aim of this study was to evaluate the KomHIT communication intervention, encompassing education to the staff and the use of pictorial supports as Universal Design for communication and information. Whether this intervention could reduce the reported pain intensity and distress in children who underwent needle-related procedures in nitrous oxide sedation was studied.

The level of pain intensity as measured by the CAS showed to be low in both groups (mean $\leq$ 1.74), which means that the nitrous oxide sedation did help the children in their pain management, regardless of the communication intervention. However, this study had no control group without nitrous oxide sedation, so no conclusions could be drawn in this regard. Comparing the two groups of children in this study, it was seen that the children who had access to the KomHIT communication intervention reported a lower intensity of pain, however, one not reaching a level of statistical significance. A future study including larger groups of participants might prove if this trend is significant. It would also be interesting to compare nitrous oxide sedation with the use of pictorial support. In another study within the KomHIT project, it was seen that the number of children who were in need of premedication during day surgery was reduced when the KomHIT communication intervention with pictorial supports was introduced [21].

The results on the FAS scale where the children reported their feelings of distress before, during, and after the procedure showed that the children's preprocedural stress was significantly reduced when the KomHIT communication intervention was implemented. The levels of distress during and after the procedure were low for both groups, which again points to a positive effect of the nitrous oxide sedation. As already has been suggested, a future study should be done that compares the use of pictorial supports to nitrous oxide sedation. The possibility of identifying groups of children who can cope well with the use of pictorial supports, and therefore do not need nitrous oxide sedation, is highly relevant due to both costs and the negative pollution effects of nitrous oxide [22].

Taken together, the results in this study showed that the KomHIT communication intervention had a positive effect in reducing distress before the nitrous oxide sedation. Some other positive trends, such as reduced pain before and after the procedure, were also seen but could not be proved significant. These results confirm the earlier positive reports of the use of pictorial supports [7, 8]. The mechanisms behind these results are not yet fully known, and, in this study, it is impossible to separate the possible effects of staff education from the effects of having access to pictorial supports. But, most possibly, pictorial supports assist a child in creating a concrete idea of what will happen and so in bringing a child a sense of control in a situation that otherwise could be frightening for him or her. Achieving a sense of control is one of the most commonly used strategies for children in a needle-related procedure [23]. The child's feeling of control is dependent on the people around him or her, and this social support will be necessary for the child to gain a sense of control [24]. In general, the use of cognitive strategies to control pain will increase with age [25]. Children can view themselves as active agents in pain relief, and, to make this possible, they have to be informed about the procedure [26].

Nurses also have to fulfill the requirements of the conventions that come from the UN and that stress that all children should have access to information about their activities at a hospital [1, 4]. Hitherto, there has been little research in the context of paediatric care that provides nurses with evidence-based strategies when it comes to pictorial supports or other AAC strategies [27]. However, this study gives an example of an AAC strategy that has an effect on children's distress, at least in regard to procedures in nitrous oxide sedation.

5.1. Methodological Considerations. This study was not a randomised clinical trial, which was a weakness in regard to scientific control. However, the type of intervention that was evaluated also included staff education and communication, which means that it would have been tricky or impossible for nurses to change behaviour between different children. Additionally, earlier research has shown small differences among the results of randomised versus nonrandomised studies [28]. Another weakness in the study design was that children with and without a communicative disability were not separated in different study groups and that the children with a communicative disability were few in total ($n = 13$). This means that the results mainly tell us something about children without a communicative disability. Furthermore, it is not possible to separate the effects of the education about communication from the use of visual supports. These two elements of the intervention need to be considered separately in a future study. Finally, the effects of the nitrous oxide sedation per se are another factor that cannot be separated from the KomHIT communication intervention. A future study controlling this factor and comparing it to communication intervention would be of great value.

6. Conclusions

The results showed that the intervention had a positive effect in significantly lowering the level of preprocedural distress. The results showed that the pain intensity was lowered however not reaching statistical significance, and children reported low levels of pain intensity. This confirms other positive research results on the use of visual supports within paediatric care, a topic that has to be further studied.

Acknowledgments

The authors would like to thank the participants of the study who generously shared their time and experiences. Grants from the Swedish Heritage Foundation supported this study.

References

[1] United Nations, "Convention on the rights of the child document," in *Proceedings of the 61st Plenary Meeting*, Contract No.: A/RES/44/25, November 1989.

[2] G. Y. Lee, J. Yamada, O. Kyololo, A. Shorkey, and B. Stevens, "Pediatric clinical practice guidelines for acute procedural pain: a systematic review," *Pediatrics*, vol. 133, no. 3, pp. 500–515, 2014.

[3] G. R. M. de Freitas, C. G. de Castro Jr., S. M. J. Castro, and I. Heineck, "Degree of knowledge of health care professionals about pain management and use of opioids in pediatrics," *Pain Medicine*, vol. 15, no. 5, pp. 807–819, 2014.

[4] United Nations, *Final Report of the Ad Hoc Committee on a Comprehensive and Integral International Convention on the Protection and Promotion of the Rights and Dignity of Persons with Disabilities*, United Nations, 2006.

[5] B. Hemsley, S. Lee, K. Munro, N. Seedat, K. Bastock, and B. Davidson, "Supporting communication for children with cerebral palsy in hospital: views of community and hospital

staff," *Developmental Neurorehabilitation*, vol. 17, no. 3, pp. 156–166, 2014.

[6] G. Thunberg, M. Buchholz, and S. Nilsson, "Strategies that assist children with communicative disability during hospital stay: parents' perceptions and ideas," *Journal of Child Health Care*, 2015.

[7] J. M. Costello, "AAC intervention in the intensive care unit: the children's hospital Boston model," *Augmentative and Alternative Communication*, vol. 16, no. 3, pp. 137–153, 2000.

[8] P. J. Mesko, A. B. Eliades, C. Christ-Libertin, and D. Shelestak, "Use of picture communication aids to assess pain location in pediatric postoperative patients," *Journal of Perianesthesia Nursing*, vol. 26, no. 6, pp. 395–404, 2011.

[9] S. Lundeberg, "Klassificering av smärta och smärtfysiologi," *Information från Läkemedelsverket*, vol. 25, no. 3, pp. 27–28, 2014.

[10] E.-L. Maunuksela and R. Korpela, "Double-blind evaluation of a lignocaine-prilocaine cream (EMLA) in children. Effect on the pain associated with venous cannulation," *British Journal of Anaesthesia*, vol. 58, no. 11, pp. 1242–1245, 1986.

[11] R. Carbajal, V. Biran, R. Lenclen et al., "EMLA cream and nitrous oxide to alleviate pain induced by palivizumab (Synagis) intramuscular injections in infants and young children," *Pediatrics*, vol. 121, no. 6, pp. e1591–e1598, 2008.

[12] V. Shah, A. Taddio, C. M. McMurtry et al., "Pharmacological and combined interventions to reduce vaccine injection pain in children and adults: systematic review and meta-analysis," *The Clinical Journal of Pain*, vol. 31, supplement 10, pp. S38–S63, 2015.

[13] C. Darby and P. Cardwell, "Restraint in the care of children," *Emergency Nurse*, vol. 19, no. 7, pp. 14–17, 2011.

[14] H. C. Shane, S. Blackstone, G. Vanderheiden, M. Williams, and F. DeRuyter, "Using AAC technology to access the world," *Assistive Technology*, vol. 24, no. 1, pp. 3–13, 2012.

[15] G. Thunberg, M. Johansson, and J. Wikholm, "Meeting the communicative rights of people with autism—using pictorial supports during assessment, intervention and hospital care," in *Autism Spectrum Disorder—Recent Advances*, M. Fitzgerald, Ed., chapter 15, InTech, Rijeka, Croatia, 2015.

[16] D. G. Altman, *Practical Statistics for Medical Research*, Chapman & Hall/CRC Press, London, UK, 1990.

[17] P. A. McGrath, C. E. Seifert, K. N. Speechley, J. C. Booth, L. Stitt, and M. C. Gibson, "A new analogue scale for assessing children's pain: an initial validation study," *Pain*, vol. 64, no. 3, pp. 435–443, 1996.

[18] K. A. Birnie, M. Noel, J. A. Parker et al., "Systematic review and meta-analysis of distraction and hypnosis for needle-related pain and distress in children and adolescents," *Journal of Pediatric Psychology*, vol. 39, no. 8, pp. 783–808, 2014.

[19] K. B. L. Lim, S. S. Tan, S. N. S. Abdullah, L.-L. Ong, M.-L. Wong, and J. C. Allen, "Percutaneous pin removal in the outpatient clinic—do children require analgesia? A randomized controlled trial," *The Journal of Bone & Joint Surgery—American Volume*, vol. 96, no. 7, pp. 597–602, 2014.

[20] S. Nilsson, K. Enskär, C. Hallqvist, and E. Kokinsky, "Active and passive distraction in children undergoing wound dressings," *Journal of Pediatric Nursing*, vol. 28, no. 2, pp. 158–166, 2013.

[21] G. Thunberg, C.-J. Törnhage, and S. Nilsson, "Evaluating the impact of AAC interventions in reducing hospitalization-related stress: challenges and possibilities," *Augmentative and Alternative Communication*, In press.

[22] F. Gilchrist, C. J. Whitters, A. M. Cairns, M. Simpson, and M.-T. Hosey, "Exposure to nitrous oxide in a paediatric dental unit," *International Journal of Paediatric Dentistry*, vol. 17, no. 2, pp. 116–122, 2007.

[23] S. Ayers, I. Muller, L. Mahoney, and P. Seddon, "Understanding needle-related distress in children with cystic fibrosis," *British Journal of Health Psychology*, vol. 16, part 2, pp. 329–343, 2011.

[24] A. Antonovsky, "Janforum: locus of control theory," *Journal of Advanced Nursing*, vol. 17, no. 8, pp. 1014–1015, 1992.

[25] R. Esteve and V. Marquina-Aponte, "Children's pain perspectives," *Child: Care, Health and Development*, vol. 38, no. 3, pp. 441–452, 2012.

[26] L. S. Franck, A. Sheikh, and K. Oulton, "What helps when it hurts: children's views on pain relief," *Child: Care, Health and Development*, vol. 34, no. 4, pp. 430–438, 2008.

[27] E. H. Finke, J. Light, and L. Kitko, "A systematic review of the effectiveness of nurse communication with patients with complex communication needs with a focus on the use of augmentative and alternative communication," *Journal of Clinical Nursing*, vol. 17, no. 16, pp. 2102–2115, 2008.

[28] J. P. A. Ioannidis, A.-B. Haidich, M. Pappa et al., "Comparison of evidence of treatment effects in randomized and nonrandomized studies," *The Journal of the American Medical Association*, vol. 286, no. 7, pp. 821–830, 2001.

17

Cost-Saving Early Diagnosis of Functional Pain in Nonmalignant Pain: A Noninferiority Study of Diagnostic Accuracy

Rafael J. A. Cámara,[1] Christian Merz,[2] Barbara Wegmann,[2] Stefanie Stauber,[3] Roland von Känel,[4,5] and Niklaus Egloff[2]

[1] *University Medical Center of the Johannes Gutenberg University, Mainz, Institute of Medical Biostatistics, Epidemiology, and Informatics, Obere Zahlbacher Straße 69, 55131 Mainz, Germany*
[2] *Department of General Internal Medicine, Division of Psychosomatic Medicine, Inselspital, Bern University Hospital, 3010 Bern, Switzerland*
[3] *Heart Failure and Transplantation, Department of Cardiology, Inselspital, Bern University Hospital, 3010 Bern, Switzerland*
[4] *Department of Psychosomatic Medicine, Clinic Barmelweid, 5017 Barmelweid, Switzerland*
[5] *Department of Neurology, Inselspital, Bern University Hospital, 3010 Bern, Switzerland*

Correspondence should be addressed to Rafael J. A. Cámara; racamara@uni-mainz.de

Academic Editor: Donald A. Simone

Objectives. We compared two index screening tests for early diagnosis of functional pain: pressure pain measurement by electronic diagnostic equipment, which is accurate but too specialized for primary health care, versus peg testing, which is cost-saving and more easily manageable but of unknown sensitivity and specificity. Early distinction of functional (altered pain perception; nervous sensitization) from neuropathic or nociceptive pain improves pain management. *Methods.* Clinicians blinded for the index screening tests assessed the reference standard of this noninferiority diagnostic accuracy study, namely, comprehensive medical history taking with all previous findings and treatment outcomes. All consenting patients referred to a university hospital for nonmalignant musculoskeletal pain participated. The main analysis compared the receiver operating characteristic (ROC) curves of both index screening tests. *Results.* The area under the ROC curve for peg testing was not inferior to that of electronic equipment: it was at least 95% as large for finger measures (two-sided $p = 0.038$) and at least equally as large for ear measures (two-sided $p = 0.003$). *Conclusions.* Routine diagnostic testing by peg, which is accessible for general practitioners, is at least as accurate as specialized equipment. This may shorten time-to-treatment in general practices, thereby improving the prognosis and quality of life.

1. Introduction

The lifetime prevalence of chronic nonmalignant musculoskeletal pain varies between 13.5% and 47% in the general population [1]. In one-third of these patients, this pain is "functional," which is defined as not explainable by lesions or inflammations of tissues or nerves [2, 3]. Because, as opposed to nociceptive and neuropathic pain, surgery and the analgesics scheme recommended by the World Health Organization are not adequate for functional pain, the distinction is clinically relevant (International Statistical Classification of Diseases and Related Health Problems: F45.40 and F45.41). Functional pain requires specialized multicomponent management involving physical exercise, activating physiotherapy, electrical, thermal, and tactile stimulation, relaxation techniques, psychological support, tricyclic antidepressants, and muscle relaxants [4]. Functional pain may occur as an isolated entity or as the dominant symptom of "central sensitivity syndromes" such as fibromyalgia [5, 6], whereby the functional alteration of the nervous system is probably involved [7, 8].

A delay of eight years on average to classify pain as either functional, nociceptive, or neuropathic increases expenditures and reduces the prognosis and the quality of life of the patients [3, 4, 9, 10]. Because imaging and laboratory findings often seem to correspond to the symptoms at the first evaluation, diagnosing functional pain by the exclusion of nociceptive and neuropathic pain is difficult [3, 8]. When pain is functional, namely, prolonged by central nervous system sensitization [5, 7], nociceptive stimuli such as whiplash-associated pain syndrome or osteoarthritis and inflammation are often mistaken for its cause [3, 11–13]. The diagnostic process involves repetitions of, for instance, computer tomographies, electromyographies, infiltrations of local anesthetics, surgery, and extensive laboratory examinations [3].

Despite the importance of distinguishing functional from nociceptive and neuropathic pain early, screening tests are still missing in primary care [4, 11–13]. Techniques to measure pressure pain sensitivity, summarized as electronic algometry, are very precise (one kilopascal), but expensive, and thus only used in specialized centers and studies [14–17]. They show that the pain threshold is reduced in many functional pain syndromes [5–7]. While electronic algometry is indispensable for research, cost-effective and more easily manageable alternatives are required for functional pain screening in primary care [18].

Our hypothesis was that peg algometry's ability to distinguish functional from nociceptive and neuropathic pain is not inferior to that of electronic algometry, which has been widely investigated but is many times more costly than peg algometry and only used by specialists. The latter is a recently introduced test performed with a pressure pain device that easily fits into a coat pocket. We had shown that peg algometry is very reliable and consistent according to criteria of the British Standards Institution [19, 20]. For instance, standardized Bland Altman repeatability coefficients were 0.96 for finger peg algometry and even 0.63 for ear peg algometry. Moreover, 95% of the differences between test and retest results were within two standard deviations from "no difference" for ear lobe, and even within one standard deviation for middle finger peg algometry, with all p values <0.001.

2. Methods

The enrolment and data collection for this noninferiority study of diagnostic accuracy comparing the two index tests, namely, peg with electronic algometry, were carried out at the Clinical Departments for Psychosomatic Medicine and for Orthopedics at the Bern University Hospital. The local ethics committee had approved the study protocol. All eligible patients were informed about the study. The main eligibility criteria were hospitalization for nonmalignant musculoskeletal pain and written informed consent. Further eligibility criteria were the absence of local lesions at the site of measurement or at an efferent innervation of this site.

Following eligibility assessment, an advanced medical student read the index tests, and the attending specialists, who ignored the readings of the index tests, assessed the reference standard. All passed their written results to the data manager. The enrolment continued until at least 60 patients with functional and 60 patients with nociceptive or neuropathic pain consented (see "analysis and presentation of data"). The STARD checklist for reporting studies on diagnostic accuracy [21] was followed for reporting the introduction, methods, and results part (see Supplementary Material 1 available online at http://dx.doi.org/10.1155/2016/5964250), and the STROBE checklist [22] was used for the discussion.

The reference standard for comparing the two index tests was a thorough review of the medical history including clinical, imaging, arthroscopic, and surgical findings and treatment outcomes according to the criteria of the International Statistical Classification of Diseases and Related Health Problems. By reviewing pain histories of eight years on average, exclusion of alternate pain causes and little effect of conventional analgesics confirmed *functional* pain [23]. The correlation of the localization and character of pain symptomatology with clinical and investigative findings from the patients' histories corroborated *nociceptive* or *neuropathic* pain. Functional pain was found, for instance, in somatoform pain, fibromyalgia, complex regional pain syndrome, chronic temporomandibular joint disorder, whiplash disorder, and chronic low back pain, as well as combinations of such disorders. However, neither the given diagnosis nor any central nervous system hypersensitivity testing was our reference standard, but rather a long and costly exclusion of lesions, degenerations, and inflammations of tissues or nerves which could have explained the pain, as well as failure of conventional pain treatment [2, 3].

Combinations of functional and nociceptive pain were classified as functional pain. Such combinations are frequent [24], and early diagnosis of the functional pain component is as important in such combinations as in isolated functional pain. Missing neither the one nor the other remains a challenge. Having said that, the focus of this study was the identification of patients requiring multicomponent pain treatment, from which most patients with functional pain might benefit, whether or not they also have nociceptive pain.

Standardized pegs of polypropylene were used for peg algometry [20], and a device that had been tested in multiple studies and is regularly employed in pain research was used for electronic algometry according to the manufacturer's instructions [25]. Whether to start with peg or with electronic algometry was determined by flipping a coin. Both algometry techniques were applied to the distal phalanx of the middle finger and then to the ear lobe. Measurements were performed at the left and the right side of the body in order to control for side-specific differences of perception [26]. A pause of one minute before each measurement aimed to minimize sensitization phenomena. Finger algometry was conducted without touching the nail fold, and ear algometry was performed in the middle of the ear lobe without touching cartilaginous structures. All algometry results were immediately documented for later calculation of the mean between the left and the right side.

The peg was left in place for 10 seconds. Before removing it, the study participants rated their pain sensitivity numerically on a scale from 0 to 10 with intervals of 0.5, where "0" was "no pain at all" and "10" was "the worst imaginable pain." Each of the four anatomical sites (left and right middle finger as well as left and right ear lobe) was measured once.

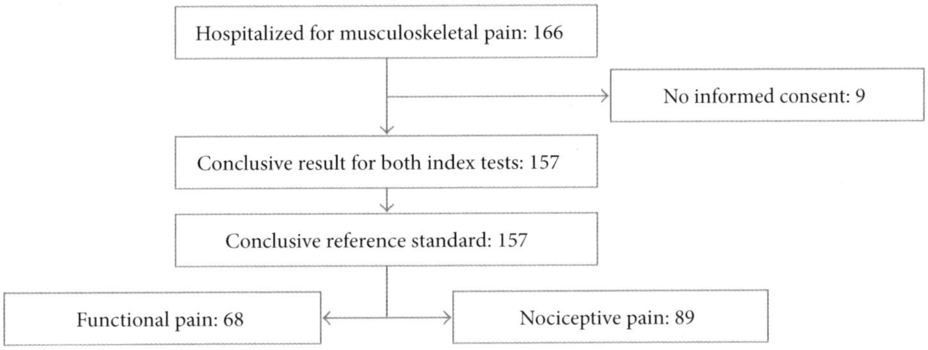

FIGURE 1: Flow of a referred sample of 166 individuals hospitalized for musculoskeletal pain. The reference standard, namely, a thorough review of the clinical pain history including past investigations and pharmacological responses, revealed 68 participants with functional and 89 participants with nociceptive pain.

In contrast to peg algometry, electronic algometry increased the pressure at 50 kilopascals per second until the study participants experienced the pressure as pain. At that moment, they pressed a button to display the pressure pain threshold in kilopascals. To proceed as recommended by the manufacturer, electronic algometry was conducted three times for each of the anatomical sites (see the previous paragraph), and the average of the three readings was computed before computing the average between the left and right sides.

In order to address potential interviewer-bias and competing interests, the reader of the index tests knew that the internal consistency of peg and electronic algometry would be investigated but ignored the reference standard and the diagnostic accuracy comparison [20]. She was involved neither in the assessment of the medical history of the study participants nor in the management of their pain. Once she had forwarded the results of peg and electronic algometry to the data manager, she was granted access to the participants' files to extract descriptive data that she sent to the data manager. To improve consistency, the index tests were performed by the same person and in the same manner across all study participants. To relax the participants, the measurements were performed in their rooms.

The areas under the receiver operating characteristic curves (AUC) enabled a direct comparison of both algometry techniques (roc, Stata SE®, version 12.1). The larger an AUC, the higher the probability of detecting functional pain if there is any and of excluding it if there is none. An AUC of 50% would correspond to an uninformative test, and an AUC of 100% to a perfectly discerning test. Graphs were drawn for visual comparison (roccomp, Stata SE, version 12.1). Statistical significance was tested by noninferiority comparisons. To compute the standard error of the difference between the AUCs of the index tests, the correction factor for the correlation between these two techniques was needed, which was computed by the functional-pain-nonfunctional-pain average of their correlation coefficients (ktau, Stata SE, version 12.1) and the average of their AUCs (roctab, Stata/SE, version 12.1) [27].

Noninferiority of peg to electronic algometry was assumed if the AUC of peg algometry was at least 80% as large as the AUC of electronic algometry against a p value smaller than 0.05 [20].

The reference variable was "functional versus nociceptive and neuropathic pain," and the two classification variables to compare were "numerical pain rating of peg algometry" and "pain threshold of electronic algometry in kilopascals."

The aim was to detect noninferiority of peg to electronic algometry, as defined above, with 80% power. Assuming a rank correlation of peg and electronic algometry of 0.4 [20] and an AUC of electronic algometry of 80% [15, 16], a minimum of 60 study participants with functional pain and 60 study participants with nociceptive pain were required for this aim [27].

The study participants were described using Stata/SE, version 12.1. The description included "peg algometry rating from 0 to 10 in 1/2 units," "electronic algometry in kilopascals," "age, sex, pain onset, and pain localization," "numeric analogue scales from 0 to 10 in 1/2 units," and medication. "Numeric analogue scales from 0 to 10 in 1/2 units" included musculoskeletal pain and mood. Medication included "analgesics," "antidepressants (yes/no)," and "antiepileptic drugs (yes/no)." Analgesics were categorized as "strong opiates," "weak opiates," "nonopiate analgesics only," and "no analgesics." A table describes these variables as counts and percentages if they are binary or categorical and other types of variables as means and standard deviations. It also provides the ranges of the index tests for the identification of outliers.

3. Results

Of 166 individuals hospitalized for musculoskeletal pain from May to August 2009 and January to March 2010, 157 consented to participate, of which none had to be excluded (Figure 1). The nociceptive pain group of 89 participants included nine patients with neuropathic rather than nociceptive pain (Figure 2). Due to the delayed process until referral to specialized therapeutic centers [3], study participants with

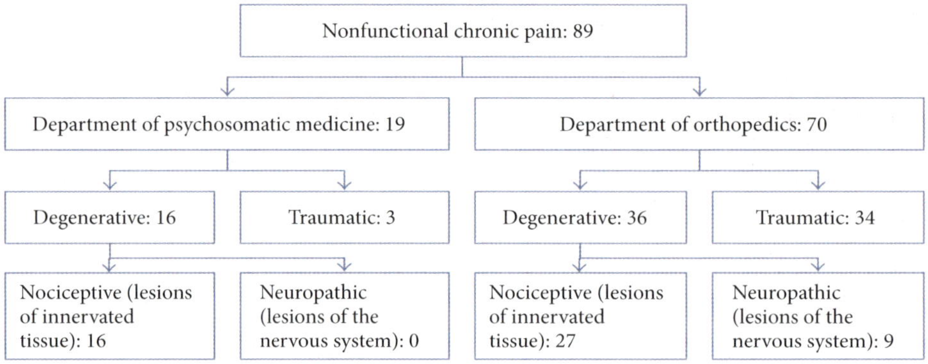

FIGURE 2: Classification of nonfunctional pain according to study site and pathology. Nine individuals of the nociceptive pain group of 89 participants had neuropathic rather than nociceptive pain. This number was too small for sensitivity analyses.

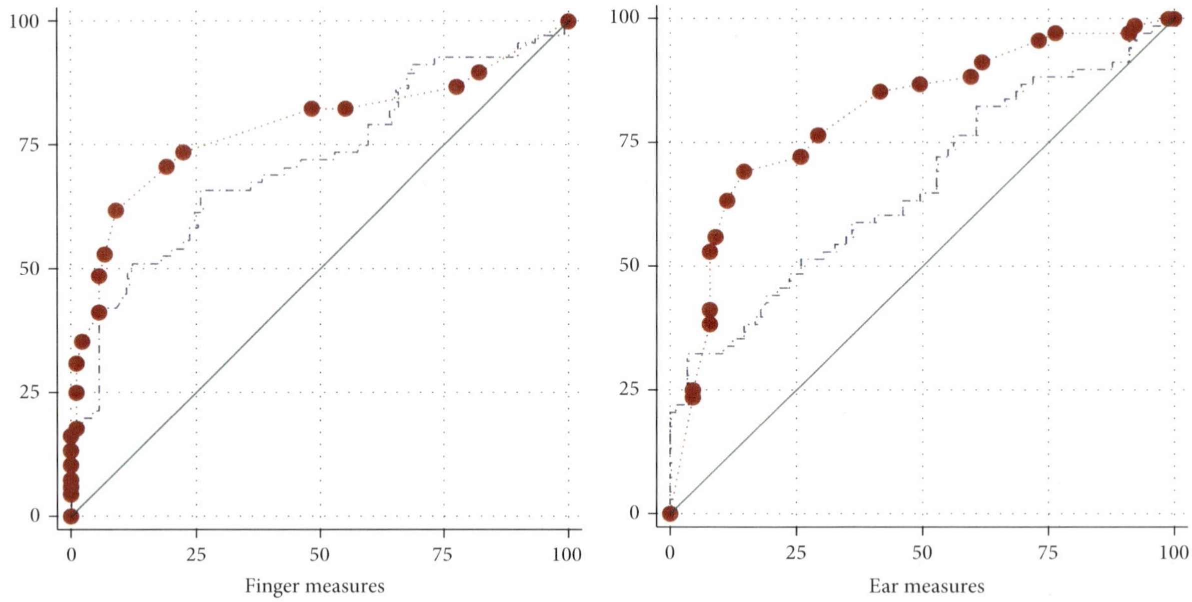

FIGURE 3: Visual comparison of peg and electronic algometry in discerning functional from nociceptive pain: receiver operating characteristic curves. Axes: x-axis = 100% − specificity in %; y-axis = sensitivity in %. Peg algometry: the red circles reflect the maximum of 21 possible test results given by the 0 to 10 pain rating at intervals of 0.5 points. Electronic algometry: the blue dashed line reflects the multitude of possible test results provided by the pressure pain measurement unit "kilopascal" with standard deviations ranging between 72 and 97 kilopascals.

this condition had experienced pain for a longer period of time and differed in medications (Table 1).

The visual comparison showed that, for finger and ear measures, the AUCs for peg algometry were larger than those for electronic algometry (Figure 3).

The noninferiority comparison in Table 2 showed that, for finger measures, the AUC for peg algometry was at least 95% as large as that for electronic algometry ($p = 0.038$), and for ear measures, the AUC for peg algometry was at least equally as large as that for electronic algometry ($p = 0.003$).

4. Discussion

Taken together, we found that finger peg algometry is at least 95% as reliable as finger electronic algometry in distinguishing functional from nociceptive and neuropathic musculoskeletal pain, and we found that ear peg algometry is even equally good or better than ear electronic algometry. Cost-effective and more easily manageable alternatives for electronic algometry were developed in the past [18], but we were the first to investigate their accuracy to differentiate functional from nociceptive musculoskeletal pain. One strength of this study is that we used identical conditions to compare a new screening test accessible for primary care with an established research test of known accuracy [14–17]. This means that most potential limitations would affect the absolute performance of both tests, thereby leaving the comparison between them only minimally affected, it at all.

A pain history of unsuccessful examinations for and treatment of assumed organic pain-sustaining factors is a strong reference standard because it has very important clinical implications for the patients [3, 4]. However, this reference standard might also include the limitation of unequal years of

TABLE 1: Cross-sectional description of study participants with functional and nociceptive pain[a].

	Functional pain	Nociceptive pain
Number of participants (denominator)	68	89
Peg algometry rating from 0 to 10 in 1/2 units		
Mean finger pressure pain (SD)	4.5 (3.0)	1.5 (1.5)
Mean ear lobe pressure pain (SD)	7.5 (2.5)	4.5 (2.5)
Range of finger pressure pain[b]	0 to 10	0 to 7
Range of ear lobe pressure pain[b]	1 to 10	0 to 10
Electronic algometry in kilopascals		
Mean finger pain threshold (SD)	156 (96)	228 (97)
Mean ear lobe pain threshold (SD)	125 (85)	164 (72)
Range of finger pain threshold[b]	12 to 467	71 to 676
Range of ear lobe pain threshold[b]	2 to 461	47 to 368
Age, sex, pain onset, and pain localization		
Mean age in years (SD)	46 (12)	57 (16)
Number of women (%)	40 (59)	37 (42)
Mean pain duration in months (SD)	98 (114)	35 (75)
Number of pain onsets before the 50th birthday (%)	59 (87)	40 (45)
Number of patients with multilocular pain (%)	56 (82)	33 (37)
Numeric analogue scales from 0 to 10 in 1/2 units		
Mean intensity of musculoskeletal pain (SD)	6.5 (2.0)	4.0 (2.0)
Mean mood (SD)	6.0 (2.5)	4.0 (2.0)
Medication		
Number of patients		
With strong opiates (%)	10 (15)	14 (16)
With weak opiates (%)[c]	12 (18)	6 (7)
With nonopiate analgesics only (%)	33 (49)	67 (75)
Without analgesics (%)	13 (19)	2 (2)
Number of patients with antidepressants (%)	58 (85)	17 (19)
Number of patients with antiepileptic drugs (%)	16 (24)	10 (11)

[a]No missing data; [b]no outliers; [c]weak opiates = tramadol and codeine.

TABLE 2: Noninferiority comparison of peg and electronic algometry in discerning functional from nociceptive pain: areas under the receiver operating characteristic curves (AUC)[a].

	AUC in % of a perfectly discerning test (95% CI)		Difference (95% CI) p value	
	Peg algometry	Electronic algometry	Crude	AUC of peg minus 95% of the AUC of electronic algometry
Finger measures	79 (71 to 86)	72 (64 to 80)	7 (−3 to 16) 0.18	11 (1 to 20) 0.04
Ear measures	81 (74 to 88)	66 (57 to 75)	15 (5 to 24) 0.003	18 (8 to 27) < 0.001

[a]No missing data.

pain history and medication between study participants with functional and nociceptive pain, as well as corroboration of the reference standard in a sample referred to specialized centers rather than in general practices. In addition, we cannot exclude that the patients spoke about their pain history to the person who performed the index tests. However, this person ignored the study objectives and had no competing interests. In addition, the pressure algometry depends on the perception of the patients but not on the perception of the tester. Prior to the results of this study, there was no good reference standard for an early pain stage [11–13], and only at an early pain stage there are patients certainly blind to their condition who do not differ substantially in terms of medication.

Since we found that an economical device is at least as good at screening for functional musculoskeletal pain as a tried and trusted device used in specialized departments, screening is also possible in primary care. This does not mean that peg algometry provides diagnostic certitude at the very onset but that it is a useful screening tool. At onset, musculoskeletal pain might result from altered function of the nervous system (functional pain) and from nociceptive or neuropathic stimuli such as injury, inflammation, or degeneration. In the event of suspected functional pain, this would make a parallel investigation of different causes mandatory [3, 7]. But as pain starts to become chronic [1], having screened for central nervous system sensitization may support general practitioners in determining whether an injury or a disease might have been overseen or inadequately treated, or whether it is more likely that the pain is functional [3, 5, 7].

It would be interesting to know how well peg algometry carried out before initiation of extensive diagnostic and therapeutic procedures predicts their success. Since we obtained our findings in a highly specialized setting, caution is appropriate when generalizing them to primary care. However, a gain in certitude regarding generalizability would require a long observation period in a primary care setting for which the expensive electronic algometry is not accessible. Then again, we found that peg algometry is at least as good as electronic algometry. We deduce that the research we suggest is possible only with peg algometry. In an upcoming third phase, we plan to investigate the difference in therapeutic success between taking into account and ignoring the screening results of peg algometry.

What we can say now is that general practitioners can start appropriate pain treatment earlier, because early separation of functional from nociceptive and neuropathic pain becomes easier. Interested general practitioners may manufacture their own peg algometers, which is also possible in countries with few resources. They may explain to their patients that a short innocuous test performed instantly with a small device of familiar appearance can help to tell if there is probably no alteration of the painful tissue behind the very frequent condition of musculoskeletal pain. If the test unmasks an enhanced reactivity of the central nervous system to pain stimuli (central nervous system sensitization) [5, 7], patients may prefer knowing this early rather than hearing that "nothing" has been found. Awareness that their central nervous system is even likely to continue reacting after removal of the initial pain stimulus might reduce insecurity if the pain becomes chronic [9]. Even if patients have a combination of functional and nociceptive pain, unmasking a hypersensitivity component might help understanding why the standard treatment remains unsatisfactory and additional treatment modalities are required.

As appropriate pain treatment can start earlier, the prognoses of functional, nociceptive, and perhaps even neuropathic pain are likely to improve [3, 4]. This might be perceived with more personal satisfaction than years of diagnostic and therapeutic incertitude [3, 9].

Acknowledgments

The authors thank Elizabeth Marti, M.D. (Bürgerspital Solothurn, Solothurn, Switzerland), for the participation of the Department of Orthopaedics. The authors further thank several colleagues in other specialties, in particular Oliver Bayer (Institute of Medical Biostatistics, Epidemiology, and Informatics, Mainz, Germany), for critically reviewing this paper during a 4-day workshop in scientific communication. Finally yet importantly, the authors thank Katherine Taylor (Institute of Medical Biostatistics, Epidemiology, and Informatics, Mainz, Germany) for linguistic assistance.

References

[1] M. A. Cimmino, C. Ferrone, and M. Cutolo, "Epidemiology of chronic musculoskeletal pain," *Best Practice & Research Clinical Rheumatology*, vol. 25, no. 2, pp. 173–183, 2011.

[2] J. L. Jackson and M. Passamonti, "The outcomes among patients presenting in primary care with a physical symptom at 5 years," *Journal of General Internal Medicine*, vol. 20, no. 11, pp. 1032–1037, 2005.

[3] F. Atzeni, M. Cazzola, M. Benucci, M. Di Franco, F. Salaffi, and P. Sarzi-Puttini, "Chronic widespread pain in the spectrum of rheumatological diseases," *Best Practice and Research: Clinical Rheumatology*, vol. 25, no. 2, pp. 165–171, 2011.

[4] D. C. Turk, H. D. Wilson, and A. Cahana, "Treatment of chronic non-cancer pain," *The Lancet*, vol. 377, no. 9784, pp. 2226–2235, 2011.

[5] M. B. Yunus, "Fibromyalgia and overlapping disorders: the unifying concept of central sensitivity syndromes," *Seminars in Arthritis and Rheumatism*, vol. 36, no. 6, pp. 339–356, 2007.

[6] N. Egloff, R. J. Cámara, R. von Känel, N. Klingler, E. Marti, and M.-L. Ferrari, "Hypersensitivity and hyperalgesia in somatoform pain disorders," *General Hospital Psychiatry*, vol. 36, no. 3, pp. 284–290, 2014.

[7] A. I. Basbaum, D. M. Bautista, G. Scherrer, and D. Julius, "Cellular and molecular mechanisms of pain," *Cell*, vol. 139, no. 2, pp. 267–284, 2009.

[8] R. J. Gatchel, Y. B. Peng, M. L. Peters, P. N. Fuchs, and D. C. Turk, "The biopsychosocial approach to chronic pain: scientific advances and future directions," *Psychological Bulletin*, vol. 133, no. 4, pp. 581–624, 2007.

[9] S. Nettleton, I. Watt, L. O'Malley, and P. Duffey, "Understanding the narratives of people who live with medically unexplained illness," *Patient Education and Counseling*, vol. 56, no. 2, pp. 205–210, 2005.

[10] L. Annemans, S. Wessely, E. Spaepen et al., "Health economic consequences related to the diagnosis of fibromyalgia syndrome," *Arthritis & Rheumatism*, vol. 58, no. 3, pp. 895–902, 2008.

[11] M.-A. Fitzcharles and P. Boulos, "Inaccuracy in the diagnosis of fibromyalgia syndrome: analysis of referrals," *Rheumatology*, vol. 42, no. 2, pp. 263–267, 2003.

[12] K. Klaus, W. Rief, E. Brähler, A. Martin, H. Glaesmer, and R. Mewes, "The distinction between 'medically unexplained' and 'medically explained' in the context of somatoform disorders," *International Journal of Behavioral Medicine*, vol. 20, no. 2, pp. 161–171, 2013.

[13] H. Dagfinrud, K. Storheim, L. H. Magnussen et al., "The predictive validity of the Örebro Musculoskeletal Pain Questionnaire and the clinicians' prognostic assessment following manual therapy treatment of patients with LBP and neck pain," *Manual Therapy*, vol. 18, no. 2, pp. 124–129, 2013.

[14] L. Arendt-Nielsen and D. Yarnitsky, "Experimental and clinical applications of quantitative sensory testing applied to skin, muscles and viscera," *Journal of Pain*, vol. 10, no. 6, pp. 556–572, 2009.

[15] N. Tastekin, K. Uzunca, N. Sut, M. Birtane, and O. B. Mercimek, "Discriminative value of tender points in fibromyalgia syndrome," *Pain Medicine*, vol. 11, no. 3, pp. 466–471, 2010.

[16] R. A. Scudds, G. B. Rollman, M. Harth, and G. A. McCain, "Pain perception and personality measures as discriminators in the classification of fibrositis," *Journal of Rheumatology*, vol. 14, no. 3, pp. 563–569, 1987.

[17] A. Y. Neziri, M. Curatolo, A. Limacher et al., "Ranking of parameters of pain hypersensitivity according to their discriminative ability in chronic low back pain," *Pain*, vol. 153, no. 10, pp. 2083–2091, 2012.

[18] T. W. Johnson and P. J. Watson, "An inexpensive, self-assembly pressure algometer," *Anaesthesia*, vol. 52, no. 11, pp. 1070–1072, 1997.

[19] British Standards Institution, "Accuracy (trueness and precision) of measurement methods and results—part 5: alternative methods for the determination of the precision of a standard measurement method," BS ISO 5725-5:1998, British Standards Institution, London, UK, 1998.

[20] N. Egloff, N. Klingler, R. von Känel et al., "Algometry with a clothes peg compared to an electronic pressure algometer: a randomized cross-sectional study in pain patients," *BMC Musculoskeletal Disorders*, vol. 12, article 174, 2011.

[21] P. M. Bossuyt and J. B. Reitsma, "Standards for reporting of diagnostic accuracy. The STARD initiative," *The Lancet*, vol. 361, no. 9351, p. 71, 2003.

[22] E. Von Elm, D. G. Altman, M. Egger, S. J. Pocock, P. C. Gøtzsche, and J. P. Vandenbroucke, "The strengthening the reporting of observational studies in epidemiology (STROBE) statement: guidelines for reporting observational studies," *The Lancet*, vol. 370, no. 9596, pp. 1453–1457, 2007.

[23] W. M. Schuepbach, R. H. Adler, and M. E. Sabbioni, "Accuracy of the clinical diagnosis of 'psychogenic disorders' in the presence of physical symptoms suggesting a general medical condition: a 5-year follow-up in 162 patients," *Psychotherapy and Psychosomatics*, vol. 71, no. 1, pp. 11–17, 2002.

[24] F. Wolfe, D. J. Clauw, M.-A. Fitzcharles et al., "Fibromyalgia criteria and severity scales for clinical and epidemiological studies: a modification of the ACR preliminary diagnostic criteria for fibromyalgia," *The Journal of Rheumatology*, vol. 38, no. 6, pp. 1113–1122, 2011.

[25] Somedic Production AB: Algometer. Somedic Production AB: Algometer, 2015, http://www.somedicprod.se/uk/algometer-uk.shtml.

[26] N. Egloff, F. Maecker, S. Stauber, M. E. Sabbioni, L. Tunklova, and R. von Känel, "Nondermatomal somatosensory deficits in chronic pain patients: are they really hysterical?" *Pain*, vol. 153, no. 9, pp. 1847–1851, 2012.

[27] J. A. Hanley and B. J. McNeil, "A method of comparing the areas under receiver operating characteristic curves derived from the same cases," *Radiology*, vol. 148, no. 3, pp. 839–843, 1983.

18

Chronic Pain and Sleep Disorders in Primary Care

Robert Jank,[1] Alexander Gallee,[2] Markus Boeckle,[1] Sabine Fiegl,[1] and Christoph Pieh[1,3]

[1]*Department of Psychotherapy and Biopsychosocial Health, Danube University Krems, Krems, Austria*
[2]*Practice for General Medicine, Vorderweißenbach, Austria*
[3]*Department of Psychosomatic Medicine, University Hospital Regensburg, Regensburg, Germany*

Correspondence should be addressed to Robert Jank; robert.jank@donau-uni.ac.at

Academic Editor: Steve McGaraughty

Background. Chronic pain (CP) and sleep disorders (SD) are highly prevalent in the general population. However, comprehensive data regarding the prevalence and characteristics of pain and SD in primary care are rare. *Methods.* From $N = 578$ patients $N = 570$ were included within 8 weeks (mean age: 50.8 ± 18.7 years, females: 289). Sociodemographic data, Insomnia Severity Index (ISI), and parts of a self-report questionnaire for pain (Multidimensional German Pain Questionnaire) were recorded and additional medical information (pain medication, sleep medication) was gathered from the patient charts. *Results.* Of the total sample, 33.2% ($n = 189$) suffer from CP (pain ≥ 6 months) and 29.1% ($n = 166$) from SD. 45.5% of the CP patients suffer from SD and 26.5% from clinical insomnia (ISI ≥ 15). SD ($\beta = 0.872$, SE = 0.191, $t = 4{,}572$, $p < 0.001$, CI [0.497; 1.246]) and older age ($\beta = 0.025$, SE = 0.005, $t = 5.135$, $p < 0.001$, CI [0.015; 0.035]) were significantly associated with pain experience. *Conclusion.* About a quarter of CP patients suffer from clinical insomnia. The suggested bidirectional relation should be considered during comprehensive assessment and treatment of patients.

1. Introduction

Chronic pain (CP) and sleep disorders (SD) have become two of the most common symptoms reported by primary care patients. The prevalence of CP ranges from 10 to 40% [1], which is similar to prevalence rates of SD (10–36% [2–8]). CP is tied to considerable personal impairment in quality of life [9, 10]. Due to the high prevalence in the general population and its prominent disabling nature, CP imposes a burden, not only for the patient but also for the society in terms of economic productivity and health care costs [11–14]. The results of an European cross-sectional survey report that 19% of CP patients lost their job and 13% had to change their jobs [15]. These indirect costs (informal caregiving, work impairment, etc.) cause significantly higher expenditures than direct health care costs alone [16]. Comparable to patients with CP, patients with SD suffer from poor quality of life and considerable health restrictions and social limitations [17, 18]. SD are well-documented risk factors for psychiatric diseases [19–21], cardiovascular diseases [22, 23], and increased mortality [24].

There is limited but growing epidemiological information on the prevalence of CP and comorbid SD in primary care. In clinical settings SD have been found to impact 50–88% of CP patients [25, 26]. Vice versa, more than 40% of patients suffering from SD report CP [4]. Cooccurring health problems are considered as the norm rather than the exception in primary care patients [27]. They increase the risk of premature death, hospitalization, loss of physical functioning, depression, poly-pharmacy, reduced quality of life, and increased health care costs [28]. The interaction of sleep and pain is complex and still not well understood [7]. A recent meta-analysis confirms a medium effect of sleep deprivation on pain perception in healthy individuals [29]. However, the occurrence and size of this effect are unclear in clinical relevant populations. There is increasing evidence suggesting a reciprocal relationship between pain and sleep. Results from studies in animal models [30–33], healthy persons [5, 34–37], and patients with different types of pain [38–42] support the reciprocal interaction of CP and SD. For example, pharmaceutical studies on eszopiclone [43, 44], triazolam [45], or pregabalin [46] show a simultaneous improvement of both pain and sleep.

The presence of comorbid SD in patients with diabetic peripheral neuropathy and postherpetic neuralgia may even predict substantial pain relief in response to pain treatment with pregabalin [47].

Patients with several SD, such as obstructive sleep apnea syndrome (OSAS) [48] and restless legs syndrome (RLS) [49], seem to be hyperalgesic. Effective treatment of the respective sleep disorder improves pain sensitivity. This improvement has been demonstrated by pharmacological interventions against pain, such as levodopa (L-DOPA) therapy for RLS [49], and in nonpharmacological interventions, such as continuous positive airway pressure (CPAP) treatment for OSAS [48]. Despite the suspected high prevalence of SD in the general population, they are often underidentified by primary care professionals and thus a large percentage of patients remain untreated [18]. Only in about half of the cases the treating general practitioner knows about sleeping problems [50]. Given the significant impact of SD on pain experience and the fact that pain is a frequent reason for primary care consultations, the focus of this study was to explore the prevalence and characteristics of CP and SD in primary care patients.

2. Methods

2.1. Participants. Participants were patients of a general practice in Austria. In this practice, patients are treated by a licensed general physician who underwent a qualification programme for psychosomatic and psychotherapeutic medicine (including, e.g., sleep and pain) at the time of the study. The practice is the only general practice for a relatively large rural region where mainly workers and agriculturalists live.

Within eight-week duration (06/01 to 07/24 2015) every patient of the general practice was asked to participate. The study nurses screened all potential participants for their eligibility and their level of cooperation in order to raise the responder rate. Subjects who were unable to complete the questionnaires due to linguistic barriers or serious physical or psychological health issues and patients younger than 10 years were excluded. After the initial information session all subjects were provided with questionnaires in the doctor's waiting room prior to the consultation. The following questions regarding pain and sleep disorders were included: "Do you suffer from pain/sleep disorders?" If this was answered by "yes" subjects were asked to proceed answering the relevant questions. In case patients did not know how to answer a question, the study nurses gave explanations.

2.2. Measures

2.2.1. Pain. Pain was assessed according to the Multidimensional German Pain Questionnaire (Deutscher Schmerzfragebogen (DSF) [51]). The items comprised type of pain ("do you have background pain, background pain with breakthrough pain, breakthrough pain?"), duration ("since when do you have pain?"), and localization ("where on your body do you feel pain?"). CP was defined by pain ≥ 6 months. The instrument is empirically evaluated [52] and also includes questions concerning age, gender, weight, and height.

2.2.2. Education. Self-reported level of education was assessed by using 4 response options. We asked for the highest educational attainment. Employment status was defined by using a 3-point categorical variable. Job seekers, person doing family work, and retired persons were assigned as "unemployed." We categorized worker, piece worker, employees, self-employed people, apprentices, volunteers, and internships as "employed." Scholars and students were categorized as "in education." The specific categories of education as well as the ones of employment status can be seen in Table 1.

2.2.3. Medical Information. The current use of prescribed pain and sleep medication was gathered from the patients' charts. The coding of the medication as medication for pain or medication for sleep was done by A.G. According to the "Pain ladder," or analgesic ladder, created by the World Health Organization (WHO) [53], nonopioids (nonsteroidal anti-inflammatory drugs) and weak opioids were coded as pain medication. Non-benzodiazepine hypnotics (Z-Drugs), benzodiazepines, and sedating antidepressants (off-label sleep aids) were coded as sleep medication. If patients were prescribed sleep medication and pain medication together, we coded as "combinations."

2.2.4. Sleep Disorders. SD were assessed by the Insomnia Severity Index (ISI), a brief self-report questionnaire consisting of seven items. Each item has to be rated on a five-point Likert scale, ranging from 0 (not at all) to 4 (extremely). The items are problems initiating sleep, problems maintaining sleep, early awake, satisfaction with current sleep patterns, impact on daytime quality of life due to SD, noticeability of sleep problems by others, distress or worry caused by SD, and interference with daytime functioning. Total scores range from 0 to 28. Higher scores indicate a greater insomnia severity (0–7: no clinically significant insomnia; 8–14: subthreshold insomnia; ≥15: clinical insomnia). The psychometric properties are considered to be sound [54, 55].

2.3. Source of Funding and Ethical Considerations. The study was conducted in accordance with the Declaration of Helsinki and approved by the local ethical committee of the Danube University of Krems.

Patients were informed about the voluntary nature of participation and informed consent was obtained from each subject. If participants were younger than 18 years also parents had to agree. This study was conducted independently of any institutional influence and was not funded externally.

2.4. Statistics. The statistical analyses were performed with SPSS 23.0. Frequencies (N, n), percentages (%), means (M), and standard deviations (Std) were calculated as descriptive statistics; Chi-squared tests were performed to compare men and women. Individuals were excluded from the statistical

TABLE 1: Sociodemographic data, body mass index, and pain and sleep medication *n* (%).

	Male	Female
Gender n (%)	281 (49.3)	289 (50.7)
Age M years (±Std*)	50.9 (18.6)	50.8 (18.8)
Education % (*n*)#		
Compulsory school 9 years $n = 181$	63 (34.8)	118 (65.2)
Apprenticeship Compulsory school and additional training of at least 2 years in a specific occupational scope $n = 276$	162 (58.7)	114 (41.3)
Matriculation equal a higher school graduation $n = 60$	31 (51.7)	29 (48.3)
University, University of Applied Science $n = 51$	24 (47.1)	27 (52.9)
Employment status n (%)+		
Unemployed/retired $n = 209$	109 (52.2)	100 (47.8)
Employed $n = 306$	146 (47.7)	160 (52.3)
In education $n = 45$	23 (51.1)	22 (48.9)
BMI Mean (±Std*) $n = 568$	27.1 (4.7)	26.2 (5.3)
Medication n (%)¯		
None $n = 387$	201 (51.9)	186 (48.1)
Pain $n = 129$	61 (47.3)	68 (52.7)
Sleep $n = 31$	11 (35.5)	20 (64.5)
Combinations $n = 18$	5 (27.8)	13 (72.2)

*Standard deviation (Std). #Education was available for $n = 568$ patients (99.6% of total sample). +Employment status was available for $n = 560$ patients (98.2% of total sample). ¯Medication was available for $n = 565$ patients (99.1% of total sample).

analysis of a variable if they had a missing value in this given variable.

We modeled predictors for pain experience and sleep disturbance with type III generalized linear models (GLM). We used standard stepwise backward model selection procedures based on AICc [56] for identification of predictor variables. The backward method and not the forward method was selected because the forward method has a higher Type II error risk [57].

3. Results

3.1. Sample. A total of $N = 570$ ($N = 289$ female) patients participated in the study. This equals a response rate of 98.6%. The mean (Std) age was 50.8 (±18.7), for women 50.8 (±18.8) and for men 50.9 (±18.6) years. The majority attended compulsory school and apprenticeship (80.2% of the total sample). About half of the patients were employed (53.7% of total sample). The mean of the body mass index in both genders is slightly increased. Not medicated were 67.9%, 22.6% took medications for pain, 5.4% received medication for sleep, and 3.2% were medicated for both pain and sleep. Further results for pain are summarized in Table 2. Detailed data are presented in Table 1.

3.2. Clinical Variables

3.2.1. Pain. Of the total sample $n = 238$ (41.8%) answered yes to the question "do you suffer from pain?" indicating pain experiences (41.3% of the men versus 42.2% of the women; $p = 0.82$). Pain duration of at least 6 months (CP) was reported by $n = 189$ (33.2% of total sample; see Table 2).

3.2.2. Sleep. One hundred and sixty-six patients of the total sample (29.1%) answered yes to the question "do you suffer from sleep disorders?" (25.6% of the men versus 32.5% of the women; $p = 0.04$) and $n = 33$ (5.8%) of the total sample suffered from a clinical insomnia (see Table 3). Of the $n = 189$ patients with CP, $n = 86$ patients (45.5%) also reported SD. Of the $n = 86$ patients with CP and SD, $n = 83$ also completed the ISI and $n = 22$ (26.5% of $n = 83$) had a clinical insomnia

TABLE 2: Pain.

	% of total sample (N = 570)	% of sample with pain experiences (n = 238)	Male (n, %% of the n given in the left column)	Female (n, %% of the n given in the left column)	p value for the comparison men versus women
*Type of pain**					
Background pain n = 85	14.9	37.6	40 (47.1)	45 (52.9)	
Background pain with breakthrough pain n = 17	3.0	7.5	9 (52.9)	8 (47.1)	p = 0.89
Breakthrough pain n = 124	21.8	54.9	61 (49.2)	63 (50.8)	
Duration of pain#					
Less than 1 month n = 17	3.0	7.2	13 (76.5)	4 (23.5)	
One to six months n = 29	5.1	12.3	13 (44.8)	16 (55.2)	
Six to twelve months n = 12	2.1	5.2	6 (50.0)	6 (50.0)	p = 0.31
One to two years n = 32	5.6	13.6	16 (50.0)	16 (50.0)	
Two to five years n = 41	7.2	17.4	20 (48.8)	21 (51.2)	
More than 5 years n = 104	18.2	44.3	47 (45.2)	57 (54.8)	
Localization of pain+					
Head n = 18	3.2	7.9	4 (22.2)	14 (77.8)	
Chest n = 6	1.1	2.6	5 (83.3)	1 (16.7)	
Abdominal n = 2	0.4	0.9	2 (100.0)	0 (0)	p = 0.02
Back n = 51	8.9	22.5	30 (58.8)	21 (41.2)	
Joints n = 56	9.8	24.7	29 (51.8)	27 (48.2)	
Multiple n = 94	16.5	41.4	42 (44.7)	52 (55.3)	

*Type of pain was available for n = 226 patients (95.0% of the n = 238 patients with pain experiences). #Duration of pain was available for n = 235 patients (98.7% of the n = 238 patients with pain experiences). +Localization of pain was available for n = 227 patients (95.4% of the n = 238 patients with pain experiences).

(ISI $\geq$ 15). Table 3 provides an overview for the patients with self-reported sleep disorders.

3.3. General Linear Model. We include 567 individuals in the full model. The full model includes age, gender, BMI, employment status, education and sleep disturbances as correlates of experience of pain. After the stepwise reduction of variables the final model includes age ($F1$, 567 = 29.123, $p < 0.001$) and SD ($F2$, 567 = 20.903, $p < 0.001$). SD was significantly associated with pain experiences ($\beta = 0.872$, SE = 0.191, t= 4,572, $p < 0.001$, CI [0.497; 1.246]).

Older age was associated with pain experience also significantly ($\beta = 0.025$, SE = 0.005, $t = 5.135$, $p < 0.001$, CI [0.015; 0.035.]).

4. Discussion

This study underlines the high prevalence of CP and SD in primary care. 33.2. % suffered from CP. Out of all participants 29.1% reported SD. 26.5% of CP patients suffered from clinical insomnia. These findings confirm results from previous studies [4, 36]. In contrast, several studies indicate a higher rate of SD in pain patients [40, 58]. These differences can be partially explained by the different types of pain (pain experienced in the last four weeks versus CP). This could be supported by Fishbain and colleagues [59], who showed that SD are significantly more prevalent in CP patients than in patients with acute pain.

In our study SD and older age were significantly associated with pain as already reported [60]. Employment status

TABLE 3: Sleep.

	% of total sample ($N = 570$)	% of sample with sleep disorders ($n = 166$)	Male (n, % of the n given in the left column)	Female (n, % of the n given in the left column)	p value for the comparison men versus women
CP and SD $n = 86$	15.1	51.8	39 (45.3)	47 (54.7)	$p = 0.33$
CP, SD, and problems falling asleep (ISI item 1 answered as mild, moderate, severe, or very severe) $n = 64$	11.2	38.6	27 (42.2)	37 (57.8)	$p = 0.18$
CP, SD, and problems maintaining sleep (ISI item 2 answered as mild, moderate, severe, or very severe) $n = 66$	11.6	39.8	30 (45.5)	36 (54.5)	$p = 0.49$
CP, SD, and early awaking (ISI item 3 answered as mild, moderate, severe, or very severe) $n = 52$	9.1	31.3	25 (48.1)	27 (51.9)	$p = 0.85$
CP, SD, and sleep dissatisfaction (ISI item 4 answered as dissatisfied and very dissatisfied) $n = 31$	5.4	18.7	13 (41.9)	18 (58.1)	$p = 0.43$
CP, SD, and impact of sleep disorder on performance (ISI item 7 answered as a little, somewhat, much, very much) $n = 76$	13.3	45.8	34 (44.7)	42 (55.3)	$p = 0.34$
CP, SD, and impact on other life areas (ISI item 5 answered as a little, somewhat, much, very much) $n = 68$	11.9	41.0	32 (47.1)	36 (52.9)	$p = 0.69$
CP, SD, and worries (ISI item 6 answered as a little, somewhat, much, very much) $n = 62$	10.9	37.3	32 (51.6)	30 (48.4)	$p = 0.79$
Clinical insomnia (ISI ≥ 15) $n = 33^{\#}$	5.8	20.8	16 (48.5)	17 (51.5)	$p = 0.41$
CP and Clinical insomnia (ISI ≥ 15) $n = 22$	3.9	13.3.	11 (50.0)	11 (50.0)	$p = 0.72$

$^{\#}$ISI score was available for $n = 159$ of the $n = 166$ patients with sleep disorders.

and education were not significantly correlated with pain. These results are not in line with earlier studies [61–63]. One possible reason might be the sample characteristics covered by the study. Our participants showed lower education attainments [64] and a higher unemployment rate [65] than Austria as a whole.

We found a higher prevalence in patients suffering from initiating sleep, maintaining sleep, early awake, and dissatisfaction with sleep in comparison to Baker et al. [60]. The most likely reasons for these differences might be that we considered longer durations of pain.

The results did not confirm existing evidence, that women experience chronic pain more often than men [66, 67]. As a recent systematic review and meta-analysis revealed, chronic pain prevalence estimations are an obvious matter of survey methods [68]. Our defining of CP (≥6 month) and data collection method might explain these differences. We found no differences in the prevalence of pain type by gender [69]. Male and female patients suffered around the same frequency from background pain, background pain with breakthrough pain, and breakthrough pain. We found gender differences in pain sites. The most common body sites in women affected by pain were 1st multiple sites, 2nd joint pain, 3rd back pain, 4th headache, and 5th chest pain. Men reported most frequent 1st multiple site pain, 2nd back pain, 3rd joints pain, 4th chest pain, 5th headache, and 6th abdominal pain. These results confirm findings from a recent Austrian study [62] that found comparable frequencies. Our result revealed that headache is significantly more common in women [62, 67].

SD are often overlooked in CP patients [70]. This is especially intriguing as treating cooccurring SD has a high potential to improve pain management outcomes [71]. About half of CP patients with SD in our study were prescribed with pain medication, about 10% to 20% with sleep medication or combinations of both. Female patients received more often sleep medications or both, sleep and pain medications. In clinical practice it would be beneficial to pharmacologically treat CP and SD jointly [7, 72]. There are several pharmacological approaches that can improve both CP and cooccurring SD. Some tricyclic antidepressants (amitriptyline, nortriptyline, trimipramine, and doxepin) show positive effects on both, CP and SD [16, 35, 40, 73, 74]. Trazodone, a serotonin modulator, has been studied in patients with various types of pain. The outcome was associated with both improved sleep quality and pain reduction [25]. Mirtazapine is effective in the treatment of SD [32] as well as for the treatment of pain [15, 71].

Gabapentin and pregabalin are also often used to treat CP and cooccurring SD [60, 75, 76]. Short term use of benzodiazepines (BRA) [45, 75, 77] and non-benzodiazepine drugs (NBRA) [43, 44, 78] has been shown to be potentially useful in improving SD in CP patients. In contrast to benzodiazepines [74], long- term efficacy trials have supported the use of NBRA [76, 79, 80].

A variety of psychological interventions have been found to be effective in both pain treatment [81–84] and insomnia treatment [73, 85]. Psychological techniques for CP management usually involve strategies for the identification of dysfunctional and/or maladaptive thoughts and specific strategies, such as distraction techniques, relaxation training, and activity pacing. These skills help patients to manage pain symptoms [70]. Psychological interventions for SD typically utilize behavioral interventions like general sleep education, stimulus control instructions, sleep hygiene education, alternation of biorhythm, and sleep restriction [71]. Given the effectiveness of these interventions, there has been growing interest in simultaneous treatments of the symptoms. Combined treatments utilize components of both interventions. In a pilot study with CP patients, Tang and colleagues [86] found a greater improvement in sleep after treatment, in comparison to a waiting group, who kept pain and sleep diaries.

The results of our study have to be interpreted with respect to its limitations. The generalizability of the results is limited as only one general practice took part in the study. Yet, some aspects speak for the generalizability of the results. First, patients were treated under the conditions of routine. Second, the practice is the only general practice in a relatively large rural region. Moreover, it is important to note that the sample is based on a cross-sectional design, which does not allow causal inferences.

Additionally, we did not assess psychiatric conditions, which are frequently associated with SD and pain [87, 88]. Another limitation is that we did not carry out comprehensive assessment of pain and sleep disorders. For example, the screening question "do you suffer from pain/sleep disorders?" was not validated before and it is not clear how children understood the questions. However, only two participants were younger than 15 years and it has been shown that even children five years old can give meaningful self-reports of pain when age-appropriate tools and training are provided [89]. While the present study has limitations, the results are based on a relatively large sample size with an extraordinary high response rate. Thus we can provide an almost complete evaluation of the cooccurrence of SD and pain experiences in patients of a general practice.

Comprehensive management of CP and SD in primary care requires an individualized assessment and treatment approach. A shift from predominantly biomedical strategies to a more biopsychosocial perspective would raise treatment outcomes. SD should be systematically evaluated in CP patients in primary care settings based on the reported high cooccurrence. A proactive diagnostic approach for these persons is needed to achieve accurate information and treatment. Coordinated multidisciplinary and interdisciplinary care has a high potential to provide this. The high influence on personal life-quality and health care costs make it important that increased efforts in experimental and clinical research are made. The aim of these efforts should be a translationally meaningful understanding of the mutual impact of CP and poor sleep.

References

[1] R. Nickel and H. H. Raspe, "Chronic pain: epidemiology and receiving treatment," *Der Nervenarzt*, vol. 72, no. 12, pp. 897–906, 2001.

[2] K. Harman, R. T. Pivik, J. L. D'Eon, K. G. Wilson, J. R. Swenson, and L. Matsunaga, "Sleep in depressed and nondepressed participants with chronic low back pain: Electroencephalographic and behaviour findings," *SLEEP*, vol. 25, no. 7, pp. 775–783, 2002.

[3] C. M. Morin, D. Gibson, and J. Wade, "Self-reported sleep and mood disturbance in chronic pain patients," *The Clinical Journal of Pain*, vol. 14, no. 4, pp. 311–314, 1998.

[4] M. M. Ohayon, "Relationship between chronic painful physical condition and insomnia," *Journal of Psychiatric Research*, vol. 39, no. 2, pp. 151–159, 2005.

[5] S. H. Onen, A. Alloui, A. Gross, A. Eschallier, and C. Dubray, "The effects of total sleep deprivation, selective sleep interruption and sleep recovery on pain tolerance thresholds in healthy subjects," *Journal of Sleep Research*, vol. 10, no. 1, pp. 35–42, 2001.

[6] I. Raymond, T. A. Nielsen, G. Lavigne, C. Manzini, and M. Choinière, "Quality of sleep and its daily relationship to pain intensity in hospitalized adult burn patients," *PAIN*, vol. 92, no. 3, pp. 381–388, 2001.

[7] T. Roehrs and T. Roth, "Sleep and pain: Interaction of two vital functions," *Seminars in Neurology*, vol. 25, no. 1, pp. 106–116, 2005.

[8] M. T. Smith, R. R. Edwards, U. D. McCann, and J. A. Haythomthwaite, "The effects of sleep deprivation on pain

inhibition and spontaneous pain in women," *SLEEP*, vol. 30, no. 4, pp. 494–505, 2007.

[9] N. Becker, A. B. Thomsen, A. K. Olsen, P. Sjogren, P. Bech, and J. Eriksen, "Pain epidemiology and health related quality of life in chronic non-malignant pain patients referred to a Danish multidisciplinary pain center," *PAIN*, vol. 73, no. 3, pp. 393–400, 1997.

[10] R. Wolff, C. Clar, C. Lerch, and J. Kleijnen, "Epidemiology of chronic non-malignant pain in Germany," *Der Schmerz*, vol. 25, no. 1, pp. 26–44, 2011.

[11] A. Becker, R. Seitz, E. Jacobi, and R. Leidl, "Cost measurement based on patient surveys - A pilot study on a cost diary," *Rehabilitation*, vol. 40, no. 1, pp. 12–20, 2001.

[12] W. Bolten, A. Kempel-Waibel, and W. Pförringer, "Analysis of cost of illness of low back pain," *Medizinische Klinik - Intensivmedizin und Notfallmedizin*, vol. 93, no. 6, pp. 388–393, 1998.

[13] C. O. Schmidt, B. Schweikert, C. M. Wenig et al., "Modelling the prevalence and cost of back pain with neuropathic components in the general population," *European Journal of Pain*, vol. 13, no. 10, pp. 1030–1035, 2009.

[14] C. M. Wenig, C. O. Schmidt, T. Kohlmann, and B. Schweikert, "Costs of back pain in Germany," *European Journal of Pain*, vol. 13, no. 3, pp. 280–286, 2009.

[15] H. Breivik, B. Collett, V. Ventafridda, R. Cohen, and D. Gallacher, "Survey of chronic pain in Europe: prevalence, impact on daily life, and treatment," *European Journal of Pain*, vol. 10, no. 4, pp. 287–333, 2006.

[16] H. Liedgens, M. Obradovic, J. De Courcy, T. Holbrook, and R. Jakubanis, "A burden of illness study for neuropathic pain in Europe," *ClinicoEconomics and Outcomes Research*, vol. 8, pp. 113–126, 2016.

[17] G. E. Simon and M. Vonkorff, "Prevalence, burden, and treatment of insomnia in primary care," *The American Journal of Psychiatry*, vol. 154, no. 10, pp. 1417–1423, 1997.

[18] E. M. Wickwire, F. T. Shaya, and S. M. Scharf, "Health economics of insomnia treatments: The return on investment for a good night's sleep," *Sleep Medicine Reviews*, vol. 30, pp. 72–82, 2016.

[19] D. E. Ford and D. B. Kamerow, "Epidemiologic study of sleep disturbances and psychiatric disorders. An opportunity for prevention?" *Journal of the American Medical Association*, vol. 262, no. 11, pp. 1479–1484, 1989.

[20] Y. J. Lee, S.-J. Cho, I. H. Cho, and S. J. Kim, "Insufficient sleep and suicidality in adolescents," *SLEEP*, vol. 35, no. 4, pp. 455–460, 2012.

[21] M. M. Ohayon, "Determining the level of sleepiness in the American population and its correlates," *Journal of Psychiatric Research*, vol. 46, no. 4, pp. 422–427, 2012.

[22] M. Li, X.-W. Zhang, W.-S. Hou, and Z.-Y. Tang, "Insomnia and risk of cardiovascular disease: A meta-analysis of cohort studies," *International Journal of Cardiology*, vol. 176, no. 3, pp. 1044–1047, 2014.

[23] F. Sofi, F. Cesari, A. Casini, C. Macchi, R. Abbate, and G. F. Gensini, "Insomnia and risk of cardiovascular disease: a meta-analysis," *European Journal of Preventive Cardiology*, vol. 21, no. 1, pp. 57–64, 2014.

[24] E. Condén and A. Rosenblad, "Insomnia predicts long-term all-cause mortality after acute myocardial infarction: A prospective cohort study," *International Journal of Cardiology*, vol. 215, pp. 217–222, 2016.

[25] I. Pilowsky, I. Crettenden, and M. Townley, "Sleep disturbance in pain clinic patients," *PAIN*, vol. 23, no. 1, pp. 27–33, 1985.

[26] M. T. Smith, M. L. Perlis, M. S. Smith, D. E. Giles, and T. P. Carmody, "Sleep quality and presleep arousal in chronic pain," *Journal of Behavioral Medicine*, vol. 23, no. 1, pp. 1–13, 2000.

[27] C. Salisbury, "Multimorbidity: redesigning health care for people who use it," *The Lancet*, vol. 380, no. 9836, pp. 7–9, 2012.

[28] C. Violan, Q. Foguet-Boreu, G. Flores-Mateo et al., "Prevalence, determinants and patterns of multimorbidity in primary care: a systematic review of observational studies," *PLoS ONE*, vol. 9, no. 7, Article ID e102149, 2014.

[29] M. Schrimpf, G. Liegl, M. Boeckle, A. Leitner, P. Geisler, and C. Pieh, "The effect of sleep deprivation on pain perception in healthy subjects: A meta-analysis," *Sleep Medicine*, vol. 16, no. 11, article no. 2861, pp. 1313–1320, 2015.

[30] S. H. Onen, A. Alloui, D. Jourdan, A. Eschalier, and C. Dubray, "Effects of rapid eye movement (REM) sleep deprivation on pain sensitivity in the rat," *Brain Research*, vol. 900, no. 2, pp. 261–267, 2001.

[31] B. C. Sutton and M. R. Opp, "Musculoskeletal Sensitization and sleep: chronic muscle pain fragments sleep of mice without altering its duration," *SLEEP*, vol. 37, no. 3, pp. 505–513, 2014.

[32] B. C. Sutton and M. R. Opp, "Sleep fragmentation exacerbates mechanical hypersensitivity and alters subsequent sleep-wake behavior in a mouse model of musculoskeletal sensitization," *SLEEP*, vol. 37, no. 3, pp. 515–524, 2014.

[33] G. Vanini, K. Nemanis, H. A. Baghdoyan, and R. Lydic, "GABAergic transmission in rat pontine reticular formation regulates the induction phase of anesthesia and modulates hyperalgesia caused by sleep deprivation," *European Journal of Neuroscience*, vol. 40, no. 1, pp. 2264–2273, 2014.

[34] J. N. Ablin, D. J. Clauw, A. K. Lyden et al., "Effects of sleep restriction and exercise deprivation on somatic symptoms and mood in healthy adults," *Clinical and Experimental Rheumatology*, vol. 31, no. 79, pp. 53–59, 2013.

[35] S. S. Odegard, P. M. Omland, K. B. Nilsen, M. Stjern, G. B. Gravdahl, and T. Sand, "The effect of sleep restriction on laser evoked potentials, thermal sensory and pain thresholds and suprathreshold pain in healthy subjects," *Clinical Neurophysiology*, vol. 126, no. 10, pp. 1979–1987, 2015.

[36] T. Roehrs, M. Hyde, B. Blaisdell, M. Greenwald, and T. Roth, "Sleep loss and REM sleep loss are hyperalgesic," *SLEEP*, vol. 29, no. 2, pp. 145–151, 2006.

[37] T. A. Roehrs, E. Harris, S. Randall, and T. Roth, "Pain sensitivity and recovery from mild chronic sleep loss," *SLEEP*, vol. 35, no. 12, pp. 1667–1672, 2012.

[38] S. M. Alsaadi, J. H. McAuley, J. M. Hush et al., "The bidirectional relationship between pain intensity and sleep disturbance/quality in patients with low back pain," *The Clinical Journal of Pain*, vol. 30, no. 9, pp. 755–765, 2014.

[39] S. M. Alsaadi, J. H. McAuley, J. M. Hush et al., "Poor sleep quality is strongly associated with subsequent pain intensity in patients with acute low back pain," *Arthritis & Rheumatology*, vol. 66, no. 5, pp. 1388–1394, 2014.

[40] T. A. Call-Schmidt and S. J. Richardson, "Prevalence of sleep disturbance and its relationship to pain in adults with chronic pain," *Pain Management Nursing*, vol. 4, no. 3, pp. 124–133, 2003.

[41] R. Marin, T. Cyhan, and W. Miklos, "Sleep disturbance in patients with chronic low back pain," *American Journal of Physical Medicine & Rehabilitation*, vol. 85, no. 5, pp. 430–435, 2006.

[42] M. T. Smith, P. H. Finan, L. F. Buenaver et al., "Cognitive-behavioral therapy for insomnia in knee osteoarthritis: a randomized, double-blind, active placebo-controlled clinical trial," *Arthritis & Rheumatology*, vol. 67, no. 5, pp. 1221–1233, 2015.

[43] H. W. Goforth, X. A. Preud'Homme, and A. D. Krystal, "A randomized, double-blind, placebo-controlled trial of eszopiclone for the treatment of insomnia in patients with chronic low back pain," *SLEEP*, vol. 37, no. 6, pp. 1053–1060, 2014.

[44] T. Roth, J. M. Price, D. A. Amato, R. P. Rubens, J. M. Roach, and T. J. Schnitzer, "The effect of eszopiclone in patients with Insomnia and coexisting rheumatoid arthritis: a pilot study," *Primary Care Companion to the Journal of Clinical Psychiatry*, vol. 11, no. 6, pp. 292–301, 2009.

[45] J. K. Walsh, M. J. Muehlbach, S. A. Lauter, N. A. Hilliker, and A. K. Schweitzer, "Effects of triazolam on sleep, daytime sleepiness and morning stiffness in patients with rheumatoid arthritis," *The Journal of Rheumatology*, vol. 23, no. 2, pp. 245–252, 1996.

[46] L. Pauer, A. Winkelmann, P. Arsenault et al., "An international, randomized, double-blind, placebo-controlled, phase III trial of pregabalin monotherapy in treatment of patients with fibromyalgia," *The Journal of Rheumatology*, vol. 38, no. 12, pp. 2643–2652, 2011.

[47] A. Vinik, B. Emir, B. Parsons, and R. Cheung, "Prediction of pregabalin-mediated pain response by severity of sleep disturbance in patients with painful diabetic neuropathy and post-herpetic neuralgia," *Pain Medicine*, vol. 15, no. 4, pp. 661–670, 2014.

[48] I. Khalid, T. A. Roehrs, D. W. Hudgel, and T. Roth, "Continuous positive airway pressure in severe obstructive sleep apnea reduces pain sensitivity," *SLEEP*, vol. 34, no. 12, pp. 1687–1691, 2011.

[49] K. Stiasny-Kolster, D. B. Pfau, W. H. Oertel, R.-D. Treede, and W. Magerl, "Hyperalgesia and functional sensory loss in restless legs syndrome," *PAIN*, vol. 154, no. 8, pp. 1457–1463, 2013.

[50] B. A. Stuck, J. T. Maurer, M. Schredl, H. Weeß, and L. Fricke-Oerkermann, *Praxis der Schlafmedizin: Schlafstörungen bei Erwachsenen und Kindern Diagnostik, Differenzialdiagnostik und Therapie*, Springer, Berlin, Germany, 2013.

[51] H. R. Casser, M. Hüppe, T. Kohlmann et al., "German pain questionnaire and standardised documentation with the KEDOQ-Schmerz. A way for quality management in pain therapy," *Der Schmerz*, vol. 26, no. 2, pp. 168–175, 2012.

[52] B. Nagel, H. U. Gerbershagen, G. Lindena, and M. Pfingsten, "Development and evaluation of the multidimensional German pain questionnaire," *Der Schmerz*, vol. 16, no. 4, pp. 263–270, 2002.

[53] J. Stjernswärd, "WHO cancer pain relief programme.," *Cancer Surveys*, vol. 7, no. 1, pp. 195–208, 1988.

[54] C. H. Bastien, A. Vallières, and C. M. Morin, "Validation of the insomnia severity index as an outcome measure for insomnia research," *Sleep Medicine*, vol. 2, no. 4, pp. 297–307, 2001.

[55] M. Gerber, C. Lang, S. Lemola et al., "Validation of the German version of the insomnia severity index in adolescents, young adults and adult workers: results from three cross-sectional studies," *BMC Psychiatry*, vol. 16, no. 1, article no. 174, 2016.

[56] K. P. Burnham and D. R. Anderson, *Model Selection and Multimodel Inference: A Practical Information-Theoretic Approach*, Springer, New York, NY, USA, 2nd edition, 2013.

[57] A. Field, Discovering Statistics Using IBM SPSS Statistics: SAGE Publications, 2013.

[58] N. K. Y. Tang, K. J. Wright, and P. M. Salkovskis, "Prevalence and correlates of clinical insomnia co-occurring with chronic back pain," *Journal of Sleep Research*, vol. 16, no. 1, pp. 85–95, 2007.

[59] D. A. Fishbain, J. Gao, J. E. Lewis, D. Bruns, L. J. Meyer, and J. M. Disorbio, "Prevalence comparisons of somatic and psychiatric symptoms between community nonpatients without pain, acute pain patients, and chronic pain patients," *Pain Medicine*, vol. 16, no. 1, pp. 37–50, 2015.

[60] S. Baker, J. McBeth, C. A. Chew-Graham, and R. Wilkie, "Musculoskeletal pain and co-morbid insomnia in adults; a population study of the prevalence and impact on restricted social participation," *BMC Family Practice*, vol. 18, no. 1, pp. 1–9, 2017.

[61] T. E. Dorner, J. Muckenhuber, W. J. Stronegger, É. Rsky, B. Gustorff, and W. Freidl, "The impact of socio-economic status on pain and the perception of disability due to pain," *European Journal of Pain*, vol. 15, no. 1, pp. 103–109, 2011.

[62] T. E. Dorner, K. V. Stein, J. Hahne, F. Wepner, M. Friedrich, and E. Mittendorfer-Rutz, "How are socio-demographic and psycho-social factors associated with the prevalence and chronicity of severe pain in 14 different body sites? A cross-sectional population-based survey," *Wiener Klinische Wochenschrift*.

[63] P. Saastamoinen, P. Leino-Arjas, M. Laaksonen, and E. Lahelma, "Socio-economic differences in the prevalence of acute, chronic and disabling chronic pain among ageing employees," *PAIN*, vol. 114, no. 3, pp. 364–371, 2005.

[64] M. Bruneforth, L. Lassnigg, S. Vogtenhuber, C. Schreiner, and S. Breit, "Nationaler bildungsbericht österreich 2015," *Band 1: Das Schulsystem im Spiegel von Daten und Indikatoren: Leykam*, 2016.

[65] K. Jäger, alt - älter - arbeitslos: Das Leben von arbeitslosen Menschen ab 50plus in Wien: Diplom.de, 2014.

[66] R. B. Fillingim, C. D. King, M. C. Ribeiro-Dasilva, B. Rahim-Williams, and J. L. Riley III, "Sex, gender, and pain: a review of recent clinical and experimental findings," *The Journal of Pain*, vol. 10, no. 5, pp. 447–485, 2009.

[67] J. S. Mogil, "Sex differences in pain and pain inhibition: multiple explanations of a controversial phenomenon," *Nature Reviews Neuroscience*, vol. 13, no. 12, pp. 859–866, 2012.

[68] Ó. A. Steingrímsdóttir, T. Landmark, G. J. Macfarlane, and C. S. Nielsen, "Defining chronic pain in epidemiological studies," *PAIN*, vol. 158, no. 11, pp. 2092–2107, 2017.

[69] B. Gerdle, J. Björk, L. Cöster, K. G. Henriksson, C. Henriksson, and A. Bengtsson, "Prevalence of widespread pain and associations with work status: a population study," *BMC Musculoskeletal Disorders*, vol. 9, article 102, 2008.

[70] M. D. Cheatle, S. Foster, A. Pinkett, M. Lesneski, D. Qu, and L. Dhingra, "Assessing and managing sleep disturbance in patients with chronic pain," *Anesthesiology Clinics*, vol. 34, no. 2, pp. 379–393, 2016.

[71] P. H. Finan, L. F. Buenaver, V. T. Runko, and M. T. Smith, "Cognitive-behavioral therapy for comorbid insomnia and chronic pain," *Sleep Medicine Clinics*, vol. 9, no. 2, pp. 261–274, 2014.

[72] H. Moldofsky, "Sleep and pain," *Sleep Medicine Reviews*, vol. 5, no. 5, pp. 387–398, 2001.

[73] C. R. Jungquist, Y. Tra, M. T. Smith et al., "The durability of cognitive behavioral therapy for insomnia in patients with chronic pain," *Journal of Sleep Disorders: Treatment & Care*, vol. 2012, Article ID 679648, 8 pages, 2012.

[74] S. A. King and J. J. Strain, "Benzodiazepine use by chronic pain patients," *The Clinical Journal of Pain*, vol. 6, no. 2, pp. 143–147, 1990.

[75] S. L. Bartusch, B. J. Sanders, J. G. D'Alessio, and J. R. Jernigan, "Clonazepam for the treatment of lancinating phantom limb pain," *The Clinical Journal of Pain*, vol. 12, no. 1, pp. 59–62, 1996.

[76] T. Roth, J. K. Walsh, A. Krystal, T. Wessel, and T. A. Roehrs, "An evaluation of the efficacy and safety of eszopiclone over 12 months in patients with chronic primary insomnia," *Sleep Medicine*, vol. 6, no. 6, pp. 487–495, 2005.

[77] L. A. Menefee, M. J. M. Cohen, W. R. Anderson, K. Doghramji, E. D. Frank, and H. Lee, "Sleep disturbance and nonmalignant chronic pain: a comprehensive review of the literature," *Pain Medicine*, vol. 1, no. 2, pp. 156–172, 2000.

[78] H. Moldofsky, F. A. Lue, C. Mously, B. Roth-Schechter, and W. J. Reynolds, "The effect of zolpidem in patients with fibromyalgia: a dose ranging, double blind, placebo controlled, modified crossover study," *The Journal of Rheumatology*, vol. 23, no. 3, pp. 529–533, 1996.

[79] M. Pollack, G. Kinrys, A. Krystal et al., "Eszopiclone coadministered with escitalopram in patients with insomnia and comorbid generalized anxiety disorder," *Archives of General Psychiatry*, vol. 65, no. 5, pp. 551–562, 2008.

[80] S. Randall, T. A. Roehrs, and T. Roth, "Efficacy of eight months of nightly zolpidem: a prospective placebo-controlled study," *SLEEP*, vol. 35, no. 11, pp. 1551–1557, 2012.

[81] J. E. Broderick, F. J. Keefe, S. Schneider et al., "Cognitive behavioral therapy for chronic pain is effective, but for whom?" *PAIN*, vol. 157, no. 9, pp. 2115–2123, 2016.

[82] D. C. Cherkin, K. J. Sherman, B. H. Balderson et al., "Effect of mindfulness-based stress reduction vs cognitive behavioral therapy or usual care on back pain and functional limitations in adults with chronic low back pain," *The Journal of the American Medical Association*, vol. 315, no. 12, pp. 1240–1249, 2016.

[83] A. Kohl, W. Rief, and J. A. Glombiewski, "Acceptance, cognitive restructuring, and distraction as coping strategies for acute pain," *The Journal of Pain*, vol. 14, no. 3, pp. 305–315, 2013.

[84] G. Liegl, M. Boeckle, A. Leitner, and C. Pieh, "A meta-analytic review of brief guided self-help education for chronic pain," *European Journal of Pain*, vol. 20, no. 10, pp. 1551–1562, 2016.

[85] B. Sivertsen, S. Omvik, S. Pallesen et al., "Cognitive behavioral therapy vs zopiclone for treatment of chronic primary insomnia in older adults: A randomized controlled trial," *Journal of the American Medical Association*, vol. 295, no. 24, pp. 2851–2858, 2006.

[86] N. K. Y. Tang, C. E. Goodchild, and P. M. Salkovskis, "Hybrid cognitive-behaviour therapy for individuals with insomnia and chronic pain: a pilot randomised controlled trial," *Behaviour Research and Therapy*, vol. 50, no. 12, pp. 814–821, 2012.

[87] L. A. McWilliams, B. J. Cox, and M. W. Enns, "Mood and anxiety disorders associated with chronic pain: an examination in a nationally representative sample," *PAIN*, vol. 106, no. 1-2, pp. 127–133, 2003.

[88] L. Palagini, U. Faraguna, M. Mauri, A. Gronchi, C. M. Morin, and D. Riemann, "Association between stress-related sleep reactivity and cognitive processes in insomnia disorder and insomnia subgroups: Preliminary results," *Sleep Medicine*, vol. 19, pp. 101–107, 2016.

[89] C. L. von Baeyer, "Children's self-reports of pain intensity: scale selection, limitations and interpretation," *Pain Research & Management*, vol. 11, no. 3, pp. 157–162, 2006.

19

Quantitative Thermal Testing Profiles as a Predictor of Treatment Response to Topical Capsaicin in Patients with Localized Neuropathic Pain

A. Serrano,[1] D. Torres,[2] M. Veciana,[3] C. Caro,[1] J. Montero,[3] and V. Mayoral[1]

[1] *Department of Anesthesiology, Critical Care and Pain Clinics, Hospital Universitari de Bellvitge, L'Hospitalet de Llobregat, 08907 Barcelona, Spain*
[2] *Department of Anesthesiology, Critical Care and Pain Clinics, Hospital Universitario de Santiago de Compostela, 15701 Santiago, Spain*
[3] *Department of Neurology and Neurophysiology, Hospital Universitari de Bellvitge, L'Hospitalet de Llobregat, 08907 Barcelona, Spain*

Correspondence should be addressed to A. Serrano; a.serrano@bellvitgehospital.cat

Academic Editor: Pierangelo Geppetti

There are no reliable predictors of response to treatment with capsaicin. Given that capsaicin application causes heat sensation, differences in quantitative thermal testing (QTT) profiles may predict treatment response. The aim of this study was to determine whether different QTT profiles could predict treatment outcomes in patients with localized peripheral neuropathic pain (PeLNP). We obtained from medical records QTT results and treatment outcomes of 55 patients treated between 2010 and 2013. Warm sensation threshold (WST) and heat pain threshold (HPT) values were assessed at baseline at the treatment site and in the asymptomatic, contralateral area. Responders were defined as those who achieved a > 30% decrease in pain lasting > 30 days. Two distinct groups were identified based on differences in QTT profiles. Most patients (27/31; 87.1%) with a homogenous profile were nonresponders. By contrast, more than half of the patients (13/24, 54.2%) with a nonhomogenous profile were responders ($p = 0.0028$). A nonhomogenous QTT profile appears to be predictive of response to capsaicin. We hypothesize patients with a partial loss of cutaneous nerve fibers or receptors are more likely to respond. By contrast, when severe nerve damage or normal cutaneous sensations are present, the pain is likely due to central sensitization and thus not responsive to capsaicin. Prospective studies with larger patient samples are needed to confirm this hypothesis.

1. Introduction

Neuropathic pain is a chronic condition that is very difficult to treat [1], and only small improvements in treatment efficacy have been achieved in the last decade. However, one of the most promising treatments for peripheral neuropathic pain (PeNP) developed in recent years is the capsaicin 8% patch (CP8%) (QutenzaTM). This patch delivers capsaicin into the skin and clinical trials have shown that it can provide up to 12 weeks of PeNP relief with a single topical patch application [2–4].

Capsaicin works by directly targeting, with a highly selective agonism, the transient receptor potential vanilloid 1 (TRPV1) receptor, which is primarily present in C-fibers and in some Aδ-fibers. High-concentration capsaicin activates TRPV1 channels by overstimulating the nociceptors, resulting in the defunctionalization of the nociceptor nerve fibers and thereby reducing spontaneous nerve activity, leading to a loss of responsiveness. After defunctionalization, patients perceive a decrease in PeNP [5–7], which is frequently referred to as "desensitization."

The European Medical Agency (EMA) has recommended that CP8% be applied by a doctor or other healthcare professionals under the supervision of a doctor [8]. However, this recommendation limits treatment options, primarily because it depends on the availability of treatment at outpatient clinics. This requirement also makes treatment more expensive. In addition, the indirect costs of personnel and other materials must be added to the direct cost of CP8% [9]. As a result, many patients who could benefit from treatment may not be treated due to affordability issues. The number-needed-to-treat (NNT) for CP8% is high [10]. Given the aforementioned high cost of treatment, the patch should be applied only to those most likely to benefit from improvement. However, to date, no clear predictors of treatment response in patients with PeNP have been identified, despite recent efforts to do so [11–13].

Given that capsaicin affects unmyelinated or slightly myelinated fibers and studies have shown that the CP8% patch involves heat sensation [6], we hypothesized that quantitative thermal testing (QTT) could be a potential predictor of treatment response. To investigate this question, we performed a retrospective study of clinical records to assess the QTT profiles of patients who underwent capsaicin treatment for PeLNP. Our main aim was to compare the baseline QTT profiles to determine whether any of these were associated with treatment response.

2. Material and Methods

This was a retrospective analysis of all patients treated with the CP8% patch for PeNP at our pain clinic between 2010 and 2013. From patient medical records, we obtained QTT results and treatment outcomes (response versus nonresponse) for all patients. All procedures were performed according to clinical protocols in place at our institution during the study period.

2.1. Patients. Since late 2010, all patients presenting at our pain clinic with a high suspicion for PeNP have been asked to complete the *Douleur Neuropathique* 4 Scale (DN4), followed by consultations with a pain physician and a neurophysiologist for complete neurological assessment. Based on this evaluation, patients are classified into one of the following pain categories: (1) postherpetic neuralgia (PHN) and (2) chronic postsurgical pain (CPSP), or type I or II complex regional pain syndrome (CRPS). PeNP is considered possible when the patient meets the criteria given in the International Association for the Study of Pain (IASP) recommendations [14]. In cases in which the PeNP is confined to a single, localized area, it is classified as localized peripheral neuropathic pain (PeLNP) [15]. Patients with PeLNP are eligible to choose either CP8% or lidocaine plaster for topical treatment.

2.2. Establishing the Area to Be Treated. Prior to treatment, a discontinuous line is drawn with a permanent-ink marker on the skin to mark the boundaries between the painful area (identified by the patient as hyperalgesia or allodynia) and the area with normal skin sensation. Transparent paper is used to copy this area and save for further patch applications.

2.3. Assessment of Pain. A numerical pain rating scale (NPRS), ranging from 0 to 10 points, is used to assess the pain level, with 0 indicating no pain and 10 indicating the worst imaginable pain. Patients are asked to rate their pain scores at the following times: at first visit, before patch application, throughout the treatment procedure (see Section 2.6), at one week after application, and at 4–6 weeks after treatment. One week after treatment, patients are contacted by telephone to assess discomfort, heat pain, and any analgesics used.

2.4. Quantitative Thermal Testing. A QTT profile is routinely obtained in all patients at the following time points: pretreatment, one to two weeks after the first consultation and at PeNP diagnosis. The QTT test is always performed in the same room under the same environmental conditions. We determine warm sensation threshold (WST) and heat pain threshold (HPT) values, first in the normal contralateral skin area and then in the affected skin area, using the limits method [16]. The QTT test is performed using the pathway 9.0 cm^2 thermode (MEDOC Ltd., Israel) [17, 18]. The baseline temperature is set at 32°C (center of neutral range), with a cut-off temperature of 50°C and a ramp rate of 1°C/s for warm threshold and 1.5°C/s for heat pain. Patients are instructed to press a button (which returns the temperature to baseline) as soon as they perceive a warm or heat pain sensation. For each threshold, the test is repeated from 3 (minimum) to 5 (maximum) times. Based on these tests, a mean threshold value and standard deviation (SD) are automatically calculated.

2.5. Treatment with Capsaicin 8% Patch. On the day of treatment, the patients are told to eat a small meal (either breakfast or lunch, as appropriate) before presenting at the outpatient clinic. Topical local anaesthetic is applied for 75–90 minutes before procedure. The anaesthetic cream is then removed and the skin washed and dried. Afterwards, the patch is cut to fit using the previously created transparent sheet and applied to the patient's skin for 30 to 60 minutes, depending on the location. Health professionals and patients are required to wear the recommended protection at all times [8]. Once the patch has been removed, the area is cleaned with the gel provided by the patch manufacturer and the patient is discharged.

2.6. Management of Treatment-Related Discomfort. As part of the treatment protocol, patients are asked to rate their actual discomfort level using the NPRS. This is reevaluated every 20 minutes for one-hour procedures and every 15 minutes for 30-minute procedures. Blood pressure is also taken after every pain rating. After the CP8% treatment has finished, patients are discharged and given two sheets of malleable frozen gel for home use. Instructions are also provided for extra treatment with nonsteroidal oral analgesics.

2.7. Efficacy. Treatment response (i.e., pain relief) was defined as a > 30% decrease in the NPRS from baseline to the posttreatment assessment at weeks 4–6. In cases in which the difference is exactly 30% or when the patient is unable to rate pain relief with the NPRS, then treatment efficacy is determined by asking the patient to estimate overall improvement and willingness to repeat treatment.

2.8. Statistical Analysis. The statistical analysis was performed with the VassarStats online software [19]. To check for differences in demographic data between responders and nonresponders, we performed a two sample t-test for independent samples for parametric values. χ^2 was calculated for responders. Given that the total sample size was barely enough to perform the chi-squared test for some groups, the Fisher exact test was also calculated in these cases.

2.9. Difference in QTT for the Target and Control Areas. The patient sample was highly heterogenous due to variability in the following factors/conditions: time elapsed from injury to treatment; the use of multiple different concomitant medications; use of drugs acting on central nervous system (CNS) (i.e., antidepressants, psychoactive, or anticonvulsants) (see Table S4 in Supplementary Material available online at https://doi.org/10.1155/2017/7425907); different pain localizations involving one or several nerve territories. For these reasons, we were unable to compare out sample to normalized data reported elsewhere [20].

Since all patients in this sample had localized pain only, we used the contralateral asymptomatic healthy area as a control. The QTT profiles at the target PeLNP area were compared to the corresponding QTT profile at the contralateral area. As part of the routine treatment procedures, both WST and HPT values were assessed at baseline in the treatment (PeLNP site) area and at the asymptomatic contralateral site. Differences between the WST and HPT values in the target and control areas were considered not significant when there was a crossover between mean results (±1.96 SD) for the measurement on both areas; when this occurred, the painful area was considered to present normal thermal sensations. By contrast, if there was no crossover, we considered the WST (or HPT) for the treatment site to be significantly different (higher or lower) from the contralateral site.

3. Results

3.1. Patients. We initially identified a total of 65 patients diagnosed with PeLNP who had been treated with CP8% during the 2010–2013 period. Of these, 10 were excluded from the study for varying reasons: five were excluded because the contralateral area was not asymptomatic (contralateral pain in 5 cases and midline pain in 2 cases). Three other patients were excluded for the following reasons: one had an interventional pain procedure between treatment and assessment, another developed a recurrence requiring radiotherapy before the follow-up visit; and QTT data was not available in the third case. As a result, the final sample consisted of 55 patients. Table 1 shows the demographic parameters organized according to responders and nonresponders. The mean age was 59 years old (range 32–82 years). There were no significant differences between the groups in terms of gender, age, DN4, or pretreatment NPRS scores. Of the 24 responders, the pain improvement lasted for > 6 months in 5 patients, where in 2 of them pain relief lasted for almost 12 months, while another patient fully recovered from the pain. For the other 19 patients (see Table 1), 7 of them had pain relief over 90 days, whereas 8 recovered between 60 and 90 days, and only 4 had recovery for less than 60 days or less (always more than 45 days). In all patients, the DN4 score was ≥ 4.

3.2. QTT Profile. Figure 1 is a flowchart of QTT profiles for WST and HPT values at the pain area versus the contralateral asymptomatic area. None of the patients presented a significantly high WST combined with a significantly low HTP, nor did any present the opposite (i.e., significantly low WST and significantly high HPT). Among the nonresponders, 4 patterns emerged.

Pattern 1. There were no significant differences in WST or HPT between the painful area and the control areal.

Pattern 2. WST is not significantly different between the control and target areas while the HPT value showed significant abnormal thermal sensations (either high or low) at the painful area.

Pattern 3. HPT presents no significant differences while the WST value shows significant abnormal thermal sensations (either high or low) in the painful area.

Pattern 4. Both WST and HPT values present significant differences between the two areas (both high or both low). Both WST and HPT show abnormal thermal sensations at the pain site.

Two distinct groups were identified based on differences in QTT profiles for responders and nonresponders (Tables S1, S2, and S3). One group presented nonhomogenous WST and HPT results while the second group had homogenous WST and HPT results (Figure 2).

(i) Homogenous Profile Group. The first group presented homogenous WST and HPT profiles, defined as either the presence of significant differences in the same direction (both high or both low) in WST and HPT values between the PeLNP region and the asymptomatic contralateral area or no significant difference in these measures (both the treatment and control sites normal).

(ii) Nonhomogenous Group. The second group consisted of patients with nonhomogenous WST and HPT profiles, defined as the presence of significant differences between the PeLNP area and the contralateral site in only one (either WST or HPT) measure but not the other.

3.3. Predictors of Response to Treatment

3.3.1. Demographics: Aetiology and Duration of Pain. There were no baseline differences between responders and nonresponders in terms of gender, age, DN4 scores, etiological diagnosis, or NPRS. There was a slightly larger number of females in the nonresponse group, but this was not statistically significant.

3.3.2. Patterns and Responders. Table 2 shows the sensitivity, specificity, positive and negative predictive values, and positive and negative probability coefficients. As Table 2 shows, 24

Table 1: Demographic data according to treatment response.

Variable	Nonresponders	Responders	p value
Gender (female/male ratio)	19/12	13/11	0.28
Age (mean)	60.26 (14.25)	58.42 (13.28)	0.62
DN4 score	5.90 (1.37)	5.39 (1.29)	0.24
Pretreatment NPRS	7.21 (1.20)	6.89 (1.75)	0.79
Posttreatment NPRS	7.08 (1.29)	2.92 (1.38)	n.a.
Duration of improvement, months (mean)	b	72.89 (24.68)[a]	n.a.
Type of PeNP			0.88[c]
CPSP	18	13	
PHN	12	8	
Posttrauma	0	1	
CRPS	1	2	

DN4 = *Douleur Neuropathique 4 Questionnaire*. NPRS = numerical pain rating scale (0–10). CPSP = chronic postsurgical pain. PHN = postherpetic neuralgia. CRPS = complex regional pain syndrome type I. n.a. = not applicable. Gender and type of PeNP for the whole patient sample. For the others, numbers are given as means. Standard deviation in parenthesis. a = calculated for 19 patients. The other 5 were excluded due to reporting > 6 months of improvement. b = nonresponders had no days of improvement, most of whom reported no improvement at all. c = posttrauma and CRPS were not taken into account for the analysis due to the small number of patients.

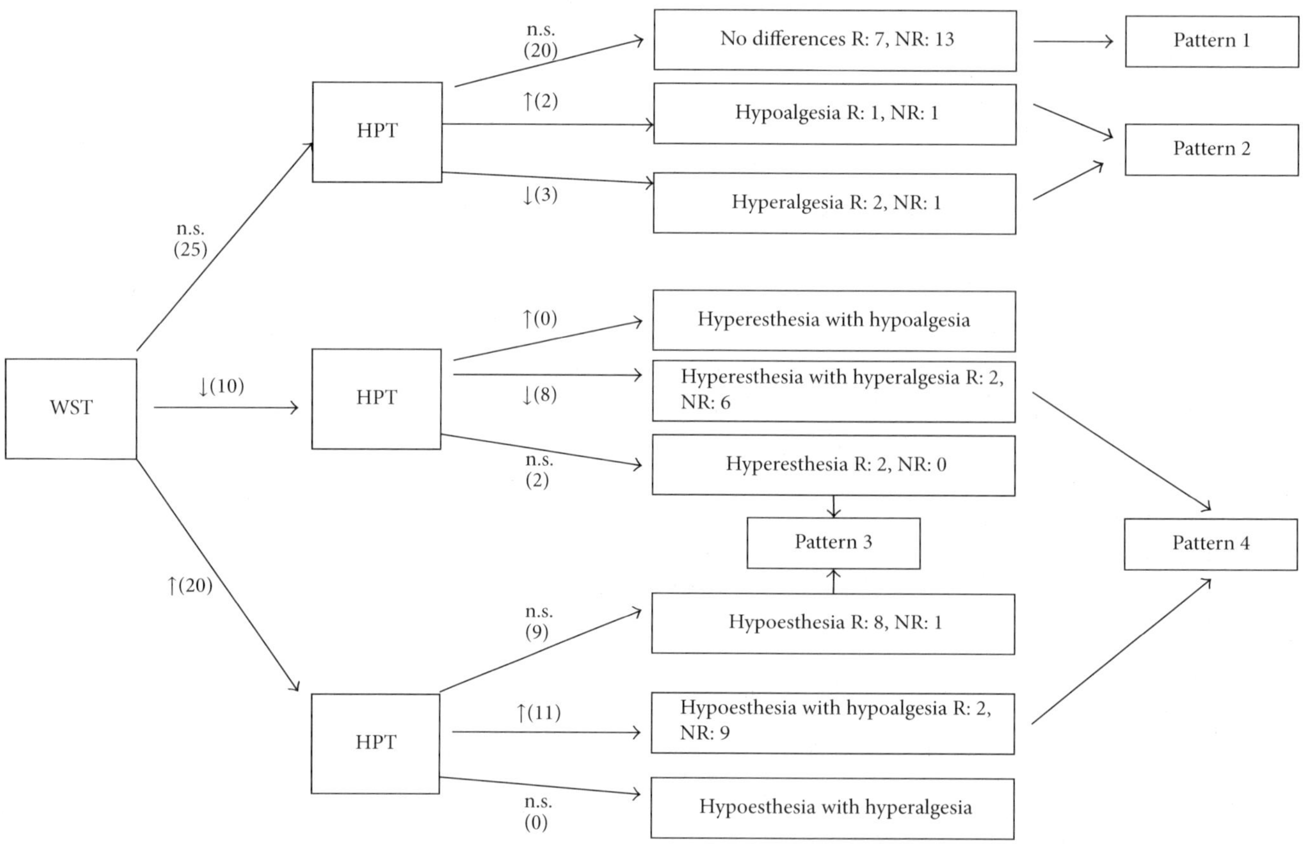

Figure 1: QTT profiles flowchart and responders/nonresponders to treatment. WST = warm sensation threshold. HPT = heat pain threshold. n.s. = not significant differences between painful and asymptomatic areas. ↑ = painful area with a significantly high difference versus the asymptomatic contralateral area. ↓ = painful area with a significantly low difference versus the asymptomatic contralateral area. In parenthesis (), number of patients with this profile. R = responders to treatment with capsaicin patch. NR = nonresponders to treatment with capsaicin patch. Clinical definitions such as hypoalgesia, hyperalgesia, hypoesthesia, and hyperesthesia are given to improve reading comprehension to understand the comparison versus the contralateral asymptomatic area; these QTT are not comparable to normalized published data.

TABLE 2: Contingency table.

	Total	No improvement	Improvement	
PPV = 76%	17	4	13[a]	Nonhomogenous (WST ≠ HPT)
NPV = 71%	38	27	11	Homogenous (WST = HPT)
	55	31	24	Total
		E = 87%	S = 54%	
		NLR = 0.52	PLR = 4.2	

Contingency table for the QTT profiles and patterns observed as a predictor of improvement after application of the capsaicin 8% patch. WST ≠ HPT: nonhomogenous results for warm sensation threshold and heat pain threshold in the peripheral neuropathic pain area versus the contralateral control area, with one measurement (either WST or HPT) showing a significant difference between the control and treatment areas while the other measurement (either WST or HPT) is not significantly different between the two sites. WST = HTP: both warm sensation threshold and heat pain threshold had homogenous test results in the pain and control areas: both were either significantly higher or lower, or neither was significantly different. S: sensibility. E: specificity. PPV: positive predictive value. NPV: negative predictive value. PLR: Positive Likelihood Ratio. NLR: Negative Likelihood Ratio. [a]$\chi^2 = 8.94$ ($p = 0.0028$). Fisher exact test $p = 0.0014$ (two tailed).

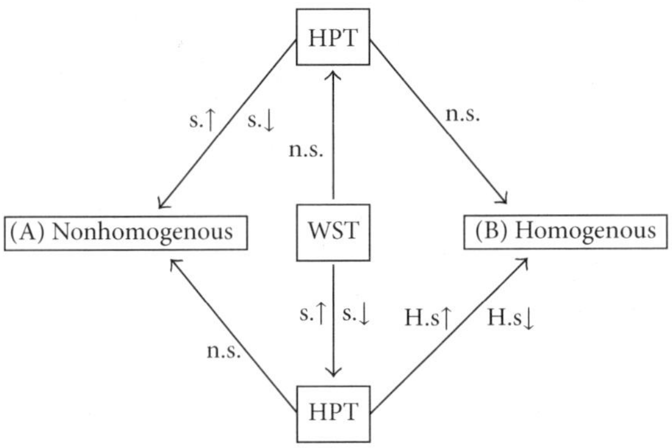

FIGURE 2: QTT profile groups identified after matching responder and nonresponders to treatment with capsaicin patch. WST: warm sensation threshold. HPT: heat pain threshold. n.s.: no significant difference between pain site and asymptomatic contralateral area for the thermal test. s.↑: the thermal test was significantly higher in the painful area versus the asymptomatic contralateral area. s.↓: the thermal test was significantly lower in the painful area versus the asymptomatic contralateral area. H.s↑/H.s↓: HPT for the painful area was significantly higher when WST was significantly higher or lower when WST was significantly lower than the asymptomatic contralateral area.

patients improved after a single application of CP8% whereas 31 did not improve. The χ^2 was 8.94 ($p = 0.0028$) and Fisher exact test (two tailed) was $p = 0.0014$ for patients who responded to treatment and had nonhomogenous WST and HPT values.

4. Discussion

At present, there are no reliable predictors of response to treatment with capsaicin for analgesia. Given that the application of capsaicin causes heat sensation, the aim of this study was to assess quantitative thermal testing (QTT) profiles in a group of patients with localized peripheral neuropathic pain (PeLNP) treated with topic capsaicin, to determine whether different QTT profiles could predict treatment outcomes. We did a retrospective analysis of 55 patients treated between 2010 and 2013 for PeLNP, where, as part of the routine treatment procedures, both warm sensation threshold (WST) and heat pain threshold (HPT) values were assessed at baseline in the treatment (PeLNP site) area and the asymptomatic contralateral site. From the analysis, two different groups were identified based on their QTT profile. The first group presented homogenous WST and HPT profiles, defined as either the presence of significant differences in the same direction (both high or both low) in WST and HPT values between the PeLNP region and the asymptomatic contralateral area or no significant difference in these measures (both the treatment and control sites normal). The second group consisted of patients with nonhomogenous WST and HPT profiles, defined as the presence of significant differences between the PeLNP area and the contralateral site in only one (either WST or HPT) measure but not the other. Most patients (27/31, 87.1%) with a homogenous profile were nonresponders. By contrast, more than half of the patients (13/24, 54.2%) with a nonhomogenous profile were responders ($p = 0.0028$). Although the reasons for this difference are not clear, we hypothesize patients with a partial loss of cutaneous nerve fibers or receptors are more likely to respond to treatment. By contrast, when severe nerve damage or normal cutaneous sensations are present, the pain is likely due to central sensitization and thus not responsive to capsaicin.

Potentially damaging mechanical, thermal, and chemical stimuli are detected by nerve endings called nociceptors found in the skin and other organs [21, 22]. The largest group of such nociceptors is the family of channels of the transient receptor potential (TRP) [23]. Within the TRP family, there are four different molecules (TRPV1, TRPV2, TRPV3, and TRPV4) that respond to different degrees of temperature increase, ranging from the perception of heat all the way up to harmful levels [24–26].

TRPV1 is a nonselective, ligand-dependent cationic channel that can be activated by a series of exogenous and endogenous physical and chemical stimuli, including temperatures above 43°C, low pH (in acid medium), endocannabinoids anandamide and N-arachidonyl-dopamine, or chemicals such as capsaicin (8-methyl-N-vanillyl-6-nonenamide) [27, 28], allowing the passage of different monovalent or divalent cations [29, 30]. TRPV1 is mainly expressed in peripheral nervous system (PNS) neurons such as the dorsal root ganglion (DRG) and in C and Aδ sensory fibers [27, 28, 31]. In patients with neuropathic pain (NP), TRPV1 is expressed through the nociceptive pathway, from unmyelinated axons in the skin to the back of the spinal cord [22]. Transduction of the signal is achieved through the influx of sodium and calcium. In this way, the neurons expressing these receptors are depolarized [32, 33]. Many of the ligands that come into contact with TRPV1 possess synergistic effects, channel them integrally, and lead to a response or signal transduction [34].

In primary afferents, the nociceptors, upon activation, trigger the release of various peptides, including glutamate, neurokinin A, substance P, and the peptide related to the calcitonin gene in the dorsal horn (DH) of the spinal cord [35–38]. These neurotransmitters then trigger a series of signals that contribute to the activation of second-order sensory neurons, such as spinothalamic tract cells (STT) [39, 40] and other projection neurons. This causes the transmission of nociceptive information to the brain. In addition, signals are released that will activate GABAergic inhibitory interneurons of the DH [40, 41]. Together, the information that reaches the central nervous system (CNS) is interpreted as a burning pain or an itch, in addition to causing the peripheral release of proinflammatory substances that sensitize other neurons and subsequently give rise to other stimuli [32].

Multiple inflammatory stimuli increase the expression of TRPV1 and even increase the density of axons positive for TRPV1 [42–46]. A priori, this suggests that TRPV1 is involved in the pathogenesis of hyperalgesia and other pathological sensations. TRPV1 antiserum reduces thermal allodynia and hyperalgesia in diabetic mice [47]. In addition, TRPV1 antagonists reduce inflammation and NP [48]. Despite these known effects, the importance of TRPV1 in the pathogenesis of NP or peripheral neuropathies remains controversial [22]. It has been suggested that TRPV1 has an effect on the pathogenesis of nerve pain secondary to nerve damage [49]. However, some studies indicate that the TRPV1 receptor is not directly involved in the pathogenesis of PeNP [28, 50] and other studies suggest that the TRPV1 receptor does not contribute to the triggered hyperalgesia in situations of nerve injury [51]. In addition, numerous studies have reported conflicting data about the density of TRPV1 and the degree of nerve damage [52–57]. Taken altogether, these facts suggest that TRPV1 is not useful as a specific marker in cases of nerve injury [22]. However, more recent studies suggest that recipients of the same TRP family present patterns suggestive of an association between NP and injury, specifically, TRPV3 [58–60] and TRPV4 [46, 61]. Despite the aforementioned controversy, TRPV1 receptors continue to offer great therapeutic possibilities [62]. Given the ongoing research in this area, it seems likely that, in the near future, we will come to better understand the pharmacological potential of TRPV1.

Capsaicin is a well-known exogenous activator of TRPV1. Its pain relief effect is believed to be due to the activation of small diameter afferent nerve fibers and specialized DRG neurons that respond to many different noxious stimuli [63]. Capsaicin also mediates some actions of the endocannabinoid CB1 anandamide, which shares the same intracellular binding site as TRPV1 [64, 65]. Thus, capsaicin stimulates nociceptors and generates signal transmission to the brain, which interprets the signal as pain [40]. As a result, the application of capsaicin can desensitize the nerve terminals of nociceptors by inducing long-term desensitization after prolonged exposure. This desensitization allows the use of capsaicin as an analgesic, and its mechanism of action is based on the destruction of axons and, ultimately, of the DRG nociceptors [66].

Cutaneous injection of capsaicin activates the TRPV1 receptors, causing an influx of sodium and calcium ions into the cytoplasm of nociceptive neurons expressing that receptor [64]. At the capsaicin injection site, primary mechanical hyperalgesia and heat develop due to desensitization of the afferents containing TRPV1 receptors [67–69]. In a larger area surrounding the injection site, secondary mechanical hyperalgesia and allodynia take place. The primary effects of mechanical hyperalgesia and heat are believed to be attributable to sensitization of the primary afferent nociceptors [70]. However, at the site of secondary mechanical hyperalgesia and allodynia, the degree of excitability of first-order neurons is normal [40, 71, 72], implying that allodynia and secondary hyperalgesia depend on the CNS, such as STT. This effect is called central sensitization (CS) [33, 37, 40, 73–81]. This suggests that NP is maintained by second- or third-order neurons without a significant effect on the peripheral nerve afferents [82].

Previous studies [13] have found that patients can be grouped into various subgroups based on their response to treatment with CP8%. This finding suggests that response variability may be related to different pain mechanisms. One patient group in that study presented high variability in pain rating scores (i.e., mixed treatment response), whereas the low variability group were nonresponders. The authors suggested that the lack of response in this group could be due to long-term chronic pain and the presence of severe central plastic changes. By contrast, high variability in pain rating scores could be due to a more recent development of chronic pain status, as occurred in the CPSP group in our study. Given that the EMA authorised treatment in Europe for any condition with PeNP (except for diabetes), we included patients with a wide variety of etiological diagnoses (Table 1). Many of our patients had a diagnosis of CPSP, which is not surprising given that this diagnosis accounts for a large percentage of patients with PeNP [83, 84]. Our findings suggest that CPSP patients may be more responsive to CP8% than other groups. Martini et al. suggested that other factors or predictors related to the treatment of patients with chronic pain could enhance the ability to predict therapeutic efficacy. Specific patterns in the QST profile may represent specific phenotypes that have a greater or lesser probability of treatment response. Indeed, several authors have already shown that specific tests in the QST profile may represent a specific population that is more likely to respond to therapy. Eisenberg et al. [10] showed that the magnitude of heat pain thresholds predicts the magnitude of the decrease in pain intensity in response to oxycodone treatment (the greater the heat pain threshold, the greater the opioid effect; $R2 = 0.17$) in healthy volunteers. Yarnitsky et al. [85] showed in a sample of patients with painful diabetic neuropathy that patients with less efficient conditioned pain modulation have greater analgesic responses to duloxetine ($R2 = 0.39$).

The present study involves a cohort of patients treated as part of routine clinical practice at a single center. We retrospectively identified patients who had been treated with CP8% and who also had a pretreatment QTT profile test available. The main aim was to determine the existence (or not) of a QTT pattern that could help identify those patients likely to respond to CP8% treatment. The main limitation to this study is its retrospective design. Other limitations include the relatively small number of patients, which precluded the use of subgroup analysis. We found no differences in demographics (gender, age, and etiological diagnosis of PeNP) between responders and nonresponders. We assume that the demographic data represent a normal distribution although this cannot be verified. Another limitation is that the number of responders in our study was larger than expected in the context of the high NNT reported in other studies [86]. There are several possible reasons for this, particularly the calculation of the NNT itself [87]. Clinical trials were not compared to placebo, but rather to low-dose capsaicin (0.075%), which has been shown to be effective for the relief of NP [88]. The NNT could have been miscalculated, making it difficult to compare NNTs from a study that used a low-dose control to NNTs in studies using inert placebos [89]. Another reason for the high response rate in our study could be the inclusion of patients with variable etiological diagnoses for PeNP, such as CPSP. In addition, a placebo effect cannot be ruled out, especially given that controlled trials have described a placebo response rate ranging from 23% to 36% [7, 90]. Another limitation is that the medical team was not blinded, and this may have introduced bias into the patient assessment at follow-up.

We found that the clinical effects of CP8% were better in patients with nonhomogenous QTT profiles. These patients showed a significantly higher response rate than patients with homogenous QTT profiles. This difference may be due to incomplete nerve damage in these patients, leading to an imbalance in the sensitive inputs to second-order neurons from peripheral receptors and to the presence of ectopic discharges on nerve endings. If so, pain in these patients may be purely peripheral, with no additional CS mechanisms. Capsaicin application in these patients could eliminate the factor resulting in dysaesthesia when they activate the remaining TRPV1 receptors, desensitizing the nerve terminals of nociceptors by destroying the remaining axons and nociceptors.

By contrast, the group of patients with homogeneous QTT profiles had little or no clinical improvement. These patients either had no peripheral damage (normally functioning nociceptors) or may have had complete peripheral nerve damage (absent or nonfunctional nociceptors). When no peripheral nerve damage is present, there should not be any receptor loss and thus there should be no differences in WST/HPT values between the painful area and the asymptomatic contralateral area. The opposite should also be true: in the case of complete peripheral nerve damage, nearly complete loss of receptors is to be expected, meaning that both warmth and heat sensations are likely to significantly differ between the painful and control areas. Thus, in both of these cases (i.e., complete peripheral nerve damage and no damage at all), the QTT tests should be homogenous, with capsaicin therapy unlikely to be efficacious in either of these two groups. Indeed, our results point in this direction. Pain in these patients could be due to CS mechanisms, with inputs multiplied at the DH as explained above; that is, the origin of the pain in these patients is probably less peripheral and more central. For this reason, the capsaicin is less effective in providing pain relief.

In the 3rd pattern identified (i.e., no significant differences in the HPT but significant differences in the WST) the hypoesthesia (high WST only) subgroup presented a better response rate (8 responders versus only 1 nonresponder). Although we were unable to perform a subgroup analysis due to the small sample size, these findings support the hypothesis developed by Malmberg et al. [6], who argued that the foremost psychophysical manifestation of topical capsaicin treatment is a reduced sensitivity to heat stimuli. This is the expression of an elevated-warmth detection threshold, corresponding to a loss of cutaneous sensory nerve fibers.

Overall, and within the aforementioned study limitations, our results seem to confirm previous reports. Höper et al. [12] evaluated sensory neuropathic abnormalities (painDETECT questionnaire), finding that the presence of burning and pressure-evoked pain was weakly associated with treatment response. They argued that thermal hyperalgesia is difficult to interpret and thus cannot serve as a predictor of response, which could be ascribed to the fact that the painDETECT questionnaire does not distinguish between cold and heat-evoked pain. Consequently, they concluded that data on heat-evoked pain, which is very likely TRPV1 receptor-dependent, would be preferable to predict treatment response to CP8%. Edwards et al. [91] found that the HPT values in the affected area and at the corresponding contralateral side predicted the effect of morphine and methadone on pain in patients with PHN. We found a similar association between certain QTT profiles and capsaicin response when we compared the pain site to the contralateral asymptomatic area. Gustorff et al. [11] identified potential differences in the sensory profiles—particularly the pressure pain threshold and degree of allodynia—of patients with PeNP who responded to CP8% and those who did not. In that study, the authors were unable to find warm hyperesthesia of heat hyperalgesia in responders, and they found similar WST/HPT profiles at baseline for both responders and nonresponders. By contrast, we looked at QTT profiles from a different point of view, using the contralateral asymptomatic area as the only control reference.

Despite the findings described above, it is possible that unilateral PeLNP may be associated with bilateral changes in PNS [92]. Thresholds measured on the contralateral side in PeLNP patients may not represent basal pain sensitivity. For this reason, we considered the homogeneity of QTT profiles rather than clinical symptoms (i.e., heat hyperalgesia). Martini et al. [13] found one group of patients with PeLNP whose pain could be attributed to a rigid and fully manifested chronic pain process with severe CS plastic changes that were unresponsive to therapy. In our study, we were aware that central or bilateral peripheral changes could occur—even though our sample consisted of patients with PeLNP—and for this reason we considered differences between the treatment and contralateral areas to be significant only when there was no crossover between mean results (±2 SD). Using these criteria, two patterns were found for responders and nonresponders when we examined profile homogeneity. For instance, a significantly differently low HPT (i.e., heat hyperalgesia) with no significant difference in WST was considered nonhomogeneous. By contrast, if the WST was also significantly different between the control and treatment areas, then the QTT profile was considered homogenous. Based on our results, it appears that patients who show a nonhomogenous profile in terms of WST and HPT values are significantly more likely to respond to capsaicin treatment, probably due to the presence of incomplete nerve damage. Nevertheless, these findings need to be confirmed in a prospective controlled blinded study, preferably with a large sample to enable subgroup analysis to better identify the QTT profile of responders.

Additional Points

What is already known about this topic? (i) There are no reliable predictors of response to treatment for localized neuropathic pain. (ii) Although some studies have attempted to identify predictors of treatment response, none have proven reliable.

What does this study add? (i) Quantitative thermal tests may help to predict which patients will respond to capsaicin patch treatment. (ii) Patients with partial damage to peripheral nerves may respond better to the mechanism of action of topical capsaicin than patients with completely damaged or undamaged peripheral nerves.

Competing Interests

A. Serrano has received honoraria for lectures from Astellas Spain, Astellas Pharma Europe Ltd., and has received payments to cover travel expenses and congress registration fees. He owns a small quantity of shares from Almirall. D. Torres has no conflict of interests. M. Veciana has no conflict of interests. C. Caro was supported with travel expenses and congress registration fees from Cardiva. J. Montero has received honoraria for consulting work from Ferrer Int. and for lectures from Medtronic and payments for travel expenses and congress registration fees from Boston Scientific. V. Mayoral has received honoraria for consulting work from Grünenthal, Almirall, and Mundipharma and for lectures from Grünenthal, Pfizer, Prostakam, Archimedes, Mundipharma, and Ferrer.

Authors' Contributions

All authors of this manuscript have read and approved all of its complete content. All authors have discussed the results previous to writing the discussion and have approved the final manuscript. Ancor Serrano Afonso treated patients as clinical pain physician, helped with data retrieval from the clinical record, performed the statistical analysis, and wrote the first draft of the manuscript. Daniel Torres Rodríguez helped with retrieval of clinical data from the patient records. Misericordia Veciana de las Heras treated patients as a clinical neurophysiologist and helped to write Material and Methods, Results, and Discussion, specifically the neurophysiological reasoning. Carmen Caro González, a registered nurse, was responsible for patient nursing care and also in charge of data retrieval. She also helped to write Material and Methods. Jordi Montero Homs helped to write Discussion. In particular, he was involved in investigating the neurophysiological underpinning for the findings. He also helped to correct other sections of the manuscript. Víctor Mayoral Rojals treated some patients as a clinical pain physician. He also helped to interpret the results and perform the statistical analysis. He also assisted with writing the discussion and abstract and correcting other sections of the manuscript.

Acknowledgments

The authors want to acknowledge the other members of the pain clinic for their support: Dr. Tomás Domingo, Dr. Cristina Vieta, Dr. Miquel Casals, Dr. Montse Fernández, and Dr. Carmen Ribes. This work was done under no extra funding sources than the routine clinical assessment. The data was obtained reviewing clinical history. The authors wish to thank Bradley Londres for his valuable assistance in editing and improving this manuscript. Finally they also want to thank IDIBELL, Institut d'Investigació Biomèdica de Bellvitge, the research institute at our working facility, for the financial support as part of its policy for publishing in Open Access Journals.

References

[1] R. H. Dworkin, A. B. O'Connor, J. Audette et al., "Recommendations for the pharmacological management of neuropathic pain: an overview and literature update," *Mayo Clinic Proceedings*, vol. 85, no. 3, pp. S3–S14, 2010.

[2] M. M. Backonja, "High-concentration capsaicin for the treatment of post-herpetic neuralgia and other types of peripheral neuropathic pain," *European Journal of Pain Supplements*, vol. 4, no. S2, pp. 170–174, 2010.

[3] M. M. Backonja, T. P. Malan, G. F. Vanhove, and J. K. Tobias, "NGX-4010, a high-concentration capsaicin patch, for the treatment of postherpetic neuralgia: a randomized, double-blind, controlled study with an open-label extension," *Pain Medicine*, vol. 11, no. 4, pp. 600–608, 2010.

[4] G. A. Irving, M. M. Backonja, E. Dunteman et al., "A multicenter, randomized, double-blind, controlled study of NGX-4010, a high-concentration capsaicin patch, for the treatment of postherpetic neuralgia," *Pain Medicine*, vol. 12, no. 1, pp. 99–109, 2011.

[5] W. R. Kennedy, G. F. Vanhove, S.-P. Lu et al., "A randomized, controlled, open-label study of the long-term effects of NGX-4010, a high-concentration capsaicin patch, on epidermal nerve fiber density and sensory function in healthy volunteers," *Journal of Pain*, vol. 11, no. 6, pp. 579–587, 2010.

[6] A. B. Malmberg, A. P. Mizisin, N. A. Calcutt, T. Von Stein, W. R. Robbins, and K. R. Bley, "Reduced heat sensitivity and epidermal nerve fiber immunostaining following single applications of a high-concentration capsaicin patch," *Pain*, vol. 111, no. 3, pp. 360–367, 2004.

[7] P. L. McCormack, "Capsaicin dermal patch: in non-diabetic peripheral neuropathic pain," *Drugs*, vol. 70, no. 14, pp. 1831–1842, 2010.

[8] European Medicines Agency, Human Medicines deailed information for Qutenza, Capsaicin, http://www.ema.europa.eu/ema/index.jsp?curl=pages/medicines/human/medicines/000909/human_med_001008.jsp&mid=WC0b01ac058001d124.

[9] E. P. Armstrong, D. C. Malone, B. McCarberg, C. J. Panarites, and S. V. Pham, "Cost-effectiveness analysis of a new 8% capsaicin patch compared to existing therapies for postherpetic neuralgia," *Current Medical Research and Opinion*, vol. 27, no. 5, pp. 939–950, 2011.

[10] E. Eisenberg, A. Midbari, M. Haddad, and D. Pud, "Predicting the analgesic effect to oxycodone by static and dynamic quantitative sensory testing in healthy subjects," *Pain*, vol. 151, no. 1, pp. 104–109, 2010.

[11] B. Gustorff, C. Poole, H. Kloimstein, N. Hacker, and R. Likar, "Treatment of neuropathic pain with the capsaicin 8% patch: quantitative sensory testing (QST) in a prospective observational study identifies potential predictors of response to capsaicin 8% patch treatment," *Scandinavian Journal of Pain*, vol. 4, no. 3, pp. 138–145, 2013.

[12] J. Höper, S. Helfert, M.-L. S. Heskamp, C. G. Maihöfner, and R. Baron, "High concentration capsaicin for treatment of peripheral neuropathic pain: effect on somatosensory symptoms and identification of treatment responders," *Current Medical Research and Opinion*, vol. 30, no. 4, pp. 565–574, 2014.

[13] C. H. Martini, A. Yassen, A. Krebs-Brown et al., "A novel approach to identify responder subgroups and predictors of response to low- and high-dose capsaicin patches in postherpetic neuralgia," *European Journal of Pain*, vol. 17, no. 10, pp. 1491–1501, 2013.

[14] M. Haanpää, N. Attal, M. Backonja et al., "NeuPSIG guidelines on neuropathic pain assessment," *Pain*, vol. 152, no. 1, pp. 14–27, 2011.

[15] G. Mick, R. Baron, N. B. Finnerup et al., "What is localized neuropathic pain? A first proposal to characterize and define a widely used term," *Pain Management*, vol. 2, no. 1, pp. 71–77, 2012.

[16] P. S. T. Chong and D. P. Cros, "Technology literature review: quantitative sensory testing," *Muscle and Nerve*, vol. 29, no. 5, pp. 734–747, 2004.

[17] H. Fruhstorfer, U. Lindblom, and W. G. Schmidt, "Method for quantitative estimation of thermal thresholds in patients," *Journal of Neurology, Neurosurgery and Psychiatry*, vol. 39, no. 11, pp. 1071–1075, 1976.

[18] D. Yarnitsky, E. Sprecher, R. Zaslansky, and J. A. Hemli, "Heat pain thresholds: normative data and repeatability," *Pain*, vol. 60, no. 3, pp. 329–332, 1995.

[19] "VassarStats: Website for Statistical Computation," http://www.vassarstats.net/.

[20] Y. Granovsky, P. Anand, A. Nakae et al., "Normative data for Aδ contact heat evoked potentials in adult population: a multicenter study," *Pain*, vol. 157, no. 5, pp. 1156–1163, 2016.

[21] P. Geppetti, R. Patacchini, and R. Nassini, "Transient receptor potential channels and occupational exposure," *Current Opinion in Allergy and Clinical Immunology*, vol. 14, no. 2, pp. 77–83, 2014.

[22] G. Lauria, M. Morbin, R. Lombardi et al., "Expression of capsaicin receptor immunoreactivity in human peripheral nervous system and in painful neuropathies," *Journal of the Peripheral Nervous System*, vol. 11, no. 3, pp. 262–271, 2006.

[23] C. Montell, K. Jones, E. Hafen, and G. Rubin, "Rescue of the Drosophila phototransduction mutation trp by germline transformation," *Science*, vol. 230, no. 4729, pp. 1040–1043, 1985.

[24] A. Patapoutian, A. M. Peier, G. M. Story, and V. Viswanath, "ThermoTRP channels and beyond: mechanisms of temperature sensation," *Nature Reviews Neuroscience*, vol. 4, no. 7, pp. 529–539, 2003.

[25] D. W. Cortright and A. Szallasi, "Biochemical pharmacology of the vanilloid receptor TRPV1: an update," *European Journal of Biochemistry*, vol. 271, no. 10, pp. 1814–1819, 2004.

[26] T. Voets, G. Droogmans, U. Wissenbach, A. Janssens, V. Flockerzi, and B. Nilius, "The principle of temperature-dependent gating in cold- and heat-sensitive TRP channels," *Nature*, vol. 430, no. 7001, pp. 748–754, 2004.

[27] M. J. Caterina, M. A. Schumacher, M. Tominaga, T. A. Rosen, J. D. Levine, and D. Julius, "The capsaicin receptor: a heat-activated ion channel in the pain pathway," *Nature*, vol. 389, no. 6653, pp. 816–824, 1997.

[28] A. Szallasi and P. M. Blumberg, "Vanilloid (Capsaicin) receptors and mechanisms," *Pharmacological Reviews*, vol. 51, no. 2, pp. 159–211, 1999.

[29] I. S. Ramsey, M. Delling, and D. E. Clapham, "An introduction to TRP channels," *Annual Review of Physiology*, vol. 68, pp. 619–647, 2006.

[30] G. Owsianik, K. Talavera, T. Voets, and B. Nilius, "Permeation and selectivity of TRP channels," *Annual Review of Physiology*, vol. 68, pp. 685–717, 2006.

[31] A. Szallasi, S. Nilsson, T. Farkas-Szallasi, P. M. Blumberg, T. Hökfelt, and J. M. Lundberg, "Vanilloid (capsaicin) receptors in the rat: distribution in the brain, regional differences in the spinal cord, axonal transport to the periphery, and depletion by systemic vanilloid treatment," *Brain Research*, vol. 703, no. 1-2, pp. 175–183, 1995.

[32] J. Ochoa and E. Torebjörk, "Sensations evoked by intraneural microstimulation of C nociceptor fibres in human skin nerves," *The Journal of Physiology*, vol. 415, no. 1, pp. 583–599, 1989.

[33] W. D. Willis, "Long-term potentiation in spinothalamic neurons," *Brain Research Reviews*, vol. 40, no. 1–3, pp. 202–214, 2002.

[34] V. Vellani, S. Mapplebeck, A. Moriondo, J. B. Davis, and P. A. McNaughton, "Protein kinase C activation potentiates gating of the vanilloid receptor VR1 by capsaicin, protons, heat and anandamide," *Journal of Physiology*, vol. 534, no. 3, pp. 813–825, 2001.

[35] L. S. Sorkin, D. J. McAdoo, and W. D. Willis, "Stimulation in the ventral posterior lateral nucleus of the primate thalamus leads to release of serotonin in the lumbar spinal cord," *Brain Research*, vol. 581, no. 2, pp. 307–310, 1992.

[36] L. S. Sorkin and D. J. McAdoo, "Amino acids and serotonin are released into the lumbar spinal cord of the anesthetized cat following intradermal capsaicin injections," *Brain Research*, vol. 607, no. 1-2, pp. 89–98, 1993.

[37] R. Sun, J. Yan, and W. D. Willis, "Activation of protein kinase B/Akt in the periphery contributes to pain behavior induced by capsaicin in rats," *Neuroscience*, vol. 144, no. 1, pp. 286–294, 2007.

[38] J.-Y. Yan, R.-Q. Sun, M. G. Hughes, D. J. McAdoo, and W. D. Willis, "Intradermal injection of capsaicin induces acute substance P release from rat spinal cord dorsal horn," *Neuroscience Letters*, vol. 410, no. 3, pp. 183–186, 2006.

[39] P. M. Dougherty, J. Palecek, V. Paleckova, L. S. Sorkin, and W. D. Willis, "The role of NMDA and non-NMDA excitatory amino acid receptors in the excitation of primate spinothalamic tract neurons by mechanical, chemical, thermal, and electrical stimuli," *Journal of Neuroscience*, vol. 12, no. 8, pp. 3025–3041, 1992.

[40] W. D. Willis Jr., "The role of TRPV1 receptors in pain evoked by noxious thermal and chemical stimuli," *Experimental Brain Research*, vol. 196, no. 1, pp. 5–11, 2009.

[41] X. Zou, Q. Lin, and W. D. Willis, "NMDA or non-NMDA receptor antagonists attenuate increased Fos expression in spinal dorsal horn GABAergic neurons after intradermal injection of capsaicin in rats," *Neuroscience*, vol. 106, no. 1, pp. 171–182, 2001.

[42] S. M. Carlton and R. E. Coggeshall, "Peripheral capsaicin receptors increase in the inflamed rat hindpaw: a possible mechanism for peripheral sensitization," *Neuroscience Letters*, vol. 310, no. 1, pp. 53–56, 2001.

[43] Y. Yiangou, P. Facer, N. H. C. Dyer et al., "Vanilloid receptor 1 immunoreactivity in inflamed human bowel," *Lancet*, vol. 357, no. 9265, pp. 1338–1339, 2001.

[44] M. Trevisani, D. Smart, M. J. Gunthorpe et al., "Ethanol elicits and potentiates nociceptor responses via the vanilloid receptor-1," *Nature Neuroscience*, vol. 5, no. 6, pp. 546–551, 2002.

[45] C. L. H. Chan, P. Facer, J. B. Davis et al., "Sensory fibres expressing capsaicin receptor TRPV1 in patients with rectal hypersensitivity and faecal urgency," *Lancet*, vol. 361, no. 9355, pp. 385–391, 2003.

[46] P. Gopinath, E. Wan, A. Holdcroft et al., "Increased capsaicin receptor TRPV1 in skin nerve fibres and related vanilloid receptors TRPV3 and TRPV4 in keratinocytes in human breast pain," *BMC Women's Health*, vol. 5, article 2, 2005.

[47] J. Kamei, K. Zushida, K. Morita, M. Sasaki, and S.-I. Tanaka, "Role of vanilloid VR1 receptor in thermal allodynia and hyperalgesia in diabetic mice," *European Journal of Pharmacology*, vol. 422, no. 1–3, pp. 83–86, 2001.

[48] K. M. Walker, L. Urban, S. J. Medhurst et al., "The VR1 antagonist capsazepine reverses mechanical hyperalgesia in models of inflammatory and neuropathic pain," *Journal of Pharmacology and Experimental Therapeutics*, vol. 304, no. 1, pp. 56–62, 2003.

[49] M. H. Rashid, M. Inoue, S. Bakoshi, and H. Ueda, "Increased expression of vanilloid receptor 1 on myelinated primary afferent neurons contributes to the antihyperalgesic effect of capsaicin cream in diabetic neuropathic pain in mice," *Journal of Pharmacology and Experimental Therapeutics*, vol. 306, no. 2, pp. 709–717, 2003.

[50] G. J. Michael and J. V. Priestley, "Differential expression of the mRNA for the vanilloid receptor subtype 1 in cells of the adult rat dorsal root and nodose ganglia and its downregulation by axotomy," *Journal of Neuroscience*, vol. 19, no. 5, pp. 1844–1854, 1999.

[51] M. J. Caterina, A. Leffler, A. B. Malmberg et al., "Impaired nociception and pain sensation in mice lacking the capsaicin receptor," *Science*, vol. 288, no. 5464, pp. 306–313, 2000.

[52] M. Polydefkis, C. T. Yiannoutsos, B. A. Cohen et al., "Reduced intraepidermal nerve fiber density in HIV-associated sensory neuropathy," *Neurology*, vol. 58, no. 1, pp. 115–119, 2002.

[53] C.-L. Pan, T.-J. Tseng, Y.-H. Lin, M.-C. Chiang, W.-M. Lin, and S.-T. Hsieh, "Cutaneous innervation in Guillain-Barré syndrome: pathology and clinical correlations," *Brain*, vol. 126, no. 2, pp. 386–397, 2003.

[54] D. N. Herrmann, J. W. Griffin, P. Hauer, D. R. Cornblath, and J. C. McArthur, "Epidermal nerve fiber density and sural nerve morphometry in peripheral neuropathies," *Neurology*, vol. 53, no. 8, pp. 1634–1640, 1999.

[55] G. Lauria, J. C. McArthur, P. E. Hauer, J. W. Griffin, and D. R. Cornblath, "Neuropathological alterations in diabetic truncal neuropathy: evaluation by skin biopsy," *Journal of Neurology Neurosurgery and Psychiatry*, vol. 65, no. 5, pp. 762–766, 1998.

[56] K. L. Petersen, F. L. Rice, F. Suess, M. Berro, and M. C. Rowbotham, "Relief of postherpetic neuralgia by surgical removal of painful skin," *Pain*, vol. 98, no. 1-2, pp. 119–126, 2002.

[57] G. Lauria, R. Lombardi, M. Borgna et al., "Intraepidermal nerve fiber density in rat foot pad: neuropathologic–neurophysiologic correlation," *Journal of the Peripheral Nervous System*, vol. 10, no. 2, pp. 202–208, 2005.

[58] A. M. Peier, A. J. Reeve, D. A. Andersson et al., "A heat-sensitive TRP channel expressed in keratinocytes," *Science*, vol. 296, no. 5575, pp. 2046–2049, 2002.

[59] S. P. Cook and E. W. McCleskey, "Cell damage excites nociceptors through release of cytosolic ATP," *Pain*, vol. 95, no. 1-2, pp. 41–47, 2002.

[60] M. D. Southall, T. Li, L. S. Gharibova, Y. Pei, G. D. Nicol, and J. B. Travers, "Activation of epidermal vanilloid receptor-1 induces release of proinflammatory mediators in human keratinocytes," *Journal of Pharmacology and Experimental Therapeutics*, vol. 304, no. 1, pp. 217–222, 2003.

[61] N. Alessandri-Haber, O. A. Dina, J. J. Yeh, C. A. Parada, D. B. Reichling, and J. D. Levine, "Transient receptor potential vanilloid 4 is essential in chemotherapy-induced neuropathic pain in the rat," *The Journal of Neuroscience*, vol. 24, no. 18, pp. 4444–4452, 2004, Erratum in *The Journal of Neuroscience*, vol. 24, no. 23, p. 5457, 2004.

[62] G. Appendino, L. De Petrocellis, M. Trevisani et al., "Development of the first ultra-potent 'capsaicinoid' agonist at transient receptor potential vanilloid type 1 (TRPV1) channels and its therapeutic potential," *Journal of Pharmacology and Experimental Therapeutics*, vol. 312, no. 2, pp. 561–570, 2005.

[63] J. Szolcsányi, J. Nagy, and G. Pethö, "Effect of CP-96,345 a non-peptide substance P antagonist, capsaicin, resiniferatoxin and ruthenium red on nociception," *Regulatory Peptides*, vol. 46, no. 1-2, pp. 437–439, 1993.

[64] V. Di Marzo, L. De Petrocellis, F. Fezza, A. Ligresti, and T. Bisogno, "Anandamide receptors," *Prostaglandins Leukotrienes and Essential Fatty Acids*, vol. 66, no. 2-3, pp. 377–391, 2002.

[65] É. Szoke, G. Czéh, J. Szolcsányi, and L. Seress, "Neonatal anandamide treatment results in prolonged mitochondrial damage in the vanilloid receptor type 1-immunoreactive B-type neurons of the rat trigeminal ganglion," *Neuroscience*, vol. 115, no. 3, pp. 805–814, 2002.

[66] G. Jancsó and M. Wollemann, "The effect of capsaicin on the adenylate cyclase activity of rat brain," *Brain Research*, vol. 123, no. 2, pp. 323–329, 1977.

[67] P. Holzer, "Capsaicin: cellular targets, mechanisms of action, and selectivity for thin sensory neurons," *Pharmacological Reviews*, vol. 43, no. 2, pp. 143–201, 1991.

[68] R. H. LaMotte, C. N. Shain, D. A. Simone, and E.-F. P. Tsai, "Neurogenic hyperalgesia: psychophysical studies of underlying

mechanisms," *Journal of Neurophysiology*, vol. 66, no. 1, pp. 190–211, 1991.

[69] C. N. Sang, R. H. Gracely, M. B. Max, and G. J. Bennett, "Capsaicin-evoked mechanical allodynia and hyperalgesia cross nerve territories: evidence for a central mechanism," *Anesthesiology*, vol. 85, no. 3, pp. 491–496, 1996.

[70] J. D. Hardy, H. G. WolV, and H. Goodell, *Pain Sensations and Reactions*, Williams and Wilkins, New York, NY, USA, 1967, reprinted by Hafner Publishing Co, New York, NY, USA, 1952.

[71] R. H. LaMotte, L. E. Lundberg, and H. E. Torebjörk, "Pain, hyperalgesia and activity in nociceptive C units in humans after intradermal injection of capsaicin," *The Journal of Physiology*, vol. 448, no. 1, pp. 749–764, 1992.

[72] M. Schmelz, R. Schmidt, M. Ringkamp, H. O. Handwerker, and H. E. Torebjörk, "Sensitization of insensitive branches of C nociceptors in human skin," *The Journal of Physiology*, vol. 480, no. 2, pp. 389–394, 1994.

[73] L. Fang, J. Wu, Q. Lin, and W. D. Willis, "Calcium-calmodulin-dependent protein kinase II contributes to spinal cord central sensitization," *Journal of Neuroscience*, vol. 22, no. 10, pp. 4196–4204, 2002.

[74] K. A. Sluka, H. Rees, P.-S. Chen, M. Tsuruoka, and W. D. Willis, "Capsaicin-induced sensitization of primate spinothalamic tract cells is prevented by a protein kinase C inhibitor," *Brain Research*, vol. 772, no. 1-2, pp. 82–86, 1997.

[75] Q. Lin, J. Wu, and W. D. Willis, "Effects of protein kinase A activation on the responses of primate spinothalamic tract neurons to mechanical stimuli," *Journal of Neurophysiology*, vol. 88, no. 1, pp. 214–221, 2002.

[76] X. Zou, Q. Lin, and W. D. Willis, "Role of protein kinase A in phosphorylation of NMDA receptor 1 subunits in dorsal horn and spinothalamic tract neurons after intradermal injection of capsaicin in rats," *Neuroscience*, vol. 115, no. 3, pp. 775–786, 2002.

[77] T. J. Coderre and R. Melzack, "The contribution of excitatory amino acids to central sensitization and persistent nociception after formalin-induced tissue injury," *Journal of Neuroscience*, vol. 12, no. 9, pp. 3665–3670, 1992.

[78] J. Palecek, V. Paleckova, P. M. Dougherty, and W. D. Willis, "The effect of phorbol esters on the responses of primate spinothalamic neurons to mechanical and thermal stimuli," *Journal of Neurophysiology*, vol. 71, no. 2, pp. 529–537, 1994.

[79] X. Zou, Q. Lin, and W. D. Willis, "Effect of protein kinase C blockade on phosphorylation of NR1 in dorsal horn and spinothalamic tract cells caused by intradermal capsaicin injection in rats," *Brain Research*, vol. 1020, no. 1-2, pp. 95–105, 2004.

[80] Q. Lin, Y. B. Peng, J. Wu, and W. D. Willis, "Involvement of CGMP in nociceptive processing by and sensitization of spinothalamic neurons in primates," *Journal of Neuroscience*, vol. 17, no. 9, pp. 3293–3302, 1997.

[81] P. Geppetti, M. Tramontana, E. Del Bianco, and B. M. Fusco, "Capsaicin-desensitization to the human nasal mucosa selectively reduces pain evoked by citric acid," *British Journal of Clinical Pharmacology*, vol. 35, no. 2, pp. 178–183, 1993.

[82] G. Lauria, M. Morbin, R. Lombardi et al., "Axonal swellings predict the degeneration of epidermal nerve fibers in painful neuropathies," *Neurology*, vol. 61, no. 5, pp. 631–636, 2003.

[83] C. Maihofner and M.-L. Heskamp, "Prospective, non-interventional study on the tolerability and analgesic effectiveness over 12 weeks after a single application of capsaicin 8% cutaneous patch in 1044 patients with peripheral neuropathic pain: first results of the QUEPP study," *Current Medical Research and Opinion*, vol. 29, no. 6, pp. 673–683, 2013.

[84] A. Montes, G. Roca, S. Sabate et al., "Genetic and clinical factors associated with chronic postsurgical pain after hernia repair, hysterectomy, and thoracotomy: a two-year multicenter cohort study," *Anesthesiology*, vol. 122, no. 5, pp. 1123–1141, 2015.

[85] D. Yarnitsky, M. Granot, H. Nahman-Averbuch, M. Khamaisi, and Y. Granovsky, "Conditioned pain modulation predicts duloxetine efficacy in painful diabetic neuropathy," *Pain*, vol. 153, no. 6, pp. 1193–1198, 2012.

[86] N. B. Finnerup, S. H. Sindrup, and T. S. Jensen, "The evidence for pharmacological treatment of neuropathic pain," *Pain*, vol. 150, no. 3, pp. 573–581, 2010.

[87] A. Moore, "What is NNT? What is... ? Series," April 2009, http://www.whatisseries.co.uk/what-is-an-nnt/.

[88] S. Derry, R. Lloyd, R. A. Moore, and H. J. McQuay, "Topical capsaicin for chronic neuropathic pain in adults," *Cochrane Database of Systematic Reviews*, no. 4, Article ID CD007393, 2009.

[89] J. Mou, F. Paillard, B. Turnbull, J. Trudeau, M. Stoker, and N. P. Katz, "Efficacy of Qutenza® (capsaicin) 8% patch for neuropathic pain: a metaanalysis of the qutenza clinical trials database," *Pain*, vol. 154, no. 9, pp. 1632–1639, 2013.

[90] M. Backonja, M. S. Wallace, E. R. Blonsky et al., "NGX-4010, a high-concentration capsaicin patch, for the treatment of postherpetic neuralgia: A Randomised, Double-Blind Study," *The Lancet Neurology*, vol. 7, no. 12, pp. 1106–1112, 2008.

[91] R. R. Edwards, J. A. Haythornthwaite, P. Tella, M. B. Max, and S. Raja, "Basal heat pain thresholds predict opioid analgesia in patients with postherpetic neuralgia," *Anesthesiology*, vol. 104, no. 6, pp. 1243–1248, 2006.

[92] A. L. Oaklander, K. Romans, S. Horasek, A. Stocks, P. Hauer, and R. A. Meyer, "Unilateral postherpetic neuralgia is associated with bilateral sensory neuron damage," *Annals of Neurology*, vol. 44, no. 5, pp. 789–795, 1998.

20

Increased Risk of Postthoracotomy Pain Syndrome in Patients with Prolonged Hospitalization and Increased Postoperative Opioid Use

Michelle A. O. Kinney,[1] Adam K. Jacob,[1] Melissa A. Passe,[2] and Carlos B. Mantilla[1]

[1]*Department of Anesthesiology, Mayo Clinic, 200 First Street SW, Rochester, MN 55905, USA*
[2]*Department of Anesthesiology, Anesthesia Clinical Research Unit, Mayo Clinic, 200 First Street SW, Rochester, MN 55905, USA*

Correspondence should be addressed to Michelle A. O. Kinney; kinney.michelle@mayo.edu

Academic Editor: Giustino Varrassi

Background. Postthoracotomy pain syndrome (PTPS) is unfortunately very common following thoracotomy and results in decreased quality of life. The purpose of this retrospective study was to determine perioperative patient, surgical, and analgesic characteristics associated with the development of PTPS. *Methods.* Sixty-six patients who presented to the Mayo Clinic Rochester Pain Clinic were diagnosed with PTPS 2 months or more after thoracotomy with postoperative epidural analgesia. These patients were matched with sixty-six control patients who underwent thoracotomy with postoperative epidural analgesia and were never diagnosed with PTPS. *Results.* Median (IQR) hospital stay was significantly different between control patients (5 days (4, 6)) compared with PTPS patients (6 days (5, 8)), $P < 0.02$. The total opioid equivalent utilized in oral morphine equivalents in milligrams for the first three days postoperatively was significantly different between control patients and PTPS patients. The median (IQR) total opioid equivalent utilized was 237 (73, 508) for controls and 366 (116, 874) for PTPS patients ($P < 0.005$). *Conclusion.* Patients with a prolonged hospital stay after thoracotomy were at an increased risk of developing PTPS, and this is a novel finding. Patients who utilize higher oral morphine equivalents for the first 3 days were also at increased risk for PTPS.

1. Introduction

Postthoracotomy pain syndrome (PTPS) is unfortunately very common. In a recent prospective trial, we determined that 68% of patients had pain three months following serratus-sparing posterolateral thoracotomy or limited thoracotomy, resulting in decreased quality of life, physical function, and vitality [1]. We have also demonstrated that preoperative gabapentin in the setting of multimodal analgesia with thoracic epidural bupivacaine and hydromorphone, along with acetaminophen, ketorolac, and intravenous fentanyl via patient-controlled analgesic (PCA pump), did not decrease acute or chronic postthoracotomy pain [2].

Various studies have made observations about predictive risk factors for PTPS. In a prospective study by Ochroch and colleagues involving 120 patients, it was demonstrated that women reported more pain than men during their hospitalization and for 48 weeks postoperatively [3]. In a separate prospective study by Ochroch and colleagues, the initiation of thoracic epidural analgesia prior to thoracotomy incision rather than at the time of rib approximation was not found to significantly decrease acute pain during hospitalization or at 48 weeks [4]. A critical review of the literature by Wildgaard et al. concluded that intercostal nerve injury is probably the most important risk factor in the development of chronic postthoracotomy pain [5]. A systematic review of randomized trials by Joshi and colleagues noted that the efficacy of thoracic epidural combining local anesthetic and opioid is established for decreasing acute postthoracotomy pain, but it remains unclear if perioperative analgesia is related to the development of PTPS [6]. Therefore, the purpose of this retrospective, case-control study was to determine perioperative characteristics for the development of PTPS.

2. Materials and Methods

Institutional Review Board approval was obtained prior to reviewing medical records. The Mayo Clinic Life Sciences System database was searched using CPT codes 32035 through 32525 to identify all patients who had undergone a noncardiac thoracic procedure from May 14, 2000, through December 31, 2010. This database is a comprehensive data storage system that stores patient information including demographics, patient characteristics, perioperative management, and details regarding complications [7]. A query-building tool called Data Discovery and Query Builder (DDQB) was used to search the Mayo database and interrogate data files (International Business Machines, Corp.). The primary outcome variable was the presence of PTPS documented within 2 months of the surgery date. Among the cohort of thoracic surgical patients, cases of PTPS were identified using the following two approaches: (1) search for International Classification of Diseases-9 code for PTPS (code 338.22) and (2) free-text query of all notes in the electronic medical record for the following terms: thoracotomy pain, thoracotomy pain syndrome, postthoracotomy syndrome, postthoracotomy pain, postthoracotomy pain syndrome, post-thoracotomy syndrome, post-thoracotomy pain, post-thoracotomy pain syndrome, post thoracotomy syndrome, post thoracotomy pain, and post thoracotomy pain syndrome. The medical records of patients identified as having one or more key words were then manually reviewed to confirm eligibility. Sixty-six patients had a thoracotomy procedure with an epidural catheter used for perioperative analgesia and were seen in the Pain Clinic 2 months or greater after their thoracotomy for ipsilateral PTPS. In cases of repeat thoracotomies, only the date of the patient's most recent thoracotomy was used to calculate the minimum 2-month interval between thoracotomy and first documentation of PTPS. Identification of false positive cases was minimized by excluding those cases identified as "no thoracotomy pain" and "denies thoracotomy pain." For each case of PTPS, a control patient who underwent thoracotomy and had their analgesia managed by a dedicated acute pain service utilizing an epidural catheter was identified. The control group patients were never diagnosed with PTPS and were matched with PTPS cases by patient age, sex, surgeon, and date of surgery. The control group patients were limited to a local residence status using a tristate area (MN, IA, and WI) to increase their chances of presenting to the Mayo Clinic Rochester Pain Clinic should PTPS have developed. All control group patients had follow-up at Mayo beyond 2 months after thoracotomy and the diagnosis was never made.

The following information was collected from the medical record: age, gender, height, weight, PTPS, side of PTPS, date of Pain Clinic visit, date of surgery, side of surgery, surgeon, surgical procedure, medications taken at Pain Clinic visit, epidural catheter placement date and time, the thoracic spinal level at which the epidural catheter was placed, the loading dose of opioid, whether the epidural had to be replaced, when the epidural was removed, why the epidural was removed, the epidural infusion rate and medications, and the dose of pain medications administered. Numeric rating scores (NRS) were collected every 4 hours of pain at rest and with movement (including coughing).

Clinical records were reviewed by the investigators on the study. Data were collected from the Mayo electronic medical record using a standardized data collection form and were then entered into the REDCap (Research Electronic Data Capture) electronic data capture tools at Mayo Clinic [9].

2.1. Statistical Analysis. Data were summarized and compared for the PTPS versus control groups. Categorical variables were compared using the Pearson chi-square test or Fisher's exact test, and continuous variables were compared using the two-sample t-test (or Rank Sum test). All analyses were two-tailed with a significance level of $P < 0.05$. All statistical analyses were conducted using JMP statistical software (version 9.0, SAS Institute Inc., Cary, North Carolina).

3. Results

Sixty-six patients were included in the postthoracotomy pain group, and sixty-six controls were matched for age, gender, surgeon, and date of surgery. There was no statistically significant difference between groups in terms of age, body mass index, gender, procedure type, or thoracotomy side (Table 1).

Overall, the age of the cohorts was 59 years, and 68 patients were male and 64 patients were female. Of the 64 females, 32 developed PTPS and 32 did not. Of the 68 males, 34 developed PTPS and 34 did not. There was no statistically significant difference between procedure types and the subsequent development of PTPS ($P < 0.54$, Pearson). Further, there was no statistical difference between patients who underwent more than one thoracic surgery and the subsequent development of PTPS (9 control patients (14%) and 16 PTPS patients (24%) underwent more than one thoracic surgery, $P < 0.12$, Pearson).

The median hospital duration was significantly different between control patients and PTPS patients. Control patients' median (IQR) hospital stay was 5 days (4, 6) compared with PTPS patients' stay of 6 days (5, 8), $P < 0.020$ (t-test). The median duration for patients having indwelling chest tubes was not significantly different between control patients and PTPS patients. Control patients' median (IQR) chest tube duration was 5 days (4, 6) compared with PTPS patients' chest tube duration of 5 days (4, 7), $P < 0.069$ (t-test).

The total opioid equivalent utilized for the first three days postoperatively was significantly different between control patients and PTPS patients. The median (IQR) total oral morphine equivalent utilized was 236.5 mg (73, 508) for controls and 365.5 mg (115.6, 874) for PTPS patients ($P < 0.005$, t-test) (Table 2).

Postoperative pain scores are summarized in Table 3. Only on POD1 did PTPS patients experience more pain with movement than control patients ($P < 0.03$). Otherwise, average reported pain scores were not significantly different between groups.

There was no statistically significant difference between groups in characteristics of epidural analgesia management. The median epidural level in the PTPS group and the control

Table 1: Patient and procedural characteristics.

Characteristic	PTPS ($N = 66$)	Control ($N = 66$)
Age (years, mean ± SD)	59.0 ± 11.7	59.2 ± 13.1
BMI (kg/m^2, mean ± SD)	27.4 ± 5.1	28.7 ± 6.8
Gender		
Male (*n*, %)	34 (52%)	34 (52%)
Female (*n*, %)	32 (48%)	32 (48%)
Procedure		
Pneumonectomy	8 (12%)	7 (11%)
Other thoracotomies	52 (79%)	55 (83%)
Combined thoracotomy and laparotomy	6 (9%)	4 (6%)
*Thoracotomy side**		
Left	33 (50%)	25 (38%)
Right	30 (45%)	41 (62%)
Bilateral	3 (5%)	0 (0%)

There were no statistically significant differences between groups. Statistical analyses were conducted using Student's *t*-test for continuous variables and Pearson chi-square test for categorical variables. * $P = 0.05$.

Table 2: Postoperative analgesic outcomes.

Characteristic	PTPS ($N = 66$)	Control ($N = 66$)	*P* value
*Total opioid equivalent**			0.005
Median (25, 75 IQ)	366 (116, 874)	237 (74, 508)	
Type of epidural opioid infusion			0.367
Fentanyl	17 (26%)	14 (21%)	
Hydromorphone	44 (67%)	42 (64%)	
Morphine	5 (8%)	10 (15%)	
Epidural bupivacaine infusion	59 (89%)	55 (83%)	0.448

P values are from Student's *t*-test.

*Opioid equivalents were calculated as oral morphine equivalents (mg) during the first three postoperative days and did not include epidural opioid [8].

Table 3: Postoperative pain scores (NRS).

Characteristic	PTPS		Control		*P* value
	N	Mean ± SD	*N*	Mean ± SD	
Rest pain					
POD1	33	4.7 ± 2.8	33	4.0 ± 3.1	0.30
POD2	37	4.1 ± 2.6	37	3.4 ± 2.3	0.25
POD3	31	2.9 ± 2.2	31	2.4 ± 2.3	0.38
Overall	44	4.1 ± 2.2	47	3.6 ± 2.6	0.38
Movement pain					
POD1	9	6.0 ± 2.5	10	3.3 ± 2.2	0.03
POD2	20	6.4 ± 2.8	26	6.1 ± 2.9	0.74
POD3	16	6.1 ± 3.1	24	5.1 ± 2.7	0.32
Overall	25	6.2 ± 2.5	30	5.0 ± 2.4	0.08

* *P* values are from ANOVA.

group was T6-7 ($P < 0.70$, Pearson). For the control group, the interquartile range was T5-6 and T8-9. For the PTPS group, the interquartile range was T5-6 and T7-8. Fifty-six patients (85%) in the control group had thoracic epidural catheters, and ten patients (15%) had lumbar epidural catheters. Fifty-seven patients (86%) in the PTPS group had thoracic epidural catheters, and nine patients (14%) had lumbar epidural catheters. There was also no statistically significant difference between groups in the type of opioid used for initial epidural loading dose ($P < 0.58$, Wilcoxon). Overall, 69 (52%) of patients received hydromorphone, 26 (20%) received fentanyl, and 13 (10%) received morphine for their epidural opioid loading dose, while 22 patients (17%) did not receive an opioid for an epidural loading dose. There was no difference in the selection of opioid medication or infusion used for epidural management, and there was no statistically significant difference between the initial epidural infusion type and the subsequent development of PTPS ($P < 0.19$, Pearson). The two most common initial epidural infusions were hydromorphone 10 mcg/mL with bupivacaine 0.075% (50 patients, 38%) and fentanyl 5 mcg/mL with bupivacaine 0.075% (30 patients, 23%). There was no statistically significant difference between groups in epidural catheter duration ($P < 0.06$, Wilcoxon Rank Sum). The median epidural catheter duration in the control group was 2.8 days (2.4–3.0, interquartile range) and was 2.9 days (2.7–3.0, interquartile range) in the PTPS group.

Median duration of last documentation of the 66 PTPS patients' diagnosis was 17 months (10–31 months, 25–75% IQR). At the time of follow-up, 13 patients (20%) were not taking any analgesic medications. Twenty-eight patients (42%) were taking one analgesic medication, 18 patients (27%) were taking two medications, and seven patients (11%) were taking three medications. Opioids were being utilized by 32 patients (48%). Antineuropathic pain medications (such as gabapentin, lidocaine transdermal patches, duloxetine, carbamazepine, and tricyclic antidepressants) were also being utilized by 32 patients (48%). Acetaminophen was utilized by eight patients (12%), and nonsteroidal anti-inflammatory medications were utilized by 13 patients (20%).

4. Discussion

Chronic PTPS remains a significant problem, despite aggressive postoperative analgesia [1, 2, 4, 10–13]. Postthoracotomy pain syndrome decreases quality of life with decreased physical function, decreased vitality, and ongoing consumption of analgesics [1, 2]. Chronic PTPS has proven to be very challenging to prevent, as it develops even following continuous thoracic epidural analgesia managed by a dedicated acute pain service utilizing multimodal adjuvant therapies including acetaminophen, nonsteroidal analgesics, opioids, and gabapentin [1, 2]. Of note, perioperative gabapentin has not been shown to prevent PTPS in prospective, randomized, controlled, and registered studies [2, 14], and gabapentinoids result in postoperative sedation and respiratory depression [15–17]. Genetic differences have not been identified as a risk factor in the development of chronic postsurgical pain [18]. Prolonged hospitalization and greater acute opioid usage are predictors for PTPS and therefore can be utilized as potential signals that a patient might benefit from closer follow-up and early referral to pain management specialists. Continued advances in surgical techniques, less traumatic chest drainage and suction equipment, and intercostal injections of liposomal local anesthetic preparations in high-risk patients may be valuable future studies to begin decreasing the incidence and severity of PTPS.

This case-control study of patients detected that the median hospital duration was significantly longer for PTPS patients. This raises the question of which contributing surgical or medical issues not only prolong hospitalization but are potentially associated with increased risk for the development of PTPS. Some preexisting medical conditions such as chronic obstructive pulmonary disease and/or postoperative complications such as infections, air or chyle leaks, and reoperations can lead to prolonged hospitalizations and prolonged causes of pain. Chest tubes are utilized following thoracotomy to evacuate air and fluid from the pleural space and promote lung expansion [19]. The presence of a chest tube is associated with an increased risk of developing PTPS [20]. The duration of chest tube drainage has also been shown to be a risk factor for the subsequent development of PTPS [21]. Chest tubes typically remain indwelling longer with prolonged chyle leaks, empyemas, air leaks, and hemothoraces and cause significant acute postoperative pain that can be challenging to treat [22]. Chest tube duration was not statistically significantly different between control and PTPS groups in this study, however.

While our thoracic epidural management and multimodal analgesic regimen produced statistically similar acute postoperative pain scores overall, the PTPS patients' opioid consumption was greater. The total opioid equivalent utilized for the first three days postoperatively was significantly greater in the PTPS patients. This suggests that patients who subsequently developed PTPS needed more opioid in the first three postoperative days and may have had greater acute pain that resulted in greater opioid usage.

We did not observe a significant difference in average rest pain or average movement pain between PTPS and control groups. A dedicated inpatient pain service managed the epidural infusions and other analgesics and helped achieve appropriate analgesia. Some authors have noted significant differences in acute postoperative pain in patients who have subsequently developed PTPS. Şentürk et al. [10] noted that 83% of patients having pain NRS ≥ 2 on the second postoperative day subsequently reported having PTPS at 6 months. This compared with 48% of patients who had NRS ≤ 2 on the second postoperative day who subsequently developed PTPS at 6 months. Ochroch et al. [4] also noted that acute pain at the first postoperative day was predictive of pain 24 weeks after surgery, but not 36 or 48 weeks after surgery. Katz et al. [23] observed virtually identical acute postoperative patient-controlled morphine usage between patients who subsequently had PTPS at 1.5 years and those who did not. Of note, epidural analgesia was not provided in the study by Katz et al. In our previous study [1], we did not note any significant difference between pain scores at rest or with coughing on the first or second morning after surgery between PTPS patients and control patients. Katz et al. found that the severity of acute postoperative pain correlated with the severity of chronic postthoracotomy pain. Pain intensity at rest and after movement on the first day after surgery was significantly greater in patients who subsequently had PTPS 1.5 years later [23]. Gotoda et al. found that early acute postoperative pain increased the probability of developing postthoracotomy pain syndrome [24], and Wang et al. [21] found that more intense wound pain predicted PTPS.

Grider et al. [25] observed that thoracic epidural analgesia (TEA) with bupivacaine and hydromorphone may improve acute postoperative analgesia compared with TEA with bupivacaine alone or paravertebral infusion alone. Epidural administration of bupivacaine and hydromorphone has been previously described [2, 26–29] and can provide significant postoperative analgesia but unfortunately has not been shown to decrease the incidence of PTPS [25].

The procedure type, thoracotomy side, repeat thoracic surgery, and the surgeon did not predict PTPS. In our previous study [1], we also did not observe a significant difference between surgical sides and PTPS. In contrast, Richardson et al. [20] found that resection of a rib decreased the probability of developing PTPS, and the left 8th intercostal incision for antireflux procedures increased the risk of developing PTPS. Ivor Lewis surgery did not change the risk of developing PTPS in Richardson's study, though.

This study is retrospective and is therefore limited in terms of the strength of our conclusions. The possibility of a type I error also exists. Preoperative opioid use was not an exclusion criterion and might have affected the total opioid utilized by a patient perioperatively. Numerous providers staff the inpatient pain service and selection of the type and rate of epidural infusion was likely subject to individual preferences. Pain scores with movement were not solicited as consistently in the beginning of our 11-year retrospective study period, and this reflects our change in clinical practice to attend to both rest and movement pain scores as a more thorough assessment of patient comfort. Our data is subject to the completeness of the record, but we utilized experienced abstractors. We limited the cases to local patients who were residents in the tristate area to maximize the likelihood of follow-up by the surgeons and referral to the Mayo Clinic Rochester Pain Clinic, and all patients were followed up at Mayo beyond 2 months after thoracotomy.

5. Conclusions

We observed that the median hospital duration was significantly different between control patients and PTPS patients. This risk factor has not been previously reported and provides a simple marker for patients who might be at increased risk for the development of PTPS. Similarly, the total opioid equivalent utilized in oral morphine mg equivalents for the first three days postoperatively was significantly different between control patients and PTPS patients. Greater opioid usage postoperatively is also a simple marker for identifying patients who might be at risk for PTPS. Early referral to pain management specialists can then occur in these patients with increased risk for PTPS.

Competing Interests

The authors declare that they have no conflict of interests regarding the publication of this paper.

Acknowledgments

Mayo Clinic's Department of Anesthesiology, Anesthesia Clinical Research Unit (ACRU), Andrew C. Hanson, and secretarial assistance by Pamela J. Fenske are acknowledged. Mayo Foundation and the project described were supported by Grant no. 1 UL1 RR024150 from the National Center for Research Resources (NCRR), a component of the National Institutes of Health (NIH), and the NIH Roadmap for Medical Research.

References

[1] M. A. O. Kinney, W. M. Hooten, S. D. Cassivi et al., "Chronic postthoracotomy pain and health-related quality of life," *Annals of Thoracic Surgery*, vol. 93, no. 4, pp. 1242–1247, 2012.

[2] M. A. O. Kinney, C. B. Mantilla, P. E. Carns et al., "Preoperative gabapentin for acute post-thoracotomy analgesia: a randomized, double-blinded, active placebo-controlled study," *Pain Practice*, vol. 12, no. 3, pp. 175–183, 2012.

[3] E. A. Ochroch, A. Gottschalk, A. B. Troxel, and J. T. Farrar, "Women suffer more short and long-term pain than men after major thoracotomy," *Clinical Journal of Pain*, vol. 22, no. 5, pp. 491–498, 2006.

[4] E. A. Ochroch, A. Gottschalk, J. Augostides et al., "Long-term pain and activity during recovery from major thoracotomy using thoracic epidural analgesia," *Anesthesiology*, vol. 97, no. 5, pp. 1234–1244, 2002.

[5] K. Wildgaard, J. Ravn, and H. Kehlet, "Chronic post-thoracotomy pain: a critical review of pathogenic mechanisms and strategies for prevention," *European Journal of Cardio-Thoracic Surgery*, vol. 36, no. 1, pp. 170–180, 2009.

[6] G. P. Joshi, F. Bonnet, R. Shah et al., "A systematic review of randomized trials evaluating regional techniques for postthoracotomy analgesia," *Anesthesia and Analgesia*, vol. 107, no. 3, pp. 1026–1040, 2008.

[7] C. G. Chute, S. A. Beck, T. B. Fisk, and D. N. Mohr, "The Enterprise Data Trust at Mayo Clinic: a semantically integrated warehouse of biomedical data," *Journal of the American Medical Informatics Association*, vol. 17, no. 2, pp. 131–135, 2010.

[8] G. W. Hanks, F. D. Conno, N. Cherny et al., "Morphine and alternative opioids in cancer pain: the EAPC recommendations," *British Journal of Cancer*, vol. 84, no. 5, pp. 587–593, 2001.

[9] P. A. Harris, R. Taylor, R. Thielke, J. Payne, N. Gonzalez, and J. G. Conde, "Research electronic data capture (REDCap)-a metadata-driven methodology and workflow process for providing translational research informatics support," *Journal of Biomedical Informatics*, vol. 42, no. 2, pp. 377–381, 2009.

[10] M. Şentürk, P. E. Özcan, G. K. Talu et al., "The effects of three different analgesia techniques on long-term postthoracotomy pain," *Anesthesia & Analgesia*, vol. 94, no. 1, pp. 11–15, 2002.

[11] C. L. Bong, M. Samuel, J. M. Ng, and C. Ip-Yam, "Effects of preemptive epidural analgesia on post-thoracotomy pain," *Journal of Cardiothoracic and Vascular Anesthesia*, vol. 19, no. 6, pp. 786–793, 2005.

[12] E. Tiippana, E. Nilsson, and E. Kalso, "Post-thoracotomy pain after thoracic epidural analgesia: a prospective follow-up study," *Acta Anaesthesiologica Scandinavica*, vol. 47, no. 4, pp. 433–438, 2003.

[13] V. Guastella, G. Mick, C. Soriano et al., "A prospective study of neuropathic pain induced by thoracotomy: incidence, clinical description, and diagnosis," *Pain*, vol. 152, no. 1, pp. 74–81, 2011.

[14] K. Grosen, A. M. Drewes, A. Højsgaard, M. Pfeiffer-Jensen, V. E. Hjortdal, and H. K. Pilegaard, "Perioperative gabapentin for the prevention of persistent pain after thoracotomy: a randomized controlled trial," *European Journal of Cardio-thoracic Surgery*, vol. 46, no. 1, Article ID ezu032, pp. 76–85, 2014.

[15] M. Myhre, L. M. Diep, and A. Stubhaug, "Pregabalin has analgesic, ventilatory, and cognitive effects in combination with remifentanil," *Anesthesiology*, vol. 124, no. 5, 2016.

[16] J. E. Chelly, "Pregabalin effective for the prevention of chronic postsurgical pain: really?" *Anesthesia & Analgesia*, vol. 116, no. 2, pp. 507–508, 2013.

[17] T. N. Weingarten, A. K. Jacob, C. W. Njathi, G. A. Wilson, and J. Sprung, "Multimodal analgesic protocol and postanesthesia respiratory depression during phase I recovery after total joint arthroplasty," *Regional Anesthesia and Pain Medicine*, vol. 40, no. 4, pp. 330–336, 2015.

[18] A. Montes, G. Roca, S. Sabate et al., "Genetic and clinical factors associated with chronic postsurgical pain after hernia repair, hysterectomy, and thoracotomy: a two-year multicenter cohort study," *Anesthesiology*, vol. 122, no. 5, pp. 1123–1141, 2015.

[19] A. Brunelli, S. D. Cassivi, J. Fibla, and L. Di Nunzio, "Pleural pressure immediately after pulmonary lobectomy: single versus double chest tubes for suction," *The Journal of Thoracic and Cardiovascular Surgery*, vol. 140, no. 3, pp. e52–e53, 2010.

[20] J. Richardson, S. Sabanathan, A. J. Mearns, C. Sides, and C. P. Goulden, "Post-thoracotomy neuralgia," *The Pain Clinic*, vol. 7, no. 2, pp. 87–97, 1994.

[21] H.-T. Wang, W. Liu, A.-L. Luo, C. Ma, and Y.-G. Huang, "Prevalence and risk factors of chronic post-thoracotomy pain in Chinese patients from peking union medical college hospital," *Chinese Medical Journal*, vol. 125, no. 17, pp. 3033–3038, 2012.

[22] J. A. Stanik-Hutt, K. L. Soeken, A. E. Belcher, D. K. Fontaine, and A. G. Gift, "Pain experiences of traumatically injured patients in a critical care setting," *American Journal of Critical Care*, vol. 10, no. 4, pp. 252–259, 2001.

[23] J. Katz, M. Jackson, B. P. Kavanagh, and A. N. Sandler, "Acute pain after thoracic surgery predicts long-term post-thoracotomy pain," *Clinical Journal of Pain*, vol. 12, no. 1, pp. 50–55, 1996.

[24] Y. Gotoda, N. Kambara, T. Sakai, Y. Kishi, K. Kodama, and T. Koyama, "The morbidity, time course and predictive factors for persistent post-thoracotomy pain," *European Journal of Pain*, vol. 5, no. 1, pp. 89–96, 2001.

[25] J. S. Grider, T. W. Mullet, S. P. Saha, M. E. Harned, and P. A. Sloan, "A randomized, double-blind trial comparing continuous thoracic epidural bupivacaine with and without opioid in contrast to a continuous paravertebral infusion of bupivacaine for post-thoracotomy pain," *Journal of Cardiothoracic & Vascular Anesthesia*, vol. 26, no. 1, pp. 83–89, 2012.

[26] R. S. Sinatra, S. Levin, and C. A. Ocampo, "Neuroaxial hydromorphone for control of postsurgical, obstetric, and chronic pain," *Seminars in Anesthesia*, vol. 19, no. 2, pp. 108–131, 2000.

[27] R. S. Sinatra, S. Eige, J. H. Chung et al., "Continuous epidural infusion of 0.05% bupivacaine plus hydromorphone for labor

analgesia: an observational assessment in 1830 parturients," *Anesthesia & Analgesia*, vol. 94, no. 5, pp. 1310–1311, 2002.

[28] S. S. Liu, M. Bieltz, B. Wukovits, and R. S. John, "Prospective survey of patient-controlled epidural analgesia with bupivacaine and hydromorphone in 3736 postoperative orthopedic patients," *Regional Anesthesia & Pain Medicine*, vol. 35, no. 4, pp. 351–354, 2010.

[29] M. J. Brown, D. J. Kor, M. S. Allen et al., "Dual-epidural catheter technique and perioperative outcomes after ivor-lewis esophagectomy," *Regional Anesthesia and Pain Medicine*, vol. 38, no. 1, pp. 3–8, 2013.

21

Interventional Pain Management in Multidisciplinary Chronic Pain Clinics: A Prospective Multicenter Cohort Study with One-Year Follow-Up

Cláudia Gouvinhas,[1] Dalila Veiga,[2] Liliane Mendonça,[3] Rute Sampaio,[1,4] Luís Filipe Azevedo,[3,5,6] and José Manuel Castro-Lopes[1,3,4]

[1]*Department of Biomedicine, Faculty of Medicine, University of Porto, Porto, Portugal*
[2]*Chronic Pain Center-Anesthesiology Department, Centro Hospitalar do Porto, Porto, Portugal*
[3]*National Observatory for Pain (NOPain), Porto, Portugal*
[4]*Institute for Molecular and Cell Biology (IBMC), University of Porto, Porto, Portugal*
[5]*Department of Community Medicine, Information and Health Decision Sciences (MEDCIDS), Faculty of Medicine, University of Porto, Porto, Portugal*
[6]*Centre for Health Technology and Services Research (CINTESIS), University of Porto, Porto, Portugal*

Correspondence should be addressed to Cláudia Gouvinhas; c.gouvinhas@gmail.com

Academic Editor: Robert L. Barkin

Background. Interventional Pain Management (IPM) is performed in multidisciplinary chronic pain clinics (MCPC), including a range of invasive techniques to diagnose and treat chronic pain (CP) conditions. Current patterns of use of those techniques in MCPC have not yet been reported. *Objective.* We aimed to describe quantitatively and qualitatively the use of IPM and other therapeutic procedures performed on-site at four Portuguese MCPC. *Methods.* A prospective cohort study with one-year follow-up was performed in adult patients. A structured case report form was systematically completed at baseline and six and 12 months. *Results.* Among 808 patients referred to the MCPC, 17.2% had been prescribed IPM. Patients with IPM were on average younger and had longer CP duration and lower levels of maximum pain and pain interference/disability. The three main diagnoses were low back pain ($n = 28$), postoperative CP, and knee pain ($n = 16$ each). From 195 IPM prescribed, nerve blocks ($n = 108$), radiofrequency ($n = 31$), and viscosupplementation ($n = 22$) were the most prevalent. Some IPM techniques were only available in few MCPC. One MCPC did not provide IPM. *Conclusions.* IPM are seldom prescribed in Portuguese MCPC. Further studies on IPM safety and effectiveness are necessary for clear understanding the role of these techniques in CP management.

1. Introduction

Chronic pain (CP) is a worldwide public health problem that causes a substantial burden on healthcare systems and society, taking into account its high prevalence, economic costs, and the quality of life impairment of the patients and their families. CP requires a multidisciplinary approach for its adequate assessment and management [1–5]. For more than twenty years, the International Association for the Study of Pain (IASP) defined chronic CP as "pain that persists beyond normal tissue healing time, which is assumed to be 3 months" [6]. Variations in the definition of CP between and within countries, differences in standards of living and healthcare resources, high prevalence of pain-generating diseases, cultural background, and local traditions can help explain the estimated CP prevalence ranging from 11% to 55% [2, 7–9]. In a recent epidemiological study, CP prevalence in Portugal was estimated at 37% [10]. CP of moderate to severe intensity has been estimated to occur in 19% of European adults and 40% of them reported inadequate management of their pain [8, 11].

CP is one of the most common reasons why people seek medical care [1]. The economic impact of CP in the USA, in 2008, ranged from $560 to $635 billion USD [12]; in Portugal, it was €4611.69 million (in 2010), corresponding to 2.71% of the Portuguese annual gross domestic product, with 42.7% direct and 57.3% indirect costs [2]. Indirect costs of CP are mainly linked to work absenteeism with reduced levels of productivity and increased risk of leaving the labor market [13].

Ideally, supported by the most recent guidelines for the CP management, these patients should have access to a multidisciplinary range of diagnostic and therapeutic modalities appropriate to their clinical condition [14–17]. The primary emphasis should be placed on pain management to improve physical and social function and minimize the disability [18–20]. Pain management includes pharmacological therapy, psychological assessment and treatment, invasive techniques, occupational therapy, and rehabilitation medicine [2, 15, 20–25]. Interventional Pain Management (IPM) encompasses a wide variety of techniques such as epidural injections [26–29], nerve blocks [18, 21, 30], joint infiltrations [31, 32], spinal cord stimulation [33, 34], botulinum toxin application [35–37], and radiofrequency denervation [38, 39]. Recent data suggests that some of the IPM techniques allow a superior improvement in physical and functional status of CP patients [18, 25, 26, 35, 38], as well as a reduction in associated work absenteeism [18]. Other therapeutic procedures (OTP) are also performed on-site at multidisciplinary chronic pain clinics (MCPC), namely, acupuncture [40–46] and infusion of parenteral drugs [47–49].

In Portugal, there is no available information regarding patterns of prescription of IPM or OTP performed on-site at MCPC. Therefore, as a part of a larger real-world outcomes research prospective cohort study on CP patients followed at MCPC, this study inquired about the utilization of those techniques and procedures. We aimed at describing quantitatively and qualitatively the patterns of prescription of IPM and OTP performed on-site at MCPC in Portugal.

2. Methods

2.1. Selection and Description of Participants. Participants were recruited at their first consultation in four MCPC from the North of Portugal, in the context of a large real-world outcomes research project. The eligible population included adult patients (≥18 years old) with chronic noncancer pain lasting more than 3 months (the standard IASP criteria for CP [50]) or with cancer pain regardless of its duration. Patients with psychiatric and/or cognitive impairment, unable to communicate verbally or not fluent in Portuguese were excluded. Participants were followed for twelve months and their clinical records were obtained at baseline and six and 12 months. From all 1343 patients eligible, 808 patients were elected to be part of this study. From these, 139 patients had IPM at least once during the one-year follow-up (Supplement 1 in Supplementary Material available online at https://doi.org/10.1155/2017/8402413).

All participating patients were previously informed of the study objectives and about the data selection and collection procedures, and questions regarding the study, posed by the patients, were properly answered by the research team. All participating patients signed an informed consent form. The study protocol was approved by institutional review boards, ethics committees of the participating hospitals, and CNPD, the Portuguese Data Protection Authority.

2.2. Instruments and Variables. A structured questionnaire was used in baseline interviews. For the purpose of the present study the following data were systematically collected: demographic characteristics, clinical and pain characteristics, and IPM and OTP performed on-site at MCPC prescribed. The Brief Pain Inventory (BPI) [51] which is recommended by consensus groups in the area of measurement and evaluation of pain [52] was used. This instrument was constructed for measuring and evaluating pain in a multidimensional perspective. It includes 15 items evaluating pain presence, severity, location, functional interference, therapeutic strategies, and efficacy of pain management. It is easily applicable, fast, and simple and with very good psychometric properties [53–56]. For the present study, only two constructs were assessed: pain severity and functional interference. Pain severity scale entails four items, maximum, minimum, on average, and at this moment, rated with a numerical scale (0 [no pain] to 10 [the worst pain]) and categorized using Serlin et al. classification [57]. The functional interference scale consists of seven items with numerical rating scale (0 [no interference] to 10 [extreme interference]) that assess pain interference in general activities, mood, mobility, work, personal relationships, sleep, and pleasure to live.

In the descriptive analysis of the sample (all patients) and subsamples (patients with and without IPM), we defined the general characteristics, including sociodemographic (sex, age, educational level, and family support), professional/occupational status, pain characteristics (duration, persistence pattern, location, severity, and interference), general health, and clinical variables (International Statistical Classification of Diseases and Related Health Problems-(ICD-) 10 diagnostic classification). The persistence pattern of pain was classified as continuous, pain present every day/always, or discontinuous (recurrent [pain present once to several times/week] and sporadic [pain present less than once to several times/month]).

2.3. Statistical Analysis. Categorical variables were described as absolute (n) and relative (%) frequencies; continuous variables were described using the median and interquartile ranges considering the tested asymmetric (not normal) distribution or mean and standard deviation otherwise. We used the Chi-square test, or the Fisher's exact test, to test hypotheses for categorical variables. In the case of continuous variables (with asymmetrical distribution) the Mann–Whitney test was used. For all hypothesis tests a significance level of $\alpha = 0.05$ was considered. The statistical analysis was performed using the software SPSS v21.0®.

3. Results

Table 1 shows the number of patients that were prescribed IPM and/or OTP throughout the study. Considering IPM,

TABLE 1: Number of patients that received a prescription of interventional pain management and other therapeutic procedures performed on-site at multidisciplinary chronic pain clinics.

	Baseline (n = 808)		Six months (n = 801)		Twelve months (n = 744)		Total throughout the one-year follow-up (n = 744)	
IPM and/or OTC performed on-site								
Yes	89		122		139		—	
No	719		679		605		—	
	n	%	n	%	n	%	n	%
IPM								
Nerve blocks	39	4.8	32	4.0	20	2.7	88	11.8
Viscosupplementation	18	2.2	1	0.1	1	0.1	16	2.2
Radiofrequency	13	1.6	11	1.4	5	0.7	28	3.8
Botulinum toxin	10	1.2	2	0.2	1	0.1	12	1.6
Epidural injections	9	1.1	9	1.1	1	0.1	17	2.3
Neurostimulation	—	—	1	0.1	—	—	1	0.1
Total	89	11.0	56	7.0	28	3.8	162	21.8
OTP performed on-site								
Acupuncture	33	4.1	20	2.5	12	1.6	52	7.0
Infusions	21	2.6	8	1.0	11	1.5	31	4.2
Mesotherapy	1	0.1	1	0.1	—	—	2	0.3
Total	55	6.8	29	3.6	23	3.1	85	11.4

At the top of the table, in each row there is the cumulative number of patients who had interventional pain management and/or other therapeutic procedures prescribed at multidisciplinary chronic pain clinics at each assessment time point. n, number of patients at each assessment time point. Furthermore, in each row there are the number of patients (n) and proportions of patients (%) that were prescribed interventional pain management or other therapeutic procedures performed on-site at multidisciplinary chronic pain clinics at each assessment time point and during the follow-up time. IPM, interventional pain management. OTP, other therapeutic procedures.

nerve blocks were the most frequently prescribed at all time points (39 patients at baseline, 32 patients at 6 months, 20 patients at 12 months, and 88 patients in total throughout the one-year follow-up). On the contrary, botulinum toxin and viscosupplementation were prescribed to a few patients and almost exclusively at baseline. Neuromodulation by neurostimulation was only prescribed to one patient at 6 months. OTP were also prescribed to a considerable number of patients. Among them, acupuncture was prescribed to 52 patients throughout the study, followed by drug infusions to 31 patients.

Sociodemographic characteristics of all patients, patients with IPM, and patients without IPM are described in Table 2. It was observed that 17.2% of the patients followed in MCPC had IPM prescribed, of which 71.9% were women and 28.1% men. Moreover, age was significantly lower in patients with IPM (54.6 (44.0–65.0) versus 59.7 (50.0–71.0) years, $p < 0.001$). Elderly patients (over 75 years) were less frequently prescribed IPM. Patients with IPM were mainly full- or part-time workers while those without IPM were mostly retirees ($p < 0.001$).

Table 3 shows pain clinical characteristics, at the inclusion time in our study, among all patients, patients with IPM, and patients without IPM. Almost 1/3 of the patients with IPM had pain for over 10 years, while almost 90% of patients with pain duration from 3 to 12 months did not have IPM ($p = 0.006$). Patients in both groups referred to almost exclusively continuous pain. Significant differences in pain intensity could only be seen for pain at its worst (8.01 without IPM versus 7.23 with IPM; $p = 0.003$). The location of the pain was heterogeneous and statistically significant differences were found; in all patients that indicated pain in unspecified bones, joints, and muscles 92.1% were patients without IPM, whereas among all cases of pain in inguinal and pelvic region 31.2% are reported by patients with IPM ($p = 0.047$). Patients with IPM had significantly lower pain interference score ($p <$ 0001). Specifically, pain-related interference was inferior in general ability (6.20 ± 3.26 versus 7.04 ± 2.71, $p = 0.015$), walking ability (5.76 ± 3.81 versus 6.67 ± 3.44, $p = 0.024$), normal work (6.09 ± 3.53 versus 7.26 ± 2.82, $p < 0.001$), relations with other people (3.17 ± 3.64 versus 4.22 ± 3.58, $p = 0.002$), and enjoyment of life (4.18 ± 3.95 versus 5.55 ± 3.79, $p < 0.001$). More than 57% of patients who had no pain interference had invasive techniques for pain management, while 88.1% of patients with severe interference did not had IPM prescribed. In general health no differences were found.

Using the ICD 10 to classify patient's pathologies, 34 diagnoses were obtained from all patients. The five most prevalent diagnoses in patients with IPM were low back pain (28 patients), chronic postoperative pain (16 patients), knee pain (16 patients), pelvic and perineal pain (13 patients), and low back with sciatica (11 patients). We only found five

TABLE 2: Sociodemographic characteristics of all patients, chronic pain patients with interventional pain management, and chronic pain patients without interventional pain management.

	All [†]CP patients		CP patients without IPM		CP patients with IPM			[*]p
	n	%	n	%	n	%	UF (%)	
Gender								
Male	265	32.8	226	33.8	39	28.1	14.7	0.199
Female	543	67.2	443	66.2	100	71.9	18.4	
Total	808	100.0	669	100.0	139	100.0	17.2	
Age								
Median (P25–P75)	60.0 (48.3–70.8)		59.7 (50.0–71.0)		54.6 (44.0–65.0)			**<0.001**
Age categories								
18–24 years	9	1.1	5	0.7	4	2.9	44.4	**0.010**
25–34 years	31	3.8	21	3.1	10	7.2	32.3	
35–44 years	108	13.4	87	13.0	21	15.1	19.4	
45–54 years	164	20.3	132	19.7	32	23.0	19.5	
55–64 years	190	23.5	156	23.3	34	24.5	17.9	
65–74 years	180	22.3	154	23.0	26	18.7	14.4	
75 years or older	126	15.6	114	17.0	12	18.6	9.5	
Total	808	100.0	669	100.0	139	100.0	17.2	
Family household								
Alone	84	10.4	69	10.3	15	10.8	17.9	0.121
With wife/husband or partner	317	39.2	262	39.2	55	39.6	17.4	
With wife/husband or partner and sons/daughters	244	30.2	192	28.7	52	37.4	21.3	
With sons/daughters	62	7.7	54	8.1	8	5.8	12.9	
In elderly care homes	2	0.2	2	0.3	—	—	—	
Other	99	12.3	90	13.5	9	6.5	9.1	
Total	808	100.0	669	100.0	139	100.0	17.2	
Professional/occupational status								
Full or part-time worker	242	30.0	180	26.9	62	44.6	25.6	**<0.001**
Student	6	0.7	5	0.7	1	0.7	16.7	
Unemployed	101	12.5	84	12.6	17	12.2	16.8	
House worker or domestic worker	33	4.1	26	3.9	7	5.0	21.2	
Retired or preretired	387	47.9	342	51.1	45	32.0	11.6	
Other	39	4.8	32	4.8	7	5.0	17.9	
Total	808	100.0	669	100.0	139	100.0	17.2	
Education level								
No education	24	3.0	24	4.1	—	—	—	0.195
1–4 years (basic 1st cycle)	401	49.8	330	56.4	71	51.1	17.7	
5–9 years (basic 2nd and 3rd cycles)	189	23.4	156	26.7	33	23.7	17.5	
10–12 years (secondary)	85	10.5	66	11.3	19	13.7	22.4	
More than 12 years (higher)	86	10.7	74	12.6	12	8.6	14.0	
Other	21	2.6	17	2.6	4	2.9	19.0	
Total	806	100.0	667	100.0	139	100.0	17.2	

Each row of the table includes absolute (n) and relative (%) frequencies of each characteristic and the utilization frequency (%) of interventional pain management by category (UF). Highlighted in bold are statistically significant results, at a 0.05 significance level. CP, chronic pain. IPM, interventional pain management. P25–P75, 25th percentile and 75th percentile (representing the interquartile range).[*] p value for statistical hypothesis tests comparing the subsample of CP subjects with IPM to CP subjects without IPM. Chi-square test or Fisher's exact test for categorical variables and Mann–Whitney test for numerical variables were used. [†]Chronic pain was defined, using the IASP standard definition, as pain present with duration ≥3 months.

TABLE 3: Clinical characteristics of all patients, chronic pain patients with interventional pain management, and chronic pain patients without interventional pain management.

Clinical characteristics of pain	All †CP patients		CP patients without IPM		CP patients with IPM			*p
	n	%	n	%	n	%	UF (%)	
Duration (categorized)								
≤3 months–≤1 year	218	27.3	196	29.7	22	15.8	10.1	**0.006**
<1-≤2 years	110	13.8	87	13.2	23	16.5	20.9	
<2–≤5 years	157	19.6	128	19.4	29	20.9	18.5	
<5–≤10 years	123	15.4	103	15.6	20	14.4	16.3	
>10 years	191	23.9	146	22.1	45	32.4	23.6	
Total	799	100.0	660	100.0	139	100.0	17.4	
‡Persistence pattern								
Continuous	754	93.4	626	93.7	128	92.1	17.0	0.455
Discontinuous	53	6.6	42	6.3	11	7.9	20.8	
Total	807	100.0	668	100.0	139	100.0	17.2	
	Mean (SD)		Mean (SD)		Mean (SD)			
Intensity								
Pain on average (0–10 NRS)	5.96	(2.13)	6.00	(2.01)	5.77	(2.50)		0.641
Pain at its least (0–10 NRS)	3.63	(2.50)	3.63	(2.44)	3.63	(2.79)		0.759
Pain at its worst (0–10 NRS)	7.88	(2.11)	8.01	(1.98)	7.23	(2.61)		**0.003**
Pain right now (0–10 NRS)	4.83	(2.99)	4.88	(2.94)	4.58	(3.23)		0.304
	n	%	n	%	n	%	UF (%)	
No pain	14	1.8	6	0.9	8	6.2	57.1	**<0.001**
§Mild	229	29.4	181	27.8	48	37.2	21.0	
§Moderate	244	31.3	215	33.0	29	22.5	11.9	
§Severe	293	37.6	249	38.2	44	34.1	15.0	
Total	780	100.0	651	100.0	129	100.0	16.5	
‖Location								
Lower limb	742	34.4	590	33.7	152	38.7	20.5	**0.047**
Dorsum and lower back	414	19.3	343	19.6	71	18.1	17.1	
Upper limb	363	16.9	288	16.4	75	19.1	20.7	
Cervical and facial region	261	12.1	224	12.8	37	9.4	14.2	
Bones/joints/muscles- unspecified	89	4.1	82	4.7	7	2.3	7.9	
Abdominal and anterior thoracic region	87	4.0	78	4.4	9	6.1	10.3	
Inguinal and pelvic region	77	3.6	53	3.0	24	4.6	31.2	
Other	115	5.6	97	5.5	18	4.6	15.7	
Total	2150	100.0	1757	100.2	393	100.0	18.3	
	Mean (SD)		Mean (SD)		Mean (SD)			
Pain-related interference								
General activity	6.90	(2.82)	7.04	(2.71)	6.20	(3.26)		**0.015**
Mood	6.25	(3.28)	6.37	(3.21)	5.64	(3.58)		0.054
Walking ability	6.52	(3.51)	6.67	(3.44)	5.76	(3.81)		**0.024**
¶Normal work	7.06	(2.98)	7.26	(2.82)	6.09	(3.53)		**<0.001**
Relations with other people	4.05	(3.60)	4.22	(3.58)	3.17	(3.64)		**0.002**
Sleep	5.64	(3.80)	5.72	(3.81)	5.20	(3.74)		0.087
Enjoyment of life	5.33	(3.84)	5.55	(3.79)	4.18	(3.95)		**<0.001**

Table 3: Continued.

Clinical characteristics of pain	All †CP patients		CP patients without IPM		CP patients with IPM			*p
	n	%	n	%	n	%	UF (%)	
£Interference								
No interference	14	1.8	6	0.9	8	6.3	57.1	
Mild	229	29.4	180	27.6	49	38.3	21.4	**<0.001**
Moderate	244	31.3	208	31.9	36	28.1	14.8	
Severe	293	37.6	258	39.6	35	27.3	11.9	
Total	780	100.0	652	100.0	128	100.0	16.4	
General health								
Excellent	13	1.6	11	1.7	2	1.4	15.4	
Very good	15	1.9	12	1.8	3	2.2	20.0	
Good	117	14.6	94	14.1	23	16.5	19.7	0.082
Fair	342	42.5	271	40.8	71	51.1	20.8	
Poor	317	39.4	277	41.7	40	28.8	12.6	
Total	804	100.0	665	100.0	139	100.0	17.3	

Each row of the table includes the absolute (n) and relative (%) frequencies of each characteristic, the utilization frequency (%) of interventional pain management by category (UF (%)), and in some cases the mean and standard deviation (SD). Highlighted in bold are statistically significant results, at a 0.05 significance level. CP, chronic pain. IPM, interventional pain management. SD, standard deviation. *p value for statistical hypothesis tests comparing the subsample of CP subjects with IPM to CP subjects without IPM. Chi-square test or Fisher's exact test for categorical variables and Mann–Whitney test for numerical variables were used. †Chronic pain was defined, using the IASP standard definition, as pain present with duration ≥3 months. ‡Persistence pattern: continuous—pain present every day/ always; discontinuous—recurrent (pain present once to several times/ week); and sporadic (pain present less than once to several times/month). $Pain intensity score was categorized taking into account the Serling classification: mild (1–4), moderate (5-6), and severe pain intensity (7–10). ||Multiple pain locations were recorded for each patient. ¶Including both work outside the home and housework. £Pain interference was categorized as mild (1–4), moderate (5-6), and severe pain interference (7–10).

significant differences between patients with and without IPM in what concerns the diagnosis. IPM was only used in 2.8% of patients with fibromyalgia ($p = 0.013$) and 4.2% of patients with cancer pain ($p < 0.001$), while it was used in 36.7% of patients with low back pain with sciatica ($p = 0.011$), 41% of patients with knee ($p < 0.001$) pain, and 46.4% of patients with pelvic or perineal pain ($p < 0.001$) (Supplement 2).

Throughout the study 420 treatments were prescribed as seen in Table 4. The most prescribed IPM in all assessment time points was nerve blocks. In one-year follow-up nerve blocks were 108 times prescribed followed by radiofrequency (31 prescriptions) and viscosupplementation (22 prescriptions). The botulinum toxin and viscosupplementation prescriptions were scarce and occurred almost exclusively at baseline. The most prescribed OTP performed on-site at MCPC at baseline were infusions (43 prescriptions) and at 6 and 12 months acupuncture (73 and 45 prescriptions, resp.).

The five most frequent diagnoses of patients that were prescribed each of the IPM and/or OTP are shown in Table 5. IPM was not exclusive to patients with a specific diagnosis. Nerve blocks, epidural, and radiofrequency were extensively used in several diagnoses, and the same occurred with acupuncture. Botulin toxin was prescribed to 69.2% of patients with pelvic and perineal pain; viscosupplementation was prescribed to 68.4% of patients diagnosed with knee pain. Considering OTP performed on-site at MCPC, drug infusions were prescribed to 57.9% of patients with cancer pain.

There was large heterogeneity in the type of treatments and prescription frequency in each MCPC. It is noted that there are techniques only prescribed in some MCPC, such as viscosupplementation, radiofrequency, botulinum toxin, and neurostimulation. One MCPC had only OTP performed on-site (Supplement 3).

4. Discussion

There are very few studies focused on IPM utilization patterns in multidisciplinary CP clinics [17, 24]. To our best knowledge, this is the first study focused on this issue in Portugal and one of the very few elsewhere.

We found that nerve blocks were the most frequent IPM prescribed in MCPC; with a total of 420 IPM or OTP prescribed during the one-year follow-up. A total of 139 patients (17.2%) in our cohort received IPM for their CP management. Of those, almost 32.4% had pain for over 10 years and 92.1% of these reported a continuous pain pattern. There was a diversity of IPM prescribed in the participating MCPC, and botulinum toxin, viscosupplementation, neurostimulation, and radiofrequency were only available in very few centers. In our cohort there is a higher prevalence of women with CP which is in accordance with the available literature [10, 20, 58], and average pain intensity was approximately 6 in a 0–10 numerical rating scale.

In general, the success of these techniques is partly dependent on the experience and skill of the provider. There is controversy over the evidence that supports these

Table 4: Prescriptions and rate of prescription of interventional pain management and other therapeutic procedures performed on-site at multidisciplinary chronic pain clinics at baseline, six months, and twelve months and during the whole follow-up period.

	Baseline (nt = 808)		Six months (nt = 801)		Twelve months (nt = 744)		Total throughout the one-year follow-up (nt = 744)	
	n	Rate	n	Rate	n	Rate	n	Rate
Interventional pain management								
Nerve blocks	41	5.1	51	6.4	37	5.0	108	14.5
Viscosupplementation	19	2.4	6	0.7	4	0.5	22	3.0
Radiofrequency	12	1.5	16	2.0	5	0.7	31	4.2
Botulinum toxin	10	1.2	2	0.2	3	0.4	14	1.9
Epidural injections	9	1.1	11	1.4	2	0.3	19	2.6
Neurostimulation	—	—	1	0.1	—	—	1	0.1
Total	91	11.3	87	10.9	51	6.9	195	26.2
OTP performed on-site								
Infusions	43	5.3	38	4.7	25	3.4	95	12.8
Acupuncture	38	4.7	73	9.1	45	6.0	128	17.2
Mesotherapy	1	0.1	1	0.1	—	—	2	0.3
Total	82	10.1	199	14.0	70	9.4	225	30.2

Each row of the table includes the number of interventional pain management or other therapeutic procedures performed on-site at multidisciplinary chronic pain clinics at each assessment time point and during the follow-up time (n), the average number of prescriptions per 100 patients at each assessment time point (rate). nt, number of patients at each assessment time point. OTP, other therapeutic procedures.

techniques [16], as there is no sufficient data to ascertain the efficacy of some procedures. In some cases, pain relief is only observed during a short period and does not essentially convert into improved function and reduced work absenteeism [59]. Moreover, there is a risk of potential complications associated, but most are transient and often subclinical [30]. IPM techniques have been used for a long time as a last option for patients when all other conservative approaches have failed. Therefore, it is understandable that patients to whom they are actuality prescribed have a much longer reported pain duration [59].

In the present study, IPM were prescribed mainly to patients that did not report significant interference of pain, as measured by the functional interference scale of the Brief Pain Inventory, while the vast majority of patients that reported severe interference were not prescribed IPM. The reasons for these unexpected results are not clear at present, and one can only speculate that patients with severe interference suffered from conditions and/or had a health status (e.g., comorbidities) less likely to be treated by IPM, but additional data is required to investigate this issue.

Among the great variety of IPM used in multidisciplinary pain management [14, 25], six techniques plus three OTP performed on-site at MCPC were prescribed in the course of our study.

Nerve blocks, the most frequently prescribed technique in the present study (88 patients), consist in anesthetics delivered to visceral and peripheral nerves in order to interrupt nociceptive input at the source of pain [16, 28]. This procedure may be understood, especially by patients, as curative, but similarly to other IPM techniques, that is not the case. However, it can be very useful, for instance, to alleviate pain and allow patient to take part in their physical therapy [30].

Viscosupplementation consists of intra-articular injection of hyaluronic acid derivatives. It is one of the more used local treatments for osteoarthritis along with corticosteroid injection. It has been used mainly in knee joint, where it shows moderate and significant pain reduction and increased function [32], but a recent meta-analysis provided no evidence that the effect remains longer than six months [31].

Radiofrequency denervation consists in nerve ablation using heat generated by a radiofrequency current [38]. Facet joints radiofrequency is one of the most prevalent indications for its use with high rates of clinical improvement. However, these effects have also a limited temporal efficacy [25, 39].

Botulinum toxin injections as well as acupuncture and dry needling techniques are effective options for myofascial pain, namely, trigger point's deactivation [36, 38]. However there is no clear evidence about long-term effectiveness of botulinum toxin treatment [35].

Epidural injection was primarily recommended for radicular pain from a herniated disc but could also be performed in patients with spinal stenosis and other low back pain conditions [25, 26]. Fair evidence of moderate benefit versus placebo injection for short-term low back pain relief was found [27], and even when compared with other pharmacological treatment, epidural injection may be better in some outcomes, but the differences are transient and modest [28]. In fact, epidural steroid injections are the most commonly performed procedure in USA, differing from what we have found in our study, yet evidence is controversial and inconclusive as to their long-term effectiveness [25, 28, 29]. The potential complications associated with neuraxial techniques

TABLE 5: Characterization of interventional pain management and other therapeutic procedures performed on-site at multidisciplinary chronic pain clinics by the five main diagnoses.

Interventional pain management	*ICD-10 diagnostic classification*				
Nerve blocks	Low back pain	Chronic postoperative pain	Low back pain with sciatica	Shoulder pain	Cervicalgia
np (%)	23 (25.7)	14 (15.4)	9 (9.9)	5 (5.5)	5 (5.5)
ni (%)	32 (20.9)	22 (14.4)	12 (7.8)	7 (4.6)	5 (3.3)
Viscosupplementation	Knee pain	Unspecified osteoarthritis, unspecified site	Chronic postoperative pain	Pain in unspecified joint	Low back pain with sciatica
np (%)	13 (68.4)	3 (15.8)	1 (5.3)	1 (5.3)	1 (5.3)
ni (%)	22 (75.9)	3 (10.3)	1 (3.4)	2 (6.9)	1 (3.4)
Botulinum toxin	Pelvic and perineal pain	Central pain syndrome	Chronic postprocedural pain	Cancer pain	Lower abdominal pain, unspecified
np (%)	9 (69.2)	1 (7.7)	1 (7.7)	1 (7.7)	1 (7.7)
ni (%)	11 (73.3)	1 (6.7)	1 (6.7)	1 (6.7)	1 (6.7)
Radiofrequency	Low back pain	Low back pain with sciatica	Shoulder pain	Knee pain	Other hereditary and idiopathic neuropathies
np (%)	7 (25.0)	5 (17.9)	3 (10.7)	3 (10.7)	2 (7.1)
ni (%)	9 (27.3)	5 (15.2)	3 (9.1)	3 (9.1)	2 (6.1)
Epidural injections	Low back pain	Low back pain with sciatica	Hip pain	Chronic postoperative pain	Radiculopathy, lumbar region
np (%)	5 (26.3)	4 (21.1)	2 (10.5)	2 (10.5)	2 (10.5)
ni (%)	5 (22.7)	4 (18.2)	2 (9.1)	2 (9.1)	3 (16.6)
Neurostimulation	Chronic postoperative pain				
np (%)	1 (100.0)				
ni (%)	1 (100.0)				
OTP performed on-site	*ICD-10 diagnostic classification*				
Infusions	Cancer pain	Disorders of trigeminal nerve	Chronic postoperative pain	Radiculopathy, lumbar region	Cervicalgia
np (%)	22 (57.9)	4 (10.5)	3 (7.9)	2 (5.3)	2 (5.3)
ni (%)	37 (45.1)	26 (31.7)	5 (6.1)	13 (15.9)	13 (15.9)
Acupuncture	Low back pain	Cervicalgia	Myalgia	Pain in unspecified joint	Fibromyalgia
np (%)	15 (23.1)	11 (16.9)	6 (9.2)	5 (7.7)	5 (7.7)
ni (%)	49 (30.4)	12 (7.5)	27 (16.8)	5 (3.1)	22 (13.7)
Mesotherapy	Low back pain	Unspecified mononeuropathy of lower limb			
np (%)	1 (50.0)	1 (50.0)			
ni (%)	1 (50.0)	1 (50.0)			

Each row of the table includes the number of patients and percentage (%) that were prescribed interventional treatments or other therapeutic procedures performed on-site at multidisciplinary chronic pain clinics (np) and the number and percentage (%) of prescribed interventional treatments or other therapeutic procedures performed on-site at multidisciplinary chronic pain clinics (ni). ICD, International Statistical Classification of Diseases and Related Health Problems. OTP, other therapeutic procedures.

performance may explain the low prevalence reported on its use.

Neuromodulation is used in some Portuguese MCPC. However, during the recruitment period of our study there was only one patient who was referred to this treatment [33]. Spinal cord stimulation has formal indication in CP conditions such as failed back surgery, complex regional pain syndrome, peripheral vascular diseases (Buerger disease, Raynaud syndrome, and limb ischemia I/II), and refractory *angina pectoris* [34].

Taking into consideration OTP performed on-site, prescribed in the MCPC, acupuncture was the most frequently prescribed. Some evidence supports acupuncture effectiveness for chronic low back pain treatment [41], fibromyalgia [42], and neck pain treatment [43]. It is increasingly prescribed [40], but the lack of strong studies that clearly prove its effectiveness has delayed its global recognition [44–46].

Pain is a common symptom in cancer patients. In spite of advances in pain management, effective pain control remains an ongoing challenge, despite high doses of opioids [47]. Drugs infusions can be used safely and should be considered to manage cancer neuropathic pain [47, 48]. Trigeminal neuralgia is the most common neuralgia in which intravenous infusion of lidocaine may be a therapeutic option when other treatments are ineffective [49]. Thus further investigation will be needed to evaluate clinical significance of infusion therapy [48].

The present findings clarify which and in what extent IPM and OTP performed on-site at MCPC are being prescribed. This study has several strengths, namely, inclusion of several MCPC, a well-structured and detailed questionnaire, telephonic interviews performed systematically, a restricted and trained team, a large sample, and a 12-month follow-up period. The data presented are unique and to the best of our knowledge there are no similar data in other MCPC that describe their current clinical practice and are useful for comparison and benchmarking.

We have a comprehensive and systematic description of IPM and OTP performed on-site, prescribed, and actually used in MCPC, constituting the clear added value of our study. However, some IPM can be performed for therapeutic or diagnostic purposes and this has not been differentiated in the present study. Further ongoing research will provide data on the evaluation of real-world effectiveness and patient's reported satisfaction by type and timing of techniques performed.

5. Conclusions

In Portugal IPM is available in most MCPC, but with marked diversity in the types of techniques and clinical indications. IPM is still seldom prescribed, with only 17.2% of patients having IPM as part of their management. Future studies focused on patient's reported effectiveness and satisfaction are needed.

Disclosure

The sponsors did not participate in the design or conduct of this study; in the collection, management, analysis, or interpretation of data; or in the preparation, review, and approval of the manuscripts or decisions to submit for publication. The authors are fully responsible for the contents of the manuscript. The present work was developed as part of the Master Thesis of Dr. Claudia Gouvinhas presented and approved with honors at the Faculty of Medicine, University of Porto, Portugal, in June 7, 2017 [60].

Acknowledgments

The authors acknowledge the patients in this study and all healthcare professionals at the participating chronic pain clinics. This work was supported by intramural funds from the Chair on Pain Medicine of the Faculty of Medicine, University of Porto. This work was also partially developed under the scope of project NanoSTIMA (NORTE-01-0145-FEDER-000016), which is financed by the North Portugal Regional Operational Programme (NORTE 2020), under the PORTUGAL 2020 Partnership Agreement, and through the European Regional Development Fund (ERDF).

References

[1] A. M. Elliott, B. H. Smith, K. I. Penny, W. C. Smith, and W. A. Chambers, "The epidemiology of chronic pain in the community," *The Lancet*, vol. 354, no. 9186, pp. 1248–1252, 1999.

[2] L. F. Azevedo, A. Costa-Pereira, L. Mendonça, C. C. Dias, and J. M. Castro-Lopes, "The economic impact of chronic pain: a nationwide population-based cost-of-illness study in Portugal," *European Journal of Health Economics*, vol. 17, no. 1, pp. 87–98, 2016.

[3] H. Breivik, E. Eisenberg, and T. O'Brien, "The individual and societal burden of chronic pain in Europe: the case for strategic prioritisation and action to improve knowledge and availability of appropriate care," *BMC Public Health*, vol. 13, no. 1, article 1229, 2013.

[4] K. F. Stein and A. Miclescu, "Effectiveness of multidisciplinary rehabilitation treatment for patients with chronic pain in a primary health care unit," *Scandinavian Journal of Pain*, vol. 4, no. 4, pp. 190–197, 2013.

[5] B. H. Smith, A. M. Elliott, W. A. Chambers, W. C. Smith, P. C. Hannaford, and K. Penny, "The impact of chronic pain in the community," *Family Practice*, vol. 18, no. 3, pp. 292–299, 2001.

[6] IASP, Classification of chronic pain, Seattle: International Association for the Study of Pain, 1994.

[7] R. L. Toblin, K. A. MacK, G. Perveen, and L. J. Paulozzi, "A population-based survey of chronic pain and its treatment with prescription drugs," *Pain*, vol. 152, no. 6, pp. 1249–1255, 2011.

[8] H. Breivik, B. Collett, V. Ventafridda, R. Cohen, and D. Gallacher, "Survey of chronic pain in Europe: prevalence, impact on daily life, and treatment," *European Journal of Pain*, vol. 10, no. 4, pp. 287–333, 2006.

[9] K. J. Reid, J. Harker, M. M. Bala et al., "Epidemiology of chronic non-cancer pain in Europe: Narrative review of prevalence, pain treatments and pain impact," *Current Medical Research and Opinion*, vol. 27, no. 2, pp. 449–462, 2011.

[10] L. F. Azevedo, A. Costa-Pereira, L. Mendonça, C. C. Dias, and J. M. Castro-Lopes, "Epidemiology of chronic pain: A population-based nationwide study on its prevalence, characteristics and associated disability in Portugal," *Journal of Pain*, vol. 13, no. 8, pp. 773–783, 2012.

[11] R. Sinatra, "Causes and consequences of inadequate management of acute pain," *Pain Medicine*, vol. 11, no. 12, pp. 1859–1871, 2010.

[12] D. Gaskin and P. Richard, "The Economic Costs of Pain in the United States. Washington: Institute of Medicine (US) Committee on Advancing Pain Research, Care, and Education. Relieving Pain in America: A Blueprint for Transforming Prevention, Care, Education, and Research," 2011.

[13] C. Phillips, "The Cost and Burden of Chronic Pain," *Reviews in Pain*, vol. 3, no. 1, pp. 2–5, 2009.

[14] J. Guzmán, R. Esmail, K. Karjalainen, A. Malmivaara, E. Irvin, and C. Bombardier, "Multidisciplinary rehabilitation for chronic low back pain: systematic review," *The British Medical Journal*, vol. 322, no. 7301, pp. 1511–1516, 2001.

[15] D. R. Fitzgibbon, K. L. Posner, K. B. Domino, R. A. Caplan, L. A. Lee, and F. W. Cheney, "Chronic Pain Management: American Society of Anesthesiologists Closed Claims Project," *Anesthesiology*, vol. 100, no. 1, pp. 98–105, 2004.

[16] S. Vasudevan, *Multidisciplinary Management of Chronic Pain—A Practical Guide for Clinicians*, Springer, Cham, Switzerland, 2015.

[17] R. Dale and B. Stacey, "Multimodal Treatment of Chronic Pain," *Medical Clinics of North America*, vol. 100, no. 1, pp. 55–64, 2016.

[18] L. Manchikanti, V. Pampati, C. E. Bakhit et al., "Effectiveness of lumbar facet joint nerve blocks in chronic lower back pain: A randomized clinical trial," *Pain Physician*, vol. 4, no. 1, pp. 101–117, 2001.

[19] "Management of Chronic Pain Syndromes: Issues and Interventions," *Pain Medicine*, vol. 6, 1, pp. S1–S21, 2005.

[20] M. J. McAllister, K. E. McKenzie, D. M. Schultz, and M. G. Epshteyn, "Effectiveness of a multidisciplinary chronic pain program for treatment of refractory patients with complicated chronic pain syndromes," *Pain Physician*, vol. 8, no. 4, pp. 369–373, 2005.

[21] Z. Zhao and D. Cope, "Nerve blocks, trigger points, and intrathecal therapy for chronic pain," in *Handbook of Pain and Palliative Care Rockville*, R. Moore, Ed., pp. 550–556, Springer, Berlin, Germany, 2013.

[22] J. Garcia and R. D. Altman, "Chronic pain states: Invasive procedures," *Seminars in Arthritis and Rheumatism*, vol. 27, no. 3, pp. 156–160, 1997.

[23] R. S. Roth, M. E. Geisser, and D. A. Williams, "Interventional pain medicine: Retreat from the biopsychosocial model of pain," *Translational Behavioral Medicine*, vol. 2, no. 1, pp. 106–116, 2012.

[24] M. A. Ashburn and P. S. Staats, "Management of chronic pain," *The Lancet*, vol. 353, no. 9167, pp. 1865–1869, 1999.

[25] H. Smith, Y. Youn, R. C. Guay, A. Laufer, and J. G. Pilitsis, "The Role of Invasive Pain Management Modalities in the Treatment of Chronic Pain," *Medical Clinics of North America*, vol. 100, no. 1, pp. 103–115, 2016.

[26] J.-P. Valat and S. Rozenberg, "Local corticosteroid injections for low back pain and sciatica," *Joint Bone Spine*, vol. 75, no. 4, pp. 403–407, 2008.

[27] R. Chou, J. D. Loeser, D. K. Owens et al., "Interventional therapies, surgery, and interdisciplinary rehabilitation for low back pain: an evidence-based clinical practice guideline from the American pain society," *Spine*, vol. 34, no. 10, pp. 1066–1077, 2009.

[28] S. P. Cohen, S. Hanling, M. C. Bicket et al., "Epidural steroid injections compared with gabapentin for lumbosacral radicular pain: Multicenter randomized double blind comparative efficacy study," *BMJ (Online)*, vol. 350, Article ID h1748, 2015.

[29] S. P. Cohen, S. Hayek, Y. Semenov et al., "Epidural steroid injections, conservative treatment, or combination treatment for cervical radicular pain: A multicenter, randomized, comparative-effectiveness study," *Anesthesiology*, vol. 121, no. 5, pp. 1045–1055, 2014.

[30] C. L. Jeng, T. M. Torrillo, and M. A. Rosenblatt, "Complications of peripheral nerve blocks," *British Journal of Anaesthesia*, vol. 105, 1, pp. i97–i107, 2010.

[31] P. Jüni, R. Hari, A. W. S. Rutjes et al., "Intra-articular corticosteroid for knee osteoarthritis," *The Cochrane database of systematic reviews*, vol. 10, p. CD005328, 2015.

[32] V. Legré-Boyer, "Viscosupplementation: techniques, indications, results," *Orthopaedics and Traumatology: Surgery and Research*, vol. 101, no. 1, pp. S101–S108, 2015.

[33] J. Cortez, F. Monteiro, M. J. Ramalho, J. M. Paulo, and J. S. Duarte, "Angor e Neuroestimulação Medular," *Dor*, vol. 13, no. 2, pp. 24–26, 2005.

[34] T. R. Deer, N. Mekhail, D. Provenzano et al., "The appropriate use of neurostimulation of the spinal cord and peripheral nervous system for the treatment of chronic pain and ischemic diseases: The neuromodulation appropriateness consensus committee," *Neuromodulation*, vol. 17, no. 6, pp. 515–550, 2014.

[35] S. Patil, O. Willett, T. Thompkins et al., "Botulinum Toxin: Pharmacology and Therapeutic Roles in Pain States," *Current Pain and Headache Reports*, vol. 20, no. 3, article no. 15, pp. 1–8, 2016.

[36] R. Kermen, "Botulinum toxin for chronic pain conditions," *Disease-a-Month*, vol. 62, no. 9, pp. 353–357, 2016.

[37] P. H. Hawley, "Botulinum toxin for severe anorectal pain," *Journal of Pain and Symptom Management*, vol. 24, no. 1, pp. 11–13, 2002.

[38] R. Chou, S. J. Atlas, S. P. Stanos, and R. W. Rosenquist, "Nonsurgical interventional therapies for low back pain: A review of the evidence for an American pain society clinical practice guideline," *Spine*, vol. 34, no. 10, pp. 1078–1093, 2009.

[39] L. Manchikanti, J. A. Hirsch, F. J. E. Falco, and M. V. Boswell, "Management of lumbar zygapophysial (facet) joint pain," *World Journal of Orthopaedics*, vol. 7, no. 5, pp. 315–337, 2016.

[40] J. Wilkinson and R. Faleiro, "Acupuncture in pain management," *Continuing Education in Anaesthesia, Critical Care & Pain*, vol. 7, no. 4, pp. 135–138, 2007.

[41] E. Manheimer, A. White, B. Berman, K. Forys, and E. Ernst, "Meta-analysis: acupuncture for low back pain," *Annals of Internal Medicine*, vol. 142, no. 8, pp. 651–663, 2005.

[42] J. Vas, K. Santos-Rey, R. Navarro-Pablo et al., "Acupuncture for fibromyalgia in primary care: A randomised controlled trial," *Acupuncture in Medicine*, vol. 34, no. 4, pp. 257–266, 2016.

[43] H. MacPherson, H. Tilbrook, S. Richmond et al., "Alexander technique lessons or acupuncture sessions for persons with chronic neck pain: A randomized trial," *Annals of Internal Medicine*, vol. 163, no. 9, pp. 653–662, 2015.

[44] A. J. Vickers and K. Linde, "Acupuncture for chronic pain," *Journal of the American Medical Association*, vol. 311, no. 9, pp. 955-956, 2014.

[45] D. C. Turk, H. D. Wilson, and A. Cahana, "Treatment of chronic non-cancer pain," *The Lancet*, vol. 377, no. 9784, pp. 2226–2235, 2011.

[46] J. Ezzo, B. Berman, V. A. Hadhazy, A. R. Jadad, L. Lao, and B. B. Singh, "Is acupuncture effective for the treatment of chronic pain? A systematic review," *Pain*, vol. 86, no. 3, pp. 217–225, 2000.

[47] S. C. Chia, A. Hum, W. Y. Ong, and A. Lee, "Parenteral lignocaine in cancer neuropathic pain: A series of case reports," *Progress in Palliative Care*, vol. 22, no. 5, pp. 253–257, 2014.

[48] B. Kosharskyy, W. Almonte, N. Shaparin, M. Pappagallo, and H. Smith, "Intravenous infusions in chronic pain management," *Pain Physician*, vol. 16, no. 3, pp. 231–249, 2013.

[49] E. Stavropoulou, E. Argyra, P. Zis, A. Vadalouca, and I. Siafaka, "The Effect of Intravenous Lidocaine on Trigeminal Neuralgia: A Randomized Double Blind Placebo Controlled Trial," *ISRN Pain*, vol. 2014, pp. 1–5, 2014.

[50] A. M. Harvey, "Classification of Chronic Pain—Descriptions of Chronic Pain Syndromes and Definitions of Pain Terms," *The Clinical Journal of Pain*, vol. 11, no. 2, p. 163, 1995.

[51] C. Cleeland and K. Ryan, "Pain assessment: global use of the Brief Pain Inventory," *Annals of the Academy of Medicine*, vol. 23, no. 2, pp. 129–138, 1994.

[52] A. Caraceni, N. Cherny, R. Fainsinger et al., "Pain measurement tools and methods in clinical research in palliative care: recommendations of an Expert Working Group of the European Association of Palliative Care," *Journal of Pain and Symptom Management*, vol. 23, no. 3, pp. 239–255, 2002.

[53] C. S. Cleeland, R. Gonin, A. K. Hatfield et al., "Pain and its treatment in outpatients with metastatic cancer," *New England Journal of Medicine*, vol. 330, no. 9, pp. 592–596, 1994.

[54] S. Keller, C. M. Bann, S. L. Dodd, J. Schein, T. R. Mendoza, and C. S. Cleeland, "Validity of the brief pain inventory for use in documenting the outcomes of patients with noncancer pain," *The Clinical Journal of Pain*, vol. 20, no. 5, pp. 309–318, 2004.

[55] G. Tan, M. P. Jensen, J. I. Thornby, and B. F. Shanti, "Validation of the brief pain inventory for chronic nonmalignant pain," *Journal of Pain*, vol. 5, no. 2, pp. 133–137, 2004.

[56] C. Cleeland, "Measurement of pain by subjective report," in *Advances in Pain Research and Therapy*, C. Hapman and J. D. Loeser, Eds., vol. 12, pp. 391–403, Raven Press, New York, NY, USA, 1989.

[57] R. C. Serlin, T. R. Mendoza, Y. Nakamura, K. R. Edwards, and C. S. Cleeland, "When is cancer pain mild, moderate or severe? Grading pain severity by its interference with function," *Pain*, vol. 61, no. 2, pp. 277–284, 1995.

[58] B. H. Smith, J. L. Hopton, and W. Alastair Chambers, "Chronic pain in primary care," *Family Practice*, vol. 16, no. 5, pp. 475–482, 1999.

[59] J. Loeser, "Multidisciplinary pain management," in *The Paths of Pain 1975–2005*, H. L. J. Merskey and R. Dubner, Eds., pp. 503–511, IASP Press, Seattle, Wash, USA, 2005.

[60] C. Gouvinhas, *Interventional pain management in multidisciplinary chronic pain clinics – A prospective multicenter cohort study with one year follow-up [M.S. thesis]*, Faculty of Medicine of the University of Porto, Porto, Portugal, 2017.

22

Chronic Neck Pain and Cervico-Craniofacial Pain Patients Express Similar Levels of Neck Pain-Related Disability, Pain Catastrophizing, and Cervical Range of Motion

Daniel Muñoz-García,[1,2] Alfonso Gil-Martínez,[1,2,3,4] Almudena López-López,[5] Ibai Lopez-de-Uralde-Villanueva,[1,2,3,4] Roy La Touche,[1,2,3,4] and Josué Fernández-Carnero[2,3,4,6]

[1] *Department of Physiotherapy, Faculty of Health Science, Centro Superior de Estudios Universitarios La Salle, Universidad Autónoma de Madrid, 28023 Madrid, Spain*
[2] *Research Group on Movement and Behavioural Science and Study of Pain, Centro Superior de Estudios Universitarios La Salle, Universidad Autónoma de Madrid, 28023 Madrid, Spain*
[3] *Institute of Neuroscience and Craniofacial Pain (INDCRAN), 28023 Madrid, Spain*
[4] *Hospital La Paz Institute for Health Research, IdiPAZ, 28046 Madrid, Spain*
[5] *Department of Psychology, Universidad Rey Juan Carlos Alcorcón, 28922 Madrid, Spain*
[6] *Department of Physical Therapy, Occupational Therapy, Rehabilitation and Physical Medicine, Universidad Rey Juan Carlos, 28922 Madrid, Spain*

Correspondence should be addressed to Daniel Muñoz-García; danimgsan@gmail.com

Academic Editor: Donald A. Simone

Background. Neck pain (NP) is strongly associated with cervico-craniofacial pain (CCFP). The primary aim of the present study was to compare the neck pain-related disability, pain catastrophizing, and cervical and mandibular ROM between patients with chronic mechanical NP and patients with CCFP, as well as asymptomatic subjects. *Methods.* A total of 64 participants formed three groups. All participants underwent a clinical examination evaluating the cervical range of motion and maximum mouth opening, neck disability index (NDI), and psychological factor of Pain Catastrophizing Scale (PCS). *Results.* There were no statistically significant differences between patients with NP and CCFP for NDI and PCS ($P > 0.05$). One- way ANOVA revealed significant differences for all ROM measurements. The post hoc analysis showed no statistically significant differences in cervical extension and rotation between the two patient groups ($P > 0.05$). The Pearson correlation analysis shows a moderate positive association between NDI and the PCS for the group of patients with NP and CCFP. *Conclusion.* The CCFP and NP patient groups have similar neck disability levels and limitation in cervical ROM in extension and rotation. Both groups had positively correlated the NDI with the PCS.

1. Introduction

Neck pain (NP) is common in the adult general population, with prevalence estimates of between 30 and 50% [1] showing an incidence rate between 146 and 213 per 1,000 patients per year. Furthermore, cervical disorders have been recognized as the possible cause of pain and disorders in distant structures [2]. Nearly half of NP patients develop chronic symptoms [3] and many will continue to exhibit moderate disability at long-term follow-up [4]. The economic burden associated with the management of NP is second only to low-back pain in annual workers compensation costs in the United States [5]. Although the etiology of insidious mechanical NP is under debate, it is clear that NP is multifactorial in nature, with both physical and psychosocial contributors [6, 7].

Many NP patients will have disability at long-term follow-up, which may lead in physical and psychosocial contributors [8].

Recent research has shown that neck pain-related disability alters the normal function of craniomandibular region [9, 10]. Furthermore, several epidemiological studies have reported that patients with NP often report pain in different conditions involving the temporomandibular joint (TMJ) and the craniofacial region [11–16]. The risk of being diagnosed with pain in both regions is higher in women than men [17]. The interaction demonstrated by the literature between neck pain and craniofacial pain [18–20] has led some researchers to consider the word "cervico-craniofacial pain" (CCFP) to integrate these conditions. The CCFP is defined as "the presence of mechanical signs of dysfunction and muscular pain (e.g., limited movement, uncoordinated movement, and weakness and lack of endurance in the neck and jaw) that were exacerbated by movement and maintained postures, and that generates pain in the cervical and craniofacial regions" [21, 22].

Moreover, it appears that an intimate functional relationship exists between the neck and the craniofacial region as suggested by their anatomical and biomechanical interrelationships [15]. The neuroanatomical basis for the relationship between the head and neck may be related to the trigeminocervical nucleus caudalis in the spinal grey matter of the spinal cord at the C1–C3 level, where there is a convergence on the nociceptive second-order neurons receiving trigeminal and cervical inputs [23]. The topographic arrangement of the trigeminal nucleus caudalis allows the interchange of nociceptive information between the cervical spine and the trigeminal nerve [24]. Several studies have demonstrated that stimulation of trigeminal-innervated structures evoked painful sensations in the neck and vice versa [25, 26]. In addition, it has been reported that injection of an inflammatory irritant into deep paraspinal tissues results in a sustained activation of both jaw and neck muscles [27, 28].

Furthermore, craniofacial pain is associated with myofascial pain and can lead to a psychophysiological disorder [29] involving central nervous system pain-regulatory systems which results in physiological and neuroendocrine responses to emotional and physical stressors. In addition, many studies have established that a substantial proportion of patients with CCFP also suffer from psychological disorders [30]. A recent cohort study found that catastrophizing contributed to the intensity and disability of pain and the progression of the disorders [31]. Other authors also reported that higher levels of catastrophizing decrease the chance of treatment success in patients [32]. Given previous evidence, this study hypothesized that patients with CCFP have higher levels of neck disability and pain catastrophizing and reduced range of motion (ROM) than patients with NP and asymptomatic subjects.

We consider that patients presenting both conditions (craniofacial pain and neck pain) could alter cervical function and produce higher levels of disability and lower ranges of cervical motion.

Therefore, the primary aim of the present study was to compare the neck pain-related disability, pain catastrophizing, and cervical and mandibular ROM between patients with chronic mechanical NP and patients with CCFP, as well as asymptomatic subjects. The secondary objective is to determine the association between neck pain-related disability and pain catastrophizing with ranges of motion in patients with NP and CCFP.

2. Methods

A cross-sectional study was developed. The study was conducted as single-blind (where the evaluator did not know the patients' conditions) study and following international recommendations for the strengthening and the reporting of observational studies in epidemiology (STROBE) [33]. The protocol was approved by the local Ethics Committee (CSEULS-PI-004/2013) and conducted following the Helsinki Declaration.

2.1. Subjects. A consecutive nonprobabilistic convenience sample of patients with NP, CCFP, and asymptomatic subjects for the control group were recruited between January 2014 and October 2015. The sample was recruited from our university campus and the local community through flyers, posters, and social media in Madrid (Spain) and they were between 18 and 65 years old. An 11-point NRS (0 = no pain, 10 = maximum pain) was used to assess pain levels [34].

Patients presenting with chronic NP and patients diagnosed with CCFP were screened for eligibility criteria if they presented at least a pain rating of 3 on NPRS during the last 3 months.

Patients for the NP group were included with symptoms isolated to the neck region with cervical mechanical pain (neck and/or shoulder pain with symptoms provoked by neck postures, neck movement, or palpation of the cervical musculature) following the recognition of cervical spinal pain based on the procedures described by Visscher et al. (2000) [35] and a Neck Disability Index (NDI) score of at least 5 [36]. Patients were included for the CCFP group if they have the inclusion criteria for the NP group and also they were a primary diagnosis of myofascial pain following Axis 1 (myofascial pain) of the Research Diagnostic Criteria for Temporomandibular Disorders (TMD) [37]; and bilateral pain of the temporal, masseter, suboccipital, and trapezius muscles.

Patients were excluded for any of the following: previous surgery for treatment of TMD pain; history of rheumatoid disease; extensive anatomical destruction or deterioration of the TMJ; being diagnosed as having pain of neuropathic or odontogenic origin; having a diagnosis of psychosis; current use of antidepressants or anxiolytics; taking narcotic pain medication; or pregnancy (due to prescription of nonsteroidal anti-inflammatory drugs).

Finally, asymptomatic controls were recruited from volunteers who responded to a local announcement and were excluded if they exhibited a history of neck, facial, or head pain (infrequent episodic tension-type headache was permitted), or any systemic disease or diagnosis compatible with the inclusion criteria.

3. Procedure

The study protocol was the same for the NP and CCFP patients and the asymptomatic control group, who all signed a consent form before participation. All examinations were done in a quiet, draught-free, temperature- and humidity-controlled laboratory (24°C ± 1°C, relative humidity 25–35%). This protocol was performed by an evaluator who had not participated in the selection and data collection procedures, to ensure blinding status of the investigation.

After consenting to the study, the recruited patients were given a battery of questionnaires to complete on the day of the evaluation. These included various self-reports for demographic data and pain-related disability variables. The sociodemographic questionnaire collected information about the following variables: age, gender, and duration of pain. Measures of pain catastrophizing were assessed using the Pain Catastrophizing Scale (PCS); neck pain-related disability was collected using the Spanish version of NDI [36]. Once patients completed all self-reports, the research proceeded to evaluate the cervical ROM and maximal mouth opening (MMO).

3.1. Primary Outcomes. NDI was used to measure perceived disability. The NDI consisted of 10 questions measured on a 6-point scale (0 = no disability, 5 = full disability). The NDI has been demonstrated to be a reliable (intraclass correlation coefficients ranging from 0.50 to 0.98) and valid self-assessment for disability in chronic NP patients [36].

Pain Catastrophizing. To evaluate participants' propensity to catastrophize about pain we used the Spanish version [38] of the Pain Catastrophizing Scale (PCS). This scale is a 13-item questionnaire designed to measure the three components of catastrophizing: rumination, magnification, and helplessness.

3.2. Secondary Outcomes. The ROM of the neck was measured with the cervical ROM (CROM). This device consists of a plastic frame that rests on the nose and ears and is attached to the head via a Velcro strap. Three angles gauges were attached to the frame and arranged perpendicular to each other, indicating the range of cervical movement of the subject. Flexion, extension, and lateral flexion of the neck were recorded with gravity goniometers. Cervical rotation was measured with a goniometer compass that works in conjunction with a magnetic magnet placed around the neck [39]. Validity [40] and reliability have been demonstrated (both as intrarater and interrater [41]), to measure cervical ROM.

Patient was seated in a chair with back to 90 degrees, with feet flat on the floor, arms along the body, and head in neutral position. Verbal commands were given to the subjects to perform the neck movements until the pain or maximal ROM. First, assess mobility in the sagittal plane, followed by the frontal plane, and finally the transverse plane. The mean of 3 trials (intraexaminer reliability) was calculated and used for the analysis.

MMO was measured in millimetres with a digital calliper [42, 43]; a reduced opening capacity has been demonstrated in TMD patients relative to asymptomatic subjects. The head of the patient was controlled in a neutral position, since it has demonstrated the influence of the position in the measurement [44]. All measurements were made between the incisal edges of the upper and lower right central incisors. These measurements were made at least within 30 seconds to avoid wind-up phenomenon.

3.3. Statistical Analysis. All data analyses were performed on SPSS for Windows, Version 21.0 (SPSS Inc., Chicago, IL). The statistical analyses were conducted at a 95% confidence level and a P value less than 0.05 was considered statistically significant. Descriptive statistics was generated for the sociodemographic, psychological, and pain-related disability variables and physical measures. Results are expressed as mean, standard deviation (SD), with 95% confidence intervals (95% CI). A normal distribution of the data was confirmed with the Kolmogorov-Smirnoff test.

For comparison of the primary outcomes (NDI and PCS) between the two patients groups, a Student's t-test for independent samples was used. Effect sizes (Cohen's d) were calculated for outcome variables. According to Cohen's method, the magnitude of the effect was classified as small (0.20 to 0.49), medium (0.50 to 0.79), or large (≥0.8) [45].

One-way ANOVA was used to analyze the group factor for ROM variables (cervical ROM and MMO). Significant ANOVA findings were followed up with post hoc test using the Bonferroni correction. Partial eta-squared (η^2_p) was calculated as a measure of effect size (strength of association) for each main effect and interaction in the ANOVAs, with 0.01–0.059 representing a small effect, 0.06–0.139 a medium effect, and >0.14 a large effect [46].

The relationship between physical measures (cervical ROM and MMO) and self-reports for pain-related disability and psychological measures was examined using Pearson correlation coefficients. A Pearson correlation coefficient greater than 0.60 indicated a strong correlation, a coefficient between 0.30 and 0.60 indicated a moderate correlation, and a coefficient below 0.30 indicated a low or very low correlation [47].

4. Results

The sample was composed of 44 patients (22 patients with NP; 20 patients with CCFP) and 22 asymptomatic controls. The patients presented a mean age of 26.22 ± 4.18 (mean ± SD) years (NP group: 25.55 ± 4.23 years; CCFP group: 26.90 ± 4.12 years) and a female percentage of 61.9% years (NP group: 50%; CCFP group: 75%), whereas these values for the asymptomatic controls were 24 ± 4.58 and 54.5%, respectively. Hence, demographic data of the groups were similar and comparable ($P > 0.05$). In addition, both patients groups showed similar outcomes for cervical pain duration with 144.27 ± 155.96 weeks in NP group and 118 ± 118.54 weeks in CCFP group. The orofacial pain duration observed in patients with CCFP was 86.55 ± 74.76 weeks.

4.1. Comparisons between Groups. There were no statistically significant differences between patients with NP and those with CCFP for NDI and PCS ($P > 0.05$) (Table 1).

Table 1: Comparisons between groups.

Outcomes	Mean ± SD NP	CCFP	CG	Mean difference (95% CI); effect size (d) (a) NP versus CCFP (b) NP versus CG (c) CCFP versus CG
NDI	21.82 ± 8.37	22.60 ± 8.24	—	(a) −0.78 (−5.97 to 4.41); d = **−0.09**
PCS	13.05 ± 10.27	17.45 ± 11.26	—	(a) −4.41 (−11.12 to 2.31); d = **−0.40**
Extension	65.48 ± 15.56	63.45 ± 17.29	80.91 ± 10.13	(a) 2.03 (−9.04 to 13.09); d = **0.12** (b) −15.43 (−26.23 to −4.63)**; d = **−1.17** (c) −17.46 (−28.53 to −6.39)**; d = **−1.23**
Lateroflexion	84.93 ± 14.41	79.38 ± 15.99	91.96 ± 12.52	(a) 5.55 (−5.34 to 16.44); d = **0.36** (b) −7.02 (−17.65 to 3.61); d = **−0.52** (c) −12.57 (−23.46 to −1.68)*; d = **−0.87**
Rotation	129.52 ± 21.09	127.70 ± 17.63	143.82 ± 14.03	(a) 1.82 (−11.74 to 15.38); d = **0.09** (b) −14.30 (−27.53 to −1.06)*; d = **−0.80** (c) −16.12 (−29.68 to −2.56)*; d = **−1.01**
MMO	47.51 ± 7.11	40.25 ± 7.49	52.35 ± 6.37	(a) 7.26 (1.95 to 12.58)**; d = **0.99** (b) −4.83 (−10.02 to 0.35); d = **−0.71** (c) −12.10 (−17.41 to −6.78)**; d = **−1.74**

NDI, neck disability index; PCS, Pain Catastrophizing Scale; MMO, maximal mouth opening; NP, neck pain group; CCFP, cervico-craniofacial pain group; CG, control group.
*$P < 0.05$.
**$P < 0.01$.

One-way ANOVA revealed significant differences for all ROM measurements [extension (F = 9.270; P < 0.001; η^2_p = 0.23); lateroflexion (F = 4.076; P = 0.022; η^2_p = 0.11); rotation (F = 5.278; P = 0.008; η^2_p = 0.14); MMO (F = 15.821; P < 0.001; η^2_p = 0.34)] except for cervical flexion (F = 2.140; P = 0.126; η^2_p = 0.06). The post hoc analysis showed no statistically significant differences in cervical extension and rotation between the two patient groups (P > 0.05); however, differences in these variables were found with the control group showing a large effect size ($d \geq 0.8$). The ROM of cervical lateral-flexion was lower in the group of CCFP in relation to the other two groups with a medium-large effect size (d = 0.52 to 0.87) (Table 1).

MMO measurement was lower in the CCFP group with respect to the data obtained in the control group and NP group and this difference was statistically significant with large effect size (P < 0.001; d > 0.8) (Table 1).

4.2. Correlations Analysis. The Pearson correlation analysis shows a moderate positive association between NDI and the PCS for the group of patients with NP and CCFP. These results are presented in Table 2.

Table 2 shows a significant negative moderate correlation between the ROMs in flexion (r = −0.452; P < 0.03) and lateroflexion (r = −0.507; P < 0.01), with PCS in patients with NP; the lower the ROM in flexion, right and left lateral flexion, and right rotation, the higher the PCS levels.

For patients with CCFP, a significant negative moderate correlation between the cervical ROM in rotation (r = −0.507; P < 0.04) with NDI is presented in Table 2.

Table 2: Correlations between patient groups.

	NDI		PCS	
	NP	CCFP	NP	CCFP
PCS	0.54**	0.48*	—	—
NDI	—	—	0.540**	0.480*
Flexion	−0.204	−0.382	−0.452*	−0.219
Extension	−0.229	−0.145	−0.334	0.079
Lateroflexion	−0.327	−0.186	−0.507*	0.168
Rotation	−0.256	−0.507*	−0.386	−0.137
MMO	−0.117	0.194	0.122	−0.055

NDI, neck disability index; PCS, Pain Catastrophizing Scale; MMO, maximal mouth opening; NP, neck pain group; CCFP, cervico-craniofacial pain group.
*$P < 0.05$.
**$P < 0.01$.

5. Discussion

This survey has the main objective of comparing the data of disability, catastrophism, and ROM between the three groups studied.

It was observed that the NP and CCFP patients presented similar neck pain-related disability and pain catastrophizing levels and cervical ROM. Although these outcomes were not statistically significantly different, the lateroflexion ROM and MMO showed a medium effect size between the NP group and asymptomatic subjects with mean difference of the 95% CI included the minimal detectable change [48, 49]; therefore, this could be clinically relevant for some patients.

Moreover, both patient groups had less cervical ROM than asymptomatic subjects. MMO was lower in the CCFP and statistically significant differences were observed with respect to the other two groups. According to the results obtained in this investigation, the null hypothesis for comparing the variables neck pain-related disability, pain catastrophizing, and cervical ROM is assumed, between the NP and CCFP group and is rejected for the comparison of the cervical ROM variable between the CCFP group and the asymptomatic subjects.

5.1. Neck Disability and ROMs. We propose a hypothesis that presenting craniofacial pain and neck pain could generate greater levels of disability of neck and lower ranges of cervical motion than in patients who had neck pain only and viewing our results this was not found. Current evidence shows that the pain and disability of neck and jaw function alter the nociceptive processing at the trigeminal level [10] even when only neck pain [9, 50–52] occurs. However, our findings can not prove that this situation can be reversed. It is necessary to further investigate the possible influence of craniofacial cervical pain on motor activity, as well as disability and neck pain, as this issue is still unclear.

We found no correlations between cervical ROM and NDI in NP patients. This is in line with the findings of Cramer et al., who reported fair correlations in a large cohort study [53].

Our results for the CCFP group are consistent with Olivo et al. [54], who reported that patients with jaw pain had a high level of disability in the neck region. However, Olivo et al. reported less level of neck disability than identified here; they reported a score of 10.87 in patients with TMD, whereas we identified a mean score of 22.60 in patients with CCFP. This difference could be because the Olivo et al.'s study included myogenic or mixed TMD patients but not TMD patients suffering from neck pain. Most of the patients with NP and CCFP had moderate disability (63%), although there was more severe disability in patients with CCFP than NP (26.3% versus 18.2%).

Disability in patients with CCFP was found to be similar to patients with only NP. Although it has been suggested that disability scores of between 15 and 24 represent a moderate disability [55], other studies have suggested that a score of between 10 and 28 points in NDI represents mild disability [56]. Therefore, in our study the NP and CCFP patients showed a mild to moderate disability of the cervical spine. Although higher NDI scores in neck pain patients than reported here have been published, this could be because their patient populations had neck pain with and without symptoms to the upper extremity and also because they recruited patients from a hospital setting (i.e., where patients seek medical care) [57].

Cervical ROMs for both groups of our study were lower than typically reported values in angular ranges for similar age groups [41]. Also, the patients with NP and CCFP showed less cervical ROM and MMO than controls accounted for the largest proportions of variance in the self-report measures. However, it is likely that these measures alone are not sufficient to predict the disability status of patients with NP. Our finding of reduced ROM for the NP group is in agreement with several other studies [58]. A recent study of NP patients reported reduced ROM in extension for the upper cervical spine and reduced ROM in flexion for the lower cervical spine [59]; therefore, it is possible that the upper cervical spine is involved in nociceptive processing of CCFP. In connection with this, in recent research the presence of limitation of ROM in the upper cervical rotation mainly in TMD patients with headaches has been observed [60]. It is important to highlight that the CCFP group showed a statistically significant negative correlation between neck pain-related disability and the cervical rotation.

Various authors have studied the association between NP and craniofacial pain and their collected findings support the existence of a functional integration of the anatomic and biomechanical aspects of the craniomandibular and craniocervical regions [61]. Thus, the potential relationship between craniofacial pain and NP may be primarily expressed as the experiencing of pain in both locations. It should be noted that experimental studies showed the existence of neurologic circuits that allow convergence of proprioceptive and nociceptive afferences from C1–C4 to the trigeminal nucleus, as well as a close functional relationship between the cervical spine and the masticatory system [62]. Several studies have also reported a neuromuscular interaction between the jaw and neck muscles during functional contraction [63].

5.2. Disability and Psychological Associations. Our results support the previously proposed association between neck pain and temporomandibular disorders and emotional well-being and catastrophic thoughts [7, 27].

Our outcomes are also in agreement with other studies that have found that patients with TMD have higher levels of pain catastrophizing than pain-free subjects [64]. In addition, our results are consistent with previous research that has shown that catastrophizing is positively associated with pain intensity and disability in patients with TMD [31], as PCS scores correlated with several measures of cervical ROM.

The positive correlation between NDI and pain catastrophizing in NP and CCFP patients identified in our survey is in line with the findings of other authors that have identified an association between catastrophizing and disability, even when controlling for depression, anxiety, and pain severity [65].

The negative correlation between most of the cervical ranges of motion and PCS in our NP patient group is similar to literature findings that describe how pain-related catastrophizing plays an important role in the physical complaints of patients with chronic whiplash-associated disorders when referred to a physical therapist [66].

5.3. Clinical Implications. Currently, catastrophic behaviours to pain appear to be closely related to depressive symptoms and chronic pain. From a clinical point of view, it is essential to differentiate between patients not only based on physical examination but also on psychological factors. Our data show that patients with chronic NP or chronic CCFP could be involved in a similar trigeminal neurophysiology and exhibit similar levels of catastrophic thoughts. Therefore, such patients could benefit from similar treatments targeting the neck or craniofacial region. As catastrophizing is related to some disability measures, we also wonder whether it might be useful to complement physiotherapy treatment with psychological interventions.

6. Limitations

This study has some limitations. First, participants were recruited through flyers, posters, and social media, without them having requested health support. Differences between those that seek and those that do not seek health support have been reported, thus potentially introducing a further selection bias. This could have influenced some of our findings, for example, explaining why there was no difference between groups for pain catastrophizing. Second, limitation was not having included patients with craniofacial pain without neck symptoms. Third, although previous surveys similar to this used akin sample size, the results of the present study should be treated with caution because the sample size was small. Finally, we did not use a specific test to measure the craniofacial disability. Future studies resolving these limitations are needed.

7. Conclusion

The CCFP and NP patient groups have similar neck disability levels and limitation in cervical ROM in extension and rotation. Both groups had positively correlated the NDI with the PCS. Longitudinal research is needed to verify these associations.

Competing Interests

The authors report no conflict of interests.

Acknowledgments

The authors thank Héctor Arribas for his help with the process of patient enrolment and for administering the tests to all the subjects in the study.

References

[1] S. Hogg-Johnson, G. van der Velde, L. J. Carroll et al., "The burden and determinants of neck pain in the general population: results of the Bone and Joint Decade 2000–2010 Task Force on Neck Pain and Its Associated Disorders," *Journal of Manipulative and Physiological Therapeutics*, vol. 32, no. 2, supplement, pp. S46–S60, 2009.

[2] J. H. Bland, *Disorders of Cervical Spine Diagnosis and Medical Management*, WB Saunders, Philadelphia, Pa, USA, 2nd edition, 1994.

[3] J. A. J. Borghouts, B. W. Koes, and L. M. Bouter, "The clinical course and prognostic factors of non-specific neck pain: a systematic review," *Pain*, vol. 77, no. 1, pp. 1–13, 1998.

[4] D. R. Gore, S. B. Sepic, G. M. Gardner, and M. P. Murray, "Neck pain: a long-term follow-up of 205 patients," *Spine*, vol. 12, no. 1, pp. 1–5, 1987.

[5] J. Selhub, P. F. Jacques, I. H. Rosenberg et al., "Serum total homocysteine concentrations in the third National Health and Nutrition Examination Survey (1991–1994): population reference ranges and contribution of vitamin status to high serum concentrations," *Annals of Internal Medicine*, vol. 131, no. 5, pp. 331–339, 1999.

[6] R. J. Gatchel, J. P. Garofalo, E. Ellis, and C. Holt, "Major psychological disorders in acute and chronic TMD: an initial examination," *Journal of the American Dental Association*, vol. 127, no. 9, pp. 1365–1374, 1996.

[7] F. J. Keefe, M. E. Rumble, C. D. Scipio, L. A. Giordano, and L. M. Perri, "Psychological aspects of persistent pain: current state of the science," *The Journal of Pain*, vol. 5, no. 4, pp. 195–211, 2004.

[8] V. Johnston, N. L. Jimmieson, G. Jull, and T. Souvlis, "Contribution of individual, workplace, psychosocial and physiological factors to neck pain in female office workers," *European Journal of Pain*, vol. 13, no. 9, pp. 985–991, 2009.

[9] M. Testa, T. Geri, L. Gizzi, F. Petzke, and D. Falla, "Alterations in masticatory muscle activation in people with persistent neck pain despite the absence of orofacial pain or temporomandibular disorders," *Journal of Oral & Facial Pain and Headache*, vol. 29, no. 4, pp. 340–348, 2015.

[10] R. La Touche, A. Paris-Alemany, A. Gil-Martínez, J. Pardo-Montero, S. Angulo-Díaz-Parreño, and J. Fernández-Carnero, "Masticatory sensory-motor changes after an experimental chewing test influenced by pain catastrophizing and neck-pain-related disability in patients with headache attributed to temporomandibular disorders," *The Journal of Headache and Pain*, vol. 16, article 20, 2015.

[11] R. Ciancaglini, M. Testa, and G. Radaelli, "Association of neck pain with symptoms of temporomandibular dysfunction in the general adult population," *Scandinavian Journal of Rehabilitation Medicine*, vol. 31, no. 1, pp. 17–22, 1999.

[12] A. de Wijer, J. R. J. de Leeuw, M. H. Steenks, and F. Bosman, "Temporomandibular and cervical spine disorders. Self-reported signs and symptoms," *Spine*, vol. 21, no. 14, pp. 1638–1646, 1996.

[13] A. de Wijer, M. H. Steenks, F. Bosman, P. J. M. Helders, and J. Faber, "Symptoms of the stomatognathic system in temporomandibular and cervical spine disorders," *Journal of Oral Rehabilitation*, vol. 23, no. 11, pp. 733–741, 1996.

[14] F. Lobbezoo, C. M. Visscher, and M. Naeije, "Impaired health status, sleep disorders, and pain in the craniomandibular and cervical spinal regions," *European Journal of Pain*, vol. 8, no. 1, pp. 23–30, 2004.

[15] S. A. Olivo, J. Bravo, D. J. Magee, N. M. R. Thie, P. W. Major, and C. Flores-Mir, "The association between head and cervical posture and temporomandibular disorders: a systematic review," *Journal of Orofacial Pain*, vol. 20, no. 1, pp. 9–23, 2006.

[16] I.-M. Nilsson, T. List, and M. Drangsholt, "Headache and comorbid pains associated with TMD pain in adolescents," *Journal of Dental Research*, vol. 92, no. 9, pp. 802–807, 2013.

[17] S. Hogg-Johnson, G. van der Velde, L. J. Carroll et al., "The burden and determinants of neck pain in the general population. results of the bone and joint decade 2000–2010 task force on neck pain and its associated disorders," *Journal of Manipulative and Physiological Therapeutics*, vol. 32, no. 2, pp. S46–S60, 2009.

[18] S. Marklund, B. Wiesinger, and A. Wänman, "Reciprocal influence on the incidence of symptoms in trigeminally and spinally innervated areas," *European Journal of Pain*, vol. 14, no. 4, pp. 366–371, 2010.

[19] B. Wiesinger, H. Malker, E. Englund, and A. Wänman, "Does a dose-response relation exist between spinal pain and temporomandibular disorders?" *BMC Musculoskeletal Disorders*, vol. 10, article 28, 2009.

[20] B. Wiesinger, H. Malker, E. Englund, and A. Wänman, "Back pain in relation to musculoskeletal disorders in the jaw-face: a matched case-control study," *Pain*, vol. 131, no. 3, pp. 311–319, 2007.

[21] R. La Touche, A. París-Alemany, J. S. Mannheimer et al., "Does mobilization of the upper cervical spine affect pain sensitivity and autonomic nervous system function in patients with cervico-craniofacial pain?: a randomized-controlled trial," *Clinical Journal of Pain*, vol. 29, no. 3, pp. 205–215, 2013.

[22] R. La Touche, I. López-de-Uralde-Villanueva, H. Beltran-Alacreu, A. Paris-Alemany, and S. Angulo-Díaz-Parreño, "Relationships between craniocervical posture and pain-related disability in patients with cervico-craniofacial pain," *Journal of Pain Research*, vol. 8, pp. 449–458, 2015.

[23] C. F. Marfurt and D. M. Rajchert, "Trigeminal primary afferent projections to 'non-trigeminal' areas of the rat central nervous system," *Journal of Comparative Neurology*, vol. 303, no. 3, pp. 489–511, 1991.

[24] P. J. Goadsby and K. L. Hoskin, "The distribution of trigeminovascular afferents in the nonhuman primate brain *Macaca nemestrina*: a c-fos immunocytochemical study," *Journal of Anatomy*, vol. 190, no. 3, pp. 367–375, 1997.

[25] T. Bartsch and P. J. Goadsby, "Stimulation of the greater occipital nerve induces increased central excitability of dural afferent input," *Brain*, vol. 125, no. 7, pp. 1496–1509, 2002.

[26] T. Bartsch and P. J. Goadsby, "Increased responses in trigeminocervical nociceptive neurons to cervical input after stimulation of the dura mater," *Brain*, vol. 126, no. 8, pp. 1801–1813, 2003.

[27] J. W. Hu, X.-M. Yu, H. Vernon, and B. J. Sessle, "Excitatory effects on neck and jaw muscle activity of inflammatory irritant applied to cervical paraspinal tissues," *Pain*, vol. 55, no. 2, pp. 243–250, 1993.

[28] X.-M. Yu, B. J. Sessle, H. Vernon, and J. W. Hu, "Effects of inflammatory irritant application to the rat temporomandibular joint on jaw and neck muscle activity," *Pain*, vol. 60, no. 2, pp. 143–149, 1995.

[29] M. Kight, R. J. Gatchel, and L. Wesley, "Temporomandibular disorders: evidence for significant overlap with psychopathology," *Health Psychology*, vol. 18, no. 2, pp. 177–182, 1999.

[30] M. A. I. Rantala, J. Ahlberg, T. I. Suvinen et al., "Temporomandibular joint related painless symptoms, orofacial pain, neck pain, headache, and psychosocial factors among non-patients," *Acta Odontologica Scandinavica*, vol. 61, no. 4, pp. 217–222, 2003.

[31] A. M. Velly, J. O. Look, C. Carlson et al., "The effect of catastrophizing and depression on chronic pain—a prospective cohort study of temporomandibular muscle and joint pain disorders," *Pain*, vol. 152, no. 10, pp. 2377–2383, 2011.

[32] A. P. Verhagen, C. H. Karels, J. M. Schellingerhout, S. P. Willemsen, B. W. Koes, and S. M. A. Bierma-Zeinstra, "Pain severity and catastrophising modify treatment success in neck pain patients in primary care," *Manual Therapy*, vol. 15, no. 3, pp. 267–272, 2010.

[33] E. von Elm, D. G. Altman, M. Egger, S. J. Pocock, P. C. Gøtzsche, and J. P. Vandenbroucke, "The Strengthening the Reporting of Observational Studies in Epidemiology (STROBE) statement: guidelines for reporting observational studies," *Journal of Clinical Epidemiology*, vol. 61, no. 4, pp. 344–349, 2008.

[34] S. Summers, "Evidence-based practice part 2: reliability and validity of selected acute pain instruments," *Journal of Perianesthesia Nursing*, vol. 16, no. 1, pp. 35–40, 2001.

[35] C. M. Visscher, F. Lobbezoo, W. de Boer, J. van der Zaag, J. G. C. Verheij, and M. Naeije, "Clinical tests in distinguishing between persons with or without craniomandibular or cervical spinal pain complaints," *European Journal of Oral Sciences*, vol. 108, no. 6, pp. 475–483, 2000.

[36] J. A. Andrade Ortega, A. D. Delgado Martínez, and R. A. Ruiz, "Validation of the Spanish version of the neck disability index," *Spine*, vol. 35, no. 4, pp. E114–E118, 2010.

[37] S. F. Dworkin and L. LeResche, "Research diagnostic criteria for temporomandibular disorders: review, criteria, examinations and specifications, critique," *Journal of Craniomandibular Disorders*, vol. 6, no. 4, pp. 301–355, 1992.

[38] J. García Campayo, B. Rodero, M. Alda, N. Sobradiel, J. Montero, and S. Moreno, "Validation of the Spanish version of the pain catastrophizing scale in fibromyalgia," *Medicina Clinica*, vol. 131, no. 13, pp. 487–492, 2008.

[39] J. W. Youdas, J. R. Carey, and T. R. Garrett, "Reliability of measurements of cervical spine range of motion—comparison of three methods," *Physical Therapy*, vol. 71, no. 2, pp. 98–106, 1991.

[40] M. Tousignant, C. Smeesters, A.-M. Breton, É. Breton, and H. Corriveau, "Criterion validity study of the cervical range of motion (CROM) device for rotational range of motion on healthy adults," *Journal of Orthopaedic and Sports Physical Therapy*, vol. 36, no. 4, pp. 242–248, 2006.

[41] D. E. Hole, J. M. Cook, and J. E. Bolton, "Reliability and concurrent validity of two instruments for measuring cervical range of motion: effects of age and gender," *Manual Therapy*, vol. 1, no. 1, pp. 36–42, 1995.

[42] S. F. Dworkin, L. LeResche, T. DeRouen, and M. Von Korff, "Assessing clinical signs of temporomandibular disorders: reliability of clinical examiners," *The Journal of Prosthetic Dentistry*, vol. 63, no. 5, pp. 574–579, 1990.

[43] M. T. John, S. F. Dworkin, and L. A. Mancl, "Reliability of clinical temporomandibular disorder diagnoses," *Pain*, vol. 118, no. 1-2, pp. 61–69, 2005.

[44] E. J. Higbie, D. Seidel-Cobb, L. F. Taylor, and G. S. Cummings, "Effect of head position on vertical mandibular opening," *Journal of Orthopaedic and Sports Physical Therapy*, vol. 29, no. 2, pp. 127–130, 1999.

[45] J. Cohen, *Statistical Power Analysis for the Behavioral Sciences*, Lawrence Erlbaum Associates, Hillsdale, Mich, USA, 1988.

[46] J. Cohen, "Eta-squared and partial eta-squared in fixed factor ANOVA designs," *Educational and Psychological Measurement*, vol. 33, no. 1, pp. 107–112, 1973.

[47] D. Hinkle, S. Jurs, and W. Wiersma, *Applied Statistics for the Behavioral Sciences*, Houghton Mifflin, Boston, Mass, USA, 2nd edition, 1988.

[48] J. P. Fletcher and W. D. Bandy, "Intrarater reliability of CROM measurement of cervical spine active range of motion in persons with and without neck pain," *Journal of Orthopaedic and Sports Physical Therapy*, vol. 38, no. 10, pp. 640–645, 2008.

[49] H. Beltran-Alacreu, I. López-de-Uralde-Villanueva, A. Paris-Alemany, S. Angulo-Díaz-Parreño, and R. La Touche, "Intra-rater and inter-rater reliability of mandibular range of motion measures considering a neutral craniocervical position," *Journal of Physical Therapy Science*, vol. 26, no. 6, pp. 915–920, 2014.

[50] R. La Touche, C. Fernández-de-las-Peñas, J. Fernández-Carnero, S. Díaz-Parreño, A. Paris-Alemany, and L. Arendt-Nielsen, "Bilateral mechanical-pain sensitivity over the trigeminal region in patients with chronic mechanical neck pain," *The Journal of Pain*, vol. 11, no. 3, pp. 256–263, 2010.

[51] B. Häggman-Henrikson, C. Österlund, and P.-O. Eriksson, "Endurance during chewing in whiplash-associated disorders and TMD," *Journal of Dental Research*, vol. 83, no. 12, pp. 946–950, 2004.

[52] P.-O. Eriksson, H. Zafar, and B. Häggman-Henrikson, "Deranged jaw-neck motor control in whiplash-associated disorders," *European Journal of Oral Sciences*, vol. 112, no. 1, pp. 25–32, 2004.

[53] H. Cramer, R. Lauche, J. Langhorst, G. J. Dobos, and A. Michalsen, "Validation of the German version of the neck disability index (NDI)," *BMC Musculoskeletal Disorders*, vol. 15, no. 1, article 91, 2014.

[54] S. A. Olivo, J. Fuentes, P. W. Major, S. Warren, N. M. R. Thie, and D. J. Magee, "The association between neck disability and jaw disability," *Journal of Oral Rehabilitation*, vol. 37, no. 9, pp. 670–679, 2010.

[55] H. T. Vernon, "Assessment of self-rated disability, impairment, and sincerity of effort in whiplash-associated disorder," *Journal of Musculoskeletal Pain*, vol. 8, no. 1-2, pp. 155–167, 2000.

[56] M. Sterling, G. Jull, and J. Kenardy, "Physical and psychological factors maintain long-term predictive capacity post-whiplash injury," *Pain*, vol. 122, no. 1-2, pp. 102–108, 2006.

[57] M. C. C. En, D. A. Clair, and S. J. Edmondston, "Validity of the Neck Disability Index and Neck Pain and Disability Scale for measuring disability associated with chronic, non-traumatic neck pain," *Manual Therapy*, vol. 14, no. 4, pp. 433–438, 2009.

[58] H. Lee, L. L. Nicholson, and R. D. Adams, "Neck muscle endurance, self-report, and range of motion data from subjects with treated and untreated neck pain," *Journal of Manipulative and Physiological Therapeutics*, vol. 28, no. 1, pp. 25–32, 2005.

[59] T. Rudolfsson, M. Björklund, and M. Djupsjöbacka, "Range of motion in the upper and lower cervical spine in people with chronic neck pain," *Manual Therapy*, vol. 17, no. 1, pp. 53–59, 2012.

[60] F. Grondin, T. Hall, M. Laurentjoye, and B. Ella, "Upper cervical range of motion is impaired in patients with temporomandibular disorders," *Cranio*, vol. 33, no. 2, pp. 91–99, 2015.

[61] R. La Touche, A. París-Alemany, H. von Piekartz, J. S. Mannheimer, J. Fernández-Carnero, and M. Rocabado, "The influence of cranio-cervical posture on maximal mouth opening and pressure pain threshold in patients with myofascial temporomandibular pain disorders," *Clinical Journal of Pain*, vol. 27, no. 1, pp. 48–55, 2011.

[62] V. Busch, W. Jakob, T. Juergens, W. Schulte-Mattler, H. Kaube, and A. May, "Functional connectivity between trigeminal and occipital nerves revealed by occipital nerve blockade and nociceptive blink reflexes," *Cephalalgia*, vol. 26, no. 1, pp. 50–55, 2006.

[63] N. N. Giannakopoulos, D. Hellmann, M. Schmitter, B. Krüger, T. Hauser, and H. J. Schindler, "Neuromuscular interaction of jaw and neck muscles during jaw clenching," *Journal of Orofacial Pain*, vol. 27, no. 1, pp. 61–71, 2013.

[64] P. J. Quartana, L. F. Buenaver, R. R. Edwards, B. Klick, J. A. Haythornthwaite, and M. T. Smith, "Pain catastrophizing and salivary cortisol responses to laboratory pain testing in temporomandibular disorder and healthy participants," *Journal of Pain*, vol. 11, no. 2, pp. 186–194, 2010.

[65] M. J. L. Sullivan, W. Stanish, H. Waite, M. Sullivan, and D. A. Tripp, "Catastrophizing, pain, and disability in patients with soft-tissue injuries," *Pain*, vol. 77, no. 3, pp. 253–260, 1998.

[66] M. A. Schmitt, N. L. van Meeteren, A. de Wijer, F. R. van Genderen, Y. D. van Graaf, and P. J. Helders, "Patients with chronic whiplash-associated disorders: relationship between clinical and psychological factors and functional health status," *American Journal of Physical Medicine and Rehabilitation*, vol. 88, no. 3, pp. 231–238, 2009.

Efficacy and Safety of Subacromial Corticosteroid Injection in Type 2 Diabetic Patients

Davide Blonna,[1] Davide Edoardo Bonasia,[1] Lorenzo Mattei,[2] Enrico Bellato,[3] Valentina Greco,[2] and Roberto Rossi[1]

[1]*AO Ordine Mauriziano Umberto I, Department of Orthopedics and Traumatology, Largo Turati 62, 10128 Turin, Italy*
[2]*University of Turin, Via Po 8, 10100 Turin, Italy*
[3]*San Luigi Gonzaga of Orbassano, Department of Orthopedics and Traumatology, Regione Gonzole 10, 100443 Orbassano, Turin, Italy*

Correspondence should be addressed to Davide Blonna; davide.blonna@virgilio.it

Academic Editor: Donald A. Simone

Purpose. In type 2 diabetic patients affected by chronic shoulder pain, subacromial injection with corticosteroid could be an effective treatment. The aim of this study was to measure the risk-benefit ratio of this treatment. *Methods.* Twenty patients with well-controlled diabetes were included in a prospective study. In a first preinjection phase, patients were asked to measure glycemia for 7 days, before breakfast and dinner, and then 2 hours after lunch and dinner. Baseline data including Constant Score (CS), Subjective Shoulder Value (SSV), and Numerical Rating Scale (NRS) for pain were collected. Patients were treated with subacromial injection with 40 mg of Methylprednisolone Acetate and 2 ml of Lidocaine. At discharge, patients were asked to remeasure glycemia for the following week. *Results.* The overall pain improved and patients graded their shoulder as "greatly improved". At 30-day follow-up, the SSV and the CS improved, considering pain but not ROM. The average daily glycemia was 136 mg/dl before injection, 161 mg/dl the day of the injection ($p<0.001$), and 170 mg/dl one day after injection ($p<0.001$). Glycemia was not statistically different 3 days after injection. *Conclusion.* Subacromial injection is an effective short-term treatment in type 2 diabetic patients affected by shoulder pain, but a closed follow-up is recommended in all these patients. This trial is registered with NCT03652480. The Protocol ID is SHOULDERDM2013.

1. Introduction

Among the conservative strategies to treat shoulder pain, the use of corticosteroids in the subacromial space has been shown to be particularly effective and safe. One of the main limitations for the use of the corticosteroid injections remains the potential effect on blood glucose levels especially in diabetic patients. On the other hand, diabetic patients with noncontrolled shoulder pain could have a major benefit from a corticosteroid injection due to the increased risk of surgical complication: they are often elderly patients, affected by other severe comorbidities, and are strongly reticent to undergo any type of surgery. Nevertheless, they often ask for a rapid, even if temporary, pain relief solution and injection with corticosteroids could be an effective option.

The use of corticosteroids in joints, other than the shoulder, has been widely documented in nondiabetic and in diabetic patients, proving to be safe and effective [1–5]. However, only two studies focused on the painful shoulder and both of them included patients affected by adhesive capsulitis treated with intra-articular corticosteroid injection: the risk of hyperglycemia after injection seemed to be negligible [6, 7].

In our clinical practice, we have observed that (1) diabetic patients with subacromial pain respond very well to subacromial corticosteroid injections in terms of pain relief, but the effect on range of motion (ROM) seems to be unpredictable; (2) some patients report high levels of blood glucose after subacromial injections, an increase that seems to be different from what has been reported after intra-articular injections. The goal of our study was to document the effect of subacromial corticosteroid injections on blood sugar levels and short-term clinical outcomes in patients affected by type-2 diabetes, not suitable for surgery and nonresponsive to other conservative treatments.

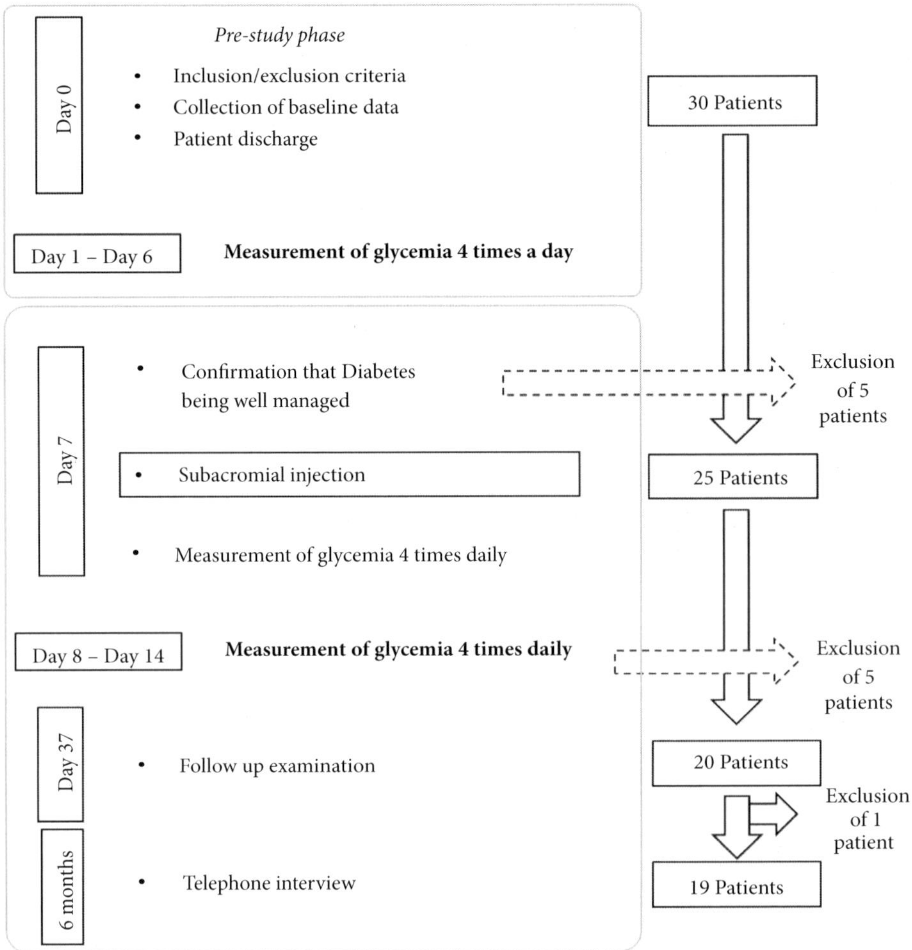

FIGURE 1: Timeline of the study protocol.

2. Methods

From 2013 to 2014, thirty consecutive type 2 diabetic patients were initially included in this analytic prospective study (level of evidence III). Patients examined in our outpatient department, complaining of chronic shoulder pain resistant to at least 6 months of conservative therapy (NSAIDs, painkillers, and physiotherapy), were considered eligible for this study (Figure 1).

To be included in the study, patients needed to have a recent (within 6 months) X-ray and an MRI or ultrasound of the affected shoulder. Other inclusion criteria were as follows:

(i) Consent to participate in the study.

(ii) Severe overall pain and night pain: Numerical Rating Scale (NRS) for pain [8] above or equal to 60/100; the scale was modified from 0-10 to 0-100 (0 = no pain 100 = unbearable pain).

(iii) No significant improvement after at least 2 courses of physiotherapy (including direct assistance from a physical therapist with specific exercises, manual therapy, and physical agents in order to reduce inflammation and pain).

(iv) Clinical signs of subacromial tendinobursitis, with or without signs of rotator cuff tear, defined as positive Neer, Yocum, and Hawkins tests [9–15]. Pain experienced during the execution of these tests needed to reproduce the type of pain that patients complained the most.

(v) No indication for surgery due to the age, concomitant comorbidities, or patient's refusal to undergo surgery.

(vi) Well-controlled type 2 diabetes, defined as follows [16]:

(a) Fasting and preprandial blood glucose levels in the range of 90-150mg/dL.

(b) HblAc <64mmol/mol (corresponding to 8%) measured within 6 months.

(vii) A device for self-measurement of blood sugar levels at home.

Exclusion criteria were as follows:

(i) Corticosteroid treatment in the past 3 months.

(ii) Complaints of shoulder stiffness more than shoulder pain.

(iii) Symptomatic glenohumeral arthritis defined as shoulder stiffness plus moderate radiographic signs of arthritis (grade >2 according to Hamada classification [17] and grade >1 according to Samilson-Prieto classification for eccentric and concentric arthritis, respectively [18]).

(iv) Shoulder trauma within 3 months of inclusion evaluation for in this study.

(v) High blood pressure values (systolic blood pressure >140mmHg, diastolic blood pressure >80mmHg [16]).

(vi) Glaucoma [19].

After an initial screening, patients were included in a prestudy phase and baseline data were recorded, including type of antidiabetes medications, range of motion (ROM), overall and night pain (NRS), Constant Score (CS) [20, 21], Oxford Shoulder Score (OSS) [22, 23], and Subjective Shoulder Value (SSV) [24].

Moreover, we asked the patients to measure their glycemia 4 times a day (before breakfast [fasting glycemia], 2 hours after lunch, before dinner [preprandial], and 2 hours after dinner) for one week after the first examination. These data were used as control values and to confirm that patients had well-controlled diabetes. In this prestudy phase patients did not receive any injection, but only NSAIDs and painkillers were prescribed. A measurement of Hb1Ac for the patients that did not have one recent blood test (within 6 months) was also prescribed.

A subsequent examination was scheduled after one week (Figure 1) when the principal investigator focused on the average fasting glycemia the week before the consultation and on the Hb1Ac. Hence, patients were either kept in the study or excluded if the diabetes was not under control. Patients with a mean fasting blood glucose of 90-150mg/dl and Hb1Ac<8% were included in the study. Patients were excluded if shoulder pain subsided after NSAIDs and painkillers previously prescribed

After discussing the risks and benefits of the therapy, a subacromial injection of Methylprednisolone Acetate 40 mg (Depo-Medrol©) and 2 ml of Lidocaine 2% was performed the morning of day 7. The same expert shoulder surgeon performed the injections using the posterior approach to the shoulder [25, 26]. The portal was located 1 cm inferior to the posterolateral border of the acromion. The needle was directed slightly superiorly, anteriorly, and medial toward the subacromial space. An ultrasound monitoring of the injection was not performed. Immediate, partial pain relief due to the Lidocaine indirectly confirmed the correct site of injection.

Patients were asked to continue the same regimen of physical activity, rehabilitation, and antidiabetes medications. Patients were informed of the probable increasing of blood glucose levels and were asked to cut down on saturated fats, salt, and sugars. Severe hyperglycemia was defined as a single value of fasting/preprandial glucose blood levels higher than 250 mg/dL or postprandial glucose blood levels higher than 300 mg/dL. Patients were also asked to report any abnormal symptoms or signs (systolic and diastolic blood pressure, respectively, over 140 mmHg and 80 mmHg [16], nausea, erythema, itching, or vomiting). Patients were requested to stay in the clinic for 30 minutes after the injection to diagnose any immediate adverse reaction. After the injection, patients were requested again to measure and record their blood sugar levels 4 times a day for the following 7 days. After 30 days, a follow-up examination was scheduled in our outpatient clinic.

At follow-up, outcomes were evaluated by using the CS, OSS, Subjective Outcome Determination (SOD) score [27, 28], and SSV. The questionnaires were filled out in the clinic. If patients reported insufficient pain relief or the recurrence of shoulder pain, a second subacromial injection was proposed. In this situation, the patient was not excluded from the study but we asked the patient to again measure their blood sugar levels 4 times a day.

Six months after the injection, a telephone interview was performed to assess pain, OSS, and SOD score.

The study was approved by the Institutional Review Board of our Hospital (Prot. CS/488) and have therefore been performed in accordance with the ethical standards laid down in the 1964 Declaration of Helsinki. All persons gave their informed consent prior to their inclusion in the study.

2.1. Statistical Analysis. A power analysis was performed. A significant reduction of the overall pain was considered as principal outcome. Eighteen patients were required for an expected reduction of 30 points of pain, with α: 0.05 and β: 0.2. The data collected were analyzed with Student's t-test, Fisher test, and the McNemar test for paired proportions. The blood glucose levels at each different time point were compared to the baseline levels (i.e., 7 days prior to the injection) using the Student's t-test. All the collected variables had a normal distribution except the SOD score. The D'Agostino-Pearson test for normal distribution rejected a normal distribution for the SOD score. The median of SOD score was therefore reported.

3. Results

Five out of 30 patients were excluded in the prestudy phase, since their diabetes was not well controlled. An additional 5 patients were excluded because they did not adequately record their glycemia after the injection (2 patients) or did not come back for the follow-up examination (3 patients). The 3 patients lost to follow-up were contacted by phone and they stated a significant improvement after injection. Twenty patients were ultimately included in the study. One patient was subsequently lost to follow-up at 6 months during the telephone interview phase. This patient was not excluded since the majority of the data important for the study were available for the analysis.

The average age was 71 years (63-83), 12 patients were female, 7 were managing their diabetes with insulin therapy, and 13 were doing so with oral diabetes medications. The average baseline CS was 43±12, the OSS 28±8, and the NRS for pain 76±11. All the patients had positive tests for subacromial tendinobursitis. Four patients had a concomitant adhesive

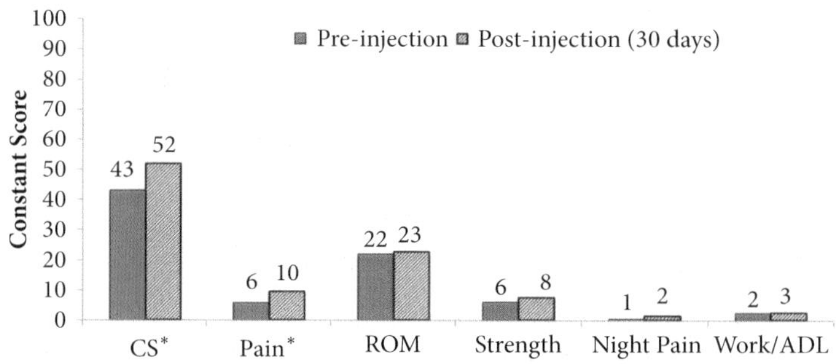

FIGURE 2: Preinjection and postinjection Constant Score (CS). The figure shows the improvement of the CS after subacromial corticosteroid injections. The improvement is significant (∗= p<0.05) for the overall CS and for the pain item. Details regarding night pain are reported in Figure 3.

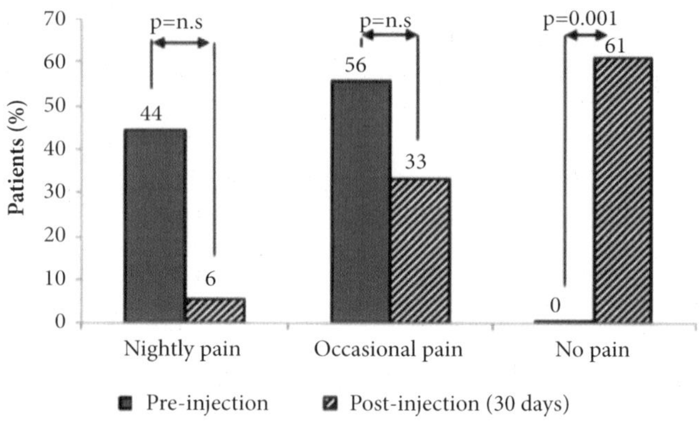

FIGURE 3: Preinjection and postinjection night pain. A significant improvement in night pain was recorded in the study. The rate of patients who experienced nightly pain decreased after the injection. Simultaneously, the rate of patients that did not have night pain increased to 61% after the injection.

capsulitis. The imaging studies showed a cuff tear involving the supraspinatus in 12 patients, a massive cuff tear involving the infraspinatus and supraspinatus in 4 patients. Four patients had mild signs of eccentric osteoarthritis (Hamada [17] stages 1 and 2).

3.1. Efficacy. At 30 days of follow-up a statistically significant improvement of the CS was reported, from 43±12 to 52±13 (p=0.008). The improvement in CS was more relevant considering the pain component of the score (Figures 2 and 3).

The variables, strength, ROM, and Work/ADL, did not improved significantly after the injection.

An improvement was also measured using the OSS but was only significant at 6 months (Figure 4).

The overall pain improved from 76±11 to 44±22 (p<0.001) at 30-day follow-up and to 38±30 at 6-month follow-up (p<0.001). However, the improvement in overall pain between 30 days and 6 months was not significant (p=n.s.). Nightly pain was reduced from 78±10 to 35±19 (p<0.001) at 30 days and to 31±25 (p<0.001) at 6-month follow-up. The improvement in nightly pain levels between 30 days and 6 months was not significant (p=n.s.).

The SSV preinjection was 49±14; it improved to 64±19 thirty days after injection (p=0.001) and to 68±25 (p<0.001) at 6-month follow-up. Again, the improvement between 30 days to 6 months was not statistically significant (p=n.s.).

One month after injection, the clinical improvement was also shown by a median SOD score of 6 points (= "Greatly Improved"). The median SOD value at 6 months remained 6 points.

During the study period, 5 patients asked for a second subacromial injection.

3.2. Safety. The average daily blood glucose levels are reported in Figure 5. Blood glucose levels were not statistically different after 3 days after injection. After 5 days blood glucose levels were normal.

Figure 6 shows that the details of the blood glucose levels increase the day of and the day after the injection. An increase of blood sugar levels was observed the day of and the day after the subacromial injection.

Five patients (25%) had severe hyperglycemia: 2 patients had one episode of fasting/preprandial glycemia >250mg/dL the day after the injection, 2 patients had a postprandial glycemia >300mg/dL (330 and 308 mg/dl), 1 patient had one episode of fasting glycemia of 265 mg/dL followed by a postprandial glycemia of 304 mg/dL. All the episodes of severe hyperglycemia were recorded the day and the day after the injection. Three out of these 5 patients were managing their diabetes with oral medications.

A posthoc analysis of the patients that experienced severe hyperglycemia revealed that they had an average preinjection fasting glycemia worse than the patients who were not affected by this complication (137mg/dl, range 113 to 150 versus 122 mg/dl, range 84 to 150).

One patient reported insomnia the night of the injection not related to shoulder pain. No other complications were reported.

4. Discussion

The aim of this prospective study was to report the short-term benefits and the effects on glucose blood levels of a subacromial injection with corticosteroids in type 2 diabetic patients affected by severe shoulder pain, not responsive to

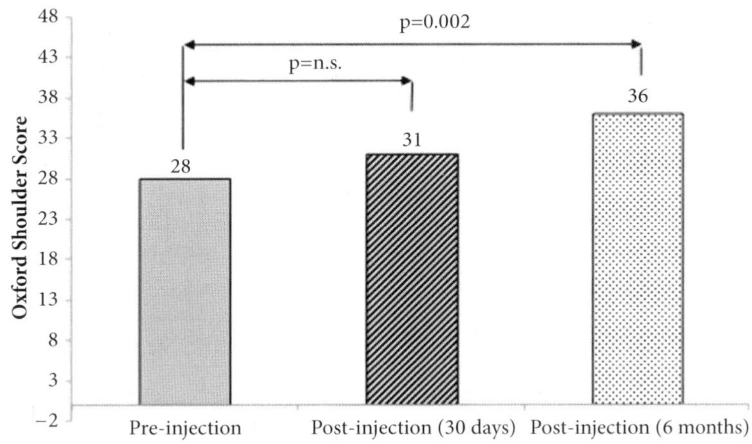

FIGURE 4: Oxford Shoulder Score (OSS) before and after injection. The improvement of the OSS was significant only after 6 months.

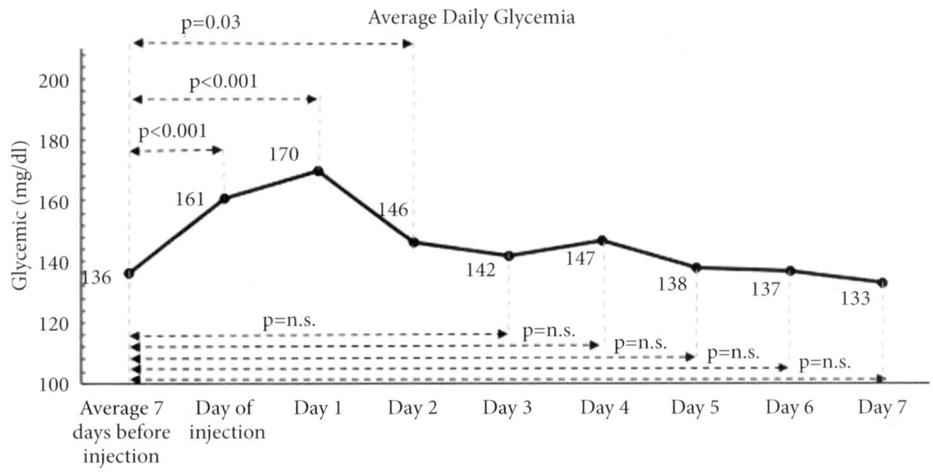

FIGURE 5: Increase of blood glucose levels after subacromial corticosteroid injections. The average daily values were 136 mg/dL (SD=28mg/dL) before the injection; they increased to 161 mg/dL (SD=25) the day of the injection ($p<0.001$) and to 170 mg/dL (SD=31) the day after the injection ($p<0.001$).

conservative treatment and not suitable for surgery. The most important finding is that the injection significantly reduced the overall pain and the night pain and most of the patients had a perception of a greatly improved shoulder at 1- and 6-month follow-up.

These data were consistent with previous reports. Yu [29] showed, in a prospective clinical study conducted on 238 shoulders, a significant improvement of the quality of life and of the ROM in 91% of cases 1 month after the injection with 1 ml of Xylocaine 2% and 1 ml of Betamethasone. One year later, the improvement was still significant in 88% of the treated patients. Akgun [30] highlighted a substantial improvement of shoulder symptoms, by using the CS 1 month after injection, due moreover to the reduction of pain at night.

In contrast to what has been reported previously, we did not observe a significant improvement in ROM and function after subacromial injection. The reason could be a difference in the patient population included in this study. We included older diabetic patients affected by shoulder pain with multiple etiologies including rotator cuff tears and mild osteoarthritis. Moreover, despite the fact that a clear diagnosis of adhesive capsulitis was present in only 4 cases, we cannot rule out the possibility that some of the patients had some minor forms of adhesive capsulitis secondary to diabetes [31, 32]. The infiltration could have improved the pain related to subacromial tendinobursitis and long head of the biceps inflammation but perhaps was unable to improve the ROM mostly due to an inflamed and tight capsule secondary to adhesive capsulitis or osteoarthritis.

The second finding was the effect of subacromial injections on blood glucose levels in type 2 diabetic patients. Overall, the infiltration increased the average glycemia for three days, with a peak the day after the injection. No hyperglycemia-related symptoms were recorded. Although these data can be considered generally a good result, they must be interpreted with extreme caution. Twenty-five percent of the patients had a transitory severe hyperglycemia. These data are in contrast with the study of Habib [6] who showed that there is no significant change in blood glucose levels after injecting 35 mg of Methylprednisolone

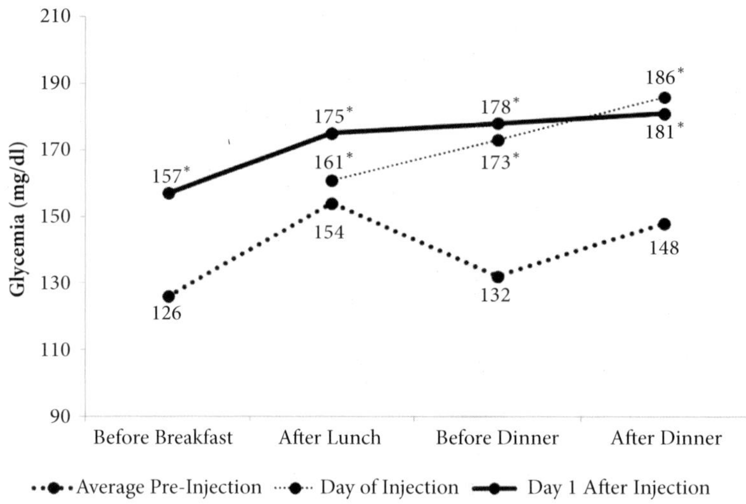

FIGURE 6: Daily glycemia the day and the days after the injection. One hour after lunch, the day of the injection (which was performed in the morning), the average glycemia was not different from the control values (161mg/dL, SD= 46.4; p=0.8). Glycemia increased significantly compared to the control values, before dinner (173mg/dL, SD=52.3 versus 132 mg/dL, SD=18.9; p=0.003) and after dinner (186mg/dL SD=54.2 versus 148 mg/dL, SD=42.2; p<0.001). The day after the injection, all glycemic values were significantly different from the control values. Before breakfast glycemia was 157 mg/dL SD= 50.7 (p=0.02), 2 hours after lunch 175 mg/dL SD=69.8 (p=0.03), before dinner 178 mg/dL SD=63.9 (p<0.001), and after dinner 181 mg/dL SD=48.5 (p=0.01).

Acetate at the shoulder joint. The reason for this difference is unknown. One potential explanation is that the effect on blood glucose levels of an intra-articular injection of Methylprednisolone Acetate is different from a subacromial injection. The absorption of the corticosteroids could be higher and faster in the inflamed subacromial bursa. Other reasons could be due to, in our study, 40 mg instead of 35 mg of Methylprednisolone Acetate being injected and that the corticosteroid was associated with Lidocaine.

Interestingly, in our series the patients that had severe hyperglycemia had had a suboptimal fasting glycemia before the injection. This data could imply that a better control of diabetes should prevent postinjection hyperglycemia and improve the safety of the treatment with corticosteroids.

The comparison of our results with other studies [1–3, 5, 6, 33] revealed that the effect of corticosteroid injections in other joints is also a variable and in some cases can significantly increase the blood glucose levels. Habib [1] reported a short glycemia increase only the first day after Celestone Chronodose in 6 knees of patients affected by type 2 diabetes. In 30 diabetic patients who underwent an injection with Triamcinolone Acetonide and Triamcinolone Esacetonide, a highly variable increase in glycemic values was reported (always below 300 mg/dL). Zufferey [5] reported no change in blood glucose levels among patients who received an epidural injection with 80 mg of Methylprednisolone Acetate, while patients who underwent an injection in their knees or shoulders with the same drug recorded an increase of glycemia, with a high individual variability.

One option for the treatment of persistent shoulder pain in diabetic patients is the injection with hyaluronic acid. However, the effect of this injection in diabetic patients has never been proven effective. Three patients in our study cohort have been injected with hyaluronic acid before being included in our study. None of them had reported a significant improvement.

Penning [34] compared subacromial Triamcinolone Acetonide, hyaluronic acid, and placebo for shoulder pain: he observed a booster effect in pain reduction after repeated Triamcinolone Acetonide injections. The hyaluronic acid and placebo group showed only slight improvements in pain reduction.

This study has some limitations. The injections were performed without use of ultrasound guidance. A study, however, showed that there is little evidence for the need of ultrasound guided needle placement [35]. Our patients reported an immediate slight to moderate benefit from the injection, indirect proof that the injection, that contained Lidocaine, was performed correctly. Another limitation is that we included diabetic patients with resistant shoulder pain, regardless the type of diagnosis. The main goal of this study was to test the short-term benefit of corticosteroid injections on pain. Shoulder pain, in old patients, has a multifactorial etiology. For this reason, we preferred to include all the patients with pain and not only those affected by a specific pathology. Future studies should address the risk-benefit ratio of corticosteroid injections in specific pathologies.

5. Conclusions

Subacromial injection with 40 mg of Methylprednisolone Acetate is effective as a short-term treatment in type 2 diabetic patients affected by shoulder pain. Patients must be informed about the possibility of transient hyperglycemia for the 3 days after injection and that 20% could have a transient severe hyperglycemia, especially the day of and the day after the injection and they must be closely followed up.

Disclosure

The study did not receive specific funding. It is self-funding and it was performed as part of the employment of all the authors.

References

[1] G. Habib and A. Safia, "The effect of intra-articular injection of betamethasone acetate/ betamethasone sodium phosphate on blood glucose levels in controlled diabetic patients with symptomatic osteoarthritis of the knee," *Clinical Rheumatology*, vol. 28, no. 1, pp. 85–87, 2009.

[2] G. S. Habib and W. Miari, "The Effect of Intra-Articular Triamcinolone Preparations on Blood Glucose Levels in Diabetic Patients," *JCR: Journal of Clinical Rheumatology*, vol. 17, no. 6, pp. 302–305, 2011.

[3] J. G. Stepan, D. A. London, M. I. Boyer, and R. P. Calfee, "Blood Glucose Levels in Diabetic Patients Following Corticosteroid Injections Into the Hand and Wrist," *The Journal of Hand Surgery*, vol. 39, no. 4, pp. 706–712, 2014.

[4] G. S. Habib, M. Bashir, and A. Jabbour, "Increased blood glucose levels following intra-articular injection of methylprednisolone acetate in patients with controlled diabetes and symptomatic osteoarthritis of the knee," *Annals of the Rheumatic Diseases*, vol. 67, no. 12, pp. 1790-1791, 2008.

[5] P. Zufferey, C. Bulliard, G. Gremion, M. Saugy, and A. So, "Systemic effects of epidural methylprednisolone injection on glucose tolerance in diabetic patients," *BMC Research Notes*, vol. 4, no. 1, p. 552, 2011.

[6] G. S. Habib and R. Abu-Ahmad, "Lack of effect of corticosteroid injection at the shoulder joint on blood glucose levels in diabetic patients," *Clinical Rheumatology*, vol. 26, no. 4, pp. 566–568, 2007.

[7] Y. H. Roh, S. R. Yi, J. H. Noh et al., "Intra-articular corticosteroid injection in diabetic patients with adhesive capsulitis: A randomized controlled trial," *Knee Surgery, Sports Traumatology, Arthroscopy*, vol. 20, no. 10, pp. 1947–1952, 2012.

[8] D. Snyder, "Pain," *Cancer Nursing*, vol. 15, no. 3, p. 211, 1992.

[9] L. A. Michener, M. K. Walsworth, W. C. Doukas, and K. P. Murphy, "Reliability and Diagnostic Accuracy of 5 Physical Examination Tests and Combination of Tests for Subacromial Impingement," *Archives of Physical Medicine and Rehabilitation*, vol. 90, no. 11, pp. 1898–1903, 2009.

[10] L. Kessel and M. Watson, "The painful arc syndrome. Clinical classification as a guide to management," *The Journal of Bone & Joint Surgery (British Volume)*, vol. 59, no. 2, pp. 166–172, 1977.

[11] F. W. Jobe and D. R. Moynes, "Delineation of diagnostic criteria and a rehabilitation program for rotator cuff injuries," *The American Journal of Sports Medicine*, vol. 10, no. 6, pp. 336–339, 1982.

[12] H. B. Park, A. Yokota, H. S. Gill, G. El Rassi, and E. G. Mcfarland, "Diagnostic accuracy of clinical tests for the different degrees of subacromial impingement syndrome," *The Journal of Bone and Joint Surgery-American Volume*, vol. 87, no. 7, pp. 1446–1455, 2005.

[13] R. J. Hawkins and J. C. Kennedy, "Impingement syndrome in athletes," *The American Journal of Sports Medicine*, vol. 8, no. 3, pp. 151–158, 1980.

[14] C. S. Neer II, "Anterior acromioplasty for the chronic impingement syndrome in the shoulder: a preliminary report.," *The Journal of Bone & Joint Surgery*, vol. 54, no. 1, pp. 41–50, 1972.

[15] L. A. Yocum, "Assessing the shoulder. History, physical examination, differential diagnosis, and special tests used.," *Clinics in Sports Medicine*, vol. 2, no. 2, pp. 281–289, 1983.

[16] M. Sue Kirkman, V. J. Briscoe, N. Clark et al., "Diabetes in older adults: a consensus report," *Journal of the American Geriatrics Society*, vol. 60, no. 12, pp. 2342–2356, 2012.

[17] K. Hamada, K. Yamanaka, Y. Uchiyama, T. Mikasa, and M. Mikasa, "A radiographic classification of massive rotator cuff tear arthritis," *Clinical Orthopaedics and Related Research*, vol. 469, no. 9, pp. 2452–2460, 2011.

[18] R. L. Samilson and V. Prieto, "Dislocation arthropathy of the shoulder," *The Journal of Bone & Joint Surgery*, vol. 65, no. 4, pp. 456–460, 1983.

[19] R. J. Casson, G. Chidlow, J. P. M. Wood, J. G. Crowston, and I. Goldberg, "Definition of glaucoma: clinical and experimental concepts," *Clinical & Experimental Ophthalmology*, vol. 40, no. 4, pp. 341–349, 2012.

[20] C. R. Constant and A. H. G. Murley, "A clinical method of functional assessment of the shoulder," *Clinical Orthopaedics and Related Research*, no. 214, pp. 160–164, 1987.

[21] D. Blonna, M. Scelsi, E. Marini et al., "Can we improve the reliability of the Constant-Murley score?" *Journal of Shoulder and Elbow Surgery*, vol. 21, no. 1, pp. 4–12, 2012.

[22] J. Dawson, R. Fitzpatrick, and A. Carr, "Questionnaire on the perceptions of patients about shoulder surgery," *The Journal of Bone & Joint Surgery (British Volume)*, vol. 78, no. 4, pp. 593–600, 1996.

[23] J. Dawson, K. Rogers, R. Fitzpatrick, and A. Carr, "The Oxford shoulder score revisited," *Archives of Orthopaedic and Trauma Surgery*, vol. 129, no. 1, pp. 119–123, 2009.

[24] M. K. Gilbart and C. Gerber, "Comparison of the subjective shoulder value and the Constant score," *Journal of Shoulder and Elbow Surgery*, vol. 16, no. 6, pp. 717–721, 2007.

[25] K. I. Gruson, D. E. Ruchelsman, and J. D. Zuckerman, "Subacromial corticosteroid injections," *Journal of Shoulder and Elbow Surgery*, vol. 17, no. 1, pp. S118–S130, 2008.

[26] G. V. Lawry and A. G. Fam, *Fam's musculoskeletal examination and joint injection techniques*, Mosby/Elsevier, Philadelphia, PA, USA, 2nd edition, 2010.

[27] D. Blonna, G. Lee, and S. W. O'Driscoll, "Arthroscopic Restoration of Terminal Elbow Extension in High-Level Athletes," *The American Journal of Sports Medicine*, vol. 38, no. 12, pp. 2509–2515, 2010.

[28] P. R. Finkbone and S. W. O'Driscoll, "Box-loop ligament reconstruction of the elbow for medial and lateral instability," *Journal of Shoulder and Elbow Surgery*, vol. 24, no. 4, pp. 647–654, 2015.

[29] C.-M. Yu, C.-H. Chen, H.-T. Liu, M.-H. Dai, I.-C. Wang, and K.-C. Wang, "Subacromial injections of corticosteroids and xylocaine for painful subacromial impingement syndrome," *Chang Gung Medical Journal*, vol. 29, no. 5, pp. 474–479, 2006.

[30] K. Akgün, M. Birtane, and Ü. Akarirmak, "Is local subacromial corticosteroid injection beneficial in subacromial impingement syndrome?" *Clinical Rheumatology*, vol. 23, no. 6, pp. 496–500, 2004.

[31] S. J. Thomas, C. McDougall, I. D. M. Brown et al., "Prevalence of symptoms and signs of shoulder problems in people with diabetes mellitus," *Journal of Shoulder and Elbow Surgery*, vol. 16, no. 6, pp. 748–751, 2007.

[32] P. E. T. Arkkila, I. M. Kantola, J. S. A. Viikari, and T. Rönnemaa, "Shoulder capsulitis in type I and II diabetic patients: Association with diabetic complications and related diseases," *Annals of the Rheumatic Diseases*, vol. 55, no. 12, pp. 907–914, 1996.

[33] A. S. Nimigan, D. C. Ross, and S. G. Bing, "Steroid injections in the management of trigger fingers," *American Journal of Physical Medicine & Rehabilitation*, vol. 85, no. 1, pp. 36–43, 2006.

[34] L. I. F. Penning, R. A. De Bie, and G. H. I. M. Walenkamp, "Subacromial triamcinolone acetonide, hyaluronic acid and saline injections for shoulder pain an RCT investigating the effectiveness in the first days," *BMC Musculoskeletal Disorders*, vol. 15, no. 1, 2014.

[35] O. M. Ekeberg, E. Bautz-Holter, E. K. Tveitå, N. G. Juel, S. Kvalheim, and J. I. Brox, "Subacromial ultrasound guided or systemic steroid injection for rotator cuff disease: Randomised double blind study," *BMJ*, vol. 338, no. 7689, pp. 273–275, 2009.

Fear Avoidance Beliefs and Risk of Long-Term Sickness Absence: Prospective Cohort Study among Workers with Musculoskeletal Pain

Kenneth Jay,[1,2] Sannie Vester Thorsen,[1] Emil Sundstrup,[1] Ramon Aiguadé,[3] Jose Casaña,[4] Joaquin Calatayud,[1,4] and Lars Louis Andersen[1,5]

[1]*National Research Centre for the Working Environment, Lersø Parkallé 105, Copenhagen, Denmark*
[2]*The Carrick Institute for Graduate studies, Institute of Clinical Neuroscience and Rehabilitation, 8910 Astronaut Blvd, Cape Canaveral, LF 32920, USA*
[3]*Departamento de Enfermería y Fisioterapia, Universidad de Lleida, Cataluña, Spain*
[4]*Exercise Intervention for Health Research Group (EXINH-RG), Department of Physiotherapy, University of Valencia, Spain*
[5]*Sport Sciences, Department of Health Science and Technology, Aalborg University, Denmark*

Correspondence should be addressed to Lars Louis Andersen; lla@nrcwe.dk

Academic Editor: Sulayman D. Dib-Hajj

Background and Objective. Musculoskeletal pain is common in the population. Negative beliefs about musculoskeletal pain and physical activity may lead to avoidance behavior resulting in absence from work. The present study investigates the influence of fear avoidance beliefs on long-term sickness absence. *Methods.* Workers of the general working population with musculoskeletal pain (low back, neck/shoulder, and/or arm/hand pain; n = 8319) from the Danish Work Environment Cohort Study were included. Long-term sickness absence data were obtained from the Danish Register for Evaluation and Marginalization (DREAM). Time-to-event analyses (cox regression) controlled for various confounders estimated the association between fear avoidance beliefs (very low, low, moderate [reference category], high, and very high) at baseline and long-term sickness absence (LTSA; ≥6 consecutive weeks) during a 2-year follow-up. *Results.* During the 2-year follow-up, 10.2% of the workers experienced long-term sickness absence. In the fully adjusted model, very high-level fear avoidance increased the risk of LTSA with hazard ratio (HR) of 1.48 (95% CI 1.15-1.90). Similar results were seen analyses stratified for occupational physical activity, i.e., sedentary workers (HR 1.72 (95% CI 1.04-2.83)) and physically active workers (HR 1.48 (95% CI 1.10-2.01)). *Conclusion.* A very high level of fear avoidance is a risk factor for long-term sickness absence among workers with musculoskeletal pain regardless of the level of occupational physical activity. Future interventions should target fear avoidance beliefs through information and campaigns about the benefits of staying active when having musculoskeletal pain.

1. Introduction

The Fifth European Working Condition Survey from 2010 shows that sickness absence is a challenge in all the Nordic countries [1]. It is estimated that employers' costs for wages of absent employees amount to about DKK 25 billion (€3.36 billion) a year, not considering the enterprises' contributions to sickness absence insurance.

Chronic musculoskeletal pain is a major cause of sickness absence [2]. However, biology alone cannot explain the occurrence of chronic pain and sickness absence, and psychological and social factors must also be considered [3]. For example, thoughts and beliefs about pain and movement may be important in the interplay between pain and the decision for a worker to either call in sick or go to work. Explained by Vlaeyen & Linton, the fear avoidance model of chronic pain states that the pain experience may in some individuals start a process of negative affect and catastrophizing thoughts that lead to defensive motivation, elevated arousal, or feeling threatened due to fear of experiencing pain [4, 5]. Thinking of the fear avoidance model in relation to work, a high level of fear avoidance can be speculated to lead to avoidance behavior in relation to work activities and thus increased risk of absence from work. Contrastingly, when pain is not considered a threat, the individual will likely remain physically active and engaged in everyday activities and therefore also work [6].

The degree of fear avoidance beliefs (FAB) is commonly assessed by the two-part Fear Avoidance Beliefs Questionnaire (FABQ) where part one focuses on fear avoidance in relation to leisure-time activities (e.g., bending, lifting, walking, or driving) and part two focuses on physical activities related to the individual's work [7]. In patients with chronic back pain, high levels of fear avoidance have been shown to increase the risk of poor work-related outcomes such as sick leave and not returning to work [8]. Fear avoidance beliefs can therefore be construed as mediators between pain and avoidance behaviors, such as sick leave, early retirement, or withdrawal from working life [9, 10]. Thus, we hypothesize that a high level of fear avoidance increases the risk of sick leave, because the worker fears that working will aggravate the pain situation and will thus be more likely to stay at home and rest.

The aim of this study is to investigate the impact of fear avoidance beliefs on register-based long-term sickness absence in the general working population.

2. Methods

2.1. Study Design. The present study uses data from the 2010 round of the Danish Work Environment Cohort Study (DWECS) a with 2-year follow-up from the Danish Register for Evaluation and Marginalization (DREAM). The DWECS consists of questionnaires assessing work environment and health in the Danish general working population. The DREAM register holds information about all social transfer payments for all citizens in Denmark, including granted sickness absence compensation. In this study, long-term sickness absence is defined as receiving sickness absence compensation of 6 weeks or more according to DREAM.

2.2. Participants. The questionnaire was distributed to a random sample drawn from the Danish Central Population Register of 30,000 people between 18 and 59 years with residence in Denmark, of which two-thirds were from the working population [11]. A total of 10,605 (~53%) from the working population replied to the 2010 questionnaire. For the present analyses, we only included currently employed wage earners with musculoskeletal pain (>= 1 scale 0-9 in the low back, neck/shoulder, and/or arm/hand; n = 8319). Characteristics of the study population are shown in Table 1.

2.3. Registration and Ethical Approval. The Danish Data Protection Agency (Datatilsynet, Denmark) has registered and journalized the DWECS (journal number 2007-54-0059). All data were deidentified and analyzed anonymously. According to Danish legislation, questionnaire- and register-based studies do not need approval by ethical and scientific committees nor informed consent.

2.4. Explanatory Variable: Fear Avoidance Beliefs. Two questions about fear avoidance beliefs from the Fear Avoidance Beliefs Questionnaire were included in the DWECS questionnaire survey. The first question was selected from the physical activity subscale (FABQPA): "Physical activity makes my pain worse"; the second question was selected from the work subscale (FABQW): "I should not do my normal work with my present pain." Participants replied on a 7-point Likert scale from completely agree to disagree. For further analyses, the responses were averaged and normalized to a scale of 0 to 100 (higher number equals higher level of disagreement) and further subdivided in 5 categories with the following score ranges: (1) "*very low fear avoidance*" [from 0 to 20], (2) "*low fear avoidance*" [from 20-40], "*moderate fear avoidance*" [from 40 to 60], "*high fear avoidance*" [from 60 to 80], and "*very high fear avoidance*" [from 80 to 100].

2.5. Outcome Variable: Long-Term Sickness Absence. Information about long-term sickness absence was obtained from the Danish Register for Evaluation and Marginalization (DREAM) and linked to DWECS by the individual social security number assigned to all Danish residents at birth or immigration. DREAM contains information on who received social transfer payments since 1991, e.g., sickness absence compensation, disability pension, and early retirement. Sickness absence compensation is given to the employer, who can apply for a refund from the state for employees after 30 calendar days of sickness absence. LTSA was defined as having at least 6 consecutive weeks in DREAM [12–14].

2.6. Control Variables. Control variables were added in two statistical models. Model 1 was a minimally adjusted model, adjusting only for age and gender. Model 2 was the fully adjusted model, adjusting for age, gender, job group (86 categories), psychosocial work environment (influence at work, emotional demands, support from colleagues, and support from leader) measured by the scales developed to COPSOQ [15], physical work demands (4 categories from sedentary to hard physical work), lifestyle (smoking, leisure physical activity, BMI), musculoskeletal pain intensity (low back, neck/shoulder, and arm/hand), previous long-term sickness absence (over the preceding two years prior to baseline), mental health, and chronic disease (depression, diabetes, cardiovascular disease, asthma, cancer, and back disease) [16].

2.7. Statistical Methods. The Cox proportional hazard models (Proc PHREG, SAS version 9.4) were applied in modelling the prospective association between fear avoidance and risk of LTSA. All events of permanent labor market drop out based on the DREAM register (i.e., statutory retirement age, early retirement, disability pension, immigration, or death) were censored at the time they occurred during the two-year follow-up. When LTSA occurred, the survival times were noncensored and referred to as event times. In addition to the main analysis, we also performed analyses stratified for occupational physical activity (1) sedentary workers and (2) physically active workers (3 subgroups combined). Proportional hazard assumptions were tested by visual inspection.

TABLE 1: Demographics, health, and work-related characteristics of the study population.

	All			Sedentary workers			Physically active workers		
	N	Mean (SD)	%	N	Mean (SD)	%	N	Mean (SD)	%
Age, years	8319	43.7 (11.4)		3753	44.3 (10.8)		4349	43.2 (11.8)	
BMI (kg.m-2)	8173	25.4 (4.4)		3698	25.3 (4.5)		4265	25.6 (4.4)	
Gender									
Women	4779		57.5	2188		58.3	2469		56.8
Men	3540		42.6	1565		41.7	1880		43.2
Smoking									
No, never	3853		46.9	1904		51.2	1868		43.6
Ex-smoker	2417		29.4	1138		30.6	1228		28.6
Yes	1950		23.7	679		18.3	1192		27.8
Physical activity, leisure									
Low	1121		13.6	458		12.3	623		14.5
Moderate	5631		68.5	2680		72.0	2826		65.9
High	1467		17.9	585		15.7	839		19.6
Physical activity at work									
Sedentary work	3753		46.3	3753		100.0	0		0.0
Physically active work	4349		53.7	0		0.0	4349		100.0
Psychosocial work factors (0-100)									
Emotional demands	8161	45.3 (25)		3707	43 (23.3)		4287	47.2 (26.2)	
Influence at work	8100	66.6 (24)		3689	71 (22.4)		4246	62.9 (24.6)	
Support from colleagues	7651	72.5 (21.5)		3425	72.2 (21)		4072	72.8 (21.8)	
Support from leader	7822	68.6 (26)		3524	69.3 (25.8)		4141	68.2 (26)	
Pain intensity (0-9)									
Neck/shoulder	8301	3 (2.3)		3746	2.9 (2.2)		4339	3 (2.3)	
Low back	8310	2.9 (2.5)		3753	2.5 (2.4)		4341	3.2 (2.5)	
Arm/hand	8302	1.8 (2.3)		3747	1.6 (2.2)		4340	1.9 (2.4)	
Back disease									
No	6699		81.0	3099		82.9	3434		79.6
Yes	1568		19.0	641		17.1	879		20.4
Previous long-term sickness absence									
No	7537		90.6	3500		93.3	3844		88.4
Yes	782		9.4	253		6.7	505		11.6
Long-term sickness absence during 2-year follow-up									
No	7475		89.9	3450		91.9	3837		88.2
Yes	844		10.2	303		8.1	512		11.8

TABLE 2: Hazard ratios (HR) and 95% confidence intervals for long-term sickness absence during the 2-year follow-up in relation to fear avoidance beliefs (FAB) at baseline.

		N	%	Model 1 HR (95% CI)	Model 2 HR (95% CI)
All	Very low FAB	1822	22.6	0.76 (0.62 - 0.93)	1.02 (0.80 - 1.29)
	Low FAB	1940	24.1	0.86 (0.71 - 1.05)	0.92 (0.73 - 1.16)
	Moderate FAB	2497	31.0	1	1
	High FAB	1042	12.9	1.31 (1.06 - 1.62)	1.13 (0.88 - 1.46)
	Very high FAB	761	9.4	1.80 (1.46 - 2.23)	1.48 (1.15 - 1.90)
Sedentary workers	Very low FAB	1049	28.8	0.70 (0.51 - 0.96)	0.86 (0.59 - 1.25)
	Low FAB	987	27.1	0.85 (0.62 - 1.16)	0.86 (0.60 - 1.23)
	Moderate FAB	1079	29.7	1	1
	High FAB	338	9.3	1.41 (0.98 - 2.04)	1.40 (0.91 - 2.15)
	Very high FAB	184	5.1	1.68 (1.08 - 2.61)	1.72 (1.04 - 2.83)
Physically active workers	Very low FAB	753	17.8	0.90 (0.68 - 1.18)	1.23 (0.89 - 1.70)
	Low FAB	925	21.9	0.91 (0.70 - 1.18)	1.00 (0.73 - 1.36)
	Moderate FAB	1344	31.9	1	1
	High FAB	660	15.6	1.21 (0.93 - 1.58)	1.08 (0.79 - 1.48)
	Very high FAB	538	12.8	1.69 (1.31 - 2.18)	1.48 (1.10 - 2.01)

Model 1: Adjusted for age and gender.
Model 2: model 1 + job group, psychosocial work environment (influence at work, emotional demands, support from colleagues, and support from leader), lifestyle (smoking, leisure physical activity, and BMI), musculoskeletal pain intensity (low back, neck/shoulder, and arm/hand), previous long-term sickness absence, mental health, and chronic disease (depression, diabetes, cardiovascular disease, cancer, and back disease).

Results are reported as hazard ratios (HR) with 95% confidence intervals (CI).

3. Results

Table 1 shows that there were slightly more women than men in the sample. Approximately half were nonsmokers and a quarter current smokers. Regarding physical activities most had a moderate level during leisure and about one-half had sedentary work and the other half had physically active work, respectively. Average pain intensity was about 3 in the neck/shoulder and low back and less than 2 in the arm/hand. 9.4% had experienced LTSA during the 2 years prior to baseline. During the 2-year follow-up, 10.2% experienced LTSA (8.1% among sedentary workers, 11.8% among physically active workers).

Table 2 shows the estimates for the minimally and fully adjusted models, as well as the analyses stratified for occupational physical activity. Moderate fear avoidance beliefs were set as reference (value = 1). In the minimally adjusted model (model 1) for all workers, very low fear avoidance was associated with reduced risk of LTSA (HR 0.76) and high (HR 1.31) and very high (HR 1.80) with increased risk. However, in the fully adjusted model (model 2), only a very high-level fear avoidance increased the risk of LTSA with hazard ratio (HR) of 1.48 (95% CI 1.15-1.90). In terms of understanding the size of this effect, a hazard ratio of 1.48 equals an increased risk of 48% ((HR-1)∗100) for long-term sickness absence in the "very high fear avoidance" compared with the "moderate fear avoidance" group. Thus, it can be considered quite a large effect. Similar results were seen analyses stratified for occupational physical activity, i.e., sedentary workers (HR 1.72 (95% CI 1.04-2.83)) and physically active workers (HR 1.48 (95% CI 1.10-2.01)), i.e., increased risks of 72% and 48%, respectively, in the "very high fear avoidance" compared with the "moderate fear avoidance" group.

4. Discussion

The main finding of this study is that a very high level of fear avoidance is a risk factor for long-term sickness absence even when adjusting to various confounders. This was seen regardless of the level of occupational physical activity, and fear avoidance can therefore be considered as a general risk factor for absence from work. Below we will discuss the present findings in relation to (1) possible underlying causes of the link between fear avoidance and sickness absence and (2) possible targets for action at the workplaces.

The present analysis showed a hazard ratio of 1.48 in fully adjusted model and 1.80 in the minimally adjusted model, corresponding to 48% and 80% increased risk in the "very high FAB" group compared with "moderate FAB group." Thus, the analyses showed that very high FAB is a risk factor for sickness absence even when adjusted to pain intensity and the physical demands in the work. Thus, FAB may not only be a mediator between the physical and psychosocial work conditions and risk of long-term sickness absence but also an independent explanatory variable. FAB is a complex phenomenon, shaped in the interplay between internal and external stressors, from competing personal goals, psychosocial factors, and daily life and workplace factors [9]. Our results fit well with the fear avoidance model; i.e., the workers with high fear avoidance are, according to the definition of fear avoidance, more likely to feel threatened due to fear of experiencing pain when moving the body [4, 5]. In this sense, work can be considered a behavior that the workers with high fear avoidance are more likely to avoid, i.e., more likely of calling in sick. In the long-term this disuse behavior may induce a vicious cycle that is difficult to break, i.e., leading to long-term sickness absence.

In relation to return to work after long-term sickness absence it may be beneficial to address FAB directly in workplace health promotion programs. For instance, Fritz & George [17] found by using the work subscale of the FABQ in patients with acute work-related low back pain that work-related FAB is the strongest predictor of return to work among the psychosocial risk factors [17].

Although the present study was not an intervention, the results suggest that future intervention targeting a reduction in FAB in the working population may have the potential to reduce sickness absence. Multifactorial intervention strategies focusing on physical activity as well as targeted physical exercise (e.g., resistance training and precise joint mobility training) and the psychological cognitive-behavioral elements of the relationship between the experience of pain-related fear have previously been reported to reduce work-related FAB in female workers with chronic musculoskeletal pain [18, 19]. Marchand and coworkers found that improvements in the work subscale of the fear avoidance questionnaire after cognitive-behavioral therapy and exercise predicted return to work within 12 months [20]. Similarly, reductions in the physical subscale of this questionnaire predicted disability at 12 months. These results highlight the relevance of being physically active to prevent disability and thus sickness absence. Further, Godges et al. [21] found that education and pain management counselling, physical activity, and exercise can reduce the number sick days in people with high fear avoidance beliefs and acute low back pain compared with standard physical therapy [21]. In addition, Frederiksen et al. [22] recently found in a cluster-randomized controlled trial that reassuring information delivered in a nonthreatening manner, about low back pain significantly, increased the odds for work participation and work ability among workers who experienced low back pain in a 12-month period [22]. These findings fit well with the biopsychosocial model first proposed by Engel [3] explaining the interconnected influence of biomedical, psychological, and social aspects of behavior in pain [3, 23]. Finding viable solutions to the immense socioeconomics costs of LTSA is a complex task as it is influenced by biomedical, psychological, and social factors and it is unlikely that any single intervention strategy will solve the problem. However, there is congruency among several studies that a high physical workload is associated with a significantly increased risk of developing work-related musculoskeletal disorders and LTSA [24–27], which should make future intervention strategies focus not only on physical activity but also include cognitive-behavioral elements to address workers' beliefs about work-related physical activity. As implementing changes in the specific working conditions (e.g. avoidance of monotonous repetitive, or heavy physical work) may be difficult or even impossible, intervention strategies focusing on the cognitive- and behavioral elements of what leads to pain reinforcement (e.g. pain catastrophizing) and subsequent FAB may contribute to a solution [28, 29]. National campaigns may also be a way forward to improve negative beliefs in relation to movement and musculoskeletal pain in the population [30, 31].

4.1. Strengths and Limitations. The present study has both strengths and limitations. Only two questions from the FABQ are included in the Danish Work Environment Cohort Study. Nevertheless, the prospective association with LTSA in the present study shows that these questions are relevant to consider in the prevention of LTSA. Another limitation is that there may be some circularity in the reasoning since the items used in the present study directly tap into physical activity and work. These items might correlate highly with self-rated "expectations" of working in the future which are not based on the fear avoidance model. Future studies should determine to what extent the full scale FABQ predicts LTSA. Further, only 53% replied to the questionnaire which could constitute a limitation. Nevertheless, a representative sample of more than 8000 workers with musculoskeletal pain from the general working population replying to the DWECS questionnaire is a large enough population to also constitute a strength of the present study. The use of register-based data on LTSA from DREAM further amplifies its strength. The validity of the DREAM register is high as the incentive for employers to report sickness absence allows them to seek compensation of employee sickness absence costs after 30 days of absence due to sickness thus reducing employer expenses. Finally, the use of sickness absence register data eliminates recall or reporting biases.

In conclusion, a very high level of fear avoidance is a risk factor for long-term sickness absence among workers with musculoskeletal pain regardless of the level of occupational physical activity. Future interventions should target fear avoidance beliefs through information and campaigns about the benefits of staying active when having musculoskeletal pain.

References

[1] C. Ardito, A. d'Errico, and R. Leombruni, *EUROfond. Health and well-being at Work - A report based on the fifth European Working Conditions Survey*, 2012.

[2] S. Bevan, *Fit For Work? Musculoskeletal Disorders in the European Workforce*, 2009.

[3] G. L. Engel, "The need for a new medical model: a challenge for biomedicine," *Science*, vol. 196, no. 4286, pp. 129–136, 1977.

[4] J. W. S. Vlaeyen and S. J. Linton, "Fear-avoidance and its consequences in chronic musculoskeletal pain: a state of the art," *PAIN*, vol. 85, no. 3, pp. 317–332, 2000b.

[5] J. W. S. Vlaeyen and S. J. Linton, "Fear-avoidance model of chronic musculoskeletal pain: 12 years on," *PAIN*, vol. 153, no. 6, pp. 1144–1147, 2012a.

[6] J. W. S. Vlaeyen and S. J. Linton, "Fear-avoidance and its consequences in chronic musculoskeletal pain: a state of the art," *PAIN*, vol. 85, no. 3, pp. 317–332, 2000a.

[7] G. Waddell, M. Newton, I. Henderson, D. Somerville, and C. J. Main, "A Fear-Avoidance Beliefs Questionnaire (FABQ) and the role of fear-avoidance beliefs in chronic low back pain and disability," *PAIN*, vol. 52, no. 2, pp. 157–168, 1993.

[8] M. M. Wertli, E. Rasmussen-Barr, S. Weiser, L. M. Bachmann, and F. Brunner, "The role of fear avoidance beliefs as a prognostic factor for outcome in patients with nonspecific low back pain: A systematic review," *The Spine Journal*, vol. 14, no. 5, pp. 816–836, 2014.

[9] G. Crombez, C. Eccleston, S. Van Damme, J. W. S. Vlaeyen, and P. Karoly, "Fear-avoidance model of chronic pain: the next generation," *The Clinical Journal of Pain*, vol. 28, no. 6, pp. 475–483, 2012.

[10] J. W. S. Vlaeyen and S. J. Linton, "Fear-avoidance model of chronic musculoskeletal pain: 12 years on," *PAIN*, vol. 153, no. 6, pp. 1144–1147, 2012b.

[11] E. Bach, L. L. Andersen, and J. B. Bjørner, *Arbejdsmiljø og helbred i Danmark*, 2010.

[12] N. H. Hjollund, F. B. Larsen, and J. H. Andersen, "Register-based follow-up of social benefits and other transfer payments: accuracy and degree of completeness in a Danish interdepartmental administrative database compared with a population-based survey," *Scandinavian Journal of Public Health*, vol. 35, no. 5, pp. 497–502, 2007.

[13] T. Lund, M. Kivimäki, M. Labriola, E. Villadsen, and K. B. Christensen, "Using administrative sickness absence data as a marker of future disability pension: the prospective DREAM study of Danish private sector employees," *Occupational and Environmental Medicine*, vol. 65, no. 1, pp. 28–31, 2008.

[14] H. Burr, J. Pedersen, and J. V. Hansen, "Work environment as predictor of long-term sickness absence: linkage of self-reported DWECS data with the DREAM register," *Scandinavian Journal of Public Health*, vol. 39, no. 7, pp. 147–152, 2011.

[15] J. H. Pejtersen, T. S. Kristensen, V. Borg, and J. B. Bjorner, "The second version of the Copenhagen Psychosocial Questionnaire," *Scandinavian Journal of Public Health*, vol. 38, no. 3, pp. 8–24, 2010.

[16] J. B. Bjorner, S. Kreiner, J. E. Ware, M. T. Damsgaard, and P. Bech, "Differential item functioning in the Danish translation of the SF-36," *Journal of Clinical Epidemiology*, vol. 51, no. 11, pp. 1189–1202, 1998.

[17] J. M. Fritz and S. Z. George, "Identifying psychosocial variables in patients with acute work-related low back pain: The importance of fear-avoidance beliefs," *Physical Therapy in Sport*, vol. 82, no. 10, pp. 973–983, 2002.

[18] K. Jay, M. Brandt, K. Hansen et al., "Effect of individually tailored biopsychosocial workplace interventions on chronic musculoskeletal pain and stress among laboratory technicians: Randomized controlled trial," *Pain Physician*, vol. 18, no. 5, pp. 459–471, 2015.

[19] K. Jay, M. Brandt, M. D. Jakobsen et al., "Ten weeks of physical-cognitive-mindfulness training reduces fear-Avoidance beliefs about work-related activity Randomized controlled trial," *Medicine (United States)*, vol. 95, no. 34, 2016.

[20] G. H. Marchand, K. Myhre, G. Leivseth et al., "Change in pain, disability and influence of fear-avoidance in a work-focused intervention on neck and back pain: A randomized controlled trial," *BMC Musculoskeletal Disorders*, vol. 16, no. 1, 2015.

[21] J. J. Godges, M. A. Anger, G. Zimmerman, and A. Delitto, "Effects of education on return-to-work status for people with fear-avoidance beliefs and acute low back pain," *Physical Therapy in Sport*, vol. 88, no. 2, pp. 231–239, 2008.

[22] P. Frederiksen, A. Indahl, L. L. Andersen, K. Burton, R. Hertzum-Larsen, and T. Bendix, "Can group-based reassuring information alter low back pain behavior? A cluster-randomized controlled trial," *PLoS ONE*, vol. 12, no. 3, 2017.

[23] G. L. Engel, "The clinical application of the biopsychosocial model," *The American Journal of Psychiatry*, vol. 137, no. 5, pp. 535–544, 1980.

[24] T. Lund, M. Labriola, K. B. Christensen, U. Bültmann, and E. Villadsen, "Physical work environment risk factors for long term sickness absence: prospective findings among a cohort of 5357 employees in Denmark," *British Medical Journal*, vol. 332, no. 7539, pp. 449–451, 2006.

[25] B. R. Da Costa and E. R. Vieira, "Risk factors for work-related musculoskeletal disorders: a systematic review of recent longitudinal studies," *American Journal of Industrial Medicine*, vol. 53, no. 3, pp. 285–323, 2010.

[26] J. Mayer, T. Kraus, and E. Ochsmann, "Longitudinal evidence for the association between work-related physical exposures and neck and/or shoulder complaints: A systematic review," *International Archives of Occupational and Environmental Health*, vol. 85, no. 6, pp. 587–603, 2012.

[27] L. L. Andersen, N. Fallentin, S. V. Thorsen, and A. Holtermann, "Physical workload and risk of long-term sickness absence in the general working population and among blue-collar workers: prospective cohort study with register follow-up," *Occupational and Environmental Medicine*, vol. 73, no. 4, pp. 246–253, 2016.

[28] G. Lorimer Moseley, "A new direction for the fear avoidance model?" *PAIN*, vol. 152, no. 11, pp. 2447-2448, 2011.

[29] G. L. Moseley and D. S. Butler, "Fifteen Years of Explaining Pain: The Past, Present, and Future," *The Journal of Pain*, vol. 16, no. 9, pp. 807–813, 2015.

[30] L. L. Andersen, N. Geisle, and B. Knudsen, "Can beliefs about musculoskeletal pain and work be changed at the national level? Prospective evaluation of the danish national job & body campaign," *Scandinavian Journal of Work, Environment & Health*, vol. 44, no. 1, pp. 25–36, 2018.

[31] R. Buchbinder, D. Jolley, and M. Wyatt, "2001 Volvo award winner in clinical studies: Effects of a media campaign on back pain beliefs and its potential influence on management of low back pain in general practice," *The Spine Journal*, vol. 26, no. 23, pp. 2535–2542, 2001.

25

Efficacy of Intrauterine Lidocaine Instillation in Reducing Pain during Endometrial Biopsy by Novak

Sawanya Benchahong,[1] Athita Chanthasenanont,[1] Densak Pongrojpaw,[1] Junya Pattaraarchachai,[2] Kornkarn Bhamarapravatana,[3] and Komsun Suwannarurk[1]

[1] *Department of Obstetrics and Gynecology, Faculty of Medicine, Thammasat University, Pathum Thani, Thailand*
[2] *Chulabhorn International College of Medicine, Thammasat University, Pathum Thani, Thailand*
[3] *Department of Preclinical Science, Faculty of Medicine, Thammasat University, Pathum Thani, Thailand*

Correspondence should be addressed to Athita Chanthasenanont; dr.athita@gmail.com

Academic Editor: Ke Ren

Abnormal uterine bleeding in women aged 35 years or over is an important clinical sign of many gynecological conditions. The diagnoses of these conditions require the pathological report of the endometrial tissue. Outpatient-based endometrial biopsy is an excellent option compared to standard fractional uterine curettage or hysteroscopy with endometrial biopsy in providing a definite diagnosis for abnormal uterine bleeding as it is less painful and does not require high potency anesthesia. This study evaluates the effect of intrauterine lidocaine on the patient's pain score during endometrial biopsy by the Novak curette. We included patients aged 35 years or more who had abnormal uterine bleeding between December 2016 and March 2018. The study was conducted at Thammasat University Hospital, Pathum Thani, Thailand. 250 patients were randomly allocated to either receive intrauterine lidocaine (study group) or normal saline (control group). Assessment of pain severity was evaluated using a visual analogue scale (VAS) score at 6 time-points, namely, before performing the procedure, when grasping the cervix by the tenaculum, during the intrauterine instillation of lidocaine or normal saline, during the uterine curettage, and then 15 minutes and 2 hours after the procedure. This study showed that there was significant pain reduction in patients who received intrauterine instillation of lidocaine compared to placebo, during uterine curettage, as well as 15 minutes and 2 hours after procedure ($p<0.0001$). Patient satisfaction was not significantly different between the two groups, while physician satisfaction significantly improved in the lidocaine group. Serious complications were not found during this study. (This research project had been approved for registration at Thai Clinical Trials Registry. TCTR identification number is TCTR20161031003.)

1. Introduction

Abnormal uterine bleeding in women aged 35 years or more is an important clinical sign of many gynecological problems such as endometrial hyperplasia, metritis, leiomyoma, endometriosis, and endometrial cancer. The gold standard for the diagnosis of abnormal uterine bleeding is endometrial histology. Endometrial tissue can be obtained from standard uterine curettage, office endometrial aspiration, or endometrial biopsy via hysteroscopy [1].

Outpatient-based endometrial biopsy is an excellent option compared to standard fractional uterine curettage or hysteroscopy with endometrial biopsy in providing a definite diagnosis for abnormal uterine bleeding. It is less painful and does not require high potency anesthesia [1], which itself can be associated with multiple complications such as paracervical or intracervical anesthetic infiltration.

Endometrial tissue aspiration devices are divided into two groups: plastic (low pressure) and metallic (high pressure) devices. Plastic devices available in Thailand include Pipelle (Unimar, CT, USA) and Endocelle (Wallach, CT, USA). Low pressure devices tend to produce less pain compared to high pressure devices [2]. However, there may be an issue of insufficient tissue sampling when using plastic devices [2].

The Novak endometrial curette is a high pressure endometrial biopsy device. It is a metallic cannula connected to a 10 ml syringe. Its diameter is larger than that of the plastic device and thus provides more pressure allowing a better tissue adequacy [2]. The Novak endometrial curette might therefore be a more suitable tool to ensure sufficient tissue sampling. However, the higher pressure can cause discomfort and pain to patients, thus reducing patient cooperation and satisfaction [2]. Therefore patients are likely to require some form of analgesia to minimize pain during this procedure.

Lidocaine, an aromatic benzene ring connected to an amide group, is a local anesthetic agent which inhibits the influx of sodium into the cell, thus preventing the occurrence of the neurotransmitter cascade. It has a rapid onset, short duration of action, low cost, minimal side effects, and good availability [3]. Recent literature showed that intrauterine lidocaine and bupivacaine instillation were appropriate methods for pain relief during intrauterine procedures [4–12].

In this study, we investigated the efficacy of intrauterine lidocaine during the endometrial biopsy in reducing pain and improving both patient and operator satisfaction.

2. Materials and Methods

This prospective double-blind randomized controlled trial was approved by the Ethics Committee, Faculty of Medicine, Thammasat University (MTU-EC-OB-2-132/59) (TCTR-20161031003). The study was conducted at Thammasat University Hospital, Pathum Thani, Thailand. Patients aged 35 years or more who had abnormal uterine bleeding between December 2016 and March 2018 were included in this study. After individual counseling, the participants signed the informed consent. Exclusion criteria include patients with underlying coagulopathy, taking medicine involved with coagulation, allergy to lidocaine, pregnancy, pelvic inflammatory disease, and cervical stenosis, as well as those who decline to participate in the study. Patients' demographics data collected include age, body weight, height, body mass index (BMI), level of education, occupation, income, underlying diseases, hormonal usage, parity, vaginal delivery, history of uterine curettage, menopausal status, and indication for endometrial biopsy. Patients were randomly assigned into two groups using a computer generated table of random number. Group allocations were concealed in sealed opaque envelopes. Nurses at the outpatient department would open the envelopes once they met the participants.

For the procedure, each patient was placed in lithotomy position. The bivalve speculum and tenaculum were applied. The Novak curette connected to a syringe containing 7 ml of either lidocaine or normal saline solution (NSS) was inserted into the uterine cavity in the intervention or control group, respectively. After three minutes [8] of lidocaine instillation, endometrial sampling was performed by aspiration and rotation at 3, 6, 9, and 12 o'clock of uterine cavity. Assessment of pain severity was evaluated by using a visual analogue scale (VAS) recorded by the assisting nurse. The VAS score was ranked from score 0 (no pain) to 10 (worst pain). The result was then categorized into mild (0-4), moderate (5-6), or severe (7-10) pain. The patients' pain was evaluated at 6 different time-points, namely, before performing the procedure, when grasping the cervix by the tenaculum, during the intrauterine instillation of lidocaine or NSS, during the uterine curettage, and then 15 minutes and two hours after the procedure. Possible side effects, i.e., nausea, vomiting, vertigo, itching, and heavy bleeding per vagina were also recorded. All tissue samples were sent for pathological report.

The pathological reports of the endometrial tissue included the proliferative phase, secretory phase, atrophic or inactive endometrium, inadequate endometrial tissue, endometrial polyp, cancer, and others. The last category included benign endometrial tissue, acute inflammation, chronic inflammation, fragment of glandular, and stromal breakdown.

The sample size in this study was calculated from the standard deviation (SD) between study and control group from Guney's literature (SD = 1.46) [9]. The alpha and beta errors were set at 0.05, which suggested that the sample size should be at least 118 cases per group.

Data were analyzed by using the statistical package for social science (SPSS Inc, Chicago, IL USA) for Windows version 17. Continuous data were analyzed using the mean and unpaired t-tests. The Chi-square test was used for categorical data. Level of statistical significance was set at p value less than 0.05.

3. Results

Out of 272 participants recruited, 250 met the inclusion criteria. Twenty-two patients were excluded from the study; 5 had cervical stenosis, 7 had pelvic inflammatory disease, and 10 declined to participate in the study. One hundred twenty-five participants were randomly assigned into either the control or the study group (Figure 1).

The patient's demographic data showed no statistical difference between the control and study groups ($p>0.05$ each) (Table 1). The minimum age was 35 years old in both groups. The maximum age was 77 years old in the study group and 73 years old in the control group, whereas the mean age was 48.5 and 47.2 years old, respectively. Around 60% of both groups (81 and 77 cases in study and control group) had previous vaginal delivery. Approximately one-third of the subjects had previous uterine curettage. There was no case that needed cervical dilatation. Indications for endometrial biopsy included menorrhagia, irregular cycle, intermenstrual bleeding, mixed symptoms, postmenopausal bleeding, and hypermenorrhea. There was no statistical difference between both groups ($p=0.194$).

In the control group, the VAS scores before performing the procedure, while grasping cervix by tenaculum, during intrauterine instillation, during uterine curettage, and 15 minutes and two hours after procedure were 0.60±1.40, 4.98±2.43, 7.08±2.23, 8.24±1.75, 2.78±2.49, and 1.19±1.79 (mean±SD), respectively, whereas the corresponding scores were 0.42±1.36, 4.67±2.38, 5.92±2.43, 6.93±2.19, 0.88±1.48, and 0.96±0.34 in the lidocaine group. There were significant pain reduction during intrauterine instillation, during uterine curettage, and 15 minutes and two hours after procedure in those who received intrauterine lidocaine compared to NSS ($p<0.0001$). The VAS pain scores before the procedure and while grasping cervix by tenaculum were

TABLE 1: Demographic character of participants (n=125 each).

	Lidocaine	Normal saline	*p* value
Age (years) *	48.53 ± 9.74	47.23 ± 8.29	0.26
BW (kg) *	60.8 ± 11.34	61.82 ± 13.04	0.51
HT (cm) *	157.26 ± 4.36	158.25 ± 5.26	0.11
BMI (kg/m^2) *	24.54 ± 4.20	24.65 ± 4.82	0.84
Education **			0.64
Below primary level	26 (20.8)	27 (21.6)	
Secondary-tertiary level	52 (41.6)	54 (43.2)	
Above bachelor	47 (37.6)	44 (35.2)	
Occupation **			0.28
House wife	22 (17.6)	26 (20.8)	
Agriculture	5 (4)	4 (3.2)	
SME	31 (24.8)	30 (24)	
Employee	43 (34.4)	43 (34.4)	
Government officer	24 (19.2)	22 (17.6)	
Income (Bath) **			0.94
<10,000	15 (12)	18 (14.4)	
10,000 - 30,000	65 (52)	61 (48.8)	
30,000 - 50,000	31 (24.8)	32 (25.6)	
>50,000	14 (11.2)	14 (11.2)	
Underlying disease **			
No	63 (50.4)	72 (57.6)	0.98
DM and HT	32 (25.6)	31 (24.8)	
Heart disease	1 (0.8)	4 (3.2)	
Anemia	2 (1.6)	2 (1.6)	
Other[a]	27 (21.6)	16 (12.8)	
Hormonal used **			0.48
No	104 (83.2)	108 (86.4)	
Tamoxifen	3 (2.4)	3 (2.4)	
DMPA	7 (5.6)	5 (4)	
OCP	10 (8)	6 (4.8)	
Other[b]	1 (0.8)	3 (2.4)	
Parous cervix **			0.6
Nulliparous	44 (35.2)	48 (38.4)	
Parous	81 (64.8)	77 (61.6)	
History of uterine curettage **	31 (24.8)	31 (24.8)	0.79
Menopausal status **			0.57
Premenopausal	93 (74.4)	89 (71.2)	
Postmenopausal	32 (25.6)	36 (28.8)	
Indication for endometrial biopsy **			0.19
Menorrhagia	30 (24)	20 (16)	
Irregular cycle	23 (18.4)	34 (27.2)	
Intermenstrual bleeding	30 (24)	31 (24.8)	
Mixed symptoms	9 (7.2)	3 (2.4)	
Postmenopausal bleeding	32 (25.6)	36 (28.8)	
Hypermenorrhea	1 (0.8)	1 (0.8)	

*: mean ± SD; **: n (%); BW: body weight; HT: height; BMI: body mass index; SME: small and medium enterprise; DM: diabetes mellitus; HT: hypertension; Other[a]: breast cancer, asthma, thyroid disease, dyslipidemia, etc.; DMPA: depot medroxyprogesterone acetate; OCP: oral contraceptive pill; Other[b]: herb, progestin only pill, and implant.

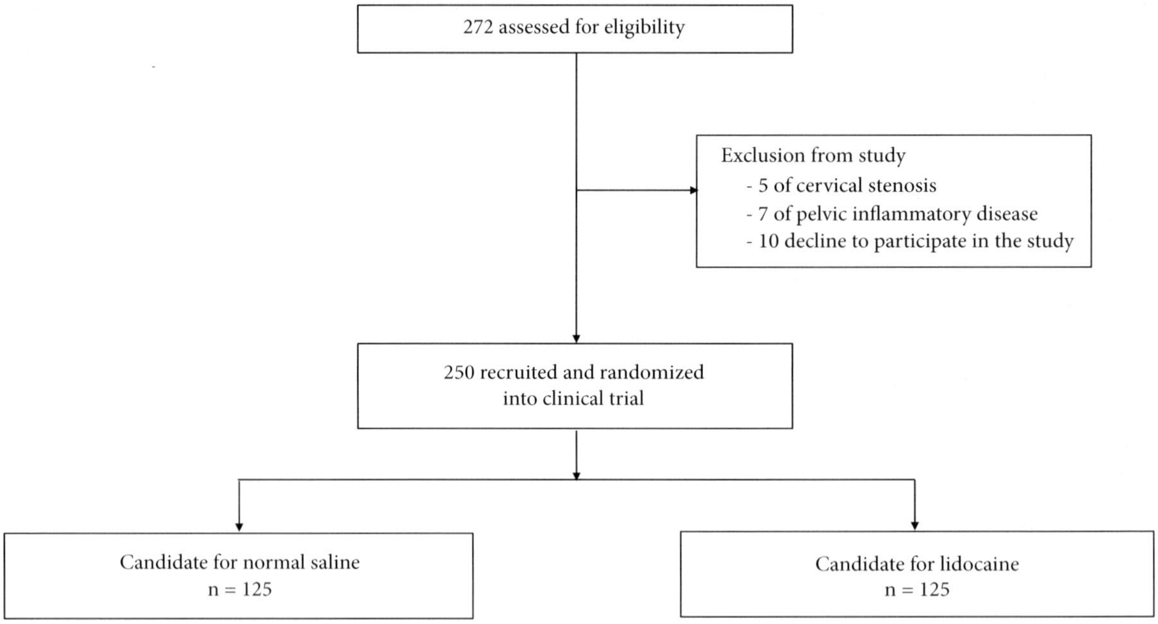

FIGURE 1: Participant flow diagram.

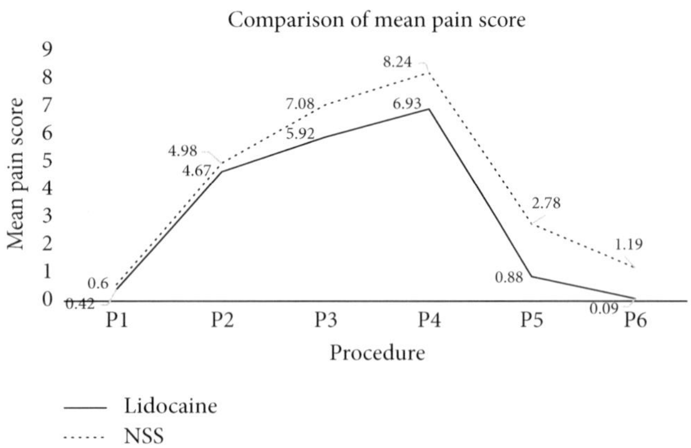

FIGURE 2: Comparison of mean pain score. P1: before procedure, P2: apply tenaculum, P3: during intrauterine infusion, P4: during aspiration, P5: 15 minutes after procedure, P6: 2 hours after procedure, NSS: normal saline.

not significantly different between the two groups (Table 2, Figure 2).

The mean duration of the procedure in study and control group were 5.12 and 5.40 minutes, respectively (p=0.13). The operative time varied from 3 to 10 minutes in the study and from 3 to 11 minutes in the control group.

Patient satisfaction was not significantly different between the two groups. Physician satisfaction was statistically superior in study group (Table 3).

Minimal cervical bleeding during tenaculum application was the only complication observed in this study. This was resolved by manual compression of the cervix with a gauze for 3-5 minutes. Serious complications, such as heavy vaginal bleeding, dizziness, and severe abdominal pain, were not found during this study.

There was no significant difference in pathological report in both groups. The two most common pathological results were proliferative phase of endometrium (24.4%) and secretory phase of endometrium (24%), respectively (Table 3). In this study, cancer prevalence was 3.2%, including one cervical cancer and 7 endometrial cancers. All cases of endometrial cancer presented with postmenopausal bleeding. The histopathological reports showed 6 endometrioid type and one clear cell type endometrial cancer. The patient with cervical cancer, however, presented with premenopausal abnormal vaginal bleeding. In this case it was the squamous cell carcinoma that was reported in the histopathology.

In patients with inadequate tissue sampling, fractional and curettage (F&C) of the endometrium was repeated. In this group, two out of 11 patients were lost during the follow-up. Six patients no longer had abnormal uterine bleeding and thus their status was changed to periodical observation. Only three patients underwent F&C. These three patients had no endometrial tissue.

4. Discussion

Endometrial biopsy has become an essential modality for obtaining the histological diagnosis of abnormal uterine bleeding [1]. It provides adequate endometrial tissue samples and can be easily performed in the gynecology outpatient departments. However, pain during the procedure may cause patients' discomfort and reduce compliance. Stovall and coworkers showed that endometrial sampling by the Pipelle caused less pain compared to the Novak, but also resulted in a higher number of insufficient tissue sampling [2]. Similarly, Kosus et al. reported that endometrial sampling was

TABLE 2: Comparison of pain score during endometrial aspiration (n=125 each).

Pain score at different stages	Lidocaine**	Normal saline**	*p* value
Before procedure			0.55
Mild	120 (96)	121 (96.8)	
Moderate	2 (1.6)	3 (2.4)	
Severe	3 (2.4)	1 (0.8)	
Apply tenaculum			0.53
Mild	54 (43.2)	49 (39.2)	
Moderate	40 (32)	37 (29.6)	
Severe	31 (24.8)	39 (31.2)	
During intrauterine infusion			0.01
Mild	29 (23.2)	14 (11.2)	
Moderate	40 (32)	31 (24.8)	
Severe	56 (44.8)	80 (64)	
During aspiration			<0.001
Mild	16 (12.8)	6 (4.8)	
Moderate	30 (24)	11 (8.8)	
Severe	79 (63.2)	108 (86.4)	
15 min after procedure			<0.001
Mild	117 (93.6)	93 (74.4)	
Moderate	7 (5.6)	18 (14.4)	
Severe	1 (0.8)	14 (11.2)	
2 hours after procedure			0.01
Mild	125 (100)	116 (92.8)	
Moderate	0	6 (4.8)	
Severe	0	3 (2.4)	

Before procedure: visual analogue scale (VAS) score before endometrial aspiration by Novak curette application; Apply tenaculum: VAS score during cervical grasping by tenaculum; During intrauterine infusion: VAS score during intrauterine lidocaine or normal saline infusion; During aspiration: VAS score during endometrial aspiration; 15 min after procedure: VAS score after 15 min of endometrial aspiration; 2 hours after procedure: VAS score after 2 hours of endometrial aspiration; **: n (%); Mild: VAS score 0-4; Moderate: VAS score 5-6; Severe: VAS score 7-10.

TABLE 3: Pathological reports and satisfaction score (n=125 each).

	Lidocaine**	Normal saline**	*p* value
Pathological reports			0.8
Proliferative phase	26 (20.8)	35 (28)	
Secretory phase	29 (23.2)	31 (24.8)	
Atrophic or inactive ET	31 (24.8)	26 (20.8)	
No or inadequate ET	7 (5.6)	4 (3.2)	
Endometrial polyp	13 (10.4)	10 (8)	
Cancer	4 (3.2)	4 (3.2)	
Other	15 (12)	15 (12)	
Satisfaction score			
Patient's*	9.00 ± 1.35	8.86 ± 1.35	0.4
Physician's*	9.27 ± 0.786	8.74 ± 1.37	< 0.001

**: n (%), ET: endometrial tissue, Other: benign endometrial tissue, acute inflammation, chronic inflammation and fragment of glandular and stromal breakdown, *: mean ± SD.

inadequate in 10% of cases when using the Pipelle curettage [4]. Moreover, the Pipelle is a single-use disposable device, whereas the Novak is nondisposable and can be sterilized for re-use during its lifetime. Therefore, the Novak is considered to be a more environmentally friendly, economical, and efficient endometrial sampling tool for the management of abnormal uterine bleeding.

Previous studies have investigated the efficacy of intrauterine lidocaine instillation for pain relief during endometrial aspiration. The studies of Kosus et al. [6], Dogan et al. [7], and Guler et al. [12] compared the intrauterine instillation of the lidocaine group to no anesthetic group while Maderak et al. [10] compared intrauterine lidocaine to sterile water during endometrial aspiration. Kosus, Trolice, and Sargin [4, 8, 11] also evaluated the efficacy of intrauterine lidocaine compared to normal saline in a similar fashion to this study. Similarly, this randomized, double-blind, controlled trial has shown that patients who received intrauterine lidocaine had significantly lower pain scores during the endometrial aspiration compared to the control group.

All previous studies used disposal plastic endometrial aspirators (Pipelle) [4, 6–12] while the present study used a metallic endometrial aspirator (Novak). We recruited a larger number of participants compared to previous studies and extended the evaluation of postoperative pain to 2 hours after the procedure. This is in contrast to previous studies [4, 6–12], which measured the patient's pain level during and up to thirty minutes after procedure. The analgesic effect of intrauterine lidocaine was still present at 15 minutes and 2 hours after the procedure. This may be explained by the inhibitory effects of lidocaine at the nerve endings located in the endometrial mucosa.

Effective analgesia during endometrial sampling is important for patient satisfaction and cooperation. In this study, although there was no statistically significant difference in patient satisfaction between the two groups, the physician satisfaction was significantly higher in the study group. This finding may be a result of improved patient compliance.

Although the Novak curette is rigid and has a larger diameter which may result in more discomfort, it has a better rate of adequate endometrial tissue sampling compared to other devices [2]. Insufficient endometrial sampling was present in only 4.4% in this study compared to 9.5% in Stovell's study [2].

In the present study, we found 8 cases of endometrial cancer. This further emphasizes the importance of adequate tissue sampling in abnormal uterine bleeding to prevent the misdiagnosis. The Novak curette used with intrauterine anesthesia serves as a good choice for obtaining the endometrial tissue.

5. Conclusion

Intrauterine lidocaine instillation during endometrial tissue sampling by the Novak curette significantly reduced patients' pain during intrauterine instillation, during uterine curettage, and 15 minutes and two hours after procedure. Cancer detection in this study was 3.2%. This showed that intrauterine lidocaine was an effective analgesia during endometrial sampling. The finding can help improve patient cooperation and operator satisfaction.

Disclosure

This manuscript is not under consideration by another journal and the final manuscript has been seen and approved by all authors.

Acknowledgments

The research was supported by Research Fund of Thammasat University, Pathum Thani, Thailand, in the year of 2016.

References

[1] C. D. Sean, M. Andrea, and R. L. John, "Uterine cancer," in *Berek & Novak's Gynecology*, J. S. Berek and D. L. Berek, Eds., pp. 1250–1304, Wolters Kluwer, Philadelphia, Pa, USA, 15th edition, 2012.

[2] T. G. Stovall, F. W. Ling, and P. L. Morgan, "A prospective, randomized comparison of the Pipelle endometrial sampling device with the Novak curette," *American Journal of Obstetrics & Gynecology*, vol. 165, no. 4, pp. 1287–1290, 1991.

[3] L. Yi and S. L. Spencer, "Local anesthetics," in *Clinical Anesthesia*, G. B. Paul and F. C. Bruce, Eds., pp. 561-79, Wolters Kluwer, Philadelphia, Pa, USA, 7th edition, 2013.

[4] N. Kosus, A. Kosus, R. I. Demircioglu et al., "Transcervical intrauterine levobupivacaine or lidocaine infusion for pain control during endometrial biopsy," *Pain Res Manag*, vol. 19, pp. 82–86, 2014.

[5] S. Tornblom-Paulander, B. K. Tingåker, A. Werner et al., "Novel topical formulation of lidocaine provides significant pain relief for intrauterine device insertion: Pharmacokinetic evaluation and randomized placebo-controlled trial," *Fertility and Sterility*, vol. 103, no. 2, pp. 422–427, 2015.

[6] N. Köşüş, A. Köşüş, A. Güler, S. A. Simavli, and N. Ö. Turhan, "Transcervical intrauterine levobupivacaine infusion or paracervical block for pain control during endometrial biopsy," *Experimental and Therapeutic Medicine*, vol. 3, no. 4, pp. 683–688, 2012.

[7] E. Dogan, M. Celiloglu, E. Sarihan, and A. Demir, "Anesthetic effect of intrauterine lidocaine plus naproxen sodium in endometrial biopsy.," *Obstetrics & Gynecology*, vol. 103, no. 2, pp. 347–351, 2004.

[8] M. P. Trolice, C. Fishburne, and S. McGrady, "Anesthetic efficacy of intrauterine lidocaine for endometrial biopsy: a randomized double-masked trial," *Obstetrics & Gynecology*, vol. 95, no. 3, pp. 345–347, 2000.

[9] M. Güney, B. Oral, and T. Mungan, "Intrauterine lidocaine plus buccal misoprostol in the endometrial biopsy," *International Journal of Gynecology and Obstetrics*, vol. 97, no. 2, pp. 125–128, 2007.

[10] E. Olad-Saheb-Madarek, M. Ghojazaeh, F. Behjati, and H. Alikhah, "The effect of different local anesthesia methods on pain relief in outpatient endometrial biopsy: randomized clinical trial," *J Caring Sci*, vol. 2, p. 211, 2013.

[11] M. A. Sargin, M. Yassa, A. Celik, E. Ergun, and N. Tug, "Lidocaine and tenoxicam effectiveness for pain relief during pipelle: Non-randomised double-blind placebo-controlled trial," *Journal of the Pakistan Medical Association*, vol. 67, no. 4, pp. 527–533, 2017.

[12] A. Guler, H. G. Sahin, Z. Kucukaydin, and E. Erdemoglu, "Comparison of the efficacy of intrauterine lidocaine, paracervical block and oral etodolac for decreasing pain in endometrial biopsy," *Journal of the Turkish German Gynecological Association*, vol. 11, no. 4, pp. 178–181, 2010.

26

Patient Satisfaction with Spanish Pain Centers: Observational Study with More than 3,000 Patients

Juan Antonio García García,[1] Patricia Hernández-Puiggròs,[2] Javier Tesedo Nieto,[3] María Pilar Acín Lázaro,[4] Alfredo Carrera González,[3] Miguel José Arranz Soler,[4] and Sergio Maldonado Vega[5]

[1]*Pain Unit, Hospital Infanta Cristina, 28981 Madrid, Spain*
[2]*Pain Unit, Hospital Son Llàtzer, 07198 Palma de Mallorca, Spain*
[3]*Pain Unit, Hospital Clínico Universitario de Valladolid, 47003 Valladolid, Spain*
[4]*Pain Unit, Hospital Royo Villanova, 50015 Zaragoza, Spain*
[5]*Pain Unit, Hospital Universitario Marqués de Valdecilla, 39008 Santander, Spain*

Correspondence should be addressed to Juan Antonio García García; jagarciag@salud.madrid.org

Academic Editor: Giustino Varrassi

Chronic pain is a serious problem in Spain. This multicenter, epidemiological 3-month follow-up study investigates pain management efficacy in Spanish centers using patient satisfaction criteria. 3,414 eligible adult patients (65,6% female) with moderate to severe chronic pain from 146 pain centers were included. Patient satisfaction was assessed based onto question 18 of Spanish healthcare barometer-CSI. Pain evolution (Brief Pain Inventory-Short Form (BPI-SF) and visual analog scale (VAS)), quality of life/EuroQol-5, and pain control expectations fulfillment were also assessed. Mean age was 61.3 years. 64.4% of participating centers employed multidisciplinary pain management approach. After 3 months, mean patient satisfaction was 7.8 (1–10) on the CIS barometer. Medical staff received the highest scores, whereas waiting for tests, appointment request to appointment date time, and waiting times at the center the lowest. Mean pain decreased from 7.4 to 4.0; BPI-SF intensity decreased from 6.5 to 3.8; pain control expectations were met in 78.7% of patients; EuroQoL-5D utility index increased from 0.37 to 0.62, $p < 0.001$, and health status (VAS) from 40.6 to 61.9, $p < 0.001$. Chronic pain patients (90%) are satisfied with Spanish centers care; 80% had their pain control expectations met. Quality of life improved remarkably: 71% felt moderately to significantly better. However, waiting times need improvement.

1. Introduction

Chronic pain is a serious public health problem in Spain. It has a prevalence of 23.4% in the Spanish general population and important health and economic repercussions [1]. The 1-year prevalence of neck, low back pain, and migraine in Spain is 19.5%, 19.9%, and 11.02%, respectively [2, 3], whereas the prevalence of incapacitating musculoskeletal pain is 6.4% [4]. All the above pain conditions occur more frequent in women than men and are associated with worse health status, depression, and other comorbidities [2, 3, 5]. Chronic pain is also very prevalent among cancer patients, ranging from 33% to 64% according to disease stage [6] and becomes a long-standing issue in many occasions [7, 8]. In a high proportion of chronic pain cases, 33% of cancer patients with pain and 46% of patients with noncancer pain in primary care [9–11], pain is neuropathic (NP) in origin. These patients with NP have the highest prevalence of insomnia, anxiety, depression, severity of pain, and also the highest healthcare-related costs among all the patients with chronic pain [12, 13].

Controlling pain becomes increasingly difficult as pain becomes chronic [14]. In addition to its association with other psychiatric and physical comorbidities (anxiety, depression, insomnia, etc.) [15], pain has an important emotional component and is associated with negative affection states, such as fear [16–18]. Moreover, cultural and environmental influences and stimuli may also affect the perception of pain [19]. Taking into account all these factors, chronic pain patients could benefit by having their condition managed in a specialized pain centers [18, 20–22], where, in addition to classical analgesic treatments, cognitive-behavioral treatments may be employed [23].

Inappropriate pain management is associated not only with increased patient suffering but also with great financial costs, in terms of loss of work time, reduced levels of productivity, and ability to function in society [24]. In Spain, previous studies have shown that a large percentage of the resources allocated by the National Health Service to fund physical treatment for back, neck, and shoulder pain in private practices are spent on treatments proven to be ineffective, or there is no clear evidence that they offer any benefits to the patients [25].

However, studies on the efficacy of pain centers or pain units in Spain are scarce.

Information regarding the effectiveness of pain management is based more on experience from routine clinical practices rather than on studies measuring the efficacy of a single drug treatment or therapeutic intervention [26]. Patient-reported outcomes (PROs) include any outcomes based on data provided by the patients and are very important for understanding the impact of treatment on patient functioning and wellbeing [27]. Healthcare results are measured in terms of satisfaction with the achieved outcome and in the literature there are studies on patient satisfaction with hospitalization or follow-up visits. On the other hand, there are hardly any studies on patient satisfaction with medical outcomes, which can be better related to clinical use [28].

The high prevalence of chronic pain with its associated allocation of resources and corresponding economic impact justifies the need to assess the effectiveness of patient management in the Spanish pain centers. Measurement of patient satisfaction was the selected method to evaluate the centers in terms of effectiveness and to identify existing gaps in management that could be further analyzed and improved.

2. Methods

A 3-month follow-up prospective, longitudinal, multicenter, descriptive, and epidemiological study was conducted among the participating Spanish pain centers. Pain observational studies in general have short follow-up times. A 3-month follow-up time was considered sufficient for valid conclusions. Patients' degree of satisfaction with such centers was assessed by means of a questionnaire, based onto the question 18 of the Spanish healthcare barometer or CIS barometer, which is related to the healthcare service. As secondary objective, we assessed the evolution of pain, according to the Brief Pain Inventory-Short Form (BPI-SF) and to a visual analog scale (VAS), and the quality of life (QoL) as well, according to EuroQol-5, in patients followed up in the pain units.

The target pain, as estimated by the participating researchers, was 2.2 based on a VAS. The target pain of 2.2 is the median value calculated for each patient by the participating physicians, according to the clinical condition of the patient and the experience of the physician. In addition, the following variables were assessed: patient satisfaction with pain control by means of a VAS, patient global clinical impression of change (PGCI-C), and compliance with patients expectations regarding pain control, based on the Patients Expectations Questionnaire (PEQ) [29].

2.1. Study Design. The study protocol was carried out in accordance with the declaration of Helsinki (Seoul, 2008). Spanish regulations were taken into account as well, including approvals by the Ethics Committee for Clinical Research of the University Hospital of Getafe (registration number E-08/018), and all other relevant Ethics Committees, as it was deemed necessary for the evaluation of the patients.

One hundred and seventy-three investigators from 146 centers throughout the Spanish national territory participated in the study. To avoid selection bias, inclusion and exclusion criteria were established. The inclusion criteria in the study were as follows: every participating researcher recruited the first 10 to 30 adult patients over the age of 18 that visited the outpatient during the agreed study period. The pain intensity was ≥ 4 (according to a 1–10 VAS), and the patients were visiting the pain center for the first time. Pain referrals (somatic, visceral, and neuropathic) from all clinical specialties, all social backgrounds, and working status were included (Table 1). Informed consent was obtained from all participating patients. The exclusion criterion was psychiatric or neurologic disorders, which could affect the patient perception of pain, as it was judged by the treating physician assessment. Patients were enrolled in the study from September 2011 to March 2012. The follow-up period ended in June 2012.

The following data were collected: medical specialties and analgesic techniques available at the pain unit; sociodemographic and clinical data of the patients, including pain origin, types of pain, and baseline pain, which was classified as moderate-intense (VAS < 7) and very intense (VAS ≥ 7). In addition, the following data were also collected at 3 months: intensity of pain and its impact on activities of everyday living (BPI-SF); current pain intensity (VAS) as assessed by the physician; quality of life (EuroQoL-5). At the 3-month follow-up visit, the following data were collected: patient satisfaction with pain control (VAS), fulfillment of expectations regarding pain control (PEQ), patient's impression of change in pain (PGCI-C), and patient satisfaction with the pain unit (CIS barometer).

The mean pain intensity (VAS) and total pain interference reductions were divided into two variable categories (mean pain reduction $<30\%$ and $\geq 30\%$ and pain interference reduction $<30\%$ and $\geq 30\%$), according to the percentage of change, following the definition of "moderately important improvement" by the Initiative on Methods, Measurement, and Pain Assessment in Clinical Trials (IMMPACT) group [30]. This group has defined the parameters and outcomes, which should be assessed in chronic pain clinical trials

TABLE 1: Baseline sociodemographic and clinical characteristics of the patients.

	N = 3,414
Women	2,239 (65.6)
Age	61.3 ± 14.4
Current pain (VAS)	7.4 ± 1.5
Referral from	
Primary care	768 (22.5)
Rheumatology	284 (8.3)
Traumatology	1,387 (40.6)
Internal medicine	79 (2.3)
Neurosurgery	306 (9.0)
Rehabilitation	221 (6.5)
Surgery	73 (2.1)
Other	296 (8.7)
Living	
Alone	425 (12.4)
With family member	2,878 (84.3)
Nursery home	71 (2.1)
Other	40 (1.2)
Care required from a third party	748 (22.0)
Ambulance use for medical visits	148 (4.3)
Working status	
Able to work	801 (23.5)
Retired	1,672 (49.0)
Unable to work	452 (13.2)
Medical leave of absence	488 (14.3)
*Pain origin**	
Somatic	2,681 (78.5)
Visceral	81 (2.4)
Neuropathic	1,996 (58.5)
Pain type	
Arthrosis/arthritis	1,867 (55.6)
Hernia/disc pathology	1,435 (42.8)
Neuropathy	527 (15.7)
Osteoporosis	456 (13.6)
Myofascial pain syndrome	418 (12.5)
Other	126 (3.8)
Visceral pain	61 (1.8)
Vascular pain	62 (1.8)
Failed back surgery syndrome	47 (1.4)
Other postsurgical pains	37 (1.1)
Vertebral compression fracture	27 (0.8)
Other posttrauma pains	25 (0.7)
Current health status as compared to last 12 months	
Better	126 (3.7)
Same	788 (23.1)
Worse	2,499 (73.2)

*Multiple answer question. Data expressed as n (%) or mean ± SD.

(pain, physical functioning, emotional functioning, participant ratings of improvement and satisfaction with treatment, symptoms and adverse events, and participant disposition), and provided the relevant recommendations to determine the clinical importance of change in these outcome measurements. Regarding pain intensity, assessed by a 0 to 10 numerical rating scale, a 10–20% decrease in pain intensity was considered as a minimally important improvement, a decrease ≥30% as a moderately important improvement, and a decrease ≥50% as a substantial improvement according to the main IMMPACT outcome recommendations [30].

2.2. Scales and Questionnaires. The Spanish healthcare barometer or CIS barometer is an annual opinion survey conducted since 1995 by the Spanish Ministry of Health (Ministerio de Sanidad y Política Social) in collaboration with the Sociological Investigation Center (CIS). Its purpose is to understand the general public perception of the public healthcare services (whether they have used them or not) [31]. The patients' degree of satisfaction with several aspects of the specialist healthcare service is presented through the answers to question 18 in 2012 [32]. In the current study, the barometer was exclusively used to measure the satisfaction of the participating chronic pain patients with the pain centers, where they were being treated, by answering all the items of question 18. Question 18 has 12 items, and each one of them should be valued by giving a score from 1 (completely unsatisfied) to 10 (totally satisfied). An average score ≥6 is considered a satisfied patient, based on data from the barometer in 2009. Usage of the barometer's data allows for a median satisfaction score of 6.35 to be calculated by averaging all the achieved median public satisfaction for the tested services [31]. Thus, the patient satisfaction with the pain unit was classified as a two-variable parameter: satisfied (score ≥ 6) and not satisfied (score < 6).

The Brief Pain Inventory (BPI) [33, 34] is a self-administered tool to assess the intensity of pain and its impact on activities in everyday living. The Spanish version has been validated [35]. The short form, which contains 11 items, was used in a recent study by de Andrés Ares et al. [36]. The items are rated on a 0 (no pain/no interference) to 10 (worst possible pain/total interference) numeric rating scale (NRS) and are grouped in two categories: pain intensity (the mean score of the first 4 items: worst, least, and average pain in the past 24 hours and pain right now) and interference with daily activities (the mean score of the last 7 items: interference with general activity, mood, walking ability, normal work, relations with others, sleep, and enjoyment of life). Pain intensity is classified as mild or no pain (0–3), moderate (4–6), and intense (≥7).

The EuroQoL-5D (EQ-5D) is a standardized, non-disease-specific instrument for describing and valuing health-related quality of life [37]. The use of the validated Spanish version [38] was approved by the EuroQoL Group Foundation. This instrument rates mobility, self-care, usual activities, pain/discomfort, and anxiety/depression and employs three severity levels (1 means no problem, 2 means some or moderate problems, and 3 means many problems). The different combinations of the EQ-D's 5 valued items provide 243 possible health status possibilities. The levels 2 (some or moderate problems) and 3 (many problems) were grouped together as "problems," as opposed to level 1 or "no problem." There is also a 100 mm VAS with two scale ends: the worst (0 or equivalent to death) and the best imaginable health status (100), where the patient indicates the perception of his own overall health. Another parameter of the EQ-5D is the index of social preference values, obtained for each health status from the overall population studies. The index varies from 1 (best health status possible) to 0 (death), although negative values exist corresponding to health status considered as worse than death.

The patient global clinical impression of change (PGCI-C) [39] is a self-administered scale assessing the experienced change in pain from no change to a great deal better.

The Patients Expectations Questionnaire (PEQ) [29] gathers information related to the fulfilled patients' expectations, scoring five entities regarding hospitalization. In the current study, the fulfillment of patients' expectations was focused on pain control. The possible answers were "as expected, somewhat or much more than expected, somewhat or much less than expected."

2.3. Statistical Analysis. Descriptive statistics were performed for every variable, including central and dispersion measurements for continuous variables, and absolute and relative frequencies for categorical variables, with 95% confidence intervals (CIs), at baseline, 1 month, and 3 months. Missing data were not included in the analyses and were considered as lost.

Continuous variables were compared between baseline and 3 months by means of the Student's t-test in case of parametric data. Categorical variables were compared by the chi-square test or by nonparametric tests (Fisher exact test, U Mann-Whitney, Wilcoxon, etc.) for parametric and nonparametric data, respectively. For the main and secondary variables, the effect size, comparing 3 months versus baseline, was calculated according to the Cohen formula [40], using the pooled standard deviation as the denominator of the equation. Logistic regression analyses were performed to assess putative factors (sex, age, and baseline pain) that might be associated with the satisfaction with the pain unit.

Statistical tests were performed with a bilateral 0.05 significance level. The SPSS software version 17.0 was used for the statistical analyses.

3. Results

Out of 3,507 patients initially enrolled, 93 patients were excluded: for 74 of them, there was no data available and 19 patients did not comply with the inclusion criteria. Out of the 3,414 eligible patients, 3,127 (91.6%) completed the study, 6 patients died, 7 withdrew their consent, 14 were discharged, 63 were lost to follow-up, and 197 did not complete the study due to other reasons (Figure 1).

Every Spanish region (Autonomous Community) had at least one pain center. Out of the 146 participating pain centers, 64.4% were multidisciplinary (more than one specialty) and 37% had at least three different specialties. In multidisciplinary pain units, medical staff from various specialties (anesthetists, psychologists, and physiotherapists) is involved in the pain management. Regarding available techniques, the most commonly used in almost every center is nerve blocking (96.6%), followed by TENS (83.6%), while spinal stimulation is provided in 50% of pain centers. Almost half of the centers (47.9%) had both spinal stimulation and intrathecal therapy techniques. One-third of the centers had every available pain controlling technique (Figure 2(b)).

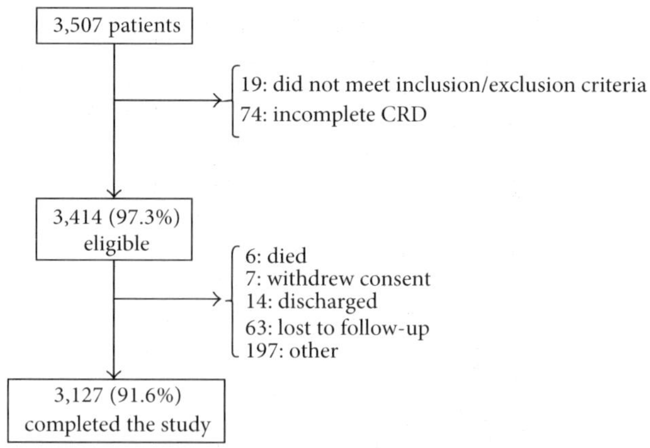

Figure 1: Patients flow chart.

Patients mean age was 61.3 years and 65.6% were female (Table 1). They were referred to the pain centers mostly from traumatology (40.6%), followed by primary care (22.5%). Most lived together with a family member (84.3%) and 22% required third-party care. Almost half of the patients were retired. About three-quarters of the patients experienced worse health status during the study period compared to the previous 12 months. Most pain was mixed in origin, and visceral pain was rare (2.4%). Main types of pain were arthritic/arthritis (55.6%) and hernia/disc pathology (42.8%). Mean pain intensity was 7.4 and the participating investigators targeted the pain intensity down to 2.2, which is, as it was mentioned earlier, the median value calculated for each patient by the participating physicians, according to the clinical condition of the patient and the experience of the physician. The most frequent areas of intense pain were the posterior lumbar (47%) and posterior sacral areas: center (49.8%), left side (44.9%), and right side (44.4%), followed by the posterior upper leg (41.6%) area.

3.1. Patient Satisfaction with the Pain Center. After three months of care, mean patient satisfaction with the pain center, as assessed by the CIS barometer, was 7.8, with more than 90% of the patients being satisfied (Table 2). The items with the highest scores were those related to the treating physicians and overall healthcare personnel, followed by the equipment and technology available at the center, while the items with the lowest scores were the waiting times for the diagnostic tests, from medical appointment request to appointment date and at the center to see the doctor, which compare similarly with the data from question 18 of the CIS barometer from 1995 to 2012 (Table 4).

3.2. Secondary Objectives. At three months, baseline mean pain (VAS) decreased from 7.4 to 4.0 (Table 3), and 67.4% of patients showed a mean decrease of pain intensity of at least 30% (data not shown). Accordingly, BPI-SF intensity summary also decreased from 6.5 to 3.8, while the percentage of patients feeling pain relief in the last 24 hours due to received treatment increased from 29.1% to 60.9%. The

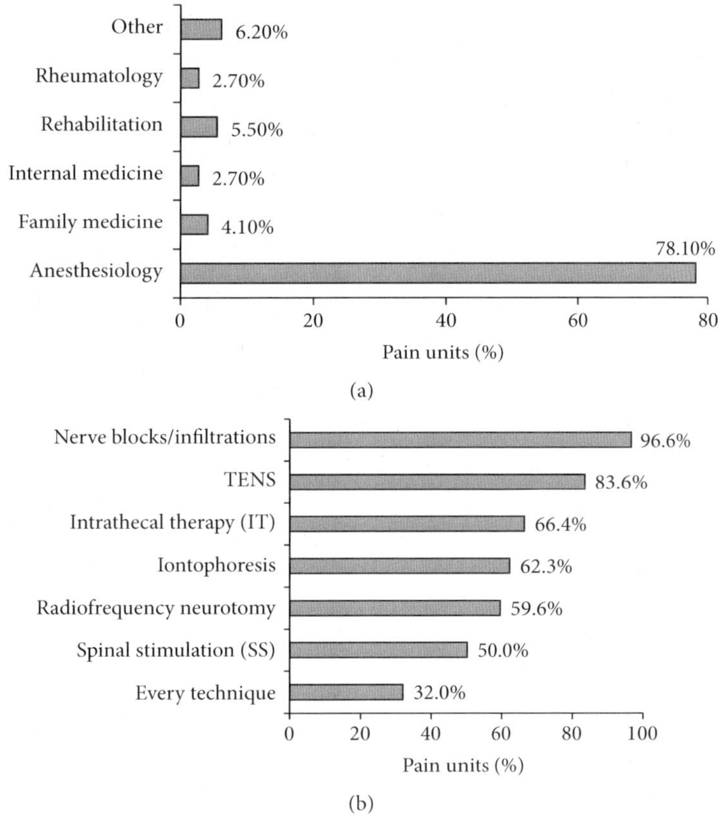

FIGURE 2: Specialties (a) and techniques (b) available in the pain centers.

TABLE 2: Patient satisfaction with the pain center at 3 months (PC) and satisfaction with the Spanish healthcare specialists' service (SH) in 2012.

Items	PC	SH 2012
Time spent by the physician with you	**8.6 ± 1.3**	6.72 ± 2.00
Number of specialists to whom you have access	7.6 ± 1.8	7.64 ± 1.82
Waiting time at the center until seeing the doctor	6.9 ± 2.2	5.72 ± 2.11
Knowledge of your medical history and follow-up of your health-related problems	**8.3 ± 1.4**	6.83 ± 2.04
Confidence and trust in your doctor	**8.6 ± 1.3**	7.29 ± 2.01
Easiness to get an appointment	7.0 ± 2.3	5.72 ± 2.47
Equipment and technological means available at the center	8.0 ± 1.6	7.54 ± 1.75
Manners of healthcare personnel	**8.7 ± 1.2**	7.42 ± 1.80
Information received about your health problem	**8.4 ± 1.4**	7.30 ± 1.95
Medical advice on diet, exercise, smoking, alcohol, and so forth	8.0 ± 1.6	7.13 ± 2.17
Time from medical appointment request to appointment date	6.9 ± 2.2	4.94 ± 2.39
Time taken by the diagnostic tests	6.5 ± 2.2	5.04 ± 2.38
Total satisfaction*	7.8 ± 1.2	
Not satisfied (<6)	200 (8.4%)	
Satisfied (≥6)	2,168 (91.6%)	

Sanitary barometer 2012 (total, three waves). Executive management of public health, quality, and innovation. Ministry of Health, Social Services and Equality and Sociological Investigation Center (CIS), Madrid, 2013.
*Average score of the 12 items.
Data expressed as mean ± SD (continuous variables) or *n* (%) (categorical variables).
Scores ranging from 0 (no satisfaction at all) to 10 (completely satisfied).
In bold: scores above 8.0.

interference summary decreased from 44.8 to 26.4, and 63% of patients showed a pain interference reduction of at least 30% (data not shown).

In addition, 70.7% of patients at three months felt moderately to much better, according to the PGCI (Figure 3), and mean satisfaction with pain control was 6.6 ± 2.2 in a visual analog scale (data not shown). Most patients (78.7%) felt that their expectations regarding pain control since their first visit to the pain center had been met as expected or more (Figure 4).

TABLE 3: Evolution of pain (VAS and BPI-SF) and quality of life (EuroQoL-5D).

	Baseline	3 months	p value
Current pain (VAS)	7.4 ± 1.5	4 ± 1.9	—
BPI-SF			
BPI-SF intensity summary	6.5 ± 1.4	3.8 ± 1.9	—
Pain relief in the last 24 h by received treatment (%)	29.1% ± 19.9%	60.9% ± 22.7%	—
BPI-SF interference summary	44.8 ± 12.5	26.4 ± 15.1	—
EuroQoL-5D			
Utility index	0.37 ± 0.21	0.62 ± 0.22	<0.001
Today's health status (VAS)	40.7 ± 20.1	61.9 ± 19.3	<0.001
Patients with problems (2 and 3) in			
Mobility	2,805 (82.2)	2,127 (65.9)	—
Self-care	2,194 (64.2)	1,224 (37.9)	—
Usual activities	3,142 (92.0)	2,091 (64.8)	—
Pain/discomfort	3,389 (99.3)	2,657 (82.4)	—
Anxiety/depression	2,650 (77.6)	1,415 (43.9)	—

Data expressed as mean ± SD for continuous variables and as n (%) for categorical variables.

TABLE 4: Data from question 18 of the CIS barometer from 1995 to 2012.

Items	1995	1998	2000*	2002*	2004*	2006*	2008*	2010	2012
Time spent by the physician with you	6.51	6.45	6.39*	5.69*	6.20*	6.23*	6.18*	6.50	6.72
Number of specialists to whom you have access	7.55	7.62	7.56	6.80*	7.40*	7.31*	7.28*	7.47	7.64
Waiting time at the center until seeing the doctor	5.79	5.77	5.62*	4.99*	5.30*	5.32*	5.40*	5.60	5.72
Knowledge of your medical history and follow-up of your health-related problems	6.71	6.69	6.61*	5.86*	6.40*	6.41*	6.41*	6.64	6.83
Confidence and trust in your doctor	7.17	7.09	7.08*	6.35*	6.90*	6.90*	6.97*	7.13	7.29
Easiness to get an appointment	5.49	5.39	5.26*	4.89*	5.20*	5.27*	5.32*	5.60	5.72
Equipment and technological means available at the center	7.69	7.78	7.69	6.88*	7.20*	7.20*	7.24*	7.40	7.54
Manners of healthcare personnel	7.56	7.44	7.37*	6.63*	7.06*	7.11*	7.09*	7.20	7.42
Information received about your health problem	7.14	7.20	7.16	6.38*	6.94*	6.94*	6.94*	7.13	7.30
Medical advice on diet, exercise, smoking, alcohol, and so forth	—	—	—	—	6.60	6.78	6.79	6.98	7.13
Time from medical appointment request to appointment date	—	—	—	—	4.70	4.68	4.67	4.89	4.94
Time taken by the diagnostic tests	—	—	—	—	—	4.73	4.65	4.87	5.04

Sanitary barometer 1995–2012. Healthcare Information Institute. Ministry of Health, Social Services and Equality Madrid, 2013.
Only the year 1995 and years ending in even number are shown.
*Scores lower than preceding years.

Regarding quality of life, the EuroQoL-5D utility index increased from 0.37 to 0.62, $p < 0.001$ (effect size $d = 1.19$) and the health status (VAS) from 40.6 to 61.9, $p < 0.001$ (effect size $d = 1.1$) (Table 3). Eighty-two percent and 79% of patients improved in EuroQoL VAS and utility index, respectively (Figures 5(a) and 5(b)), while the proportion of patients with problems (level 2 or 3) decreased across all 5 parameters at three months (Figure 5(c)).

Logistic regression analysis showed that patient satisfaction with the pain unit (satisfied VAS ≥ 6 and not satisfied VAS < 6) was affected ($p < 0.005$) by the baseline pain intensity (moderate-intense VAS < 7 and very intense VAS ≥ 7).

4. Discussion

Chronic pain is a complex psychosocial entity, whose management can be very challenging [14]. Its impact on quality of life can be extremely negative [18]. Chronic pain can result in depressed mood, poor-quality or nonrestorative sleep, fatigue, reduced activity and libido, excessive use of drugs and

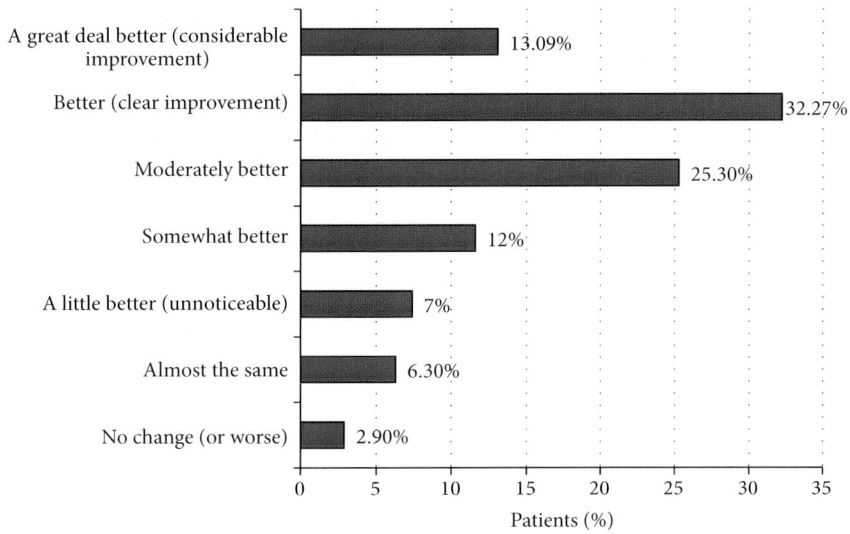

FIGURE 3: Patients global clinical impression (PGCI) of the change at month 3.

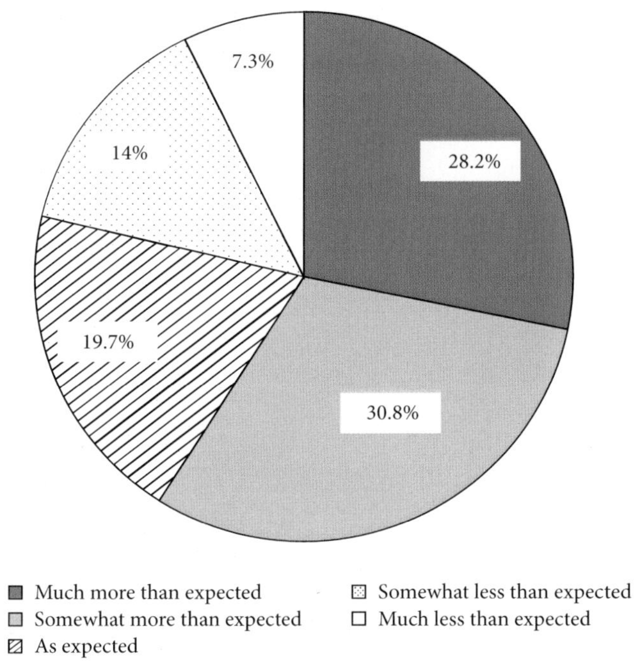

FIGURE 4: Pain control degree according to patients' expectations.

alcohol, dependent behavior, and disability out of proportion with impairment. This combination of chronic pain and the resultant problems is what we call Chronic Pain Syndrome (CPS).

A recent European survey on noncancer chronic pain showed poor management of the condition in Spain, with more than half of patients (55%) not being satisfied with their treatment [41]. However, the current study, conducted in 146 pain centers distributed along the Spanish national territory, has shown that more than 90% of patients were satisfied with the care provided by the pain centers.

In 64% of the centers, a multidisciplinary approach to the pain management was employed. Patients managed at multidisciplinary pain centers have shown to have better outcomes when compared to those managed by nonmultidisciplinary rehabilitation, usual care, or other strategies [42–48]. Improvement in negative emotional cognitive functions seems to be the key mechanism of the observed change in the multidisciplinary treatment approach of chronic widespread pain [49]. In a study conducted with injured workers of Washington state, patients showed similar clinical outcomes, regardless of their treatment being administered in a pain center or not [50]. However, those patients had experienced more than three years of disability before their admission to the multidisciplinary program. It has been shown that treating chronic pain as early as possible is very important, and prompt treatment following injury is a significant predictor of successful return to work [51].

The most recent data of the Spanish CIS Barometer are those of 2012 [32], showing that 70.6% of the population believes that the Spanish healthcare system works pretty well to well, although some changes are needed. Comparing these general outcomes of 2012 (Table 4), the year in which our study ended, taking into account the findings of our study (Table 2), it can be seen that chronic pain patients are more satisfied with the care received in the Spanish pain centers than the overall public with the care received in the Spanish healthcare specialists services. It is important to take into account that the barometer surveys the overall population, regardless of whether or not they had used the healthcare services.

The 146 pain centers participating in the study were distributed across the entire Spanish territory. Every Spanish region (Autonomous Community) had at least one center, which is an improvement from 2002, when only 11 of the 17 Autonomous Communities had at least one [52]. In addition, 64.4% were multidisciplinary in 2012 versus 53.6% in 2002.

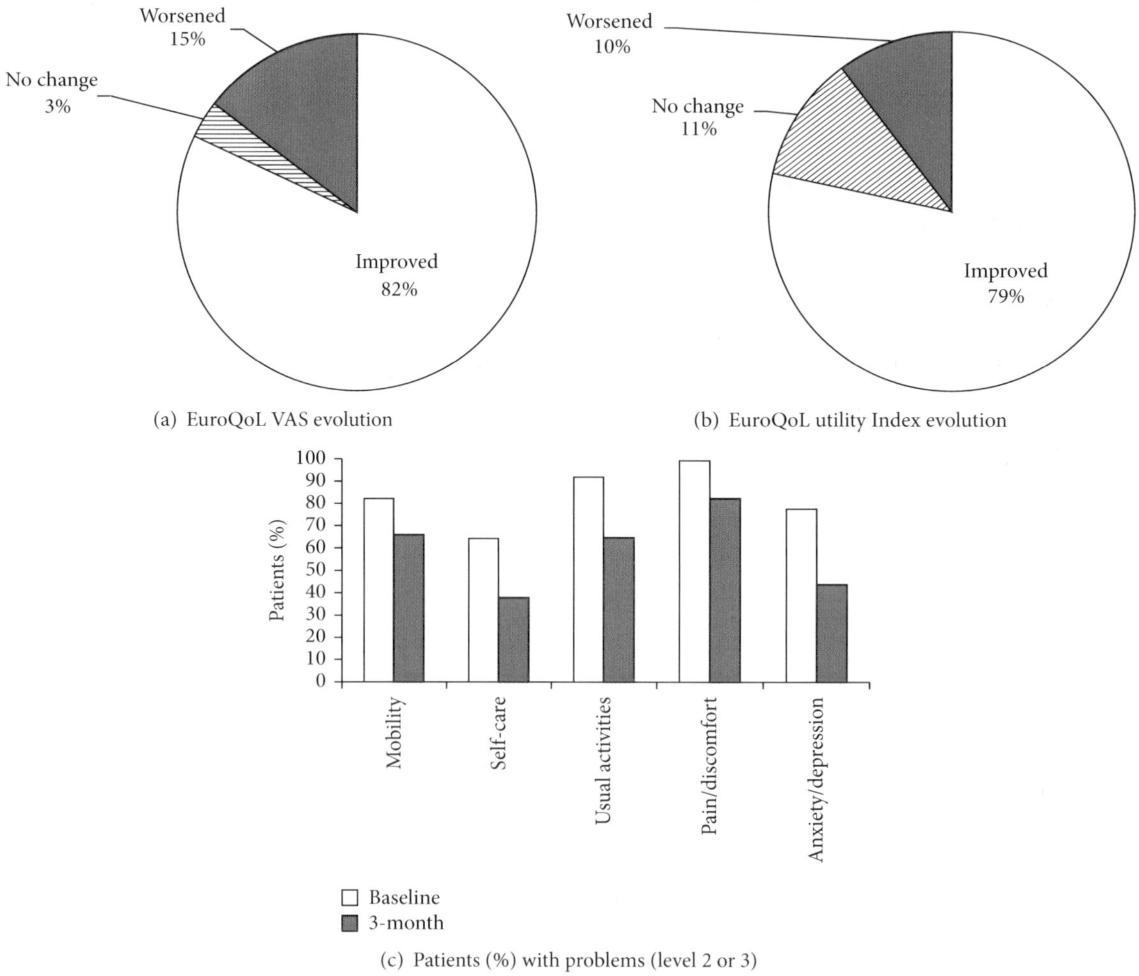

FIGURE 5: Change in EuroQoL VAS (a) and utility index (b) at 3 months and proportion of patients with problems (level 2 or 3) in the EuroQoL dimensions at baseline and 3 months (c).

Patients are satisfied with the management of their painful condition at three months of treatment and studies have shown that the positive effects of the multidisciplinary approach to chronic pain persist long after the cessation of the intervention [53, 54]. It is important to point out that patients were most satisfied with the treating physicians, followed closely by the rest of the personnel. A good interaction between the patient and the service professionals is of great importance for the success of chronic pain rehabilitation [55]. A study by Trentman et al. [56] showed that time spent with the physician, thoroughness, and listening were factors associated with the patient's perception of quality of care. Thoroughness, punctuality, listening, and clear instructions were the drivers of "very good" versus "excellent" patient's perception of the overall provider quality. Such high quality patient-professional relationship has positive repercussions on treatment outcomes in the setting of a multidisciplinary rehabilitation program for chronic pain. In fact, a previous study had also shown that changes in pain was a less important predictor of treatment satisfaction, whereas the patients perception that their evaluation was complete, the satisfaction that they experienced from a detailed and accurate explanation of the therapeutic procedures, and the realization that the treatment helped them to improve their daily activity, were the strongest predictors [57].

On the other hand, the waiting time for the diagnostic tests results, from the clinic appointment date and to actually seeing the doctor once at the center, was the item with which, patients were satisfied the least. Other studies have shown a negative association between waiting time for pain clinic appointment and healthcare system grade [58]. Therefore, improvements in this area could have a significant positive effect on the opinion of patients regarding pain centers.

As expected, there were more female patients than male, since several chronic pain conditions are more prevalent in women [2–4], and, overall, the demographic characteristics of the patients agreed with the Spanish data from the recent European noncancer chronic pain survey [41]. The most frequent location of intense pain (lumbar) corresponded to the low back, which is an extremely common problem that most people experience at some point in their lives [59]. In the European survey, the commonest diagnosis was joint pain (40%), followed by back pain (32%), but patients were recruited and managed mostly by general practitioners and other specialists instead of being treated at pain centers. At three months, not only patients were satisfied with the pain center, but their clinical symptoms had improved significantly in that period of time as well. In fact, almost 80% of patients felt their expectations regarding pain control had been met as expected or more. The pain intensity VAS score decreased from a mean 7.4 to 4.0. Although it did not reach the desired target of 2.2, the mean change (3.4) greatly exceeded the minimal important change, which, by consensus, is 1.5 in patients with low back pain [60]. A previous study conducted with Spanish chronic pain patients suffering motor disability and subjected to an intensive multidisciplinary treatment of 4 weeks in duration showed a similar significant improvement in pain intensity VAS points, from 7.4 to 3.2 ($p < 0.01$) [61].

As it was discussed already BPI-SF intensity summary decreased from 6.5 to 3.8 and interference summary decreased from 44.8 to 26.4. Sixty-three percent of patients showed a pain interference reduction of at least 30%. The BPI-SF is used to evaluate the severity of a patient's pain and the impact of this pain on the patient's daily functioning. The psychometric properties of the tool have been analyzed with acceptable reliability in various populations suffering from cancer and noncancer related pain. Various studies have shown that a two-factor model has better validity for noncancer pain patients [62, 63], as opposed to the three- or one-factor approach.

The quality of life of the patients also improved remarkably as it was tested by the Spanish version of the EQ-5D, which is a simple, valid, and practical measure and can be used as an outcome variable for research purposes and in the allocation of resources. Its ability to discriminate between healthy population and chronic patients is considered to be good [38]. The mean utility index and health status were higher than one standard deviation compared with their respective mean values at baseline; these effect size values (utility index $d = 1.2$ and health status $d = 1.1$) are quite significant, according to Cohen's results for effect size interpretation (large $d \geq 0.80$) [40]. Seventy-one percent of the patients felt moderately to much better (PGCI), which is a higher proportion than the 53% reported among the chronic low back pain patients by a long term study, which also showed that patients are doing better or much better regarding their general wellbeing after completing a multidisciplinary rehabilitation program [53].

Various other studies have shown that in general Spanish patients are satisfied with their pain management. Malouf et al. conducted a study with the aim to document the satisfaction with pain management in a Spanish inpatient population. The study showed that patients were satisfied with the received treatment, even when they were in pain, and that patient dissatisfaction was related to the pain intensity and satisfaction with caregivers [64]. On the other hand, an epidemiology survey of chronic nonmalignant pain in Spain showed that a significant percentage of patients might be inadequately treated. In this survey, it was stated that up to 60% of patients are dissatisfied with their treatment. They concluded that the variability in the collected data reflects an inconsistency in the definition of the condition and the measurement approach to assess its impact [65].

In a survey of chronic pain in Europe across 16 countries (Spain included), interesting differences between countries were observed, possibly because of different cultural backgrounds and local therapeutic preferences. The authors concluded that chronic pain occurs in 19% of adult Europeans with serious effects on the quality of their lives. Only few patients were managed by pain specialists, nearly 50% were treated inadequately and about 60% were satisfied with the effect of treatment [66]. When patients were asked to respond to the question "would you say your pain is being adequately controlled," 33% of the Spanish responders replied "no" and 67% "yes," which compares equally to the findings of this study.

5. Conclusions

In conclusion, chronic pain patients are satisfied with the management provided by Spanish pain centers more than the overall population with the hospital specialist services. Ninety percent of patients were satisfied with the management of their pain. Almost 70% of patients experienced a decrease of their pain intensity and a pain interference reduction of at least 30%. They said that at three months they felt better and that their pain control expectations were met.

There is some area for improvement regarding waiting times: time needed for diagnostic tests, time from medical appointment request to appointment date, and waiting time at the center until seeing the doctor. Waiting time shortening will provide better care to patients and higher rates of satisfaction. Many healthcare institutions use methods like revamping of the front-line scheduling process, incorporation of patient preferences, considering alternate ways of care delivery, and making the reduction of waiting times part of the hospital's culture.

Chronic pain management can have important economic repercussions. Pain management in a multidisciplinary setting may decrease the chronic pain-associated costs, since it can reduce pension expenditures, sick leave days, and usage of healthcare resource. The care provided by the Spanish pain centers seems to be successful, and, thus, although expensive, it might save costs in the long run, which should be the objective of another study.

Disclosure

J. Tesedo Nieto currently works at Hospital Universitario Río Hortega, Valladolid.

Competing Interests

The authors have no relevant affiliations or financial involvement with any organization or entity with interest in or conflict with the subject matter discussed in the paper.

Acknowledgments

The authors would like to thank the participating patients and the study Principal Investigators and Collaborators, listed by states as follows: *A Coruña*: Dr. Carceller, Dr. Cordeiro, and Dra. Ulloa; *Albacete*: Dr. Arcas and Dr. Jiménez; *Alicante*: Dr. Castillo and Dr. García; *Almería*: Dr. Cortiñas and Dr. Salmerón; *Asturias*: Dra. Brid, Dra. Jamart, and Dr. Palacio; *Badajoz*: Dr. Alcántara, Dra. Costillo, and Dr. Rodríguez; *Barcelona*: Dra. Busquets, Dra. Barcelo, Dr. Cordero, Dr. Candela, Dra. Carreras, Dr. De Sanctis, Dr. Echevarria, Dr. Fabo, Dr. Folch, Dra. Ferrándiz, Dr. Guitart, Dra. Landaluze, Dra. Lombán, Dr. López, Dr. Mañero, Dr. Moreno, Dr. Malouf, Dra. Mesas, Dra. Márquez, Dra. Paños, Dra. Ribera, Dra. Sintes, Dr. Tomàs, Dr. Vázquez, Dra. Vargas, and Dra. Vidal; *Cádiz*: Dr. Aragón, Dr. Calderón, Dr. Gómez, Dr. Martínez, Dr. Sánchez, and Dr. Ventura; *Cantabria*: Dr. Sarabia and Dra. Santillán; *Castellón*: Dra. Carro, Dr. Gómez, and Dr. Vila; *Girona*: Dr. Beltrán, Dra. Charry, Dr. Morales, Dra. Mariñansky, and Dra. Samaniego; *Granada*: Dr. Gálvez, Dr. Heredia, Dr. Muñoz, Dr. Maldonado, and Dr. Ruiz; *Guadalajara* Dr. Martínez and Dr. Palomeque; *Guipuzcoa*: Dr. Marín; *Huesca* Dr. Carrión, Dr. García, Dr. Paricio, and Dr. Sánchez; *Illes Balears*: Dr. Carbayo, Dra. Fernández, Dr. Glenny, Dr. Mata, Dr. Mirasol, Dr. Moya, Dra. Peláez, Dr. Salazar, and Dr. Valentí; *La Rioja*: Dr. Saenz; *Las Palmas*: Dra. Medina; *Lugo*: Dra. Alborés; *Lleida*: Dr. Montero and Dra. Matute; *Madrid*: Dra. Aranda, Dra. Acedo, Dra. Álvarez, Dr. Alonso, Dra. Blanco, Dra. Barrantes, Dra. Bedmar, Dra. Castro, Dr. Del Saz, Dra. Díaz, Dr. Estrada, Dra. Fernández, Dra. Guinaldo, Dr. García, Dr. González, Dra. Infante, Dr. Leal, Dra. López, Dra. Llaurado, Dr. Manzano, Dr. Ortega, Dra. Pérez, Dr. Puente, Dr. Ruiz, Dra. Ruiz, Dra. Riquelme, Dr. Sante, Dra. Solera, Dr. Vidal, Dra. Wojcikiewicz, and Dra. Zueras; *Málaga*: Dr. Aldaya, Dra. Del Valle, Dr. Fernández, Dr. González, Dr. Herva, Dra. Márquez, and Dra. Otero; *Murcia*: Dr. Alfaro, Dr. Giménez, Dr. Mendoza; *Navarra*: Dr. Ayechu, Dr. Ceberio, and Dr. Rotinen; *Ourense*: Dra. Cánovas and Dra. Gómez; *Pontevedra*: Dr. Cruces, Dr. Carregal, Dra. Cabanas, Dra. Corujeira, Dra. Fernández, Dr. Illodo, Dr. Refojos, and Dr. Sobrino; *Salamanca*: Dr. Santos; *Santa Cruz De Tenerife*: Dr. De Moraga, Dra. Oliva, Dra. Ruiz, Dr. Santos, and Dr. Walter; *Sevilla*: Dr. Bordas, Dr. Campuzano, Dr. Cobos, Dra. De La Calle, and Dr. Torres; *Tarragona*: Dr. Fuentes, Dr. Fos, Dra. Ferre, Dra. Gómez, and Dra. Roca; *Teruel*: Dra. Escartín; *Toledo*: Dr. Cid, Dr. Díaz, Dr. De Andrés, Dra. Gómez-Caro, Dra. López, and Dra. Penide; *Valencia*: Dr. Alegre, Dr. Arriete, Dr. Alcañiz, Dra. Bononad, Dr. Castillo, Dr. Chisbert, Dra. Canos, Dr. De La Cruz, Dr. Domingo, Dr. Escuder, Dr. Fenollosa, Dr. Fenollosa, Dr. Gómez-Cambronero, Dra. Izquierdo, Dr. Ibor, Dr. Moreno, Dr. Muñoz, Dr. Mora, Dra. Muñoz, Dr. Orovitg, Dr. Pérez, Dr. Sánchez, Dr. Santamaría, and Dr. Zavala; *Valladolid*: Dr. Alonso, Dr. Hernández, and Dr. Vaca; *Vizcaya*: Dr. Alava, Dra. Callejo, Dr. Castresana, Dr. Duruelo, Dra. Gómez, Dra. Lasuen, Dra. López, Dra. Mozas, Dr. Ortiz, Dra. Ortiz, Dra. Torralba, Dr. Torre, and Dra. Urtusagasti; *Zaragoza*: Dr. Cía, Dr. García, Dr. Navarro, Dra. Peralta, and Dr. Quero. The authors would also like to acknowledge Susana Traseira for participating in the study design, Nuria Pajuelo and Alfonso Casado for performing statistical analysis, Lorenzo Domínguez for organizational assistance, and Almudena Pardo for medical writing. This work was funded by Mundipharma Pharmaceuticals S.L.

References

[1] E. Català, E. Reig, M. Artés, L. Aliaga, J. S. López, and J. L. Segú, "Prevalence of pain in the Spanish population: telephone survey in 5000 homes," *European Journal of Pain*, vol. 6, no. 2, pp. 133–140, 2002.

[2] C. Fernández-de-las-Peñas, V. Hernández-Barrera, C. Alonso-Blanco et al., "Prevalence of neck and low back pain in community-dwelling adults in Spain: a population-based national study," *Spine*, vol. 36, no. 3, pp. E213–E219, 2011.

[3] C. Fernández-de-Las-peñas, V. Hernández-Barrera, P. Carrasco-Garrido et al., "Population-based study of migraine in Spanish adults: relation to socio-demographic factors, lifestyle and co-morbidity with other conditions," *Journal of Headache and Pain*, vol. 11, no. 2, pp. 97–104, 2010.

[4] S. Jiménez-Sánchez, R. Jiménez-García, V. Hernández-Barrera, M. Villanueva-Martínez, A. Ríos-Luna, and C. Fernández-de-las-Peñas, "Has the prevalence of invalidating musculoskeletal pain changed over the last 15 years (1993–2006)? A Spanish population-based survey," *The Journal of Pain*, vol. 11, no. 7, pp. 612–620, 2010.

[5] S. Jiménez-Sánchez, C. Fernández-de-las-Peñas, P. Carrasco-Garrido et al., "Prevalence of chronic head, neck and low back pain and associated factors in women residing in the Autonomous Region of Madrid (Spain)," *Gaceta Sanitaria*, vol. 26, no. 6, pp. 534–540, 2012.

[6] M. H. J. van den Beuken-van Everdingen, J. M. de Rijke, A. G. Kessels, H. C. Schouten, M. van Kleef, and J. Patijn, "Prevalence of pain in patients with cancer: a systematic review of the past 40 years," *Annals of Oncology*, vol. 18, no. 9, pp. 1437–1449, 2007.

[7] A. W. Burton, G. J. Fanciullo, R. D. Beasley, and M. J. Fisch, "Chronic pain in the cancer survivor: a new frontier," *Pain Medicine*, vol. 8, no. 2, pp. 189–198, 2007.

[8] V. Sun, T. Borneman, B. Piper, M. Koczywas, and B. Ferrell, "Barriers to pain assessment and management in cancer survivorship," *Journal of Cancer Survivorship*, vol. 2, no. 1, pp. 65–71, 2008.

[9] M. L. Garcia de Paredes, F. del Moral González, P. M. del Prado et al., "First evidence of oncologic neuropathic pain prevalence after screening 8615 cancer patients. Results of the on study," *Annals of Oncology*, vol. 22, no. 4, pp. 924–930, 2011.

[10] C. Garzón-Rodríguez, L. Lyras, L. O. Gayoso et al., "Cancer-related neuropathic pain in out-patient oncology clinics: a European survey," *BMC Palliative Care*, vol. 12, no. 1, article 41, 2013.

[11] E. Blanco, R. Galvez, E. Zamorano, V. López, and M. Pérez, "Prevalence of neuropathic pain according to the NP4 test in primary care," *Semergen*, vol. 38, no. 4, pp. 203–210, 2012.

[12] P. C. Langley, C. Van Litsenburg, J. C. Cappelleri, and D. Carroll, "The burden associated with neuropathic pain in Western Europe," *Journal of Medical Economics*, vol. 16, no. 1, pp. 85–95, 2013.

[13] C. O. Schmidt, B. Schweikert, C. M. Wenig et al., "Modelling the prevalence and cost of back pain with neuropathic components in the general population," *European Journal of Pain*, vol. 13, no. 10, pp. 1030–1035, 2009.

[14] M. C. Bushnell, M. Čeko, and L. A. Low, "Cognitive and emotional control of pain and its disruption in chronic pain," *Nature Reviews Neuroscience*, vol. 14, no. 7, pp. 502–511, 2013.

[15] P. Alföldi, T. Wiklund, and B. Gerdle, "Comorbid insomnia in patients with chronic pain: a study based on the Swedish quality registry for pain rehabilitation (SQRP)," *Disability and Rehabilitation*, vol. 36, no. 20, pp. 1661–1669, 2014.

[16] V. Neugebauer, W. Li, G. C. Bird, and J. S. Han, "The amygdala and persistent pain," *Neuroscientist*, vol. 10, no. 3, pp. 221–234, 2004.

[17] A. Stancak and N. Fallon, "Emotional modulation of experimental pain: a source imaging study of laser evoked potentials," *Frontiers in Human Neuroscience*, vol. 7, article 552, 2013.

[18] T. Ojala, A. Häkkinen, J. Karppinen, K. Sipilä, T. Suutama, and A. Piirainen, "The dominance of chronic pain: a phenomenological study," *Musculoskeletal Care*, vol. 12, no. 3, pp. 141–149, 2015.

[19] B. K. Cheon, D.-M. Im, T. Harada et al., "Cultural modulation of the neural correlates of emotional pain perception: the role of other-focusedness," *Neuropsychologia*, vol. 51, no. 7, pp. 1177–1186, 2013.

[20] B. C. Neher, "Chronic pain intervention: promoting return to function," *Work*, vol. 9, no. 2, pp. 163–175, 1997.

[21] E. J. Messelink, "The pelvic pain centre," *World Journal of Urology*, vol. 19, no. 3, pp. 208–212, 2001.

[22] J. Pergolizzi, K. Ahlbeck, D. Aldington et al., "The development of chronic pain: physiological CHANGE necessitates a multidisciplinary approach to treatment," *Current Medical Research and Opinion*, vol. 29, no. 9, pp. 1127–1135, 2013.

[23] M. den Hollander, J. R. de Jong, S. Volders, M. E. Goossens, R. J. Smeets, and J. W. Vlaeyen, "Fear reduction in patients with chronic pain: a learning theory perspective," *Expert Review of Neurotherapeutics*, vol. 10, no. 11, pp. 1733–1745, 2010.

[24] C. J. Phillips and C. Harper, "The economics associated with persistent pain," *Current Opinion in Supportive and Palliative Care*, vol. 5, no. 2, pp. 127–130, 2011.

[25] P. Serrano-Aguilar, F. Kovacs, J. Cabrera-Hernńndez, J. Ramos-Gõi, and L. García-Pérez, "Avoidable costs of physical treatments for chronic back, neck and shoulder pain within the Spanish National Health Service: a cross-sectional study," *BMC Musculoskeletal Disorders*, vol. 12, article 287, 2011.

[26] C. Bombardier and A. Maetzel, "Pharmacoeconomic evaluation of new treatments: efficacy versus effectiveness studies?" *Annals of the Rheumatic Diseases*, vol. 58, supplement 1, pp. I82–I85, 1999.

[27] C. Acquadro, R. Berzon, D. Dubois et al., "Incorporating the patient's perspective into drug development and communication: an ad hoc task force report of the patient-reported outcomes (PRO) Harmonization Group meeting at the food and drug administration, February 16, 2001," *Value in Health*, vol. 6, no. 5, pp. 522–531, 2003.

[28] J. J. Mira and J. Aranaz, "Patient satisfaction as an outcome measure in health care," *Medicina Clinica*, vol. 114, supplement 3, pp. 26–33, 2000.

[29] J. Pujiula-Masó, R. Suñer-Soler, M. Puigdemont-Guinart et al., "Satisfaction among hospitalized patients as an indicator of quality of care," *Enfermeria Clinica*, vol. 16, no. 1, pp. 19–26, 2006.

[30] D. C. Turk, R. H. Dworkin, R. R. Allen et al., "Core outcome domains for chronic pain clinical trials: IMMPACT recommendations," *Pain*, vol. 106, no. 3, pp. 337–345, 2003.

[31] "Barómetro sanitario," in *Social MdSyP*, Instituto de Información Sanitaria, Madrid, Spain, 2010.

[32] Dirección General de Salud Pública, "Barómetro Sanitario 2012 (Total, tres oleadas)," Ministerio de Sanidad, Servicios Sociales e Igualdad y Centro de Investigaciones Sociológicas (CIS), Madrid, Spain, 2013.

[33] R. L. Daut, C. S. Cleeland, and R. C. Flanery, "Development of the Wisconsin Brief Pain Questionnaire to assess pain in cancer and other diseases," *Pain*, vol. 17, no. 2, pp. 197–210, 1983.

[34] C. S. Cleeland and K. M. Ryan, "Pain assessment: global use of the Brief Pain Inventory," *Annals of the Academy of Medicine Singapore*, vol. 23, no. 2, pp. 129–138, 1994.

[35] X. Badia, C. Muriel, A. Gracia et al., "Validation of the Spanish version of the Brief Pain Inventory in patients with oncological pain," *Medicina Clinica*, vol. 120, no. 2, pp. 52–59, 2003.

[36] J. de Andrés Ares, L. M. Cruces Prado, M. A. Canos Verdecho et al., "Validation of the short form of the brief pain inventory (BPI-SF) in Spanish patients with non-cancer-related pain," *Pain Practice*, vol. 15, no. 7, pp. 643–653, 2015.

[37] R. Brooks, "EuroQol: the current state of play," *Health Policy*, vol. 37, no. 1, pp. 53–72, 1996.

[38] X. Badia, M. Roset, S. Montserrat, M. Herdman, and A. Segura, "The Spanish version of EuroQol: a description and its applications," *Medicina Clínica*, vol. 112, supplement 1, pp. 79–85, 1999.

[39] H. Hurst and J. Bolton, "Assessing the clinical significance of change scores recorded on subjective outcome measures," *Journal of Manipulative and Physiological Therapeutics*, vol. 27, no. 1, pp. 26–35, 2004.

[40] J. Cohen, *Statistical Power Analysis for the Behavioral Sciences*, Lawrence Erlbaum, New Jersey, NJ, USA, 2nd edition, 1988.

[41] C. Pérez, C. Margarit, and M. Serrano, "Survey of European patients assessing their own noncancer chronic pain: results from Spain," *Current Medical Research and Opinion*, vol. 29, no. 6, pp. 643–651, 2013.

[42] N. Becker, P. Sjøgren, P. Bech, A. K. Olsen, and J. Eriksen, "Treatment outcome of chronic non-malignant pain patients managed in a Danish multidisciplinary pain centre compared to general practice: a randomised controlled trial," *Pain*, vol. 84, no. 2-3, pp. 203–211, 2000.

[43] J. Guzmán, R. Esmail, K. Karjalainen, A. Malmivaara, E. Irvin, and C. Bombardier, "Multidisciplinary rehabilitation for chronic low back pain: systematic review," *The British Medical Journal*, vol. 322, no. 7301, pp. 1511–1516, 2001.

[44] J. Guzmán, R. Esmail, K. Karjalainen, A. Malmivaara, E. Irvin, and C. Bombardier, "Multidisciplinary bio-psycho-social rehabilitation for chronic low back pain," *Cochrane Database of Systematic Reviews*, no. 1, Article ID CD000963, 2002.

[45] J. Guzmán, R. Esmail, K. Karjalainen, A. Malmivaara, E. Irvin, and C. Bombardier, "WITHDRAWN: multidisciplinary bio-psycho-social rehabilitation for chronic low-back pain," *Cochrane Database of Systematic Reviews*, no. 3, Article ID CD000963, 2007.

[46] D. Merrick, G. Sundelin, and B.-M. Stålnacke, "An observational study of two rehabilitation strategies for patients with chronic pain, focusing on sick leave at one-year follow-up," *Journal of Rehabilitation Medicine*, vol. 45, no. 10, pp. 1049–1057, 2013.

[47] A.-S. Steiner, M. Sartori, S. Leal et al., "Added value of an intensive multidisciplinary functional rehabilitation programme for chronic low back pain patients," *Swiss Medical Weekly*, vol. 143, Article ID w13763, 2013.

[48] M. E. Nazzal, M. A. Saadah, L. M. Saadah et al., "Management options of chronic low back pain. A randomized blinded clinical trial," *Neurosciences*, vol. 18, no. 2, pp. 152–159, 2013.

[49] A. de Rooij, M. R. de Boer, M. van der Leeden, L. D. Roorda, M. P. Steultjens, and J. Dekker, "Cognitive mechanisms of change in multidisciplinary treatment of patients with chronic widespread pain: a prospective cohort study," *Journal of Rehabilitation Medicine*, vol. 46, no. 2, pp. 173–180, 2014.

[50] J. P. Robinson, D. Fulton-Kehoe, G. M. Franklin, and R. Wu, "Multidisciplinary pain center outcomes in Washington State Workers' compensation," *Journal of Occupational and Environmental Medicine*, vol. 46, no. 5, pp. 473–478, 2004.

[51] H. Hamer, R. Gandhi, S. Wong, and N. N. Mahomed, "Predicting return to work following treatment of chronic pain disorder," *Occupational Medicine*, vol. 63, no. 4, pp. 253–259, 2013.

[52] M. J. Martínez Zapata, E. Català, and M. Rigola, "Análisis descriptivo en el año 2001 de las Unidades de Tratamiento del Dolor Crónico en España," *Revista Española de Anestesiología y Reanimación*, vol. 52, pp. 141–148, 2005.

[53] T. C. Lanes, E. F. Gauron, K. F. Spratt, T. J. Wernimont, E. M. Found, and J. N. Weinstein, "Long-term follow-up of patients with chronic back pain treated in a multidisciplinary rehabilitation program," *Spine*, vol. 20, no. 7, pp. 801–806, 1995.

[54] K. Pieber, M. Herceg, M. Quittan, R. Csapo, R. Müller, and G. F. Wiesinger, "Long-term effects of an outpatient rehabilitation program in patients with chronic recurrent low back pain," *European Spine Journal*, vol. 23, no. 4, pp. 779–785, 2014.

[55] B. Oosterhof, J. H. M. Dekker, M. Sloots, E. A. C. Bartels, and J. Dekker, "Success or failure of chronic pain rehabilitation: the importance of good interaction—a qualitative study under patients and professionals," *Disability and Rehabilitation*, vol. 36, no. 22, pp. 1903–1910, 2014.

[56] T. L. Trentman, E. G. Cornidez, L. L. Wilshusen et al., "Patient satisfaction in an academic chronic pain clinic," *Pain Practice*, vol. 13, no. 5, pp. 372–379, 2013.

[57] L. M. McCracken, D. Evon, and E. T. Karapas, "Satisfaction with treatment for chronic pain in a specialty service: preliminary prospective results," *European Journal of Pain*, vol. 6, no. 5, pp. 387–393, 2002.

[58] P. Triva, M. Jukić, and L. Puljak, "Access to public healthcare services and waiting times for patients with chronic nonmalignant pain: feedback from a tertiary pain clinic," *Acta Clinica Croatica*, vol. 52, no. 1, pp. 79–85, 2013.

[59] D. Hoy, P. Brooks, F. Blyth, and R. Buchbinder, "The Epidemiology of low back pain," *Best Practice and Research: Clinical Rheumatology*, vol. 24, no. 6, pp. 769–781, 2010.

[60] R. W. J. G. Ostelo, R. A. Deyo, P. Stratford et al., "Interpreting change scores for pain and functional status in low back pain: towards international consensus regarding minimal important change," *Spine*, vol. 33, no. 1, pp. 90–94, 2008.

[61] A. Collado Cruz, X. Torres i Mata, A. Arias i Gassol et al., "Efficiency of multidisciplinary treatment of chronic pain with locomotor disability," *Medicina Clinica*, vol. 117, no. 11, pp. 401–405, 2001.

[62] G. Tan, M. P. Jensen, J. I. Thornby, and B. F. Shanti, "Validation of the brief pain inventory for chronic nonmalignant pain," *The Journal of Pain*, vol. 5, no. 2, pp. 133–137, 2004.

[63] K. L. Lapane, B. J. Quilliam, C. Benson, W. Chow, and M. Kim, "One, two, or three? constructs of the brief pain inventory among patients with non-cancer pain in the outpatient setting," *Journal of Pain and Symptom Management*, vol. 47, no. 2, pp. 325–333, 2014.

[64] J. Malouf, O. Andión, R. Torrubia, M. Cañellas, and J.-E. Baños, "A survey of perceptions with pain management in spanish inpatients," *Journal of Pain and Symptom Management*, vol. 32, no. 4, pp. 361–371, 2006.

[65] K. Soares, I. Sola, E. Aromataris et al., *Epidimiology of Chroni Non-Malignant Pain in Spain*, Fundación Grünenthal, 2010.

[66] H. Breivik, B. Collett, V. Ventafridda, R. Cohen, and D. Gallacher, "Survey of chronic pain in Europe: prevalence, impact on daily life, and treatment," *European Journal of Pain*, vol. 10, no. 4, pp. 287–333, 2006.

27

The Role of Nurses' Uncertainty in Decision-Making Process of Pain Management in People with Dementia

Mohammad Rababa

Assistant Professor, Jordan University of Science and Technology, Jordan

Correspondence should be addressed to Mohammad Rababa; mjrababa@just.edu.jo

Academic Editor: Marina De Tommaso

Pain in people with dementia (PWD) is underassessed and undertreated. Treatment of pain in people with dementia goes awry because of poor assessment, poor treatment, and factors related to nursing decision-making skills. Several theoretical models addressed the role of nurses' critical thinking and decision-making skills in pain treatment, like the cognitive continuum theory (CCT) and the adaptive pain management (APT). Only the Response to Certainty of Pain (RCP) model was the first model to posit relationships between nurses' uncertainty, pain assessment, and patient outcomes. Gilmore-Bykovskyi and Bowers developed the RCP, which incorporates the concept of uncertainty and how it relates to the problem of unrelieved pain in PWD. The RCP model has the potential to provide good understanding of the problem of unrelieved pain in people with dementia. It also could help to develop a research study that brings comfort to an often neglected and vulnerable population.

1. Introduction

Pain is one of the most prevalent problems in the elderly; pain affects approximately 20% of the elderly population [1]. Chronic pain in patients aged 85 years or older is a common problem, occurring in 40-79% of individuals [2]. Fifty-six of community-dwelling older adults and 70% of nursing home residents have pain [3]. This high prevalence of pain among older adult patients is explained in part by physiological age-related changes and comorbid problems that happen in later life (Gibson and Lussier, 2012; [2, 4]). According to Achterberg et al. [5], elderly people are more prone to receive poor pain management.

Despite the high prevalence of pain among older adults, people with dementia (PWD) appear to be at great risk of poor treatment of pain because they have difficulty communicating their unmet comfort needs [6]. According to Husebo et al. [7], pain affects 50% to 80% of nursing home (NH) residents with dementia. Several studies have also consistently shown the high prevalence of poor assessment and treatment of pain in NH residents with dementia [8–10]. For example, it has been reported that PWD are prescribed significantly less scheduled analgesics as well as receiving less analgesics than cognitively intact older adults even with controlling for number of painful situations [5, 11].

Treatment of pain in PWD goes awry because of many reasons. However, in this paper three reasons are chosen and will be discussed separately. These reasons include (a) poor assessment, (b) poor treatment, or (c) factors relating to nurses' critical thinking and decision-making skills. The purpose of this paper is to provide a brief overview of evidence related to poor assessment and poor treatment of pain in PWD and then to describe in more detail nurses' critical thinking and decision-making, with a description and explanation of how the Response to Certainty of Pain (RCP) model [12] may help elucidate how nurse uncertainty regarding suspected pain drives assessment and predicts patient outcomes. The RCP model may help researchers to understand factors that predict poor pain management and may aid in the development of interventions to improve treatment.

1.1. Assessment. There cannot be effective treatment without accurate assessment of pain [13]. Nurse scientists need to give much more attention to developing assessment tools that could improve practice and eliminate barriers to optimal pain management [14]. A study done by Kovach et al. [15]

identified the need to develop more critical ways to properly assess pain in PWD. It is important that healthcare professionals conduct more appropriate and accurate pain assessment in order to accurately identify pain and provide effective treatment using a range of comforting interventions [15, 16]. With a better understanding of the problem of pain, healthcare providers may be able to improve the quality of life for PWD. Over the past few years, scientists have made significant progress in this area by developing, evaluating, and introducing a variety of observational assessment tools used to detect pain in PWD [17]. However, pain is still unrelieved in PWD [13].

Because of the complexity of pain assessment in PWD and the time needed to assess pain in this population, nurses may spend a few hours rather than minutes to assess their patients' pain (Prkachin, Solomon, and Ross, 2007). Nurses may be reluctant to perform a thorough assessment. Instead, these nurses may overly simplify the assessment process by relying on the rapid data processing evident when using intuition to discern pain sufferers from others [18].

1.2. Treatment. Unrelieved pain in PWD could also be explained in part by poor treatment [19]. Nurses are often concerned about drug addiction and other consequences of analgesic use, such as respiratory depression [19]. Also, nurses may have both knowledge deficits and misconceptions regarding the use of analgesics and pain in PWD [20]. Nurses often struggle with understanding the nature of pain in PWD [21]. They cannot differentiate between the pure sensation of pain and other unpleasant emotions [21]. Even if nurses identify suspected pain in a PWD, determining pain intensity, duration, and location is far from a simple exercise [11]. According to a recent study, 30% of PWD residing in nursing homes report pain daily, but 25% of those NH residents with pain do not receive analgesics [22]. Even if analgesics are prescribed and available for PWD, nurses often fail to administer those medications or tend to administer only a portion of the prescribed amount [12]. Moreover, a recent study showed that nurses' analgesic choices are mainly determined by the ability of patients to self-report their pain. As a result, nonverbal patients like PWD have little effect on the choice of analgesics [23].

Pharmacological treatment is considered to be the first option for pain management [19]. However, nurses may start with nonpharmacological treatment to address pain in PWD and delay analgesics. The reason for this is that nurses may have misconceptions about behavioral symptoms of pain in PWD. Nurses may conceptualize these behavioral symptoms from a psychological perspective rather than physical perspective. As a result, nurses may not prioritize treatment of physical problems and try instead to treat the nonphysical underlying cause of behavioral changes, such as psychosocial causes [11, 21].

In addition, even though nurses use the pharmacological treatment to manage pain in PWD, they may use antipsychotic drugs instead of analgesics. The use of antipsychotic drugs is often associated with decreased level of functioning, unmet care needs, increased serious cardiovascular events, and decreased quality of life [24]. Furthermore, some nurses are not sure whether PWD truly have pain or just want to be medicated. Despite nurses' efforts to treat pain in PWD, they may feel frustrated with this group of older adults who have difficulty verbalizing their pain [25].

2. Critical Thinking and Decision-Making

The underestimation of pain assessments and the undertreatment of pain in PWD are well known. Little is known about how nurses think about and make their decision about pain assessment and management in PWD. The problem of pain in PWD may be explained partly by poor critical thinking and decision-making skills on the part of nurses. To make an accurate decision about pain management in PWD, nurses should clearly identify the behavioral indicators of pain, such as facial grimacing, withdrawal, restless behaviors, and negative vocalizations. However, nurses do not have a clear understanding of what the behavior indicators in PWD should look like even in those who could self-report their pain. Instead, nurses often think of autonomic nervous system changes in vital signs, evident in acute pain conditions, and observable physical changes as cues to pain in PWD who are having acute or chronic pain [26].

Nursing homes in the US have a high percentage of unlicensed nurses in relation to licensed nurses [27]. According to the same study, 80% to 90% of care in nursing homes is delivered by Certified Nursing Assistants (CNAs). CNAs often do not receive high quality education and clinical training. Furthermore, the problem of a lack of staffing in nursing homes overwhelms many CNAs and CNAs are not responsible for assessment or clinical decision-making [28]. Consistently, a recent study by Kovach et al. [16] showed that the majority of nursing staff working in nursing homes are Licensed Practical Nurses (LPNs) and associate-degree registered nurses (RNs). Those nurses may have knowledge deficit and poor experience, which make them unqualified to deal with the complexity of pain assessment in PWD and make appropriate decisions regarding pain treatment.

According to Kaasalainen et al. [11], nurses acknowledged that a major problem of pain management in PWD lies in the decision-making process they undergo until they get analgesics prescribed. Nurses believe that the way they interact with pain in PWD is mainly based on a trial and error approach. Nurses often became confused when they were uncertain regarding suspected pain in PWD.

To overcome uncertainty regarding suspected pain in PWD, it has been recommended that nurses identify a variety of behavioral indicators to make their decisions about pain assessment. These indicators are based on the nurses' understanding of the usual behaviors of PWD [11]. Unfortunately current pain assessment strategies rarely incorporate formalized decision-making processes. Nurses often look at pain symptoms in PWD as just a manifestation of a behavior change associated with the dementing illness. Regardless of how different PWD show pain, it is discussed as and responded to as a sign of a dementing illness. The current body of evidence suggests that nurses often do not have a clear understanding of what pain looks like in PWD, which then leads to a state of uncertainty. This uncertainty impacts the nurses' decision-making as regards pain treatment [11]. This paper will present theoretical and empirical evidence supporting the premise that nurses' uncertainty regarding suspected pain in PWD may explain inadequate assessment, which then leads to undertreatment of pain.

3. Background of Decision-Making Theory

3.1. Background of Field of Healthcare Decision-Making. Decision-making about treatment is an essential part of modern healthcare [29]. Dementia causes a gradual decline in decision-making ability. Therefore, PWD may be unable to make decisions related to their treatment [30]. Healthcare providers play a significant role in making decisions about different treatment options, based on information regarding risks and benefits [29]. In the case of dementia, the role of healthcare providers is even more significant. Many researchers have described how nurses learn, apply what they learned in clinical settings, derive new knowledge from clinical experience, and demonstrate their decision-making skills to translate theoretical knowledge into practice [30]. In the following paragraphs, this paper will provide an overview of some of the main decision-making models used in the field dementia of healthcare.

3.2. Overview of Core Nurse Decision-Making Models in Pain Management. The implementation of evidence-based interventions in healthcare settings has increased the importance of understanding the nursing decision-making process. A thorough review of the literature regarding research studies previously conducted among nursing home residents with dementia was completed in the following databases: CINAHL plus with full text, Medline, ERIC, Education Research Complete, and Psychology and Behavioral Sciences Collection. The search was limited between 2000 and 2017 using the following combination of search terms: "nursing home residents" "dementia", "decision-making", and "pain". Articles relatedness to the focus of describing nurse decision-making models on pain treatment in NH residents with dementia was evaluated. The retrieved articles discussed only three main theoretical models including cognitive continuum theory (CCT) [31], adaptive pain management (APM) [32], Shields et al. [33] model, and RCP model [12].

Cognitive Continuum Theory. The CCT is a descriptive theory that explains the relationship between a decision-making task and an individual's cognition. According to it the individuals' cognition is a continuum ranging from intuition to analysis. Analysis has been defined as slow processing of data with high consciousness and high certainty. Intuition is defined as a quick processing of data with low consciousness and low certainty. Quasi-rationality is considered to be the central area in the cognitive continuum that moderates the interaction between the other two modes of cognition: intuition and analysis [31]. Also according to the CCT, there are two types of decision-making tasks including well-structured and ill-structured tasks. Well-structured tasks induce an analytical thought process through decomposing the tasks into many sections. Although this process takes time to resolve the task, it has a high degree of certainty. On the other hand, ill-structured tasks induce intuitive process through decomposing the task into a very few sections. Although this process does not take time to resolve the task, it has a low level of certainty [31].

While the CCT theory gives a very good explanation of the difference between analytical and intuitive processes needed to make decisions, the processes described are quite linear and simple and fail to accommodate the multifactorial or complex nature of pain in PWD. Although the analytical process is justifiable, it is complicated. Also, although intuitive process is quick and flexible, it is imprecise and irretraceable. Intuitive errors happen unexpectedly and are often hard to be identified (Dhami and Thomson, 2012). Also, the mode of cognition that the CCT uses lacks rationality and overly relies on intuition, which has been presented as the origin of irrationality or guessing. The complexity of nurses' decision-making process suggests that intuition is insufficient for nursing intervention. Furthermore, the model does not account for or capture uncertain or ambiguous thinking in the decision-making process [34]. Research using the CCT has involved small samples with weak designs and no research has examined the association between the nurses' decision-making certainty and assessment type with agitation and pain levels in PWD.

Adaptive Pain Management (APM). The APM is a decision-making framework that aims to frequently review past and current information of patients to determine the best choice of treatment [32]. The APM demonstrates a decision-making process based on dynamic programming (DP) to create an adaptive treatment of pain. The APM has two main stages that end with DP formulation and solution process presentation. The first stage, prior to treatment, includes an evaluation of the characteristics of pain, related health parameters and medical history, and ends with the determination of a treatment regime. The second stage determines whether an adjustment in the treatment should be made or not and comes up with the final outcomes. The final decision in both stages is the on-hand treatment plans, which could be a combination of a number of different pharmacological or nonpharmacological interventions [32].

While the APM theory identifies the best choice of pain treatment in elderly patients and demonstrates a decision support system based on dynamic programming process, the process implies that nurse should continually adapt and readapt the treatment to the patient [32]. This continuous adaptation and readaptation of treatment rely on patient feedback which means that patients should be able to verbalize their unmet needs. Therefore, the model does not account for cognitive impairment and communication deficit in PWD [35]. Also, the model does not account for or capture uncertain or ambiguous thinking in the decision-making process. Research using the APM has involved small samples, with weak designs, and no research has examined the association between the nurses' decision-making certainty and assessment type with agitation and pain levels in PWD [35].

4. Uncertainty and Pain Assessment

Two theories have directly addressed the role of uncertainty in pain management in PWD. A model by Shields et al. [33] states that the decision-making process is a complex intellectual process of clinical reasoning or judgment that includes making explanations regarding what level of certainty nurses have in taking action. Action means the implementations the nurse decides or does not decide to do. Not taking action means not initiating an intervention. Both actions and nonactions are the result of the decision-making process, and both involve a process of making explanations [33]. While the work of Shields et al. posits that when recall of nurses' academic education and clinical experience, attitudes, values, beliefs, and culture to the situation may increase or decrease the level a nurse's level of certainty about pain in PWD, explanations within the model are not well developed and lack direct applicability to clinical situations of complex assessment of pain in PWD.

4.1. Introduction to the Response to Certainty of Pain (RCP) Model. The Response to Certainty of Pain (RCP) model by Gilmore-Bykovskyi and Bowers [12] illustrates two trajectories for nurses' assessment and management of pain for NH residents: one when the nurse is certain the patient is in pain and one when the nurse is uncertain whether the patient is in pain. When the nurse is certain that the patient is in pain, the trajectory moves in a timely fashion from suspected pain to treatment. When the nurse is uncertain, the patient is in pain the trajectory from suspected pain to treatment is delayed or never accomplished [12].

The uncertainty trajectory is often slowed down by a time-consuming assessment process based on trial and error. Certainty of pain is quickly confirmed by prompt treatment in the certainty trajectory. In the uncertainty trajectory, although various treatments may be tried, the nurse may never be certain that the patient was in pain because the path from suspected pain to treatment is more convoluted. Furthermore, in many cases the path never leads to treatment so there is no treatment outcome to confirm the presence of pain [12].

Gilmore-Bykovskyi and Bowers' model of how certainty and uncertainty create different trajectories for nurses' decision-making in pain management for nursing home patients could lay the foundation for much needed translational research to improve nursing practice for patients with dementia [12]. The RCP model demonstrates that the role of certainty would be a key nursing factor in future gerontological pain research. The RCP model is the first model to posit relationships between nurses' uncertainty, pain assessment, and patient outcomes of pain and agitation in PWD. The RCP model has been tested in a correlational study among a convenience sample of 78 NH residents with dementia and all study's hypotheses derived from the model were supported [2, 4].

4.2. Nurses' Certainty Trajectory. When nurses are certain regarding suspected pain they do a brief self-report assessment and provide timely pain management. According to the RCP model, nurses implement timely pain management if residents do not have dementia because their behaviors are highly suggestive of pain. In addition, nurses respond with a high level of certainty regarding suspected pain in patients with a short-term stay in the nursing home, even though nurses know that not all residents staying for short period of time are cognitively intact.

According to Gilmore-Bykovskyi and Bowers [12], nurses try to confirm suspected pain in older adult patients who do not have dementia by asking the patient for a self-report. In case of PWD, nurses become more certain regarding suspected pain and provide timely treatment if PWD show obvious pain indicators. When nurses feel a high level of certainty about pain in their PWD they are more likely to quickly validate their assessments by interviewing family members, contacting a physician, taking vital signs, or checking medical records and to confirm their certainty about the presence of pain.

4.3. Nurses' Uncertainty Trajectory. Nurses are uncertain regarding suspected pain in PWD for a number of reasons. The complexity of pain assessment in PWD does not enable nurses to suspect pain in their patients. Furthermore, the severity of dementia strongly affects the level of a nurse's certainty. As the severity of dementia increases, a nurse's level of certainty regarding suspected pain decreases [12]. Moreover, nurses may not suspect pain in PWD because of the inconsistency of their behavior and because pain may not be the primary cause of their behavior.

According to the RCP model, when nurses are uncertain regarding suspected pain in PWD, they do not confirm certainty and evaluate the effectiveness of the pain treatment given to PWD. Nurses do not try to ease their uncertainty by asking PWD if they are in pain, because PWD cannot verbalize their pain. Instead, nurses try to ease their uncertainty by conducting additional assessment to increase certainty and doing trial and error process. In this case, treatment is focused on reversing behavioral changes and consequently the treatment of pain may be delayed or not provided at all. Also, according to the model, nurses are consistently uncertain regarding suspected pain in elderly with long-term stays. Those elderly usually have many comorbid problems that make nurses unable to suspect pain because they believe pain generally is not anticipated in a long-term stay [2, 4]. In this situation, nurses also do further assessments and include additional decision-making processes. As a result, the treatment of pain may be delayed. Also, according to Gilmore-Bykovskyi and Bowers [12], nurses sometimes were not allowed by physicians and administrators to make their own decisions to select the type of pain assessment tools used for PWD. Actually, it could be a disadvantage of the RCP model that it puts the nurse in a central role to change poor pain management into good pain management, although in practice there might be other factors of influence beyond her reach.

4.4. Other Theoretical References. PWD might be unable to provide meaningful and clear verbal information about their pain experience. Therefore, they are unable to confirm nurses' certainty or uncertainty regarding suspected pain. As a result, nurses might refer to their interpretations of subjective and objective data of pain, evaluating behavioral indicators of pain. Pain cues are defined as changes in behaviors such as aggression and restlessness/agitation, sounds such as vocalization, or appearance such as facial expressions [36]. Recognizing these behavioral changes needs additional pain assessment and more decision-making steps. The nurses' ability to interpret these changes is limited, impeding them to make certain decisions about pain treatment (Parke, 1998).

Nurse also may be unable to discriminate between pain and dementia [11]. Nurses acknowledge that they are often uncertain about pain in PWD, as they are unsure whether behavioral changes are pain-related or dementia-related. In most cases, nurses believed these behavioral changes are caused by something other than pain. Indeed, the last thing that nurses think about when they care for PWD who show change in behaviors is pain. Consequently, nurses would try to manage these behavioral changes based on a pragmatic approach rather than theoretical considerations. As nurses often do not have a definitive diagnosis of pain in PWD, they struggle with treatment options and frequently question their decisions about chosen treatment of pain.

When nurses are uncertain regarding suspected pain in PWD, they tend to use their intuition. In this case, nurses not only cannot recognize the behavioral changes in PWD but also are unable to clearly translate their intuition into meaningful data, facilitating clinical decisions about pain [37]. For example, nurses may report that they just feel inside something is wrong because the patients are not being themselves. In this example, nurses' intuition is not enough to develop certainty regarding suspected pain in PWD [37]. When nurses use their intuition to assess pain in PWD, they are uncertain if the behavioral changes they observe represent pain.

In addition, nurses do not have clear understanding of decision-making processes and other relevant information. Understanding other relevant information includes medical diagnoses, pathophysiology, and the nurses' personal pain experiences. The decision-making process involves recognizing the PWD's specific pain cues, effectively assessing pain, administering analgesic in a timely manner, and evaluating the effectiveness of the intervention. However, nurses use a process of trial and error instead. This process involves administering nonpharmacological intervention and observing PWD's responses to these interventions or just looking for the reversal of behavioral changes [33].

4.5. Evidence That Relates to Uncertainty and Pain Treatment. Because healthcare providers are uncertain regarding suspected pain in PWD, PWD are prescribed significantly fewer analgesics [5]. For example, when physicians prescribe analgesics for PWD after hip fracture surgery, they put them at a dosage that is one-third of that prescribed for cognitively intact patients [5]. Furthermore, when physicians are uncertain about pain in PWD, they start with a very low dose of analgesics and then increase the dosage if a low dose does not work. However, physicians and nurses are not sure of whether and how much they should increase the dosage of analgesics. They may start to think that maybe it is not actually pain; maybe this is part of dementia, not pain [11].

Furthermore, even though physicians may prescribe analgesics for PWD, nurses may sometimes be uncertain about pain, and consequently PWD may not receive adequate pain treatment. A recent study by Kaasalainen et al. [11] found that nurses' uncertainty regarding suspected pain in PWD influenced the choice of opioid analgesics dose and contributed to poor treatment of pain. The same study found that nurses were not always certain about their ratings of pain, which were not significantly correlated with the administration of analgesics. Consequently, even though PWD have pain in the past, they do not always receive analgesics [11].

When nurses are uncertain about pain in PWD, they feel uncomfortable and hesitant to use analgesics to treat pain. They tend to administer analgesics only after all other nonpharmacological interventions have been tried and proven ineffective. According to a recent study, nurses who were uncertain whether a patient's behavior indicated pain were less likely to start pharmacological treatment than nurses who had higher levels of certainty [5]. Nurses who were uncertain about their patient's pain chose other pain interventions, delaying more effective pharmacological treatment. These other pain interventions include toileting, changing the room to fit resident preferences, providing acetaminophen, changing position, regulating the temperature of environment, reducing stimulation, doing outdoor activities, and providing food. Nurses and physicians are not willing to take the risks to treat pain with opioid analgesics. This reluctance to use analgesics results from their uncertainty regarding suspected pain in PWD [11].

5. Conclusion

PWD are at great risk of unrelieved pain due to poor assessment, inadequate management, or problems with decision-making process. Many decision-making theories including the CTT and APM have been developed on pain management recently. However, the RCP is the only theoretical framework that has examined the association between the nurses' decision-making certainty and assessment type with agitation and pain levels in PWD. The RCP provides an understanding of treatment decisions regarding pain in PWD. This article would suggest that nurses' uncertainty might explain poor treatment of pain in PWD.

References

[1] S. J. Gibson and D. Lussier, "Prevalence and relevance of pain in older persons," *Pain Medicine*, vol. 13, no. s2, pp. S23–S26, 2012.

[2] M. Rababa, "The association of nurses' assessment and certainty to pain management and outcomes for nursing home residents in Jordan," *Geriatric Nursing*, vol. 39, no. 1, pp. 66–71, 2018.

[3] Y. Takai, N. Yamamoto-Mitani, Y. Okamoto, K. Koyama, and A. Honda, "Literature review of pain prevalence among older residents of nursing homes," *Pain Management Nursing*, vol. 11, no. 4, pp. 209–223, 2010.

[4] M. Rababa, "Association of comorbid burden and patient outcomes of residents with dementia in jordanian nursing homes," *Journal of Gerontological Nursing*, vol. 44, no. 7, pp. 50–58, 2018.

[5] W. P. Achterberg, M. J. C. Pieper, A. H. van Dalen-Kok et al., "Pain management in patients with dementia," *Clinical Interventions in Aging*, vol. 8, pp. 1471–1482, 2013.

[6] K. Harrison Dening, "Palliative and end of life care for people with dementia," *Nursing standard (Royal College of Nursing (Great Britain) : 1987)*, vol. 30, no. 23, pp. 42–49, 2016.

[7] B. S. Husebo, C. Ballard, and D. Aarsland, "Pain treatment of agitation in patients with dementia: A systematic review," *International Journal of Geriatric Psychiatry*, vol. 26, no. 10, pp. 1012–1018, 2011.

[8] A.-G. Mamhidir, B.-M. Sjölund, B. Fläckman, A. Wimo, A. Sköldunger, and M. Engström, "Systematic pain assessment in nursing homes: a cluster-randomized trial using mixed-methods approach," *BMC Geriatrics*, vol. 17, no. 1, p. 61, 2017.

[9] T. B. Monroe, S. K. Misra, R. C. Habermann, M. S. Dietrich, R. L. Cowan, and S. F. Simmons, "Pain reports and pain medication treatment in nursing home residents with and without dementia," *Geriatrics & Gerontology International*, vol. 14, no. 3, pp. 541–548, 2014.

[10] J. N. Hunnicutt, C. M. Ulbricht, J. Tjia, and K. L. Lapane, "Pain and pharmacologic pain management in long-stay nursing home residents," *Pain*, vol. 158, no. 6, pp. 1091–1099, 2017.

[11] S. Kaasalainen, E. Coker, L. Dolovich et al., "Pain management decision making among long-term care physicians and nurses," *Western Journal of Nursing Research*, vol. 29, no. 5, pp. 561–580, 2007.

[12] A. L. Gilmore-Bykovskyi and B. J. Bowers, "Understanding nurses' decisions to treat pain in nursing home residents with dementia," *Research in Gerontological Nursing*, vol. 6, no. 2, pp. 127–138, 2013.

[13] T. Hadjistavropoulos, K. Herr, K. M. Prkachin et al., "Pain assessment in elderly adults with dementia," *The Lancet Neurology*, vol. 13, no. 12, pp. 1216–1227, 2014.

[14] E. Gosselin, P. Bourgault, S. Lavoie, R.-M. Coleman, and A. Méziat-Burdin, "Development and validation of an observation tool for the assessment of nursing pain management practices in intensive care unit in a standardized clinical simulation setting," *Pain Management Nursing*, vol. 15, no. 4, pp. 720–730, 2014.

[15] C. R. Kovach, B. R. Logan, P. E. Noonan et al., "Effects of the serial trial intervention on discomfort and behavior of nursing home residents with dementia," *American Journal of Alzheimer's Disease & Other Dementias*, vol. 21, no. 3, pp. 147–155, 2006.

[16] C. R. Kovach, M. R. Simpson, L. Joosse et al., "Comparison of the effectiveness of two protocols for treating nursing home residents with advanced dementia," *Research in Gerontological Nursing*, vol. 5, no. 4, pp. 251–263, 2012.

[17] K. Herr, H. Bursch, M. Ersek, L. L. Miller, and K. Swafford, "Use of pain-behavioral assessment tools in the nursing home: expert consensus recommendations for practice," *Journal of Gerontological Nursing*, vol. 36, no. 3, pp. 18–31, 2010.

[18] K. M. Prkachin, P. E. Solomon, and J. Ross, "Underestimation of pain by health-care providers: towards a model of the process of inferring pain in others," *Canadian Journal of Nursing Research*, vol. 39, no. 2, pp. 88–106, 2007.

[19] A. J. McLachlan, S. Bath, V. Naganathan et al., "Clinical pharmacology of analgesic medicines in older people: Impact of frailty and cognitive impairment," *British Journal of Clinical Pharmacology*, vol. 71, no. 3, pp. 351–364, 2011.

[20] S. M. Zwakhalen, J. P. Hamers, R. H. Peijnenburg, and M. P. Berger, "Nursing staff knowledge and beliefs about pain in elderly nursing home residents with dementia," *Pain Research and Management*, vol. 12, no. 3, pp. 177–184, 2007.

[21] N. Krumm, P. Larkin, M. Connolly, P. Rode, and F. Elsner, "Improving dementia care in nursing homes: Experiences with a palliative care symptom-assessment tool (MIDOS)," *International Journal of Palliative Nursing*, vol. 20, no. 4, pp. 187–192, 2014.

[22] D. K. Y. Miu and K. C. Chan, "Under-detection of pain in elderly nursing home residents with moderate to severe dementia," *Journal of Clinical Gerontology and Geriatrics*, vol. 5, no. 1, pp. 23–27, 2014.

[23] E. Gustavsson and L. Sandman, "Health-care needs and shared decision-making in priority-setting," *Medicine, Health Care and Philosophy*, vol. 18, no. 1, pp. 13–22, 2015.

[24] C. Salzman, D. V. Jeste, R. E. Meyer et al., "Elderly patients with dementia-related symptoms of severe agitation and aggression: Consensus statement on treatment options, clinical trials methodology, and policy," *Journal of Clinical Psychiatry*, vol. 69, no. 6, pp. 889–898, 2008.

[25] J. Y. W. Liu, M. Briggs, and S. J. Closs, "The psychometric qualities of four observational pain tools (OPTs) for the assessment of pain in elderly people with osteoarthritic pain," *The Journal of Clinical Psychiatry*, vol. 40, no. 4, pp. 582–598, 2010.

[26] K. Herr, P. J. Coyne, M. McCaffery, R. Manworren, and S. Merkel, "Pain assessment in the patient unable to self-report: position statement with clinical practice recommendations," *Pain Management Nursing*, vol. 12, no. 4, pp. 230–250, 2011.

[27] L. Clark, K. Jones, and K. Pennington, "Pain assessment practices with nursing home residents," *Western Journal of Nursing Research*, vol. 26, no. 7, pp. 733–750, 2004.

[28] M. D. Buffum and M. Haberfelde, "Moving to new settings: Pilot study of families' perceptions of professional caregivers' pain management in persons with dementia," *Journal of Rehabilitation Research and Development*, vol. 44, no. 2, pp. 295–303, 2007.

[29] J. Lally and E. Tullo, "Engaging older people in decisions about their healthcare: The case for shared decision making," *Reviews in Clinical Gerontology*, vol. 22, no. 2, pp. 99–107, 2012.

[30] K. L. Smebye, M. Kirkevold, and K. Engedal, "How do persons with dementia participate in decision making related to health and daily care? A multi-case study," *BMC Health Services Research*, vol. 12, no. 1, article no. 241, 2012.

[31] R. Cader, S. Campbell, and D. Watson, "Cognitive continuum theory in nursing decision-making," *Journal of Advanced Nursing*, vol. 49, no. 4, pp. 397–405, 2005.

[32] C.-F. Lin, A. K. LeBoulluec, L. Zeng, V. C. P. Chen, and R. J. Gatchel, "A decision-making framework for adaptive pain management," *Health Care Management Science*, vol. 17, no. 3, pp. 270–283, 2014.

[33] C. G. Shields, M. A. Finley, C. M. Elias et al., "Pain assessment: the roles of physician certainty and curiosity," *Health Communication*, vol. 28, no. 7, pp. 740–746, 2013.

[34] M. Offredy, S. Kendall, and C. Goodman, "The use of cognitive continuum theory and patient scenarios to explore nurse prescribers' pharmacological knowledge and decision-making," *International Journal of Nursing Studies*, vol. 45, no. 6, pp. 855–868, 2008.

28

Chronic Pelvic Pain: Assessment, Evaluation, and Objectivation

Maria Beatrice Passavanti, Vincenzo Pota, Pasquale Sansone, Caterina Aurilio, Lorenzo De Nardis, and Maria Caterina Pace

Department of Woman, Child, General and Specialized Surgery, University of Campania L. Vanvitelli, Naples, Italy

Correspondence should be addressed to Maria Beatrice Passavanti; beatrice.passavanti@libero.it

Academic Editor: Steve McGaraughty

Chronic Pelvic Pain (CPP) and Chronic Pelvic Pain Syndrome (CPPS) have a significant impact on men and women of reproductive and nonreproductive age, with a considerable burden on overall quality of life (QoL) and on psychological, functional, and behavioural status. Moreover, diagnostic and therapeutic difficulties are remarkable features in many patients. Therefore evaluation, assessment and objectivation tools are often necessary to properly address each patient and consequently his/her clinical needs. Here we review the different tools for pain assessment, evaluation, and objectivation; specific features regarding CPP/CPPS will be highlighted. Also, recent findings disclosed with neuroimaging investigations will be reviewed as they provide new insights into CPP/CPPS pathophysiology and may serve as a tool for CPP assessment and objectivation.

1. Introduction

Pain is an unpleasant sensory and emotional experience associated with actual or potential tissue damage or described in terms of such damage [1]. Chronic Pelvic Pain (CPP) is defined by the European Association of Urology (EAU) as "chronic or persistent pain perceived in structures related to the pelvis of either men or women. It is often associated with negative cognitive, behavioural, sexual and emotional consequences as well as with symptoms suggestive of lower urinary tract, sexual, bowel, pelvic floor or gynaecological dysfunction. In the case of documented nociceptive pain that becomes chronic/persistent through time, pain must have been continuous or recurrent for at least 6 months. If non-acute and central sensitization pain mechanisms are well documented, then the pain may be regarded as chronic, irrespective of the time period" [2]. The American College of Obstetricians and Gynaecologists similarly defines CPP as "non-cyclic pain lasting for 6 or more months, that localizes to the anatomic pelvis, anterior abdominal wall at or below the umbilicus, the lumbosacral back, or the buttocks and is of sufficient severity to cause functional disability or lead to medical care" [3]. The EAU further defines Chronic Pelvic Pain Syndrome (CPPS) as "the occurrence of CPP when there is no proven infection or other obvious local pathology that may account for the pain. It is often associated with negative cognitive, behavioural, sexual or emotional consequences, as well as with symptoms suggestive of lower urinary tract, sexual, bowel or gynaecological dysfunction. CPPS is a sub-division of CPP. [...] Pain perception in CPPS may be focused within a single organ, more than one pelvic organ and even associated with systemic symptoms such as Chronic Fatigue Syndrome (CFS), Fibromyalgia (FM) or Sjögren's Syndrome. When the pain is localized to a single organ, some specialists may wish to consider using an end organ term such as Bladder Pain Syndrome (BPS). The use of such a phrase with the terminology 'syndrome' indicates that, although peripheral mechanisms may exist, CNS neuromodulation may be more important and systemic associations may occur. When the pain is localized to more than one organ site, the term CPPS should be used." [2]. "End organ" terminology reflects the site in which pain presents, and therefore specific terms for the involved organ (such as Bladder Pain Syndrome and Prostate Pain Syndrome) are classified in EAU guidelines. In more detail, the guidelines distinguish Urological, Gynaecological, Gastrointestinal, and Musculoskeletal Pain Syndromes [2]. Urological Pain Syndromes include Bladder Pain Syndrome, which is often termed as "Interstitial Cystitis" by several authors, and Prostate Pain Syndrome, which is often termed "Chronic Prostatitis/Chronic Pelvic Pain Syndrome" instead by many authors according to the NIH Classification of Chronic Prostatitis [4]. Moreover, Scrotal Pain Syndrome, Testicular Pain Syndrome, Epididymal Pain Syndrome, Post-vasectomy Scrotal Pain Syndrome, Penile Pain Syndrome, and Urethral Pain Syndrome are all classified as Urological Pain Syndromes. Again, in many articles authors refer to these syndromes as "Chronic Orchialgia" or "Chronic Scrotal Syndrome" [5, 6]. Gynaecological Pain Syndromes include Vulvar Pain Syndrome (also termed "Vulvodynia"), Vestibular Pain Syndrome, Clitoral Pain Syndrome, Dysmenorrhea, and Endometriosis-Associated Pain Syndrome. Irritable Bowel Syndrome and Pelvic Floor Muscle Pain Syndrome are the most widespread Gastrointestinal and Musculoskeletal Pain Syndromes, respectively.

Notably, EAU guidelines underscore the fact that central sensitization mechanisms and Central Nervous System (CNS) neuromodulation and neuroplasticity are relevant pathophysiological mechanisms in CPP/CPPS, and indeed many patients (up to 50% in some cohorts) report neuropathic pain symptoms [7–10]. In particular, Endometriosis appears to be deeply connected to sensitization and neuroplasticity mechanisms [9, 11], although neuropathic pain features may occur in virtually any CPP/CPPS patient [12, 13]. Specific questionnaires for neuropathic pain assessment will be discussed later in this review, and dedicated laboratory tools to assess neuropathic features will be discussed as well. Moreover, since central neuroplasticity and neuromodulation are relevant features of CPP, the role of functional brain neuroimaging in CPP/CPPS patients will also be discussed in a dedicated section.

While acute pelvic pain is considered as the fifth vital sign [14, 15] in the same way as other acute pain conditions, CPP is generally considered to be a description of a clinical condition [16] rather than a diagnosis. Nevertheless, CPP has a significant impact on women of reproductive and nonreproductive age, with a considerable burden on overall quality of life (QoL) and on psychological, functional, and behavioural status. CPP prevalence varies in a wide range, according to different cohort sampling, from 5,6% to 30,9% [17–20]. Notably, the reported prevalence varies according to the country in which the sample is enrolled: in a recent epidemiology-based study prevalence ranged from 6,4% in Mexico to 25,4% in New Zealand [21]. This wide range of reported prevalence may reflect sociocultural differences in the investigated countries with a possible resilience to the admission of urogynaecological troubles. The prevalence of CPP/CPPS in men is also variable in different studies, although lower than their prevalence in women; the reported prevalence of CPP symptoms in men ranges between 2% and 17% [19, 22–24]. Prostate Pain Syndrome/Chronic Prostatitis and Scrotal Pain/Orchialgia are the most common syndromes male patients complain of. Prostate Pain Syndrome/Chronic Prostatitis is a high prevalent syndrome (prevalence ranges between 4,5 and 9% in different cohorts, although the effective prevalence is likely underestimated) [25], which is often accompanied by psychosocial burdening symptoms, Voiding Cycle Lower Urinary Trait Symptoms and Bladder Pain [26], Postejaculatory Pain [27], Erectile Dysfunction [28], and Pelvic Floor Muscle Pathology [29]. In a recent survey regarding young Canadian and African males with age ranging from 16 to 19 years [30, 31], Chronic Prostatitis-like symptoms were assessed, and also sexual, psychological, and overall QoL features were investigated; 8–13,3% of mild symptoms and 3–5,4% of moderate to severe symptoms were identified in the two cohorts, respectively. In both the cohorts, pain, urinary, and psychological symptoms were predictive of a worsened QoL.

Chronic Scrotal Pain is as well a likely underestimated syndrome, with reported prevalence ranging between 2,5 and 5% [5, 6, 32, 33]. It is as well accompanied by poor psychosocial, sexual, and QoL outcomes and thus represents a considerable burden for patients.

Pelvic Floor Muscle Pathology and widespread muscle tenderness deserve particular mention; they are recurrent features both in men and women affected by CPP/CPPS, as well being internal and external Pelvic Tender Points [34–38]. Objectivation tools for these relevant features of CPP/CPPS patients such as Quantitative Sensory Testing and Algometry will be further discussed in a dedicated section.

Although epidemiologic data vary in this great magnitude, CPP represents a significant socioeconomic problem, since Pelvic Pain Syndromes do have an impact on QoL and often result in depression, anxiety, impaired emotional functioning, and fatigue [39–44]. Sexual behaviour and intercourses are often impaired and disturbed by painful syndromes both in men and women. Some patients, both male and female, can even present pain catastrophizing features, which are exaggerated negative responses to imagined pain or actual pain, affecting an individual's belief system and coping strategies [45]. Pain catastrophizing has been recognized as an essential risk factor for chronic pain and could also serve as an important predictor of cognitive distress, pain-related disability, analgesic use, and dysfunctional adjustment to pain in clinical situations [46–50].

Pelvic pain affects women more frequently than men because of genetic, hormonal, sociocultural, environmental, and anthropological aspects. From an evolutionary perspective, men have always been "warriors and hunters" and consequently they more often experienced somatic pain, which is qualitatively and quantitatively different from visceral pain. Otherwise, visceral pain has always been reported mostly by women because of menstrual-related pain and painful delivery experiences.

From a biological and pathophysiological point of view, women complain of pelvic pain more than men because of both qualitative and quantitative differences in pain modulation pathways. In fact, women are more sensitive to opioid κ receptor mediated analgesia than men (qualitative aspect). Furthermore, they are less sensitive to pain modulation, and female pain threshold is lower than that of men (quantitative aspect) [15, 16, 51]. The reason for such differences probably depends on sex hormones levels with related pharmacodynamic and pharmacokinetic (opioids absorption, distribution, and metabolism) implications. Several studies reported an estrogen-related modulation of cerebral opioid peptides levels, cerebral opioids mRNA concentration, and opioid receptor density and signalling [16, 51, 52]. Furthermore, estrogens can attenuate endogenous and exogenous opioids effects through a direct link to opioid receptors [52] and can interfere with long term pain modifications in both Central and Peripheral Nervous System. As inflammatory and neuromodulating mediators received growing attention in recent years [53] in order to disclose acute (inflammatory) and chronic pain mechanisms, several researches have been assessed sex-related differences in the modulation of pain pathways. Recent investigations showed that female sex hormones, in particular 17β-estradiol and progesterone, are able to influence the levels of PGE2 and CGRP in the Periaqueductal Gray (PAG) [54]; moreover, a lower level of 17β-estradiol and/or progesterone augments PGE2 and its EP3 receptor, and PGE2 plays a role in regulating the expression of CGRP in the PAG. Different levels of 17β-estradiol were also able to influence the release of CGRP from murine F11 cells [55]. Moreover, a relationship between 17β-estradiol and pain mediators was documented in a female mice model of temporomandibular Joint arthritis [56]. It was found that 17β-estradiol upregulates both NGF and TRPV1 in a dose-dependent manner, and, in particular, synovial TRPV1 is involved in allodynia of temporomandibular joints and was responsible for COX-2 overexpression in inflamed joints. Such results seem to be relevant both for pathophysiological mechanisms of pain and also for the future development of new therapeutic pharmacological targets. Testosterone, on the other hand, is also known to be relevant in both behavioural development and pain modulation mechanisms, as it has been demonstrated in murine models that opioid analgesic sensitivity is influenced by testosterone levels even in early life in parallel with sexual differentiation of the reproductive system [57]. Other more recent researches assessed sex differences in analgesic response to antiandrogen and antiestrogen drugs in mice models of urethral calculus [58], and it was also underscored that estrogens and testosterone can interfere differently with visceral pain-related behavioural response in female and male rats [59], thus confirming that sex hormones in the two genders can act differently in enhancing/inhibiting pain perception and modulation. Pregnancy and delivery also appear to be relevant triggers to pain pathways modifications: animal studies performed in mice suggest an increased pain threshold in pregnancy, in particular immediately before delivery. Spinal opioid κ and δ receptors and the pain modulating descending noradrenergic pathways seem to be implicated [51]. Moreover, the same studies demonstrate sex-related specificity of neural pathways in the spinal cord, in the Periaqueductal Gray (PAG), and in the rostral ventromedial medulla. Sex differences in pain perception and pain modulation may thus have been maintained throughout evolution in mammalians, as sex hormones influence on neural pathways, menstruations, pregnancy, and delivery is shared among species and extends, although slightly differently, also to humans [60–62]. Despite the recent advances in research, further investigations are necessarily warranted to better evaluate both physiological and pathological mechanisms of sex-related differences in pain perception/modulation, as better understanding of this intricated arras may lead to better tailored clinical management and therapeutic strategies for male and female CPP/CPPS patients.

As mentioned earlier, CPP and CPPS are a major burden for patients and moreover imply diagnostic and therapeutic difficulties in many cases: that is, up to 55% of women with CPP/CPPS have no clear and definite pathological findings even after laparoscopic evaluation [10, 63]. Notably, pain intensity and quality reflect pathophysiological mechanisms underlying the symptoms, and therefore evaluation, assessment, and objectivation tools are often necessary to properly address each patient and consequently his/her clinical needs. Nevertheless, objectivation of pain is often a troublesome task, as pain is a subjective experience and different patients complain of it in several ways according to age, gender, and education beyond pain intensity and qualities themselves. Pain evaluation key points are patient's anamnestic interview and clinical examination, pain intensity and characteristics evaluation, patient psychological evaluation, and finally the planning of a therapeutic protocol with daily evaluation of the effects. Interview and clinical examination are still unneglectable tools for pain evaluation, as they allow the physician to know the characteristics of the painful experience of the patient and in some cases the distinction between different pain features. Nevertheless, in many times a clinical assessment based only on the examination may not yield a satisfactory diagnosis even when experienced physicians are involved, and diagnostic tools for a better assessment of pain characteristics and a complete evaluation of patient's symptoms are often warranted. A suitable qualitative and quantitative pain analysis allows, indeed, a faster and more complete diagnosis. The usefulness of these methods is of remarkable importance for CPP especially in case of difficult diagnosis and less experienced physicians [64]. Pelvic pain measurement includes both verbal and instrumental methods to choose from according to pain duration (acute or chronic), pain pathophysiology, gender, age, and education. Instrumental methods allow better objectivation of pain and may be useful to document an unspecific and subjective symptom such as pain, thus converting it into a well demonstrable sign. Here we review the different tools for pain assessment, evaluation, and objectivation; specific features regarding CPP/CPPS will be highlighted in each section.

Take-Home Message. Many patients, both male and female, suffer from CPP/CPPS during their life span. CPP/CPPS is accompanied by psychosocial and mood disturbances, worsened sexual functioning, decreased overall QoL, and occasionally even catastrophizing features. Despite this, CPP and CPPS are subtle, underestimated, and underdiagnosed clinical conditions; also, as different features are often present in the same patient (i.e., pain, muscle tenderness, urinary tract symptoms), correct and satisfied management of patients is seldom feasible. Moreover, as in other pain syndromes, objectivation and evaluation of pain are often troublesome both for patients and physicians.

2. CPP/CPPS Assessment and Objectivation Tools

2.1. Pain Scales and Questionnaires. Besides anamnestic interview and clinical examinations, pain scales and questionnaires are useful and reliable tools to assess pain intensity, and moreover some questionnaires also allow the distinction between nociceptive and neuropathic pain in patients presenting with more complex painful syndromes. Notably, several scales and questionnaires have been developed over years and the choice for the proper one depends on clinical settings; patient's gender, age, and education; and physician's personal experience. We also will review some QoL and psychological assessment questionnaires, as CPP and CPPS often have a detrimental impact on patients' daily activity and represent a considerable burden on emotional and psychological processing. Moreover, as discussed above, patients presenting with associated psychological features besides CPP/CPPS often have poorer pain control and worse clinical course than patients without these features. Recently, some criteria for the reevaluation of scales and questionnaires in chronic pain patients have been proposed [65]. The proposed criteria are content validity (scales should really measure the most important symptoms associated with pathology), test–retest reliability (a patient should give the same answer concerning the same type of pain in case of repeated administration of the same test), and responsiveness (scales results and patient conditions should change in the same way). Below we will review the most widespread scales and questionnaires that might be useful for CPP/CPPS assessment and evaluation.

2.1.1. Monodimensional Pain Scales. Monodimensional pain scales are a simple yet useful tool for a "raw" first assessment of pain. As they merely consist of a value of patient's experienced pain, they are not suitable to reveal the quality of the painful experience or to differentiate nociceptive from neuropathic features of pain. Nevertheless, they are still useful for both acute [15] and chronic pain evaluation, as they are quickly administrable in inpatient and/or outpatient service. The most widespread monodimensional pain scales are the Visual Analogical Scale (VAS) and the Numerical Rating Scale (NRS), which assess pain with an increasing number from 0 (no pain) to 10 (the worst pain imaginable). Another commonly used scale is the Verbal Numerical Rating Scale (VNRS), in which the patient is asked to match pain with an adjective (and a corresponding number). Since they consist in numeric values, monodimensional pain scales are still often used as an outcome measure for clinical trials [66], both for measuring treatment effectiveness [67] and for validating new developed diagnostic tools [68]. All the three scales are comparable in pain evaluation, although different authors may prefer one to the others [69–72]. Wong–Baker Faces Pain Rating Scale is instead a scale which is suitable for speechless patients, as they are asked to indicate a drawn face that is representative of the pain; the drawings are then matched again with corresponding numbers. Lastly, a pain intensity score may also be obtained with a behavioural index, which is the esteem of pain evinced from patient's behaviour. A specific behavioural index, which also included psychological and neurovegetative signs, has been designed for gynaecologic pain evaluation in emergency settings [15].

2.1.2. Multidimensional Pain Scales. These questionnaires allow a more complex pain evaluation beyond asking the patient to merely evaluate the intensity of the painful experience; other relevant features are investigated. The nature and location of pain are assessed, along with the esteem of the impact of pain on daily life activities and mood. Multidimensional pain scales are therefore a useful tool for chronic pain evaluation.

Mc Gill Pain Questionnaire (MPQ) is a widespread multidimensional pain questionnaire. MPQ assesses the intensity of the present pain with a 0–5 scale; moreover, it allows examining pain distribution with a picture representing the human body on ventral and dorsal planes suitable for pain distribution mapping. Further, pain qualities and psychological processing are described by the patient by answering a series of specific questions divided into clusters (sensory discriminative, cognitive evaluative, and motivational affective) [73]. As MPQ, despite being a reliable and useful tool for chronic pain, is very time consuming, a short form of Mc Gill Pain Questionnaire (SF-MPQ), with strong and significant correlation with MPQ, has been developed [74]. It is an easier and more rapidly administrable version of MPQ, consisting of 15 descriptors (11 sensory, 4 affective) which are rated on an intensity scale from 0 to 3. Both the questionnaires have been translated into several languages to make them more suitable in different sociocultural environments. The Brief Pain Inventory (BPI) [75] is another multidimensional questionnaire which assesses the severity of pain and its interference with patients' daily activities. Pain localization, drugs intake, and pain relief are also evaluated. This test could be carried out as a self-report, an interview, or an interactive vocal response system (IVR). The Brief Pain Inventory (BPI) is available in two formats: the BPI short form, which is used for clinical trials and is the version used for foreign-language translations, and the BPI long form, which contains additional descriptive items that may be clinically useful (descriptors of pain, such as "burning" or "tingling").

2.1.3. Neuropathic Pain Assessment Questionnaires. In order to distinguish nociceptive from neuropathic pain features, properly tailored, adequate therapy and screening tools for neuropathic pain are also useful in CPP/CPPS patients; besides the interviews, some tools also include physical tests and examinations. The Neuropathic Pain Scale [76] examines dysesthetic features of pain; it is administrable in an average time of 10 minutes but may be restricted by the level of education of the patient (if lower) and in the experience of the examiner (if limited). PainDETECT [77] is a self-report questionnaire which includes a schematic drawing of pain distribution and esteem of pain fluctuations in time. It, therefore, allows the patient to describe the timing, localization, and radiation of pain, along with any other pain characteristics. PainDETECT is a reliable screening tool with high (around 80%) sensitivity and specificity. The Leeds assessment of neuropathic symptoms and signs (LANSS Pain Scale) [78] is another questionnaire that allows the differentiation between nociceptive and neuropathic pain and the evaluation of the qualitative characteristics of the neuropathic pain itself; compared to clinical diagnosis, its sensitivity and specificity are 82–91 and 80–94%. ID Pain [79] can distinguish nociceptive and neuropathic pain features, with satisfactory accuracy. It is a six-item questionnaire, and for each item the patient is asked to give an affirmative or negative answer and a numeric value from −1 to 5. The total score, resulting from the sum of the scores for each item, will allow discriminating the type of pain. Neuropathic Pain Symptoms Inventory (NPSI) [80] is a questionnaire composed of 12 items (for spontaneous ongoing pain, paroxysmal pain, evoked pain, and paresthesia/dysesthesia). Each of these items is quantified on a 0–10 numerical scale. The discrimination and quantification of five distinct clinically relevant dimensions of neuropathic pain syndromes and their sensitivity to treatment are also assessed. New Neuropathic Pain Diagnostic Questionnaire (DN4) [81] is very easy to administer (only 4 questions) and to evaluate (patient is asked to generate a positive/negative sentence). If the score is equal to 4 or higher, the pain is likely to be neuropathic. The comparison between the diagnostic accuracy of the LANSS Pain Scale and the DN4 for the detection of peripheral neuropathic pain showed that, although both questionnaires are good screening tools, the DN4 questionnaire is particularly recommended for identifying patients with neuropathic pain in clinical practice and research studies [82]. Neuropathic Pain Questionnaire [83] includes 12 different items which help the physician to distinguish neuropathic from nonneuropathic pain. The questionnaire allows assessing negative sensory symptoms (i.e., numbness), positive sensory symptoms such as paresthesia and dysesthesia (often referred to as "tingling pain"), and eventual increase of pain after tactile stimulation. It does not include physical examination measures and is, therefore, not highly recommended.

2.1.4. CPP/CPPS Specific Questionnaires. Specific questionnaires for assessment and evaluation of CPP/CPPS have also been developed, both for diagnostic and therapeutic purposes. Pelvic Pain and Urgency/Frequency Questionnaire (PUF) is a self-report questionnaire designed to investigate the presence of urinary urgency/frequency, pelvic pain, or sexual dysfunction in both sexes and specifically developed by C. Lowell Parsons for the study and diagnosis of Interstitial Cystitis (IC/PBS: Interstitial Cystitis/Painful Bladder Syndrome). It examines both a symptom score (which measures how often a patient experiences problems) and a bother score (how much symptoms bother the patient); combination of both scores is the total PUF score. Score range is between 0 and 35 and a score equal to or greater than 12 is suggestive for the disease in question even if further diagnostic urological, gynaecological, or urogynaecological evaluations are needed. It was, in fact, demonstrated that high scores may be compatible with different diagnoses such as urinary tract infections or overactive bladder syndrome [84]. To date, however, the PUF questionnaire is mainly used in the followup of patients already being treated for urological disorders. Several other scales and questionnaires have been developed in order to assess and evaluate Interstitial Cystitis/Painful Bladder Syndrome patients. One of the most widespread is the O'Leary-Sant Interstitial Cystitis Symptom Index and Problem Index [85] which consist in two self-administrable indices that measure pain and urinary symptoms and their impact (the problem index) on overall QoL and daily activities. Psychometric performance of both the indices was reported to be good, with the symptom index being able to distinguish between patients' and controls' characteristics [86]. The indices also showed good responsiveness [87]. Both indices should be useful in the evaluation and management of patients with IC/PBS; accordingly, they were able to predict treatment outcomes in clinical trials [88]. Similarly, the Bladder Pain/Interstitial Cystitis Symptom score, developed by Humphrey and colleagues [89], was validated in order to properly evaluate IC/PBS patients and correctly allocate them in clinical trials. The examined items are focused on bladder and urinary issues: bladder pain, persistent urge to urinate, and high urinary frequency. The University of Wisconsin Interstitial Cystitis Scale [90] is a symptom scale originally developed for women with Interstitial Cystitis. The scale contains 7 questions directly related to bladder symptoms (bladder pain, bladder discomfort, burning bladder sensation, nycturia, sleep difficulties due to nycturia, polyuria, and urinary urgency) in the last 24 hours. The Pelvic Pain Assessment Form is another gender-specific scale designed for women and developed by the International Pelvic Pain Society [91] and is composed of two parts: the first should be filled out by the patient and the last by the physician. The form allows complete registration of information about the patient's pain (causes, duration of pain, Visual Analogue Scale score, pain medications, and pain distribution maps), patient's past and recent clinical history (including surgical, obstetrical, family, medical, menstrual, and gastrointestinal history; eating and health habits; genitourinary symptoms; coping mechanisms; sexual and physical abuse history), and eventual former evaluations performed by other physicians. The form also includes a short form of Mc Gill Pain Questionnaire and a section dedicated to a pelvic varicosity pain syndrome specific questionnaire. The physician will also provide a physical examination, a gynaecological examination, and lastly a diagnostic and therapeutic plan. Notably, this form does not have a diagnostic value. The National Institute of Health Chronic Prostatitis Symptom Index (NIH-CPSI) Questionnaire [92] is a 13-item index developed to assess symptoms and quality of life in men with Chronic Prostatitis/Chronic Pelvic Pain Syndrome (CP/CPPS) [93]. It has demonstrated good reliability, validity, and responsiveness to change [94], and it has been used as the primary outcome variable in multiple large-scale studies of CP/CPPS treatments. It has also been translated into multiple languages for international use [95, 96]. It is indicated for patients complaining of CPP, probably caused by Chronic Prostatitis or CPPS. Pain, voiding symptoms, and any interference of the symptoms with the quality of life are evaluated. The Genitourinary Pain Index (GUPI) is a more recent symptom index developed from NIH-CPSI [97] in order to assess genitourinary pain in both men and women. The GUPI included items dealing with urinary symptoms, localization and intensity of pain symptoms, and overall quality of life. Total scores range from 0 to 45; individual scores for the domains of pain, urinary symptoms, and quality of life impact can also be derived. Similarly, another questionnaire, the CPPQ-Mohedo, has been developed by Díaz Mohedo and colleagues [98]. It is also derived from NIH-CPSI score for male patients, with the purpose of editing a feasible questionnaire for both male and female patients with the same analysed items.

Recently, a novel phenotyping system for urological CPPS has been developed, the UPOINT system [99]. The acronym UPOINT stands for urinary, psychosocial, organ-specific, infection, neurological/systemic, and tenderness. It has been developed to stratify Interstitial Cystitis/Bladder Pain Syndrome and Chronic Prostatitis/Prostate Pain Syndrome according to six domains that allow patients' better assessment and evaluation, clustering and analysing the parts (i.e., the domains) of the acronym [100–102]. The UPOINT system is feasible for both genders and allows reliable and accurate match with severity of symptoms in each domain. Furthermore, several researches based patients' selection and treatment outcome measurement on UPOINT system scores [103], as the multidomain allocation of any symptom experienced by a patient allows a consequent multitargeted therapeutic strategy that is specially tailored for that patient and actually improves the various therapeutic outcomes in different trials [104–107].

Finally, a dedicated questionnaire has also been proposed for Vulvodynia patients [108], which might be helpful in assessing patients' symptoms and therefore recommending an adequate therapy.

2.1.5. QoL and Psychological Assessment. CPP and CPPS are, according to their definition, usually associated with detrimental effects on overall QoL and with psychological comorbidities. Moreover, it has been shown that psychological impairment per se is responsible for worsened symptoms and is a predictor for bad therapeutic outcome (see Section 1). Therefore, for an exhaustive evaluation of CPP/CPPS patients, both QoL and psychological status should be assessed.

Several questionnaires explore the impact of pain symptoms on QoL in order to provide more complete management of the Chronic Pelvic Pain. Quality of life is best defined as patients perception of and reaction to their health status and nonmedical aspects of their lives (i.e., physical, functional, emotional, mental, and social wellbeing). QoL is measured with a collection of items, scales, domains, and instruments. In particular, instruments are classified as generic (i.e., SF-36), disease-specific, site- or region-specific, dimension-specific (i.e., Mc Gill Pain Questionnaire), or utility measures (i.e., EuroQoL EQ-5D). To ensure an appropriate evaluation, the use of a disease-specific instrument in combination with a generic instrument should be recommended [109]. Short Form Health Survey (SF-36) evaluates different items of quality of life in various areas through 36 questions and is extremely reproducible and reliable. It is the most commonly used questionnaire for pelvic pain assessment [109]. There is also a shrunk version of SF-36, SF-12, which only examines 12 questions. EuroQoL (EQ-5D) is another reliable questionnaire [110], not disease specific, which meets internationally accepted standards. This simple and short questionnaire allows measuring the health status of the patients and their quality of life in order to evaluate overall health status. It consists of two distinct sections: The first is composed of five items (mobility, self-care, usual activities, pain/discomfort, and anxiety/depression) that affect the actual health status of the patient. Each item provides the possibility to choose between three (or more, recently five) different levels of severity. The second section of the questionnaire includes the EQ-VAS, thus allowing also pain assessment. The Pain Disability Index [111] is a psychometric assessment tool designed to help patients to measure the impact of chronic pain on daily activities. The patient is shown a form composed of various daily activities grouped into seven categories and is asked to indicate (through a 0 to 10 score) the perceived impairment. The PIQ-6 Pain Impact Questionnaire Package [112] is another tool which analyses the interference of pain with physical, mental, and social features. Pain Disability Questionnaire focuses on pain localization and radiation; time of the first episode of pain; previous events; pain description through adjectives; interference of pain with work, school, social life, family, sport, and or any other daily activity; previous therapies or medical examinations; efficacy of medication intake. Sexual functioning self-assessment is also available for both male and female patients [113, 114]; it might be worth evaluating this feature as well, as sexual function abnormalities are relatively frequent in CPP/CPPS patients of both genders.

Regarding psychological status, anxiety, depression, and catastrophizing may be assessed with proper questionnaires as well [115]. Patients with CPP/CPPS have an increased risk of developing psychological-psychiatric disorders even if the latter may preexist CPP/CPPS. We suggest that easy tools for psychological screening such as the Behaviour Illness Questionnaire, the Hamilton Psychiatric Rating Scale for Depression, and the Hospital Anxiety and depression Scale (HADS) should be used in order to provide a more complete and careful evaluation for CPP/CPPS patients. Also, catastrophizing may be assessed with a dedicate questionnaire [116].

Take-Home Message. Pain scales and questionnaires are fundamental tools when approaching, assessing, and evaluating CPP/CPPS patients. Mono- and Multidimensional scales are useful tools for patient assessment, for trials enrolment, and for therapeutic outcomes. CPP/CPPS specific questionnaires and indices are as well unneglectable tool for CPP/CPPS evaluation, as assessment and therapeutic interventions are better guided by scoring systems such as the UPOINT system. Finally, psychosocial and QoL scales as well should be borne in mind, as several patients report detrimental effects of CPP/CPPS on psychosocial functioning and overall QoL.

2.2. Pain Objectivation: Quantitative Sensory Testing and Electrophysiology. As mentioned above (see Section 1), neuropathic pain features are commonly found in many CPP/CPPS patients. Recognizing such cluster of patients has remarkable diagnostic and therapeutic value, as a proper therapy may be prescribed to those patients that experience dysesthetic/neuropathic symptoms. The objectivation of neuropathic pain features, although screening tools like questionnaires are helpful, is still a challenge for physicians. Quantitative Sensory Testing (QST) is a tool that measures the perception of mechanical, thermal, and painful stimuli delivered to determine the perceptive threshold for each sensation. Stimuli are delivered at increasing and decreasing intensities. Specific devices (i.e., von Frey hairs, weighted needles, vibrometers, and thermodes) are used to assess each sensory threshold. Several studies assessed QST changes in CPP/CPPS patients. A recent investigation comparing Neuropathic Pain Questionnaires and QST findings demonstrated [10] that only a few female CPP patients in the examined cohort have no changes in pain thresholds. Also, a positive correlation was found when matching QST results with questionnaires. QST assessment has been performed in several cohorts of CPP/CPPS patients with different techniques used to deliver the painful stimulation. Another recent investigation compared bladder sensitivity between patients with pelvic pain and patients who were pain-free by noninvasive and controlled bladder distension [37]. Reproductive-age women with nonbladder CPP, those with Painful Bladder Syndrome (PBS), and those who are healthy controls were enrolled. Participants were compared on cystometric capacity, pelvic floor PPTs, and pelvic muscle function. Participants with PBS exhibited higher bladder distension pain than those with CPP, with both groups reporting higher pain levels than controls. No significant associations were found between bladder distension pain and pelvic muscle structure or pain sensitivity measures; however, bladder distension pain positively correlated with both vaginal PPTs adjacent to the bladder and pain with transvaginal bladder palpation. Similar findings were also found in a previous study comparing CPP/PBS patients to healthy controls [117]: women with CPP or PBS exhibited enhanced pain sensitivity with lower PPTs than pain-free participants; also, prolonged pain aftersensation was documented in CPP/PBS patients. PPTs were also evaluated in male CPP patients affected by Urological Chronic Pelvic Pain Syndrome [118]; PPTs on 10 genitopelvic sites and one control site (deltoid) were measured, and UCPPS men had reliably lower pain thresholds compared to controls in all locations, including the deltoid. UCPPS men also demonstrated consistently lower overall pain thresholds regardless of location. Besides assessing a reduced PPT in pelvic area, this study also underscored widespread alteration in pain perception, shedding light on possible central mechanisms of pain perception in CPP/CPPS patients. This study assessed PPTs with a specific algometer, which is a dedicated device that administers a determined pressure to patients in order to evaluate pain thresholds. QST evaluation has also been performed in a cohort of men suffering from Erectile Dysfunction [119], which may often complicate the clinical history of men suffering from CPPS as discussed in Section 1; vibration, pressure, spatial perception, and warm and cold thermal thresholds were evaluated in 107 patients. It has been found that warm thermal thresholds were altered in Erectile Dysfunction patients versus controls, thus demonstrating a neurophysiological alteration in these patients.

Algometers have previously been used for the definition of the Myofascial Pain Syndrome (which may be responsible for CPP) [120] with the registration of PPTs, despite the lack of a gold standard in the definition of such syndrome. The study confirmed the usefulness of the pressure algometer for a more correct definition of Myofascial Pain Syndrome with the stimulation of the muscles of the anterior abdominal wall. In order to measure genital PPTs in CPP/CPPS patients, a specific algometer has been developed. It was suggested that pain threshold values measured through an internal (transvaginal) algometer can be considered a reliable and valid measures of pain sensitivity of the pelvic muscles compared with NRS values [121, 122]. Pain threshold values could be useful in the formulation of the diagnostic criteria for any disease associated with somatic and/or visceral pelvic pain. The authors found an association between pain threshold and the applied pressure value bringing on pain. The recordings were performed in 10 specific points: pubococcygeus, iliococcygeus, coccygeus, and obturator for each side as well as the anterior and posterior vaginal wall. The structure of a vaginal algometer includes a polyethylene terephthalate glycol housing, resembling a thin thimble, and fits on the distal tip of the examiner's finger as a thin shell. This fits underneath an examination glove and anatomical design minimizes any additional discomfort resulting from a normal musculoskeletal examination of the pelvis. The signal, originating from the palpation, is amplified and passes through a digital converter. A recent research investigated the relationship between nongenital tender point tenderness and intravaginal muscle pain intensity [123] in Vulvodynia patients with or without fibromyalgia. A significant correlation was found between numeric rating scale pain scores on the nongenital tender point tenderness exam and algometer testing on the iliococcygeus region and the posterior vaginal wall. Subjects with fibromyalgia by tender point tenderness had significantly higher iliococcygeal pain and posterior vaginal wall pain than women without fibromyalgia. Further, in order to measure external genitals PPT, a dedicated Vulvalgesiometer was also developed [124]. The authors performed a trial investigating different outcomes. First of all, they established that the Vulvalgesiometer was able to distinguish between women affected by Provoked Vestibulodynia (PVD) and healthy controls. Indeed, when comparing external genitals PPTs of the two cohorts, women affected by PVD showed significantly lower vestibular PPTs than unaffected women. Another assessed outcome was interrater reliability, which was assessed by PPTs measurement performed by two different investigators. As the Vulvalgesiometer also showed good interrater reliability, the authors concluded that it might serve as a tool for both clinical and research purposes. A more recent investigation evaluated PPTs in two groups of PVD patients, in order to assess differences between primary (PVD1) and secondary (PVD2) PVD patients by eliciting PPTs with a Vulvalgesiometer [125]. Also, questionnaires, psychophysical testing, and neuroimaging (both structural and functional) were examined as outcomes in order to disclose intergroup differences. Women with PVD1 showed lower PPTs compared with PVD2 patients. Moreover, PVD1 patients also exhibited higher anxiety and catastrophizing scores as demonstrated by questionnaires results. Further, neuroimaging differences between the two cohorts of patients were also confirmed. Gray matter (GM) density measured with neuroimaging differed between groups: Women with PVD1 showed significant GM density reduction in the left anterior cingulate cortex, parahippocampal gyrus, left inferior temporal gyrus, bilateral precuneus, right superior frontal gyrus, and some cerebellar areas. Women with PVD2 also showed GM density reduction, but of a minor magnitude and in fewer brain areas (the right superior occipital gyrus and the left inferior parietal cortex). In the same way, functional MRI scans documented more pronounced activation of pain-related areas (the postcentral gyrus, midcingulate cortex, insula, and thalamus) in PVD1 than PVD2 patients. The role of brain neuroimaging in CPP patients will be better elucidated in the next section (see Section 3). Another recent investigation further assessed neurophysiological modifications in a cohort of Provoked Vestibulodynia [126], as Pelvic Floor Muscle abnormalities were detected and matched with a surface Electromyographic evaluation. Pelvic Floor Muscles of the patients were stiff and more prone to increased resting and activated muscle tone (during stretching) than control subjects; all these abnormalities were documented by surface Electromyographic recording of anomalies. Recently, a new algometer for vestibular pain has been developed [127]; when compared with the Vulvalgesiometer for PPTs and Pain Pressure Tolerance (PPTol) outcomes, this new developed algometer was found to be a reliable and valid instrument for measuring PPTs and PPTols in the vestibular area in women with PVD, and therefore this technology may be promising for pinpointing treatment mechanisms and efficacy. Lastly, thermal algometry for CPP assessment has been proposed [128, 129] in men with CPP. Two series of fast trains of perineal and front thigh thermal painful stimuli through a small thermal electrode were administered to the patients, in association with a computerized VAS registration. A lower thermal pain threshold was detected, and the authors speculated that these results were related to central sensitization processes; this idea was also supported by some studies regarding pudendal somatosensory evoked potentials (SEP) recordings. SEP evaluation was also recently performed in Chronic Prostatitis/Chronic Pelvic Pain Syndrome (CP/CPPS) patients [130]. For SEP recording, electrical stimuli were applied with penile ring electrodes for dorsal penile nerve stimulation; N50 latencies were significantly shortened in the patient group compared to the healthy controls, thus demonstrating a pathogenetic neural mechanism related to central sensitization processes underlying CP/CPPS. CP/CPPS patients were also examined by investigating both SEP and Electromyography (EMG) [131]. Intramuscular EMG, right and left bulbocavernosus reflex, and cortical SEP during stimulation of pudendal nerve were evaluated, and a high frequency of abnormal neurophysiological patterns in the absence of clinical neurological disease was found in these patients.

Some authors investigated CPP/CPPS patients with Neurometer Current Perception Threshold (CPT) analysis in order to objectivate neuropathic features in such patients. Neurometer evaluations were firstly performed in male and female healthy subjects in order to assess Current Perception Thresholds in the lower urinary tract [132]. Neurometer CPT can quantify the functional integrity of myelinated (with both large or small diameter) and unmyelinated sensory fibers. Patients with Painful Bladder Syndrome/Interstitial Cystitis or overactive bladder have been evaluated [133–135] with stimuli delivered in the form of alternating currents with different stimulation frequency in order to evaluate Aß, Aδ, and C fibers and producing threshold values for the current perception in such bladder afferent fibers. Men suffering from CPPS were also evaluated using Neurometer CPT [136] although no significative differences were found between CPPS patients and matched healthy controls.

Unfortunately, only a limited number of investigations have been performed in order to reveal neurophysiological abnormalities in CPP/CPPS patients. Laser Evoked Potentials (LEPs) are one of the most reliable laboratory tools to objectivate and diagnose neuropathic pain [137], but no studies investigating CPP/CPPS have been performed so far.

Take-Home Message. QST provides integration for the regular neurological examination, giving the opportunity to better objectivate neurophysiological abnormalities in CPP/CPPS patients by establishing pain thresholds. Algometry allows optimal standardization of QST, as it gives reliable and precise quantification of the administered stimulus and the subsequent threshold. Electrophysiological evaluation, with SEP and/or EMG, may further help to objectivate neurophysiological anomalies in CPP/CPPS patients. Despite these promising features, only a few studies have been performed, and therefore further investigations are warranted to elucidate the real importance of these tools when evaluating CPP/CPPS patients.

3. New Perspectives: The Role of Brain Neuroimaging

In recent years, Magnetic Resonance Imaging (MRI) and functional MRI (fMRI) have been suggested as tools to diagnose and objectivate chronic pain, as characteristic abnormalities have been detected in several chronic pain syndromes [138–141].

In the same manner, several studies assessed brain abnormalities with fMRI protocols in different CPP/CPPS patients both for pathophysiological and for therapeutic meanings. In particular, Endometriosis patients were evaluated with different neuroimaging protocols. Proton spectroscopy and seed-based resting functional connectivity MRI were used to determine whether women with Endometriosis display differences in insula excitatory neurotransmitter concentrations or intrinsic brain connectivity to other pain-related brain regions [142]. Compared to age-matched pain-free controls, women with Endometriosis-associated CPP displayed increased levels of combined glutamine-glutamate (Glx) within the anterior insula and greater anterior insula connectivity to the medial prefrontal cortex (mPFC). Increased connectivity between these regions was positively correlated with anterior insula Glx concentrations and also with psychopathological outcomes. The same group previously investigated changes in regional Gray Matter (GM) volume in women with Endometriosis-related CPP [143] with voxel-based morphometry, which is a neuroimaging tool that allows brain volumetric comparison between two groups of patients. Different groups of patients with CPP and/or Endometriosis were compared with healthy controls. Women with Endometriosis-associated CPP displayed decreased GM volume in several brain regions when compared with healthy women: the left thalamus, left cingulate gyrus, right putamen, and right insula showed significant volume loss. The areas discovered to be relatively "atrophic" are involved in pain processing, and pain cognitive/emotional cortical pathways (the so-called "pain matrix") are often affected in CPP patients as shown by several structural and functional neuroimaging investigations. Women with CPP without Endometriosis were also evaluated and indeed showed GM volume loss in the left thalamus when compared with the healthy controls group. Notably, women with Endometriosis without CPP symptoms showed no volumetric differences in comparison with healthy women. The authors therefore speculated that different physiopathological mechanisms underlie the different MRI findings, as CPP alone (in women without Endometriosis) appeared to be responsible for volumetric GM decrease although of less magnitude than CPP accompanied by Endometriosis.

Furthermore, brain connectivity was evaluated in Endometriosis patients with resting-state fMRI imaging, before and after psychotherapeutic protocols [144]. It was identified as a cortical network comprising the right anterolateral hippocampus (a region modulating the hypothalamic-pituitary-adrenal axis and somatosensory, viscerosensory, and interoceptive brain regions), and a reduction in connectivity predicted therapy-induced improvement in patients' anxiety.

Besides patients with Endometriosis, patients with urologic CPP were evaluated in several neuroimaging protocols. The Multidisciplinary Approach to the Study of Chronic Pelvic Pain (MAPP) Research Network (http://www.mappnet-http://www.mappnetwork.org/) is a multicenter collaborative research group established to conduct integrated studies on participants with urologic Chronic Pelvic Pain Syndrome (UCPPS) [145]. The aim of the group was to evaluate etiology; natural history; and clinical, demographic, and behavioural characteristics of urological CPP patients. A branch of the MAPP Network compared resting-state brain activity analysis, which is a functional neuroimaging tool that provides estimation of brain functional connectivity (FC), between women with urological CPPS and healthy women. Several FC abnormalities were observed in the CPPS cohort. First of all, significantly decreased FC was reported in 2 regions of the posterior medial cortex (the posterior cingulate cortex and the left precuneus) [146]. The left precuneus also showed decreased FC to several prefrontal and parietal cortical regions involved in cognitive tasks, executive functioning, set-shifting processes, and reward processes. Furthermore, increased FC between the posterior cingulate cortex and insular cortex, dorsolateral prefrontal cortex, thalamus, globus pallidus, putamen, amygdala, and hippocampus was detected in the CPPS group. Notably, these involved areas are part of a cortical network that processes cognitive and emotional characteristics of several kinds of sensory information, including pain. These results show how CPPS affects brain connectivity in different regions and pathways and provide new insights into pathophysiological CPP/CPPS mechanisms. Another branch of the MAPP study compared UCPPS patients with healthy controls and Irritable Bowel Syndrome (IBS) patients [147, 148]. White Matter differences were examined, with specific neuroimaging tools developed to investigate axonal and White Matter abnormalities such as Fractional Anisotropy (FA), Generalized Anisotropy (GA), Mean Diffusivity (MD), and Track Density. All the investigations documented remarkable differences between CPPS patients and healthy controls. Reduced FA was reported in the genu and splenium of the corpus callosum of UCPPS patients compared with healthy women. Conversely, increased FA was documented in some thalamic and basal ganglia regions, as well as in a tract included in the left somatosensory cortex, which may be associated with somatosensory integration of pelvic stimuli. MD and GA also were altered in CPPS patients, as higher MD in the basal ganglia, right frontal lobe, bilateral corona radiata fibers, and genu of the corpus callosum was detected in CPPS women when compared to controls; moreover, GA analysis showed decreased GA in several brain regions, mostly in corpus callosum and corona radiata [147]. Similar results were obtained by another MAPP group of investigators, as reduced FA was observed in several regions involved in pain perception, processing, modulation, and emotional integration such as right corticospinal tract and right anterior thalamic radiation [148]. Both research groups moreover distinguished these abnormalities from the IBS group MRI findings, as neuroimaging findings appear to be more pronounced and widespread in UCPPS patients when compared with IBS patients. Thus, the authors speculated that different pain syndromes may elicit different changes in brain structure and functioning.

The MAPP study group also enrolled men with Chronic Prostatitis/Chronic Pelvic Pain Syndrome comparing them to healthy controls. With resting-state FC analysis, significant group difference was observed in the functional connectivity between pelvic-motor and the right posterior insula [149]. It was therefore speculated that brain networks controlling Pelvic Floor Muscles reflected altered resting Pelvic Floor Muscle activity in men with CP/CPPS compared to healthy controls. Another recent functional neuroimaging investigation [150] revealed alterations in Regional Homogeneity of resting-state cerebral activity in patients with Chronic Prostatitis/Chronic Pelvic Pain Syndrome. Regional Homogeneity is a voxel-based measure of brain activity which evaluates the similarity or synchronization between a voxel (of a given brain region) and its nearest neighbors, based on the hypothesis that intrinsic brain activity is manifested by clusters of voxels rather than single voxels. It was found that CP/CPPS patients had significantly decreased Regional Homogeneity in the bilateral anterior cingulate cortices, insulae, and right medial prefrontal cortex; on the other hand, significantly increased Regional Homogeneity in the brainstem and right thalamus was detected by comparing CP/CPPS values with those of healthy controls. All these structures are thought to be relevant to pain processing and modulation. Notably, left anterior cingulate cortex, bilateral insular cortices, and brainstem abnormalities also correlated with pain symptoms and pain scale scores. CP/CPPS patients were also evaluated with another functional neuroimaging technique, Arterial Spin Labelling, which allows investigating slow varying changes in brain function [151].

Therapy-related longitudinal modifications in Arterial Spin Labelling were assessed after a cycle of sono-electromagnetic therapy or placebo. It was found that responders and nonresponders to the therapeutic protocol showed different Cerebral Blood Flow (CBF) modifications as documented by Arterial Spin Labelling. In detail, nonresponder patients showed CBF upregulation in the hippocampus, whereas responders underscored CBF downregulation in the prefrontal cortex and anterior cingulate cortex and upregulation in the dorsolateral prefrontal cortex. Responders therefore, according to the positive therapeutic outcome, showed a modulation in CBF in regions involved in pain processing and modulation. Moreover, structural brain modifications have also been investigated in CP/CPPS patients [152, 153], and a significative reduction of relative Gray Matter volume in the anterior cingulate cortex of the dominant hemisphere, compared to healthy controls, was documented [152]. Also, density alterations of Gray Matter in pain relevant regions (anterior insula and anterior cingulate cortices) were evident in a different cohort of CP/CPPS patients [153]; the findings positively correlated with pain intensity and duration of chronic pain.

Vulvodynia patients have also been recently investigated with fMRI scanning (resting-state analysis) [154], and alterations in resting-state were compared with those of HCs and a chronic pain control group (IBS). Intrinsic connectivity of regions comprising sensorimotor, salience, and default mode resting-state networks was examined, and subjects with Vulvodynia showed substantial alterations in the intrinsic connectivity of these networks compared with both healthy controls and Irritable Bowel Syndrome patients. The intrinsic connectivity of many of the regions showing group differences during rest was moderately associated with clinical symptom reports in CPP patients.

Primary Dysmenorrhea (PDM) women were also enrolled in several neuroimaging protocols. Voxel-based morphometry analysis showed abnormal volumetric decreases in regions involved in pain transmission and higher level sensory processing and affected regulation, while volumetric increases were found in regions involved in pain modulation and in regulation of endocrine function [155]. The same authors also investigated PDM patients using fluorodeoxyglucose positron emission tomography [156]. Results showed increased activity in prefrontal/orbitofrontal regions and left ventral posterior thalamus, while decreased activity was mainly observed in sensorimotor regions of the left hemisphere at onset compared to offset of PDM. These results were specific to menstrual pain and were not found in menstrual matched controls. Orbitofrontal activities were positively related to subjective pain ratings, while somatosensory activities were negatively related to these ratings. Another recent study investigated PDM patients with FC analysis; also, the analysis of Single Nucleotide Polymorphism (SNP) of mu-opioid receptor was performed and matched with fMRI results [157]. It was found that G allele SNP carriers, in comparison to AA homozygotes, exhibited functional hypoconnectivity between the anterior cingulate cortex (ACC) and Periaqueductal Gray (PAG). Furthermore, G allele carriers lost the correlation with spontaneous pain experience and exhibited dysfunctional Descending Pain Modulating System as confirmed by PAG-seeded FC dynamics. Similar mismatches with the Descending Pain Modulating System were already previously detected in Brain-Derived Neurotrophic Factor (BDNF) Val66Met SNP carriers by the same authors [158] using resting-state FC examinations.

All these investigations document how CPP and CPPS, rather than being merely urogynaecological syndromes, have fundamental neural pathophysiological mechanisms, as neuroimaging abnormalities have been identified in several cohorts of patients. These alterations may possibly reflect sensitization processes and neuroplastic modifications in Central Nervous System, which are subsequent to the chronic painful stimulation arising from the periphery. It is also possible that some patients, that is, SNP carriers, have alterations in cortical circuitry that predispose them to the development of chronic pain syndromes such as CPP. Of course, other researches are warranted to better understand the alterations in CPP patients' brain and to properly match the neuroradiological findings with clinical and possibly genetic assessments. Nevertheless, brain neuroimaging in CPP patients appears to be a promising field as it offers the future possibility of a reliable noninvasive marker of CPP and CPP severity.

Take-Home Message. Being similar to other patients with chronic pain conditions, CPP/CPPS patients showed several structural and functional brain neuroimaging abnormalities. Anomalies were found in both male and female CPP/CPPS patients. Therefore, brain neuroimaging appears to be a promising tool for further evaluation of CPP/CPPS patients both for pathophysiological and for diagnostic/assessment purposes, although further researches are surely warranted to fully understand the correlations between CPP/CPPS symptoms and brain functional and structural anomalies.

4. Conclusions

Despite the development of several screening and diagnostic tools, pain evaluation and objectivation still remain not seldom troublesome in CPP/CPPS. Nevertheless, a full and correct assessment of patients' painful experience can help physicians to properly develop appropriate therapeutic protocols specially tailored for those patients, taking into account pain symptoms as well as eventual comorbidities, psychological features, and functional QoL status. Future investigations are warranted to ameliorate diagnostic tools accuracy and to correlate instrumental findings.

References

[1] http://www.iasp-pain.org/Education/Content.aspx?ItemNumber=1698.

[2] D. S. Engeler, A. P. Baranowski, P. Dinis-Oliveira et al., "The 2013 EAU guidelines on chronic pelvic pain: Is management of chronic pelvic pain a habit, a philosophy, or a science? 10 years of development," *European Urology*, vol. 64, no. 3, pp. 431–439, 2013.

[3] ACOG Practice Bulletin No. 51, "Chronic pelvic pain. ACOG Committee on Practice Bulletins-Gynecology," *Obstetrics & Gynecology*, vol. 103, no. 3, pp. 589–605, 2004.

[4] L. M. Nyberg, J. N. Krieger, and J. C. Nickel, "Textbook of Prostatitis," in *National Institutes of Health Classification of Chronic Prostatitis*, J. C. Nickel, Ed., vol. 28, CRC Press, London, UK, 1999.

[5] J. T. Sigalos and A. W. Pastuszak, "Chronic orchialgia: epidemiology, diagnosis and evaluation," *Translational Andrology and Urology*, vol. 6, Supplement 1, pp. S37–S43, 2017.

[6] A. Aljumaily, H. Al-Khazraji, A. Gordon, S. Lau, and K. A. Jarvi, "Characteristics and etiologies of chronic scrotal pain: A common but poorly understood condition," *Pain Research & Management*, vol. 2017, Article ID 3829168, 2017.

[7] V. Anaf, P. Simon, I. El Nakadi et al., "Hyperalgesia, nerve infiltration and nerve growth factor expression in deep adenomyotic nodules, peritoneal and ovarian endometriosis," *Human Reproduction*, vol. 17, no. 7, pp. 1895–1900, 2002.

[8] A. P. Malykhina, "Neural mechanisms of pelvic organ cross-sensitization," *Neuroscience*, vol. 149, no. 3, pp. 660–672, 2007.

[9] J. Brawn, M. Morotti, K. T. Zondervan, C. M. Becker, and K. Vincent, "Central changes associated with chronic pelvic pain and endometriosis," *Human Reproduction Update*, vol. 20, no. 5, Article ID dmu025, pp. 737–747, 2014.

[10] L. H. R. Whitaker, J. Reid, A. Choa et al., "An exploratory study into objective and reported characteristics of neuropathic pain in women with chronic pelvic pain," *PLoS ONE*, vol. 11, no. 4, Article ID e0151950, 2016.

[11] G. Wang, N. Tokushige, R. Markham, and I. S. Fraser, "Rich innervation of deep infiltrating endometriosis," *Human Reproduction*, vol. 24, no. 4, pp. 827–834, 2009.

[12] A. K. George, M. A. Sadek, S. S. Saluja, J. Y. Fariello, K. E. Whitmore, and R. M. Moldwin, "The impact of neuropathic pain in the chronic pelvic pain population," *The Journal of Urology*, vol. 188, no. 5, pp. 1783–1787, 2012.

[13] E. Dargie, I. Gilron, and C. F. Pukall, "Self-Reported Neuropathic Pain Characteristics of Women With Provoked Vulvar Pain: A Preliminary Investigation," *The Journal of Sexual Medicine*, vol. 14, no. 4, pp. 577–591, 2017.

[14] http://www.americanpainsociety.org.

[15] A. Fauconnier, E. Dallongeville, C. Huchon, Y. Ville, and B. Falissard, "Measurement of acute pelvic pain intensity in gynecology: A comparison of five methods," *Obstetrics & Gynecology*, vol. 113, no. 2, pp. 260–269, 2009.

[16] P. Vercellini, E. Somigliana, P. Viganò, A. Abbiati, G. Barbara, and L. Fedele, "Chronic pelvic pain in women: etiology, pathogenesis and diagnostic approach," *Gynecological Endocrinology*, vol. 25, no. 3, pp. 149–158, 2009.

[17] A. Ahangari, "Prevalence of chronic pelvic pain among women: An updated review," *Pain Physician*, vol. 17, no. 2, pp. E141–E147, 2014.

[18] E. Díaz Mohedo, J. Wärnberg, F. J. Barón López, S. Mera Velasco, and A. Cabello Burgos, "Chronic pelvic pain in Spanish women: Prevalence and associated risk factors. A cross-sectional study," *Clinical and Experimental Obstetrics & Gynecology*, vol. 41, no. 3, pp. 243–248, 2014.

[19] E. Díaz-Mohedo, F. Hita-Contreras, A. Luque-Suárez, C. Walker-Chao, D. Zarza-Luciáñez, and J. Salinas-Casado, "Prevalence and risk factors of pelvic pain," *Actas Urológicas Españolas*, vol. 38, no. 5, pp. 298–303, 2014.

[20] A. A. Ayorinde, S. Bhattacharya, K. L. Druce, G. T. Jones, and G. J. Macfarlane, "Chronic pelvic pain in women of reproductive and post-reproductive age: a population-based study," *European Journal of Pain*, vol. 21, no. 3, pp. 445–455, 2017.

[21] A. A. Ayorinde, G. J. Macfarlane, L. Saraswat, and S. Bhattacharya, "Chronic pelvic pain in women: An epidemiological perspective," *Women's Health Journal (WHJ)*, vol. 11, no. 6, pp. 851–864, 2015.

[22] A. M. Suskind, S. H. Berry, B. A. Ewing, M. N. Elliott, M. J. Suttorp, and J. Q. Clemens, "The prevalence and overlap of interstitial cystitis/bladder pain syndrome and chronic prostatitis/chronic pelvic pain syndrome in men: Results of the rand interstitial cystitis epidemiology male study," *The Journal of Urology*, vol. 189, no. 1, pp. 141–145, 2013.

[23] A. E. Bharucha and T. H. Lee, "Anorectal and Pelvic Pain," *Mayo Clinic Proceedings*, vol. 91, no. 10, pp. 1471–1486, 2016.

[24] H. Hedelin, H. Johannisson, and L. Welin, "Prevalence of the chronic prostatitis/chronic pelvic pain syndrome among 40-69-year-old men residing in a temperate climate," *Scandinavian Journal of Urology*, vol. 47, no. 5, pp. 390–392, 2013.

[25] A. S. Polackwich and D. A. Shoskes, "Chronic prostatitis/chronic pelvic pain syndrome: a review of evaluation and therapy," *Prostate Cancer and Prostatic Diseases*, vol. 19, no. 2, pp. 132–138, 2016.

[26] J. B. Forrest and S. Schmidt, "Interstitial cystitis, chronic nonbacterial prostatitis and chronic pelvic pain syndrome in men: A common and frequently identical clinical entity," *The Journal of Urology*, vol. 172, no. 6, pp. 2561-2562, 2004.

[27] D. A. Shoskes, J. R. Landis, Y. Wang, J. C. Nickel, S. I. Zeitlin, and R. Nadler, "Impact of post-ejaculatory pain in men with category III chronic prostatitis/chronic pelvic pain syndrome," *The Journal of Urology*, vol. 172, no. 2, pp. 542–547, 2004.

[28] Y. Zhang, T. Zheng, X. Tu et al., "Erectile dysfunction in chronic prostatitis/chronic pelvic pain syndrome: Outcomes from a multi-center study and risk factor analysis in a single center," *PLoS ONE*, vol. 11, no. 4, Article ID e0153054, 2016.

[29] D. A. Shoskes, R. Berger, A. Elmi, J. R. Landis, K. J. Propert, and S. Zeitlin, "Muscle tenderness in men with chronic prostatitis/chronic pelvic pain syndrome: The chronic prostatitis cohort study," *The Journal of Urology*, vol. 179, no. 2, pp. 556–560, 2008.

[30] D. A. Tripp, J. C. Nickel, S. Ross, C. Mullins, and N. Stechyson, "Prevalence, symptom impact and predictors of chronic prostatitis-like symptoms in Canadian males aged 16-19 years," *BJU International*, vol. 103, no. 8, pp. 1080–1084, 2009.

[31] D. A. Tripp, J. C. Nickel, J. L. Pikard, and L. Katz, "Chronic prostatitis-like symptoms in African males aged 16-19 years," *Canadian Journal of Urology*, vol. 19, no. 1, pp. 6081–6087, 2012.

[32] R. T. Strebel, T. Leippold, T. Luginbuehl, M. Muentener, V. Praz, and D. Hauri, "Chronic scrotal pain syndrome: management among urologists in Switzerland," *European Urology*, vol. 47, no. 6, pp. 812–816, 2005.

[33] H. Ciftci, M. Savas, E. Yeni, A. Verit, and U. Topal, "Chronic orchialgia and associated diseases," *Current Urology Reports*, vol. 4, no. 2, pp. 67–70, 2010.

[34] R. E. Berger, M. A. Ciol, I. Rothman, and J. A. Turner, "Pelvic tenderness is not limited to the prostate in chronic prostatitis/chronic pelvic pain syndrome (CPPS) type IIIA and IIIB:

Comparison of men with and without CP/CPPS," *BMC Urology*, vol. 7, article no. 17, 2007.

[35] H. H. Lai, T. Jemielita, S. Sutcliffe et al., "Characterization of Whole Body Pain in Urological Chronic Pelvic Pain Syndrome at Baseline: A MAPP Research Network Study," *The Journal of Urology*, vol. 198, no. 3, pp. 622–631, 2017.

[36] R. U. Anderson, T. Sawyer, D. Wise, A. Morey, and B. H. Nathanson, "Painful Myofascial Trigger Points and Pain Sites in Men With Chronic Prostatitis/Chronic Pelvic Pain Syndrome," *The Journal of Urology*, vol. 182, no. 6, pp. 2753–2758, 2009.

[37] F. F. Tu, J. N. Kane, and K. M. Hellman, "Noninvasive experimental bladder pain assessment in painful bladder syndrome," *BJOG: An International Journal of Obstetrics & Gynaecology*, vol. 124, no. 2, pp. 283–291, 2017.

[38] S. Loving, T. Thomsen, P. Jaszczak, and J. Nordling, "Pelvic floor muscle dysfunctions are prevalent in female chronic pelvic pain: A cross-sectional population-based study," *European Journal of Pain*, vol. 18, no. 9, pp. 1259–1270, 2014.

[39] H. Breivik, B. Collett, V. Ventafridda, R. Cohen, and D. Gallacher, "Survey of chronic pain in Europe: prevalence, impact on daily life, and treatment," *European Journal of Pain*, vol. 10, no. 4, pp. 287–333, 2006.

[40] A. P. Baranowski, "Chronic pelvic pain," *Best Practice & Research Clinical Gastroenterology*, vol. 23, no. 4, pp. 593–610, 2009.

[41] B. Riegel, C. A. Bruenahl, S. Ahyai, U. Bingel, M. Fisch, and B. Löwe, "Assessing psychological factors, social aspects and psychiatric co-morbidity associated with Chronic Prostatitis/Chronic Pelvic Pain Syndrome (CP/CPPS) in men—a systematic review," *Journal of Psychosomatic Research*, vol. 77, no. 5, pp. 333–350, 2014.

[42] J. N. Krieger, A. J. Stephens, J. R. Landis et al., "Relationship between chronic nonurological associated somatic syndromes and symptom severity in urological chronic pelvic pain syndromes: Baseline evaluation of the MAPP study," *The Journal of Urology*, vol. 193, no. 4, pp. 1254–1262, 2015.

[43] C. Bryant, R. Cockburn, A.-F. Plante, and A. Chia, "The psychological profile of women presenting to a multidisciplinary clinic for chronic pelvic pain: High levels of psychological dysfunction and implications for practice," *Journal of Pain Research*, vol. 9, pp. 1049–1056, 2016.

[44] B. D. Naliboff, A. J. Stephens, N. Afari et al., "Widespread psychosocial difficulties in men and women with urologic chronic pelvic pain syndromes: Case-control findings from the multidisciplinary approach to the study of chronic pelvic pain research network," *Urology*, vol. 85, no. 6, pp. 1319–1327, 2015.

[45] I. L. Flink, K. Boersma, and S. J. Linton, "Pain Catastrophizing as Repetitive Negative Thinking: A Development of the Conceptualization," *Cognitive Behaviour Therapy*, vol. 42, no. 3, pp. 215–223, 2013.

[46] C. E. Martin, E. Johnson, M. E. Wechter, J. Leserman, and D. A. Zolnoun, "Catastrophizing: A predictor of persistent pain among women with endometriosis at 1 year," *Human Reproduction*, vol. 26, no. 11, pp. 3078–3084, 2011.

[47] J. K. Kwon and I. H. Chang, "Pain, catastrophizing, and depression in chronic prostatitis/chronic pelvic pain syndrome," *International Neurourology Journal*, vol. 17, no. 2, pp. 48–58, 2013.

[48] A. Yosef, C. Allaire, C. Williams et al., "Multifactorial contributors to the severity of chronic pelvic pain in women," *American Journal of Obstetrics & Gynecology*, vol. 215, no. 6, pp. 760–760.e14, 2016.

[49] L. A. Payne, A. J. Rapkin, K. C. Lung, L. C. Seidman, L. K. Zeltzer, and J. C. I. Tsao, "Pain catastrophizing predicts menstrual pain ratings in adolescent girls with chronic pain," *Pain Medicine*, vol. 17, no. 1, pp. 16–24, 2016.

[50] D. A. Tripp, J. C. Nickel, Y. Wang et al., "Catastrophizing and Pain-Contingent Rest Predict Patient Adjustment in Men With Chronic Prostatitis/Chronic Pelvic Pain Syndrome," *The Journal of Pain*, vol. 7, no. 10, pp. 697–708, 2006.

[51] R. M. Craft, J. S. Mogil, and A. M. Aloisi, "Sex differences in pain and analgesia: the role of gonadal hormones," *European Journal of Pain*, vol. 8, no. 5, pp. 397–411, 2004.

[52] P. Bajaj, L. Arendt-Nielsen, and H. Madsen, "Sensory changes during the ovulatory phase of the menstrual cycle in healthy women," *European Journal of Pain*, vol. 5, no. 2, pp. 135–144, 2001.

[53] M. C. Pace, L. Mazzariello, M. B. Passavanti, P. Sansone, M. Barbarisi, and C. Aurilio, "Neurobiology of pain," *Journal of Cellular Physiology*, vol. 209, no. 1, pp. 8–12, 2006.

[54] D. Wang, J. Zhao, J. Wang, J. Li, S. Yu, and X. Guo, "Deficiency of female sex hormones augments PGE2 and CGRP levels within midbrain periaqueductal gray," *Journal of the Neurological Sciences*, vol. 346, no. 1-2, pp. 107–111, 2014.

[55] V. Pota, V. Quagliariello, E. Armenia et al., "CGRP and Visceral Pain: The Role of Sex Hormones in In Vitro Experiment," *Journal of Cellular Biochemistry*, vol. 118, no. 3, pp. 510–517, 2017.

[56] Y.-W. Wu, T. Hao, X.-X. Kou, Y.-H. Gan, and X.-C. Ma, "Synovial TRPV1 is upregulated by 17-β-estradiol and involved in allodynia of inflamed temporomandibular joints in female rats," *Archives of Oral Biolog*, vol. 60, no. 9, pp. 1310–1318, 2015.

[57] R. M. Craft and C. Ulibarri, "Sexual differentiation of rat reproductive versus opioid antinociceptive systems," *Gender Medicine*, vol. 6, no. 2, pp. 208–224, 2009.

[58] G. Affaitati, I. Ceccarelli, P. Fiorenzani et al., "Sex differences in the analgesic effects of ICI 182,780 and Flutamide on ureteral calculosis in rats," *Hormones and Behavior*, vol. 59, no. 1, pp. 9–13, 2011.

[59] A. M. Aloisi, G. Affaitati, I. Ceccarelli et al., "Estradiol and testosterone differently affect visceral pain-related behavioural responses in male and female rats," *European Journal of Pain*, vol. 14, no. 6, pp. 602–607, 2010.

[60] J. D. Greenspan, R. M. Craft, L. LeResche et al., "Studying sex and gender differences in pain and analgesia: a consensus report," *PAIN*, vol. 132, supplement 1, pp. S26–S45, 2007.

[61] D. R. Loyd and A. Z. Murphy, "The neuroanatomy of sexual dimorphism in opioid analgesia," *Experimental Neurology*, vol. 259, pp. 57–63, 2014.

[62] S. Pieretti, A. Di Giannuario, R. Di Giovannandrea et al., "Gender differences in pain and its relief," *Annali Dell'Istituto Superiore Di Sanità*, vol. 52, no. 2, pp. 184–189, 2016.

[63] J. Daniels, R. Gray, R. K. Hills et al., "Laparoscopic uterosacral nerve ablation for alleviating chronic pelvic pain: A randomized controlled trial," *Journal of the American Medical Association*, vol. 302, no. 9, pp. 955–961, 2009.

[64] J. S. McDonald, "Diagnosis and treatment issues of chronic pelvic pain," *World Journal of Urology*, vol. 19, no. 3, pp. 200–207, 2001.

[65] J. F. Steege, "Pelvic pain phenotyping: The key to progress," *Obstetrics & Gynecology*, vol. 113, no. 2, pp. 258-259, 2009.

[66] C. Staikou, P. Kokotis, A. Kyrozis et al., "Differences in pain perception between men and women of reproductive age: A laser-evoked potentials study," *Pain Medicine*, 2016.

[67] Y. C. Cheong, G. Smotra, and A. C. D. C. Williams, "Non-surgical interventions for the management of chronic pelvic pain," *Cochrane Database of Systematic Reviews*, vol. 3, article CD008797, 2014.

[68] M. Lapotka, M. Ruz, A. Salamanca Ballesteros, and O. Ocón Hernández, "Cold pressor gel test: A safe alternative to the cold pressor test in fMRI," *Magnetic Resonance in Medicine*, 2016.

[69] N. Bourdel, J. Alves, G. Pickering, I. Ramilo, H. Roman, and M. Canis, "Systematic review of endometriosis pain assessment: How to choose a scale?" *Human Reproduction Update*, vol. 21, no. 1, pp. 136–152, 2015.

[70] C.-W. Chien, K. S. Bagraith, A. Khan, M. Deen, and J. Strong, "Comparative responsiveness of verbal and numerical rating scales to measure pain intensity in patients with chronic pain," *The Journal of Pain*, vol. 14, no. 12, pp. 1653–1662, 2013.

[71] H. Mohan, J. Ryan, B. Whelan, and A. Wakai, "The end of the line? The Visual Analogue Scale and Verbal Numerical Rating Scale as pain assessment tools in the emergency department," *Emergency Medicine Journal*, vol. 27, no. 5, pp. 372–375, 2010.

[72] A. Williamson and B. Hoggart, "Pain: a review of three commonly used pain rating scales," *Journal of Clinical Nursing*, vol. 14, no. 7, pp. 798–804, 2005.

[73] R. Melzack, "The McGill pain questionnaire: from description to measurement," *Anesthesiology*, vol. 103, no. 1, pp. 199–202, 2005.

[74] R. Melzack, "The short-form McGill pain questionnaire," *PAIN*, vol. 30, no. 2, pp. 191–197, 1987.

[75] A. Caraceni, T. R. Mendoza, E. Mencaglia et al., "A validation study of an Italian version of the brief pain inventory (Breve questionario per la valutazione del dolore)," *PAIN*, vol. 65, no. 1, pp. 87–92, 1996.

[76] B. S. Galer and M. P. Jensen, "Development and preliminary validation of a pain measure specific to neuropathic pain: the Neuropathic Pain Scale," *Neurology*, vol. 48, no. 2, pp. 332–338, 1997.

[77] R. Freynhagen, R. Baron, U. Gockel, and T. R. Tölle, "painDETECT: a new screening questionnaire to identify neuropathic components in patients with back pain," *Current Medical Research and Opinion*, vol. 22, no. 10, pp. 1911–1920, 2006.

[78] M. I. Bennett, B. H. Smith, N. Torrance, and J. Potter, "The S-LANSS score for identifying pain of predominantly neuropathic origin: validation for use in clinical and postal research," *The Journal of Pain*, vol. 6, no. 3, pp. 149–158, 2005.

[79] R. Portenoy, "Development and testing of a neuropathic pain screening questionnaire: ID Pain," *Current Medical Research and Opinion*, vol. 22, no. 8, pp. 1555–1565, 2006.

[80] D. Bouhassira, N. Attal, J. Fermanian et al., "Development and validation of the Neuropathic Pain Symptom Inventory," *Pain*, vol. 108, no. 3, pp. 248–257, 2004.

[81] D. Bouhassira, N. Attal, H. Alchaar et al., "Comparison of pain syndromes associated with nervous or somatic lesions and development of a new neuropathic pain diagnostic questionnaire (DN4)," *PAIN*, vol. 114, no. 1-2, pp. 29–36, 2005.

[82] A. Hamdan, J. D. Luna, E. Del Pozo, and R. Gálvez, "Diagnostic accuracy of two questionnaires for the detection of neuropathic pain in the Spanish population," *European Journal of Pain*, vol. 18, no. 1, pp. 101–109, 2014.

[83] M.-M. Backonja and S. J. Krause, "Neuropathic pain questionnaire—short form," *The Clinical Journal of Pain*, vol. 19, no. 5, pp. 315-316, 2003.

[84] J. Quaghebeur and J. Wyndaele, "Comparison of questionnaires used for the evaluation of patients with chronic pelvic pain," *Neurourology and Urodynamics*, vol. 32, no. 8, pp. 1074–1079, 2013.

[85] M. P. O'Leary, G. R. Sant, F. J. Fowler Jr., K. E. Whitmore, and J. Spolarich-Kroll, "The interstitial cystitis symptom index and problem index," *Urology*, vol. 49, no. 5, pp. 58–63, 1997.

[86] D. P. Lubeck, K. Whitmore, G. R. Sant, S. Alvarez-Horine, and C. Lai, "Psychometric validation of the O'Leary-Sant Interstitial Cystitis Symptom Index in a clinical trial of pentosan polysulfate sodium," *Urology*, vol. 57, no. 6, pp. 62–66, 2001.

[87] K. J. Propert, R. D. Mayer, Y. Wang et al., "Responsiveness of symptom scales for interstitial cystitis," *Urology*, vol. 67, no. 1, pp. 55–59, 2006.

[88] Y.-C. Kuo and H.-C. Kuo, "O'leary-sant symptom index predicts the treatment outcome for onabotulinumtoxin a injections for refractory interstitial cystitis/bladder pain syndrome," *Toxins*, vol. 7, no. 8, pp. 2860–2871, 2015.

[89] L. Humphrey, R. Arbuckle, R. Moldwin et al., "The bladder pain/interstitial cystitis symptom score: Development, validation, and identification of a cut score," *European Urology*, vol. 61, no. 2, pp. 271–279, 2012.

[90] J. E. Goin, D. Olaleye, K. M. Peters, B. Steinert, K. Habicht, and G. Wynant, "Psychometric analysis of the university of wisconsin interstitial cystitis scale: Implications for use in randomized clinical trials," *The Journal of Urology*, vol. 159, no. 3, pp. 1085–1090, 1998.

[91] http://www.pelvicpain.org/Professional/Documents-and-Forms.aspx.

[92] M. S. Litwin, M. McNaughton-Collins, F. J. Fowler Jr. et al., "The National Institutes of Health chronic prostatitis symptom index: Development and validation of a new outcome measure," *The Journal of Urology*, vol. 162, no. 2, pp. 369–375, 1999.

[93] S. N. P. Davis, Y. M. Binik, R. Amsel, and S. Carrier, "A subtype based analysis of urological chronic pelvic pain syndrome in men," *The Journal of Urology*, vol. 190, no. 1, pp. 118–123, 2013.

[94] K. J. Propert, M. S. Litwin, Y. Wang et al., "Responsiveness of the National Institutes of Health Chronic Prostatitis Symptom Index (NIH-CPSI)," *Quality of Life Research*, vol. 15, no. 2, pp. 299–305, 2006.

[95] J. Q. Clemens, E. A. Calhoun, M. S. Litwin et al., "Rescoring the NIH chronic prostatitis symptom index: Nothing new," *Prostate Cancer and Prostatic Diseases*, vol. 12, no. 3, pp. 285–287, 2009.

[96] F. M. E. Wagenlehner, J. W. O. Van Till, V. Magri et al., "National Institutes of Health Chronic Prostatitis Symptom Index (NIH-CPSI) symptom evaluation in multinational cohorts of patients with chronic prostatitis/chronic pelvic pain syndrome," *European Urology*, vol. 63, no. 5, pp. 953–959, 2013.

[97] J. Q. Clemens, E. A. Calhoun, M. S. Litwin et al., "Validation of a Modified National Institutes of Health Chronic Prostatitis Symptom Index to Assess Genitourinary Pain in Both Men and Women," *Urology*, vol. 74, no. 5, pp. 983–e3, 2009.

[98] E. Díaz Mohedo, F. J. Barõn Lõpez, C. Pineda Galán, M. S. Dawid Milner, C. Suárez Serrano, and E. Medrano Sánchez, "Discriminating power of CPPQ-Mohedo: A new questionnaire for chronic pelvic pain," *Journal of Evaluation in Clinical Practice*, vol. 19, no. 1, pp. 94–99, 2013.

[99] http://www.upointmd.com/.

[100] D. A. Shoskes, J. C. Nickel, R. Dolinga, and D. Prots, "Clinical Phenotyping of Patients With Chronic Prostatitis/Chronic Pelvic Pain Syndrome and Correlation With Symptom Severity," *Urology*, vol. 73, no. 3, pp. 538–542, 2009.

[101] J. C. Nickel, D. Shoskes, and K. Irvine-Bird, "Clinical Phenotyping of Women With Interstitial Cystitis/Painful Bladder Syndrome: A Key to Classification and Potentially Improved Management," *The Journal of Urology*, vol. 182, no. 1, pp. 155–160, 2009.

[102] M. K. Samplaski, J. Li, and D. A. Shoskes, "Clustering of UPOINT domains and subdomains in men with chronic prostatitis/chronic pelvic pain syndrome and contribution to symptom severity," *The Journal of Urology*, vol. 188, no. 5, pp. 1788–1793, 2012.

[103] D. A. Shoskes and J. C. Nickel, "Classification and treatment of men with chronic prostatitis/chronic pelvic pain syndrome using the UPOINT system," *World Journal of Urology*, vol. 31, no. 4, pp. 755–760, 2013.

[104] A. S. Polackwich, J. Li, and D. A. Shoskes, "Patients with pelvic floor muscle spasm have a superior response to pelvic floor physical therapy at specialized centers," *The Journal of Urology*, vol. 194, no. 4, pp. 1002–1006, 2015.

[105] D. A. Shoskes, J. C. Nickel, and M. W. Kattan, "Phenotypically directed multimodal therapy for chronic prostatitis/chronic pelvic pain syndrome: a prospective study using UPOINT," *Urology*, vol. 75, no. 6, pp. 1249–1253, 2010.

[106] X. Guan, C. Zhao, Z.-Y. Ou et al., "Use of the UPOINT phenotype system in treating Chinese patients with chronic prostatitis/chronic pelvic pain syndrome: a prospective study," *Asian Journal of Andrology*, vol. 17, no. 1, pp. 120–123, 2015.

[107] V. Magri, E. Marras, A. Restelli, F. M. E. Wagenlehner, and G. Perletti, "Multimodal therapy for category III chronic prostatitis/chronic pelvic pain syndrome in UPOINTS phenotyped patients," *Experimental and Therapeutic Medicine*, vol. 9, no. 3, pp. 658–666, 2015.

[108] A. T. Goldstein, C. F. Pukall, C. Brown, S. Bergeron, A. Stein, and S. Kellogg-Spadt, "Vulvodynia: Assessment and Treatment," *The Journal of Sexual Medicine*, vol. 13, no. 4, pp. 572–590, 2016.

[109] D. Neelakantan, F. Omojole, T. J. Clark, J. K. Gupta, and K. S. Khan, "Quality of life instruments in studies of chronic pelvic pain: A systematic review," *Journal of Obstetrics & Gynaecology*, vol. 24, no. 8, pp. 851–858, 2004.

[110] R. Rabin and F. De Charro, "EQ-5D: a measure of health status from the EuroQol Group," *Annals of Medicine*, vol. 33, no. 5, pp. 337–343, 2001.

[111] R. C. Tait, J. T. Chibnall, and S. Krause, "The pain disability index: psychometric properties," *PAIN*, vol. 40, no. 2, pp. 171–182, 1990.

[112] D. Amtmann, K. F. Cook, M. P. Jensen et al., "Development of a PROMIS item bank to measure pain interference," *PAIN*, vol. 150, no. 1, pp. 173–182, 2010.

[113] J. M. Schober, H. F. L. Meyer-Bahlburg, and C. Dolezal, "Self-ratings of genital anatomy, sexual sensitivity and function in men using the 'Self-Assessment of Genital Anatomy and Sexual Function, Male' questionnaire," *BJU International*, vol. 103, no. 8, pp. 1096–1103, 2009.

[114] J. M. Schober, H. F. L. Meyer-Bahlburg, and P. G. Ransley, "Self-assessment of genital anatomy, sexual sensitivity and function in women: Implications for genitoplasty," *BJU International*, vol. 94, no. 4, pp. 589–594, 2004.

[115] C. A. Brünahl, B. Riegel, J. Höink, A. Kutup, E. Eichelberg, and B. Löwe, "Psychosomatic aspects of chronic pelvic pain syndrome. Psychometric results from the pilot phase of an interdisciplinary outpatient clinic," *Der Schmerz*, vol. 28, no. 3, pp. 311–318, 2014.

[116] M. J. L. Sullivan, S. R. Bishop, and J. Pivik, "The pain catastrophizing scale: development and validation," *Psychological Assessment*, vol. 7, no. 4, pp. 524–532, 1995.

[117] K. M. Hellman, I. Y. Patanwala, K. E. Pozolo, and F. F. Tu, "Multimodal nociceptive mechanisms underlying chronic pelvic pain Presented in poster format at the 21st annual meeting of the International Pelvic Pain Society, Orlando, FL, Oct. 18-19, 2013.," *American Journal of Obstetrics & Gynecology*, vol. 213, no. 6, pp. 827–827.e9, 2015.

[118] S. N. P. Davis, C. A. Maykut, Y. M. Binik, R. Amsel, and S. Carrier, "Tenderness as measured by pressure pain thresholds extends beyond the pelvis in chronic pelvic pain syndrome in men," *The Journal of Sexual Medicine*, vol. 8, no. 1, pp. 232–239, 2011.

[119] C. B. Bleustein, H. Eckholdt, J. C. Arezzo, and A. Melman, "Quantitative somatosensory testing of the penis: Optimizing the clinical neurological examination," *The Journal of Urology*, vol. 169, no. 6, pp. 2266–2269, 2003.

[120] B. W. Fenton, P. A. Palmieri, C. Durner, and J. Fanning, "Quantification of abdominal wall pain using pain pressure threshold algometry in patients with chronic pelvic Pain pnet," *The Clinical Journal of Pain*, vol. 25, no. 6, pp. 500–505, 2009.

[121] F. F. Tu, C. M. Fitzgerald, T. Kuiken, T. Farrell, and H. R. Norman, "Comparative measurement of pelvic floor pain sensitivity in chronic pelvic pain," *Obstetrics & Gynecology*, vol. 110, no. 6, pp. 1244–1248, 2007.

[122] F. F. Tu, C. M. Fitzgerald, T. Kuiken, T. Farrell, and R. Norman Harden, "Vaginal pressure-pain thresholds: Initial validation and reliability assessment in healthy women," *The Clinical Journal of Pain*, vol. 24, no. 1, pp. 45–50, 2008.

[123] N. Phillips, C. Brown, G. Bachmann et al., "Relationship between nongenital tender point tenderness and intravaginal muscle pain intensity: ratings in women with provoked vestibulodynia and implications for treatment," *American Journal of Obstetrics & Gynecology*, vol. 215, no. 6, pp. 751–751.e5, 2016.

[124] C. F. Pukall, R. A. Young, M. J. Roberts, K. S. Sutton, and K. B. Smith, "The vulvalgesiometer as a device to measure genital pressure-pain threshold," *Physiological Measurement*, vol. 28, no. 12, pp. 1543–1550, 2007.

[125] K. Sutton, C. Pukall, C. Wild, I. Johnsrude, and S. Chamberlain, "Cognitive, Psychophysical, and Neural Correlates of Vulvar Pain in Primary and Secondary Provoked Vestibulodynia: A Pilot Study," *The Journal of Sexual Medicine*, vol. 12, no. 5, pp. 1283–1297, 2015.

[126] M. Morin, Y. M. Binik, D. Bourbonnais, S. Khalifé, S. Ouellet, and S. Bergeron, "Heightened Pelvic Floor Muscle Tone and Altered Contractility in Women With Provoked Vestibulodynia," *The Journal of Sexual Medicine*, vol. 14, no. 4, pp. 592–600, 2017.

[127] M.-P. Cyr, D. Bourbonnais, A. Pinard, O. Dubois, and M. Morin, "Reliability and convergent validity of the algometer for vestibular pain assessment in women with provoked vestibulodynia," *Pain Medicine*, vol. 17, no. 7, pp. 1220–1228, 2016.

[128] J. C. Lee, C. C. Yang, B. G. Kromm, and R. E. Berger, "Neurophysiologic testing in chronic pelvic pain syndrome: A pilot study," *Urology*, vol. 58, no. 2, pp. 246–250, 2001.

[129] C. C. Yang, J. C. Lee, B. G. Kromm, M. A. Ciol, and R. E. Berger, "Pain sensitization in male chronic pelvic pain syndrome: Why are symptoms so difficult to treat?" *The Journal of Urology*, vol. 170, no. 3, pp. 823–826, 2003.

[130] S. Korkmaz, M. A. Karadag, K. Hamamcioglu, M. Sofikerim, and M. Aksu, "Electrophysiological identification of central

sensitization in patients with chronic prostatitis," *Urology Journal*, vol. 12, no. 4, pp. 2280–2284, 2015.

[131] M. I. Kogan, I. I. Belousov, and P. V. Shornikov, "Neurophysiologic evaluation of patients with chronic prostatitis (III B chronic pain syndrome)," *Urologiia*, vol. 4, pp. 37–42, 2012.

[132] K. De Laet, S. De Wachter, and J.-J. Wyndaele, "Current perception thresholds in the lower urinary tract: Sine- and square-wave currents studied in young healthy volunteers," *Neurourology and Urodynamics*, vol. 24, no. 3, pp. 261–266, 2005.

[133] A. Fujihara, O. Ukimura, T. Iwata, and T. Miki, "Neuroselective measure of the current perception threshold of A-delta and C-fiber afferents in the lower urinary tract," *International Journal of Urology*, vol. 18, no. 5, pp. 341–349, 2011.

[134] H.-C. Kuo, Y.-C. Chuang, and B. Michael, "Chancellor Neurourology, Diet, and Painful Bladder Highlights," *Reviews in Urology*, vol. 10, no. 1, pp. 70–72, 2008, Highlights of the 37th Annual Conference of the International Continence Society, August 20–24, 2007, Rotterdam, Netherlands.

[135] O. Ukimura, S. Ushijima, H. Honjo et al., "Neuroselective Current Perception Threshold Evaluation of Bladder Mucosal Sensory Function," *European Urology*, vol. 45, no. 1, pp. 70–76, 2004.

[136] U. Yilmaz, M. A. Ciol, R. E. Berger, and C. C. Yang, "Sensory Perception Thresholds in Men With Chronic Pelvic Pain Syndrome," *Urology*, vol. 75, no. 1, pp. 34–37, 2010.

[137] S. La Cesa, S. Tamburin, V. Tugnoli et al., "How to diagnose neuropathic pain? The contribution from clinical examination, pain questionnaires and diagnostic tests," *Neurological Sciences*, vol. 36, no. 12, pp. 2169–2175, 2015.

[138] K. T. Martucci and S. C. Mackey, "Imaging Pain," *Anesthesiology Clinics*, vol. 34, no. 2, pp. 255–269, 2016.

[139] E. A. Mayer, A. Gupta, L. A. Kilpatrick, and J.-Y. Hong, "Imaging brain mechanisms in chronic visceral pain," *PAIN*, vol. 156, no. 4, pp. S50–S63, 2015.

[140] T. Schmidt-Wilcke, "Neuroimaging of chronic pain," *Best Practice & Research Clinical Rheumatology*, vol. 29, no. 1, article no. 1145, pp. 29–41, 2015.

[141] M. C. Lee, I. Tracey, L. Colvin, and D. J. Rowbotham, "Imaging pain: A potent means for investigating pain mechanisms in patients," *British Journal of Anaesthesia*, vol. 111, no. 1, pp. 64–72, 2013.

[142] S. As-Sanie, J. Kim, T. Schmidt-Wilcke et al., "Functional Connectivity Is Associated with Altered Brain Chemistry in Women with Endometriosis-Associated Chronic Pelvic Pain," *The Journal of Pain*, vol. 17, no. 1, pp. 1–13, 2016.

[143] S. As-Sanie, R. E. Harris, V. Napadow et al., "Changes in regional gray matter volume in women with chronic pelvic pain: a voxel-based morphometry study," *PAIN*, vol. 153, no. 5, pp. 1006–1014, 2012.

[144] F. Beissner, C. Preibisch, A. Schweizer-Arau, R. M. Popovici, and K. Meissner, "Psychotherapy With Somatosensory Stimulation for Endometriosis-Associated Pain: The Role of the Anterior Hippocampus," *Biological Psychiatry*, 2016.

[145] J. R. Alger, B. M. Ellingson, C. Ashe-Mcnalley et al., "Multisite, multimodal neuroimaging of chronic urological pelvic pain: Methodology of the MAPP Research Network," *NeuroImage: Clinical*, vol. 12, pp. 65–77, 2016.

[146] K. T. Martucci, W. R. Shirer, E. Bagarinao et al., "The posterior medial cortex in urologic chronic pelvic pain syndrome: Detachment from default mode network - A resting-state study from the MAPP Research Network," *PAIN*, vol. 156, no. 9, pp. 1755–1764, 2015.

[147] D. Woodworth, E. Mayer, K. Leu et al., "Unique microstructural changes in the brain associated with urological chronic pelvic pain syndrome (UCPPS) revealed by diffusion tensor MRI, super-resolution track density imaging, and statistical parameter mapping: A MAPP network neuroimaging study," *PLoS ONE*, vol. 10, no. 10, Article ID e0140250, 2015.

[148] L. Huang, J. J. Kutch, B. M. Ellingson et al., "Brain white matter changes associated with urological chronic pelvic pain syndrome: Multisite neuroimaging from a MAPP case-control study," *PAIN*, vol. 157, no. 12, pp. 2782–2791, 2016.

[149] J. J. Kutch, M. S. Yani, S. Asavasopon et al., "Altered resting state neuromotor connectivity in men with chronic prostatitis/chronic pelvic pain syndrome: A MAPP: Research Network Neuroimaging Study," *NeuroImage: Clinical*, vol. 8, pp. 493–502, 2015.

[150] Y. Lin, Y. Bai, P. Liu et al., "Alterations in regional homogeneity of resting-state cerebral activity in patients with chronic prostatitis/chronic pelvic pain syndrome," *PLoS ONE*, vol. 12, article e0184896, no. 9, 2017.

[151] "Therapy-related longitudinal brain perfusion changes in patients with chronic pelvic pain syndrome," *Swiss Medical Weekly*, vol. 147, no. 3132, 2017.

[152] L. Mordasini, C. Weisstanner, C. Rummel et al., "Chronic pelvic pain syndrome in men is associated with reduction of relative gray matter volume in the anterior cingulate cortex compared to healthy controls," *The Journal of Urology*, vol. 188, no. 6, pp. 2233–2237, 2012.

[153] M. A. Farmer, M. L. Chanda, E. L. Parks, M. N. Baliki, A. V. Apkarian, and A. J. Schaeffer, "Brain functional and anatomical changes in chronic prostatitis/chronic pelvic pain syndrome," *The Journal of Urology*, vol. 186, no. 1, pp. 117–124, 2011.

[154] A. Gupta, A. J. Rapkin, Z. Gill et al., "Disease-related differences in resting-state networks: A comparison between localized provoked vulvodynia, irritable bowel syndrome, and healthy control subjects," *PAIN*, vol. 156, no. 5, pp. 809–819, 2015.

[155] C.-H. Tu, D. M. Niddam, H.-T. Chao et al., "Brain morphological changes associated with cyclic menstrual pain," *PAIN*, vol. 150, no. 3, pp. 462–468, 2010.

[156] C.-H. Tu, D. M. Niddam, H.-T. Chao et al., "Abnormal cerebral metabolism during menstrual pain in primary dysmenorrhea," *NeuroImage*, vol. 47, no. 1, pp. 28–35, 2009.

[157] S.-Y. Wei, L.-F. Chen, M.-W. Lin et al., "The OPRM1 A118G polymorphism modulates the descending pain modulatory system for individual pain experience in young women with primary dysmenorrhea," *Scientific Reports*, vol. 7, Article ID 39906, 2017.

[158] S.-Y. Wei, H.-T. Chao, C.-H. Tu et al., "The BDNF Val66Met polymorphism is associated with the functional connectivity dynamics of pain modulatory systems in primary dysmenorrhea," *Scientific Reports*, vol. 6, Article ID 23639, 2016.

29

Load Handling and Repetitive Movements Are Associated with Chronic Low Back Pain among Jute Mill Workers in India

S. Goswami,[1] S. Dasgupta,[1] A. Samanta,[1] G. Talukdar,[1] A. Chanda,[2] P. Ray Karmakar,[3] A. Majumdar,[4] D. Bhattacharya,[1] and A. Chakrabarti[5]

[1] *ESI Institute of Pain Management, ESI Hospital, Sealdah, 301/3A, A. P. C. Road, Kolkata, West Bengal 700009, India*
[2] *Department of Mechanical Engineering, Jadavpur University, 188 Raja S. C. Mallick Road, Kolkata 700032, India*
[3] *Department of Community Medicine, R. G. Kar Medical College & Hospital, 1 Kshudiram Bose Sarani, Kolkata 700004, India*
[4] *The Jute Corporation of India Ltd., 15N Nellie Sengupta Sarani, Kolkata 700087, India*
[5] *Regional Occupational Health Centre (Eastern), Indian Council of Medical Research (ICMR), Block DP1, Sector V, Salt Lake, Kolkata 700091, India*

Correspondence should be addressed to A. Chakrabarti; amitchakrabarti@hotmail.com

Academic Editor: Giustino Varrassi

Introduction. WHO recognizes low back pain as one of the most important ergonomic stressors. Therefore, the present study was designed to find out the magnitude of the problem among jute mill workers in India and identify possible associations. *Methodology*˙ This cross-sectional workplace based study was conducted among eight (8) selected jute mills of India. Subjects with self-reported back pain for at least last 12 weeks were included and $n = 717$ male jute mill workers actively engaged in work entered the study and completed all assessments. *Results.* Among all participants 55% ($n = 392$) had current chronic low back pain. Age was an important association with subjects in the age group of 40–59 years more likely to have pain ($p = 0.02$, OR 1.44). Regarding ergonomic risk factors lifting of load of more than 20 kg ($p = 0.04$, OR 1.42) and repetitive movements of limbs ($p = 0.03$, OR 0.67) were significant associations of chronic low back pain. *Conclusion.* This study identified a significant prevalence of current chronic low back pain among jute mill workers. Regarding ergonomic risk factors the present study has identified two significant associations: lifting of load above 20 kg and repetitive movements of limbs. Therefore, this study has identified need for workplace interventions in this occupational group employing approximately 3,50,000 workers in India.

1. Introduction

Low back pain refers to pain or stiffness in muscle localized below the costal margin and above the inferior gluteal folds, with or without leg pain, and is defined as chronic when it persists for 12 weeks or more [1, 2]. The 2013 Global Burden of Disease Study estimated that globally low back pain is the leading cause of disability with a mean of 72.3 million Years Lived with Disability (YLD) resulting in an approximate 57% increase in YLD from low back pain compared to 1990 [3]. Low back pain has been identified as an important cause of disability among occupational groups and has emerged as an important occupational health issue [4, 5]. World Health Organization (WHO) recognizes low back pain as one of the most important ergonomic stressors and estimates that 37% of all low back pain is of occupational origin resulting in morbidity and work absence with consequent economic loss [6]. Studies from different regions of the world have uniformly identified presence of significant chronic low back pain among manual workers, for example, among manual lifting workers in Thailand [7], among farmers in the US with a 33.2% prevalence [8], in a cohort of male workers in the Swedish construction industry with a 16.5% prevalence [9], and among Chinese workers in a foundry factory of an automobile company [10]. Studies have also identified prolonged bending of trunk, manual handling of heavy objects, lifting from squatting positions, and handling of load as important physical risk factors of chronic low back pain [10, 11].

TABLE 1: Number of jute mill workers participating in the study from each mill (n = 717).

Name of mill	Total number of workers	Number of workers enrolled	% of total workers	% of enrolled workers
Hukumchand, WB	12,031	260	2.0	36.3
Prabartak, WB	2,005	68	3.4	9.5
Shyamnagar, WB	5,032	89	1.8	12.4
Assam Co-operative, Assam	775	58	7.5	8.1
Budge Budge, WB	3,058	52	1.7	7.3
Ludlow, WB	4,639	101	2.2	14.1
Howrah, WB	2,886	49	1.7	6.8
Sri Krishna, AP	2,908	40	1.4	5.5

India has one of the largest work forces in the world and is expected to have problem of chronic low back pain among manual workers with significant economic consequences. Limited studies from India have identified association of significant sickness related absence with low back pain among tannery workers [12]; a 59% prevalence of chronic low back pain among brick kiln workers in rural Southern India [13]; and significant chronic low back pain among female brick workers due to awkward posture, repetitive work, and load handling [14]. However, the problem of chronic low back pain among industrial workers requiring heavy manual work has not been investigated in the Indian context. Jute industry in India with a turnover of approximately Rs. 100 billion (US$ 1.5 billion) employs approximately 3,50,000 workers with 75% of the jute processing units (mills) being located in the state of West Bengal [15]. However, little investigation regarding chronic low back pain has been focused among jute mill workers in India, although such workers encounter heavy physical workload and only one study from India has investigated musculoskeletal disorders among jute mill workers and identified presence of significant musculoskeletal pain lasting many hours after work [16] without specifically investigating chronic low back pain. Considering that an approximate 3,50,000 workers are engaged in jute mills in India the problem of chronic low back pain is likely to have a significant public health impact.

Since inception of the pain clinic at the newly initiated (since 2013) ESI Institute of Pain Management, West Bengal, India, which serves as the referral centre for chronic pain, almost 50%–60% of patients with chronic low back pain were found to be workers from jute mills. In most cases such patients require prolonged treatment resulting in long periods of laying off with consequent economic losses. Therefore, in this context there was a need to investigate the problem of chronic low back pain among jute mill workers and the present study was designed to find out the magnitude of the problem and identify possible associations so that effective prevention and treatment strategies can be developed.

2. Subjects and Methods

This cross-sectional workplace based study was conducted in six (6) matched jute mills from West Bengal (WB), with each jute mill from the states of Andhra Pradesh (AP) and Assam. Therefore, participants for the study were selected from a pool of eight (8) jute mills of India. A jute mill is a factory for processing jute. Out of 93 jute mills in India, West Bengal has 70 jute mills, the highest in India, with Andhra Pradesh having 9 mills and Assam two (2) mills [15]. Therefore, jute mills from the states of West Bengal, Andhra Pradesh, and Assam were chosen as sites for this study. Jute mills for participation in the study were chosen by convenience sampling considering ease of access, willingness of the mill owners to participate in the study, and presence of most of the main divisions in the factory for jute processing (namely, jute handling, batching, drawing, spinning, winding, beaming, weaving, and finishing). Workers from following jute mills participated in the study (Table 1). Baseline information for total worker strength for each mill was considered for the year 2013-2014.

For inclusion in the study jute mill workers from the selected mills who are in continuous employment for at least one (1) year and are of 18 completed years of age were eligible for entry in the study. Further, workers currently on active duty in the mills with self-reported back pain for at least last 12 weeks in or near the lumbosacral spine with or without radiating leg pain were considered to be suffering from chronic low back pain (cLBP) and included in the study. Exclusion criteria were presence of pain for less than 3 months and worker currently on sick leave or absent from work or not working continuously for more than one year. Other exclusion criteria were other illnesses with low back pain, for example, infection/malignancy/fracture/metabolic disease/inflammatory disorders and age less than 18 years or above 60 years. All participants were assessed clinically for confirmation of presence or absence of chronic low back pain and ascertained eligibility for inclusion in the study. Inclusion of subjects for the study was carried out by a random screening procedure for presence/absence of chronic low back pain following the employment ID of all available workers on that particular day. Each mill had workers currently on leave due to low back pain, but such workers were not included in the study. Although the intention of the study was to include adequate number of female workers, jute mills mostly employ male workers due to requirement of heavy manual work. Therefore, this study identified only n = 14 female workers across all sites and to avoid introduction of bias in analyses exclusively n = 717 male jute mill workers from all sites entered the study and completed all assessments.

Data was collected by trained research staffs by face-to-face interview with the selected workers following a predesigned schedule after explaining to the workers the nature, benefits, and risks, if any, of the study and taking their signed informed consent for participation in the study. Information regarding age, family history of musculoskeletal disorders, body weight, height, smoking status and duration in occupation, nature of the job of the worker including ergonomic postures, use of machines and instruments, units of weights lifted, and so forth were recorded on a predesigned schedule. Still and video photographs were taken when considered helpful for the problem analysis and data recording. All questionnaires were validated before use in the study. Following questionnaires constituted the predesigned schedule for assessment of participants in the study.

(1) Demographic questionnaire: recorded information on religion, ethnicity, age, gender, marital status, average monthly income, level of education, occupation, and so forth from each participant. This questionnaire is modified from the routine clinical case record form used in the pain clinic of the hospital.

(2) Brief Pain Inventory (BPI): long-collected information on pain status at this current time period. BPI assessed average, worst, and least pain intensity at the time of interview as well as over the last 24 hours using 0 ("no pain") to 10 ("pain as bad as you can imagine") numeric rating scale. Participants identified location of pain on body map indicating 31 locations. A numeric rating scale from 0 ("does not interfere") to 10 ("completely interferes") was used to find out degree at which pain interfered with seven activities (such as general activity, mood, walking ability, sleep, enjoyment of life, normal work, and relations with others) over the past 24 hours [17]. The BPI measures both the intensity of pain and interference of pain in the patient's life along with generating information on pain relief, pain quality, and patient perception about cause of pain. BPI has demonstrated both reliability and validity across different cultures and languages and has been adopted in many countries for clinical pain assessment and in epidemiological studies [18].

(3) Ergonomic and workplace questionnaire: adapted from a Chinese study among occupational population and enquired about ergonomic risk factors, namely, load handling categorized by weight, repetitive movements, bending and twisting, standing and sitting, insufficient height or space, use of vibrating tools, and so forth [19].

Information on quality of life of all participants was also collected. The content validity of the instruments was checked by translation to local language (Bengali) and retranslation, as well as review by the investigators of the study. Brief Pain Inventory (BPI) has undergone validation in a number of countries and cultural settings and has also been validated in India [20, 21]. The reliability of the instruments has been ensured by administration of the questionnaires by trained research staff, independent cross-checking of the responses encoded, and random retesting of the questionnaire in approximately 10% of the subjects.

Data collection for estimating parameters based on sample statistic in industries needs to be based on the logic of homogeneity or heterogeneity of the respondents. In most of the industry related studies 90% to 95% confidence level is good enough in most of the situations with an error estimate for the parameter between 5% and 10%. With this assumption the necessary statistical analyses depending on the nature of variables can be conducted to suit the study objectives. In our study we decided to have a 90% confidence interval with an error width within 0.07. With this assumption our $Z_{\alpha/2}$ (confidence coefficient) = 1.64 and e (half the desired interval width) = 0.07/2 = 0.035. Therefore, the required sample size $n = [(Z_{\alpha/2})^2 p(1-p)]/e^2 = [(1.64)^2(0.35)(0.65)]/(0.035)^2 = [3.6896 \times 0.2275]/0.001225 = 0.8393/0.001225 = 685$; that is, approximately $n = 700$.

The study commenced after obtaining necessary approval from competent authority and approval from Institutional Ethics Committee. For ethical reasons, other workers suffering from low back pain, outside the sample chosen for the study, were also examined by the clinician and their treatment was organized at ESI Hospital, Sealdah.

Before analysis all entries were checked and cleaned by ignoring or putting missing value codes for inconsistent or ambiguous values. As variables were mostly categorical and/or ordinal, nonparametric tests were used. Frequency distribution was used to describe demographic variables; participant characteristics; characteristics of pain; workplace characteristics; and quality of life variables. Effects of independent variables on patterns of chronic low back pain and their associations were analyzed using Chi-square test for nonparametric data. Estimate of risk was expressed by Odds Ratio (OR) with 95% confidence interval (CI). Acceptable level of significance was set at $p < 0.05$. Data was analyzed by IBM SPSS Statistics 22.0 (IBM Corporation, New York, USA).

3. Results

This study was conducted to find out the magnitude of the problem of chronic low back pain among jute mill workers in India and included $n = 717$ male workers from eight (8) jute mills from three states of India. Almost all workers worked for eight hours/day. The schedule of work each day was split into two halves of four and a half hours and three hours. Most workers were engaged in work for six days/week, that is, 48 hours per week. The main departments in each jute mill included jute handling (processing of raw jute), batching (run spreader machine and soften raw jute), drawing (processing of jute to reduce sliver width and thickness), spinning (process of producing jute yarn), winding (convert yarn to spools and cops), beaming (weaving of jute cloth from yarn), weaving (operation of the loom and producing jute fabric of desired quality), and finishing (improve quality of jute product). Apart from the main departments, a jute mill has supporting departments, for example, maintenance, where workers from main departments are rotated. Mills included in the study had all main departments apart from

Assam Co-operative Jute Mill, Assam, which did not have handling and drawing departments.

Almost 47% ($n = 333$) belonged to the age group of 20 to 39 years and the rest were above 40 years of age. In general, the sample had low levels of education with approximately 8% ($n = 56$) completing school education. Only 7% ($n = 48$) workers had a monthly earning of at least INR 12,000 (US$ 182). Almost 58% ($n = 413$) worked for less than 20 years in a jute mill, while the remaining worked for more than 20 years; and almost 51% ($n = 363$) worked for 48 h/week and the rest worked for 40 h/week. Almost 33% had either a parent or a sibling working in a jute mill. More than half of the workers consume tobacco (66%, $n = 475$).

Chronic low back pain was defined as back pain for at least last 12 weeks in or near the lumbosacral spine with or without radiating leg pain. Among the sample of jute mill workers enrolled for the present study, 31% ($n = 223$) were identified to be having current chronic low back pain for at least last 12 weeks. However, 55% ($n = 392$) subjects had current chronic low back pain with or without radiating leg pain for at least past 12 weeks satisfying laid down inclusion criteria for chronic low back pain. There was no difference in prevalence of chronic low back pain among jute mill workers by site, that is, participating jute mills ($\chi^2 = 4.30$, df = 7, $p = 0.75$). The prevalence of chronic low back pain by department across all jute mills was in handling 56%, $n = 13$, batching 48%, $n = 34$, drawing 55%, $n = 30$, spinning 49%, $n = 56$, winding 52%, $n = 32$, beaming 62%, $n = 23$, weaving 61%, $n = 134$, and finishing 58%, $n = 49$; $n = 21$ workers with chronic low back pain were from supporting departments. Approximately 26% ($n = 185$) of all workers also had a family history of chronic low back pain. Regarding intensity of pain among workers with chronic low back pain during the current week 66% ($n = 233$) had mild pain, 28% ($n = 100$) had moderate pain, and 6% ($n = 21$) had severe pain. When associations of subject characteristics were considered with presence or absence of chronic low back pain, age was identified as an important factor with subjects in the age group of 40–59 years more likely to have pain ($\chi^2 = 5.83$, df = 1, $p = 0.02$, OR 1.44, 95% CI (1.07–1.93)). Although sanitation emerged as a significant factor, this is unlikely to have a real effect as almost no worker used western system of sanitation. No other participant characteristics had a significant relation with chronic low back pain (Table 2).

Ergonomic risk factors considered for the present study were lifting load above 20 kg, carrying load above 20 kg, pulling load above 20 kg, standing or sitting for long duration, twisting or bending trunk awkwardly, maintaining the same posture for long duration, repetitive movements of limbs, and position of the work station. When associations of ergonomic risk factors were considered with presence or absence of chronic low back pain, lifting of load of more than 20 kg ($\chi^2 = 4.02$, df = 1, $p = 0.04$, OR 1.42, 95% CI (1.0–2.0)) and repetitive movements of limbs ($\chi^2 = 4.92$, df = 1, $p = 0.03$, OR 0.67, 95% CI (0.50–1.0)) were identified as significant associations of chronic low back pain. No other workplace characteristic had any association with chronic low back pain (Table 3).

4. Discussion

In keeping with pattern of jute industry in India, most mills for the study were chosen from the West Bengal, where maximum numbers of jute mills in India are located. Although the study aimed to recruit both male and female workers, female subjects were few as jute mills mostly employ male workers due to demand of heavy physical work. Similar kind of subject selection has also been observed from other studies on jute mill workers in India [16, 22] as well as Nepal [23].

This study identified a significant 55% prevalence of current chronic low back pain among jute mill workers. Although not investigated among jute mill workers, the problem of chronic low back pain has been investigated in various other occupational settings requiring heavy manual work. Using strict diagnostic criteria for low back pain a South African study among steel industry workers has identified a point prevalence of 35.8% [24]. Among agricultural workers in the American Midwest low back pain was the commonest musculoskeletal pain (33.2%) [4]. Among studies from India tannery workers from Kanpur had high prevalence of low back pain (61%) [12]. The same study also identified that 44% workers had at least one period of sickness related absence over past 12 months. Brick kiln workers from Southern India with heavy physical demand also had a [13] high prevalence of chronic low back pain (59%). Higher prevalence (70%) of low back pain was reported from female brick field workers from West Bengal, India [14]. However, our study did not include jute mill workers who are either on leave or laid-off from job due to chronic low back pain. If the prevalence is considered taking into account such workers, chronic low back pain among jute mill workers is expected to have higher magnitude.

Regarding ergonomic risk factors the present study has identified two significant associations: lifting of load above 20 kg and repetitive movements of limbs. Load carriage (OR = 1.54) and lifting (OR = 4.61) were significant risk factors for low back pain among South African manganese factory workers [11]. Similarly lifting (OR = 2.08) and moving heavy objects (OR = 1.95) were significant risk factors of low back pain among Chinese foundry workers in an automobile factory [10]. Significant association of lifting load above 20 kg (OR = 3.5) has also been reported among tannery workers from Kanpur, India [12]. A study among handloom weavers in West Bengal identified a 68% prevalence of chronic low back pain and also observed that repetitive movements of limbs to operate the looms are a likely risk factor of such pain [25]. Jute mill workers, particularly those engaged in beaming and weaving, employ significant repetitive movements of the limbs and, therefore, such workers are expected to develop chronic low back pain. However other studies also identified other ergonomic risk factors for low back pain, which were not associated with chronic low back pain in the current study, namely, bending heavily with trunk and using the same posture for prolonged periods among Chinese workers [19]; bending trunk heavily among Chinese foundry workers [10]; and prolonged trunk flexion among South African manganese factory workers [11]. Different ergonomic risk

Table 2: Relationship between chronic low back pain (cLBP) and participant characteristics ($n = 717$).

Participant characteristics	With cLBP n (%)	Without cLBP n (%)	χ^2 (p)
Age			
20–39 years	166 (49.8%)	167 (50.2%)	
40–59 years	226 (58.9%)	158 (41.1%)	$\chi^2 = 5.84$ ($p = 0.02$) OR 1.44 (1.07–1.93)
BMI			
≤25	295 (53.5%)	256 (46.5%)	
>25	97 (58.4%)	69 (41.6%)	$\chi^2 = 1.23$ ($p = 0.27$) OR 1.22 (0.86–1.73)
Education			
Illiterate	53 (57.6%)	39 (42.4%)	
Primary	86 (52.1%)	79 (48.0%)	
Middle school	125 (57.3%)	93 (42.7%)	$\chi^2 = 1.87$ ($p = 0.76$)
Secondary	97 (52.2%)	89 (47.8%)	
HS & above	31 (55.4%)	25 (44.6%)	
Tobacco			
No	121 (50.0%)	121 (50.0%)	$\chi^2 = 3.22$ ($p = 0.07$)
Yes	271 (57.1%)	204 (43.0%)	OR 1.33 (0.98–1.81)
Sanitation			
Indian	380 (54.1%)	323 (45.9%)	$\chi^2 = 5.55$ ($p = 0.02$)
Western	12 (85.7%)	2 (14.3%)	OR 5.10 (1.13–22.95)
Experience			
<20 years	211 (51.1%)	202 (48.9%)	
20 to 40 years	170 (59.4%)	116 (40.6%)	$\chi^2 = 5.06$ ($p = 0.08$)
>40 years	11 (61.1%)	7 (38.9%)	
Parent working in jute mill			
No	252 (52.9%)	224 (47.1%)	
Yes	140 (58.1%)	101 (41.9%)	$\chi^2 = 1.71$ ($p = 0.20$) OR 1.22 (0.89–1.66)
Working hr per week			
40 hr	189 (52.5%)	171 (47.5%)	
48 hr	213 (57.4%)	158 (42.6%)	$\chi^2 = 1.78$ ($p = 0.18$) OR 1.23 (0.90–1.68)

factors from different occupational groups from different countries are expected as each kind of occupation requiring heavy physical demand puts different kinds of demand on the musculoskeletal system depending on the nature of work.

The present study is an initial attempt to identify the magnitude of the problem of chronic low back pain among jute mill workers in India. The main strength of the study is to fill a knowledge gap as there is no available information with low back pain among jute mill workers in India where a significant work force is engaged and with low back pain being already identified as a major occupational stressor. Jute mill workers are an important occupational group, particularly in the eastern part of India employing approximately 3,50,000 workers. The study identified a significant 55% prevalence of chronic low back pain in this population with lifting of load above 20 kg and repetitive movements of limbs being significant associations. Therefore, this study has identified need for workplace interventions in this occupational group. Work in jute mills requires prolonged activity with awkward postures with repetitive movements handling heavy loads. Workers are also not conditioned for such musculoskeletal activity and the job requirement also does not permit adequate rest periods. As preventive interventions conditioning of musculoskeletal system for repetitive movement with exercise as well as workstation modification keeping in mind the anthropometric characteristics of the workers can be useful. Further, job rotation through different departments

TABLE 3: Relationship between chronic low back pain and ergonomic characteristics encountered by the participants ($n = 717$).

Ergonomic factors	With cLBP n (%)	Without cLBP n (%)	χ^2 (p)
Lifting load			
Up to 20 kg	255 (47.5%)	282 (52.5%)	
>20 kg	70 (38.9%)	110 (61.1%)	$\chi^2 = 4.02$ ($p = 0.04$) OR 1.42 (1.0–2.0)
Carrying load			
Up to 20 kg	356 (54.3%)	300 (45.7%)	
>20 kg	36 (59.0%)	25 (41.0%)	$\chi^2 = 0.51$ ($p = 0.48$) OR 1.21 (0.71–2.07)
Pulling load			
Up to 20 kg	317 (54.1%)	269 (45.9%)	
>20 kg	75 (57.3%)	56 (42.7%)	$\chi^2 = 0.43$ ($p = 0.51$) OR 1.13 (0.77–1.67)
Standing long hours			
No	37 (60.7%)	24 (39.3%)	
Yes	355 (54.1%)	301 (45.9%)	$\chi^2 = 0.96$ ($p = 0.33$) OR 0.76 (0.45–1.31)
Sitting long hours			
No	351 (54.3%)	296 (45.7%)	
Yes	41 (58.6%)	29 (41.4%)	$\chi^2 = 0.48$ ($p = 0.49$) OR 1.19 (0.72–1.97)
Twisting of body			
No	126 (52.5%)	114 (47.5%)	
Yes	266 (55.8%)	211 (44.2%)	$\chi^2 = 0.69$ ($p = 0.41$) OR 1.14 (0.83–1.56)
Bending of body			
No	39 (45.9%)	46 (54.1%)	
Yes	353 (55.9%)	279 (44.1%)	$\chi^2 = 3.01$ ($p = 0.08$) OR 1.49 (0.95–2.35)
Prolonged same posture			
No	253 (55.7%)	201 (44.3%)	
Yes	139 (52.9%)	124 (47.1%)	$\chi^2 = 0.56$ ($p = 0.46$) OR 0.89 (0.66–1.21)
Repetitive movements			
No	288 (57.4%)	214 (42.6%)	
Yes	104 (48.4%)	111 (51.6%)	$\chi^2 = 4.92$ ($p = 0.03$) OR 0.67 (0.50–0.96)
Work station position			
Too high	20 (60.6%)	13 (39.4%)	
Too low	156 (57.4%)	116 (42.6%)	$\chi^2 = 3.65$ ($p = 0.30$)
Away from body	19 (63.3%)	11 (36.7%)	
Others	197 (51.6%)	185 (48.4%)	

in the workplace and optimum breaks during the work hours can also reduce incidence of chronic low back pain in this population. The observations have also identified the need for a larger study with a higher sample size. Limitations of the study lie in the facts that often there is crossover of workers across different departments in a mill, which makes identification of a particular occupational pattern as possible association difficult. Further, proper definition of sites (mills) by identification of available workplace facilities and recruitment of subjects keeping a balance among departments in a mill would have further improved the quality of observations generated by this study.

Competing Interests

There are no competing interests.

Authors' Contributions

S. Goswami, S. Dasgupta, G. Talukdar, A. Chanda, P. Ray Karmakar, A. Majumdar, and A. Chakrabarti designed and supervised the study. S. Goswami, S. Dasgupta, A. Samanta, G. Talukdar, P. Ray Karmakar, D. Bhattacharya, and A. Chakrabarti carried out and supervised primary data collection and interim analyses. S. Goswami, G. Talukdar, P. Ray Karmakar, D. Bhattacharya, and A. Chakrabarti accomplished data management and statistical analyses. S. Goswami and A. Chanda drafted the primary paper. S. Dasgupta, G. Talukdar, A. Samanta, A. Chanda, P. Ray Karmakar, and A. Majumdar provided critical intellectual input.

Acknowledgments

The authors acknowledge help and support of local administration, managers, staff, and workers of Hukumchand, Prabartak, Shyamnagar, Budge Budge, Ludlow, and Howrah Jute Mill in West Bengal, Sri Krishna Jute Mill in Andhra Pradesh, and Assam Co-operative Jute Mill in Assam and also from Mr. S. K. Chandra, Chief Executive (Works) of Hukumchand Jute Mill and assistance from Dr. T. Ghosh, Ms. D. Mukherjee, Mr. S. Pramanik, Ms. S. Shaw, Ms. B. Bhaduri, Ms. S. Sinha, Mr. S. Sarkar, and Mr. M. Chatterjee in implementation of the project. The authors also acknowledge help and support from Mr. M. S. Kar, IAS, Director, ESI MB Scheme, Government of West Bengal, Dr. P. K. Bhattacharjee, Director, ESI Institute of Pain Management, and other administrators of the ESI MB Scheme and Department of Labour, Government of West Bengal. The authors acknowledge the help from the Secretary and the Assistant Secretary of National Jute Board, Ministry of Textiles, Government of India, and Indian Jute Mills Association (IJMA) for their assistance in implementation of the project. This study was supported by a research grant from National Jute Board, Ministry of Textiles, Government of India.

References

[1] G. B. J. Andersson, "Epidemiological features of chronic low-back pain," *The Lancet*, vol. 354, no. 9178, pp. 581–585, 1999.

[2] S. Rozenberg, "Chronic low back pain: definition and treatment," *Revue du Praticien*, vol. 58, no. 3, pp. 265–272, 2008.

[3] Global Burden of Disease Study 2013 Collaborators, "Global, regional, and national incidence, prevalence, and years lived with disability for 301 acute and chronic diseases and injuries in 188 countries, 1990–2013: a systematic analysis for the Global Burden of Disease Study 2013," *The Lancet*, vol. 386, no. 9995, pp. 743–800, 2015.

[4] A. Garg and J. S. Moore, "Epidemiology of low-back pain in industry," *Occupational Medicine*, vol. 7, no. 4, pp. 593–608, 1992.

[5] A. Petit and Y. Roquelaure, "Low back pain, intervertebral disc and occupational diseases," *International Journal of Occupational Safety and Ergonomics*, vol. 21, no. 1, pp. 15–19, 2015.

[6] World Health Organization, *Global Health Risks: Mortality and Burden of Disease Attributable to Selected Major Risks*, World Health Organization, Geneva, Switzerland, 2009.

[7] N. Kurustien, K. Mekhora, W. Jalayondeja, and S. Nanthavanij, "Trunk muscle performance and work-related musculoskeletal disorders among manual lifting with back belt wearing workers," *Journal of the Medical Association of Thailand*, vol. 98, supplement 5, pp. S74–S80, 2015.

[8] N. B. Fethke, L. A. Merlino, F. Gerr, M. C. Schall, and C. A. Branch, "Musculoskeletal pain among midwest farmers and associations with agricultural activities," *American Journal of Industrial Medicine*, vol. 58, no. 3, pp. 319–330, 2015.

[9] L. Burstrom, B. Jarvholm, T. Nilsson, and J. Wahlstrom, "Back and neck pain due to working in a cold environment: a cross-sectional study of male construction workers," *International Archives of Occupational and Environmental Health*, vol. 86, no. 7, pp. 809–813, 2013.

[10] J.-Z. Sun, R.-J. Ling, Z.-L. Wang et al., "Risk factors analysis of low back pain among workers in a foundry factory of the automobile company," *Zhonghua Lao Dong Wei Sheng Zhi Ye Bing Za Zhi*, vol. 29, no. 2, pp. 108–111, 2011.

[11] B. van Vuuren, H. J. van Heerden, P. J. Becker, E. Zinzen, and R. Meeusen, "Lower back problems and work-related risks in a South African Manganese factory," *Journal of Occupational Rehabilitation*, vol. 17, no. 2, pp. 199–211, 2007.

[12] F. G. Ory, F. U. Rahman, V. Katagade, A. Shukla, and A. Burdorf, "Respiratory disorders, skin complaints, and low-back trouble among tannery workers in Kanpur, India," *American Industrial Hygiene Association Journal*, vol. 58, no. 10, pp. 740–746, 1997.

[13] L. R. Inbaraj, O. J. Haebar, F. Saj et al., "Prevalence of musculoskeletal disorders among brick kiln workers in rural Southern India," *Indian Journal of Occupational and Environmental Medicine*, vol. 17, no. 2, pp. 71–75, 2013.

[14] B. Das, "An evaluation of low back pain among female brick field workers of West Bengal, India," *Environmental Health and Preventive Medicine*, vol. 20, no. 5, pp. 360–368, 2015.

[15] Indian Jute Mills Association, 2016, http://www.ijma.org/industry-at-a-glance.html.

[16] M. Sett and S. Sahu, "Study on work load and work-related musculoskeletal disorders amongst male jute mill workers of West Bengal, India," *Work*, vol. 42, no. 2, pp. 289–297, 2012.

[17] G. Tan, M. P. Jensen, J. I. Thornby, and B. F. Shanti, "Validation of the brief pain inventory for chronic nonmalignant pain," *Journal of Pain*, vol. 5, no. 2, pp. 133–137, 2004.

[18] C. S. Cleeland and K. M. Ryan, "Pain assessment: global use of the brief pain inventory," *Annals of the Academy of Medicine Singapore*, vol. 23, no. 2, pp. 129–138, 1994.

[19] J. Y. Li, S. Wang, L. H. He et al., "Risk factors of low back pain among the Chinese occupational population: a case-control study," *Biomedical and Environmental Sciences*, vol. 25, no. 4, pp. 421–429, 2012.

[20] V. Rajmohan and S. K. Kumar, "Psychiatric morbidity, pain perception, and functional status of chronic pain patients in palliative care," *Indian Journal of Palliative Care*, vol. 19, no. 3, pp. 146–151, 2013.

[21] A. Saxena, T. Mendoza, and C. S. Cleeland, "The assessment of cancer pain in North India: the validation of the Hindi Brief Pain Inventory—BPI-H," *Journal of Pain and Symptom Management*, vol. 17, no. 1, pp. 27–41, 1999.

[22] K. Bose, A. Ghosh, S. Roy, and S. Gangopadhyay, "The relationship of age, body mass index and waist circumference with blood pressure in Bengalee Hindu male jute mill workers of Belur, West Bengal, India," *Anthropologischer Anzeiger*, vol. 63, no. 2, pp. 205–212, 2005.

[23] P. K. Das and N. Jha, "Occupational exposure and pulmonary function of jute mill workers in Sunsari, Nepal," *Nepal Medical College Journal*, vol. 11, no. 4, pp. 275–277, 2009.

[24] B. van Vuuren, E. Zinzen, H. J. van Heerden, P. J. Becker, and R. Meeusen, "Work and family support systems and the prevalence of lower back problems in a South African steel industry," *Journal of Occupational Rehabilitation*, vol. 17, no. 3, pp. 409–421, 2007.

[25] S. Durlov, S. Chakrabarty, A. Chatterjee et al., "Prevalence of low back pain among handloom weavers in West Bengal, India," *International Journal of Occupational and Environmental Health*, vol. 20, no. 4, pp. 333–339, 2014.

Permissions

All chapters in this book were first published in PRT, by Hindawi Publishing Corporation; hereby published with permission under the Creative Commons Attribution License or equivalent. Every chapter published in this book has been scrutinized by our experts. Their significance has been extensively debated. The topics covered herein carry significant findings which will fuel the growth of the discipline. They may even be implemented as practical applications or may be referred to as a beginning point for another development.

The contributors of this book come from diverse backgrounds, making this book a truly international effort. This book will bring forth new frontiers with its revolutionizing research information and detailed analysis of the nascent developments around the world.

We would like to thank all the contributing authors for lending their expertise to make the book truly unique. They have played a crucial role in the development of this book. Without their invaluable contributions this book wouldn't have been possible. They have made vital efforts to compile up to date information on the varied aspects of this subject to make this book a valuable addition to the collection of many professionals and students.

This book was conceptualized with the vision of imparting up-to-date information and advanced data in this field. To ensure the same, a matchless editorial board was set up. Every individual on the board went through rigorous rounds of assessment to prove their worth. After which they invested a large part of their time researching and compiling the most relevant data for our readers.

The editorial board has been involved in producing this book since its inception. They have spent rigorous hours researching and exploring the diverse topics which have resulted in the successful publishing of this book. They have passed on their knowledge of decades through this book. To expedite this challenging task, the publisher supported the team at every step. A small team of assistant editors was also appointed to further simplify the editing procedure and attain best results for the readers.

Apart from the editorial board, the designing team has also invested a significant amount of their time in understanding the subject and creating the most relevant covers. They scrutinized every image to scout for the most suitable representation of the subject and create an appropriate cover for the book.

The publishing team has been an ardent support to the editorial, designing and production team. Their endless efforts to recruit the best for this project, has resulted in the accomplishment of this book. They are a veteran in the field of academics and their pool of knowledge is as vast as their experience in printing. Their expertise and guidance has proved useful at every step. Their uncompromising quality standards have made this book an exceptional effort. Their encouragement from time to time has been an inspiration for everyone.

The publisher and the editorial board hope that this book will prove to be a valuable piece of knowledge for researchers, students, practitioners and scholars across the globe.

List of Contributors

Kathleen C. Light, Ronald W. Hughen and Alan R. Light
Department of Anesthesiology, University of Utah, Salt Lake City, UT 84112, USA

Andrea T. White
Department of Anesthesiology, University of Utah, Salt Lake City, UT 84112, USA
Department of Exercise and Sport Science, University of Utah, Salt Lake City, UT 84112, USA

Lucinda Bateman
Department of Anesthesiology, University of Utah, Salt Lake City, UT 84112, USA
Bateman Horne Center of Excellence, Salt Lake City, UT 84102, USA

Timothy A. Vanhaitsma
Department of Exercise and Sport Science, University of Utah, Salt Lake City, UT 84112, USA
Department of Kinesiology, Westmont College, Santa Barbara, CA 93108, USA

Andri M. T. Lubis and Rangga B. V. Rawung
Department of Orthopaedic and Traumatology, Cipto Mangunkusumo National Central Hospital and Faculty of Medicine, Universitas Indonesia, Jalan Diponegoro No. 71, Central Jakarta, Jakarta 10430, Indonesia

Aida R. Tantri
Department of Anesthesiology and Intensive Care, Cipto Mangunkusumo National Central Hospital and Faculty of Medicine, Universitas Indonesia, Jalan Diponegoro No. 71, Central Jakarta, Jakarta 10430, Indonesia

Padma Gulur, Katharine Koury, Paul Arnstein, Hang Lee, Patricia McCarthy, Christopher Coley and Elizabeth Mort
Massachusetts General Hospital, Boston, MA, USA

Edward A. Shipton and Elspeth E. Shipton
Department of Anaesthesia, University of Otago, Christchurch, Corner of Riccarton and Hagley Avenues, Christchurch 8042, New Zealand

Tamara J. Somers, Sarah A. Kelleher, Rebecca A. Shelby and Francis J. Keefe
Department of Psychiatry and Behavioral Sciences, Duke University Medical Center, Durham, NC, USA

Kelly W. Westbrook and Gretchen G. Kimmick
Department of InternalMedicine, Duke Cancer Institute, Duke University Medical Center, Durham, NC, USA

Amy P. Abernethy
Duke University School of Medicine, Durham, NC, USA

Andrew D. Vigotsky
Kinesiology Program, Arizona State University, Phoenix, AZ 85004, USA

Ryan P. Bruhns
College of Medicine, University of Arizona, Tucson, AZ 85724, USA

Afshin Farhanchi, Behrouz Karkhanei and Negar Amani
Department of Anesthesiology, Hamadan University of Medical Sciences, Hamadan, Iran

Mashhood Aghajanloo
Department of Neurosurgery, Hamadan University of Medical Sciences, Hamadan, Iran

Elham Khanlarzadeh
Department of Community Medicine, Hamadan University of Medical Sciences, Hamadan, Iran

Zahra Emami
Bu-Ali Sina University, Hamadan, Iran

K. Ekbom
Division of Paediatrics, Department for Clinical Science Intervention and Technology, Karolinska Institute, Karolinska University Hospital, 141 86 Stockholm, Sweden
Division of Endocrinology, Diabetes and Metabolism, National Childhood Obesity Centre, Karolinska University Hospital, 141 86 Stockholm, Sweden

Forough Zamanian and Seyed Mojtaba Aghili
Department of Emergency Medicine, Imam Khomeini Hospital, Tehran University of Medical Sciences, Tehran, Iran

Mohammad Jalili
Emergency Medicine Department, Tehran University of Medical Sciences, Tehran, Iran

Maziar Moradi-Lakeh
Department of Community Medicine, Iran University of Medical Sciences, Tehran, Iran

Maryam Kia
Department of Internal Medicine, Dr. Ziaeian Hospital, Tehran University of Medical Sciences, Tehran, Iran

Rokhsareh Aghili
Endocrine Research Center, Institute of Endocrinology and Metabolism, Iran University of Medical Sciences, Tehran, Iran

Emil Sundstrup, Markus D. Jakobsen and Kenneth Jay
National Research Centre for theWorking Environment, 2100 Copenhagen, Denmark
Institute for Sports Science and Clinical Biomechanics, University of Southern Denmark, 5230 Odense, Denmark

Mikkel Brandt and Lars L. Andersen
National Research Centre for theWorking Environment, 2100 Copenhagen, Denmark
Physical Activity and Human Performance Group, SMI, Department of Health Science and Technology, Aalborg University, 9220 Aalborg, Denmark

Roger Persson
Department of Psychology, Lund University, 221 00 Lund, Sweden

Marianne Mustajoki
Department of General Practice and Primary Health Care, University of Helsinki, Kiskontie 23 B, 00280 Helsinki, Finland

Tom Forsén and Timo Kauppila
Department of General Practice and Primary Health Care, University of Helsinki, PB 20 (Tukholmankatu 8 B), 00014 Helsinki, Finland

Dalila R. Veiga
Anesthesiology Department, Chronic Pain Center, Centro Hospitalar Universit´ario do Porto, Largo do Prof. Abel Salazar, 4099-001 Porto, Portugal

Liliane Mendonça
Centro Nacional de ObservaçãoemDor, OBSERVDOR, Alameda Prof. Hernâni Monteiro, 4200-319 Porto, Portugal

José C. Lopes
Centro Nacional de ObservaçãoemDor, OBSERVDOR, Alameda Prof. Hernâni Monteiro, 4200-319 Porto, Portugal
Departamento de Biomedicina, Unidade de Biologia Experimental, Faculdade de Medicina da Universidade do Porto, Portugal
i3S, Instituto de Investigação e Inovaçãoem Saúde, Universidade do Porto, Portugal
Alameda Prof. Hernâni Monteiro, 4200-319 Porto, Portugal
Instituto de Biologia Molecular e Celular (IBMC), Universidade do Porto, Portugal Faculty of Medicine University of Porto, Department of Biomedicine, Porto, Portugal

Rute Sampaio
Departamento de Biomedicina, Unidade de Biologia Experimental, Faculdade de Medicina da Universidade do Porto, Portugal
i3S, Instituto de Investigação e Inovaçãoem Saúde, Universidade do Porto, Portugal
Instituto de Biologia Molecular e Celular (IBMC), Universidade do Porto, Portugal
Alameda Prof. Hernâni Monteiro, 4200-319 Porto, Portugal

Luís F. Azevedo
Center for Health Technology and Services Research (CINTESIS); Faculdade deMedicina da Universidade do Porto, Departamento deMedicina da Comunidade Informação e Decisãoem Saúde (MEDCIDS); Faculdade deMedicina da Universidade do Porto, Alameda Prof. Herñani Monteiro, 4200-319 Porto, Portugal

Jennifer M. Hah, Sean C. Mackey and Ian R. Carroll
Division of PainMedicine, Department of Anesthesiology, Perioperative, and PainMedicine, Stanford University, Palo Alto, CA, USA

Yasamin Sharifzadeh, Bing M. Wang and Matthew J. Gillespie
Stanford Systems Neuroscience and Pain Lab (SNAPL), Stanford University, Palo Alto, CA, USA

Stuart B. Goodman
Department of Orthopaedic Surgery, Stanford University, Palo Alto, CA, USA

Irene Campa-Moran and Etelvina Rey-Gudin
Faculty of Health Science, Department of Physiotherapy, The Center for Advanced Studies University La Salle, Faculty of Health Science, The Autonomous University of Madrid, Aravaca, Madrid, Spain

Alba Paris-Alemany, Alfonso Gil-Martinez and Roy La Touche
Faculty of Health Science, Department ofPhysiotherapy, The Center for Advanced Studies University La Salle, Faculty of Health Science, The Autonomous University of Madrid, Aravaca, Madrid, Spain
Hospital La Paz Institute for Health Research, IdiPAZ, Madrid, Spain

Motion in Brains Research Group, The Center for Advanced Studies University La Salle, The Autonomous University ofMadrid, Spain
Institute of Neuroscience and Craniofacial Pain (INDCRAN), Madrid, Spain

Sergio Lerma Lara
Faculty of Health Science, Department of Physiotherapy, The Center for Advanced Studies University La Salle, Faculty of Health Science, The Autonomous University of Madrid, Aravaca, Madrid, Spain
Motion in Brains Research Group, The Center for Advanced Studies University La Salle, The Autonomous University ofMadrid, Spain
Movement Analysis Laboratory, University Hospital Ni˜no Jesus, Madrid, Spain

Josué Fernández-Carnero
Department of Physical Therapy, OccupationalTherapy, Rehabilitation and Physical Medicine, King Juan Carlos University, Alcor ćon, Madrid, Spain
Hospital La Paz Institute for Health Research, IdiPAZ, Madrid, Spain
Motion in Brains Research Group, The Center for Advanced Studies University La Salle, The Autonomous University of Madrid, Spain

Almudena Prieto-Baquero and José Luis Alonso-Perez
Department of Physiotherapy, European University of Madrid, Villaviciosa de Od´on, Madrid, Spain

Nikolai Kornilov, Alexander Saraev and Konstantin Muniz
Department of Knee Surgery N 17, Russian Research Institute of Traumatology and Orthopaedics n.a. R.R. Vreden, Saint Petersburg 195427, Russia

Maren Falch Lindberg
Department of Surgery, Lovisenberg Diakonale Hospital, 0440 Oslo, Norway
Department of Nursing Science, Institute of Health and Society, Faculty of Medicine, University of Oslo, 0318 Oslo, Norway

Anners Lerdal
Department of Nursing Science, Institute of Health and Society, Faculty of Medicine, University of Oslo, 0318 Oslo, Norway
Department of Research and Development, Lovisenberg Diakonale Hospital, 0440 Oslo, Norway

Caryl Gay
Department of Family Health Care Nursing, University of California, San Francisco, CA 94143-0606, USA
Department of Research and Development, Lovisenberg Diakonale Hospital, 0440 Oslo, Norway

Taras Kuliaba
Department of Knee Surgery N 10, Russian Research Institute of Traumatology and Orthopaedics n.a. R.R. Vreden, Saint Petersburg 195427, Russia

Leiv Arne Rosseland
Department of Research and Development, Division of Emergencies and Critical Care, Oslo University Hospital, 0424 Oslo, Norway
Institute of Clinical Medicine, University of Oslo, 0316 Oslo, Norway

Merja Vantaa Benjaminsson
Södra Älvsborg Hospital, 504 55 Bor˚as, Sweden

Gunilla Thunberg
DART-Center for AAC and AT, The Queen Silvia Children's Hospital, Sahlgrenska University Hospital, 411 04 Gothenburg, Sweden

Stefan Nilsson
Faculty of Caring Science, Work Life and SocialWelfare, University of Borås, 501 90 Borås, Sweden
Institute of Health and Care Sciences, University of Gothenburg, 405 30 Gothenburg, Sweden

Rafael J.A.Cámara
University Medical Center of the Johannes Gutenberg University, Mainz, Institute of Medical Biostatistics, Epidemiology, and Informatics, Obere Zahlbacher Straße 69, 55131 Mainz, Germany

Christian Merz, Barbara Wegmann and Niklaus Egloff
Department of General Internal Medicine, Division of Psychosomatic Medicine, Inselspital, Bern University Hospital, 3010 Bern, Switzerland

Stefanie Stauber
Heart Failure and Transplantation, Department of Cardiology, Inselspital, Bern University Hospital, 3010 Bern, Switzerland

Roland von Känel
Department of Psychosomatic Medicine, Clinic Barmelweid, 5017 Barmelweid, Switzerland
Department of Neurology, Inselspital, Bern University Hospital, 3010 Bern, Switzerland

Robert Jank, Markus Boeckle and Sabine Fiegl
Department of Psychotherapy and Biopsychosocial Health, Danube University Krems, Krems, Austria

Christoph Pieh
Department of Psychotherapy and Biopsychosocial Health, Danube University Krems, Krems, Austria
Department of Psychosomatic Medicine, University Hospital Regensburg, Regensburg, Germany

Alexander Gallee
Practice for General Medicine, Vorderweißenbach, Austria

A. Serrano, C. Caro and V.Mayoral
Department of Anesthesiology, Critical Care and Pain Clinics, Hospital Universitari de Bellvitge, L'Hospitalet de Llobregat, 08907 Barcelona, Spain

D. Torres
Department of Anesthesiology, Critical Care and Pain Clinics, Hospital Universitario de Santiago de Compostela, 15701 Santiago, Spain

M. Veciana and J. Montero
Department of Neurology and Neurophysiology, Hospital Universitari de Bellvitge, L'Hospitalet de Llobregat, 08907 Barcelona, Spain

Michelle A. O. Kinney, Adam K. Jacob and Carlos B. Mantilla
Department of Anesthesiology, Mayo Clinic, 200 First Street SW, Rochester, MN 55905, USA

Melissa A. Passe
Department of Anesthesiology, Anesthesia Clinical Research Unit, Mayo Clinic, 200 First Street SW, Rochester, MN55905, USA

Cláudia Gouvinhas
Department of Biomedicine, Faculty of Medicine, University of Porto, Porto, Portugal

José Manuel Castro-Lopes
Department of Biomedicine, Faculty of Medicine, University of Porto, Porto, Portugal
National Observatory for Pain (NOPain), Porto, Portugal
Institute for Molecular and Cell Biology (IBMC), University of Porto, Porto, Portugal

Rute Sampaio
Department of Biomedicine, Faculty of Medicine, University of Porto, Porto, Portugal
Institute for Molecular and Cell Biology (IBMC), University of Porto, Porto, Portugal

Dalila Veiga
Chronic Pain Center-Anesthesiology Department, Centro Hospitalar do Porto, Porto, Portugal

Liliane Mendonça
National Observatory for Pain (NOPain), Porto, Portugal

Luís Filipe Azevedo
National Observatory for Pain (NOPain), Porto, Portugal
Department of Community Medicine, Information and Health Decision Sciences (MEDCIDS), Faculty of Medicine, University of Porto, Porto, Portugal
Centre for Health Technology and Services Research (CINTESIS), University of Porto, Porto, Portugal

Daniel Muñoz-García
Department of Physiotherapy, Faculty of Health Science, Centro Superior de Estudios Universitarios La Salle, Universidad Aut´onoma de Madrid, 28023 Madrid, Spain
Research Group on Movement and Behavioural Science and Study of Pain, Centro Superior de Estudios Universitarios La Salle, Universidad Aut´onoma de Madrid, 28023 Madrid, Spain

Alfonso Gil-Martínez, Ibai Lopez-de-Uralde-Villanueva and Roy La Touche
Department of Physiotherapy, Faculty of Health Science, Centro Superior de Estudios Universitarios La Salle, Universidad Aut´onoma de Madrid, 28023 Madrid, Spain
Research Group on Movement and Behavioural Science and Study of Pain, Centro Superior de Estudios Universitarios La Salle, Universidad Aut´onoma de Madrid, 28023 Madrid, Spain
Institute of Neuroscience and Craniofacial Pain (INDCRAN), 28023 Madrid, Spain
Hospital La Paz Institute for Health Research, IdiPAZ, 28046 Madrid, Spain

Josué Fernández-Carnero
Research Group on Movement and Behavioural Science and Study of Pain, Centro Superior de Estudios Universitarios La Salle, Universidad Aut´onoma de Madrid, 28023 Madrid, Spain
Institute of Neuroscience and Craniofacial Pain (INDCRAN), 28023 Madrid, Spain
Hospital La Paz Institute for Health Research, IdiPAZ, 28046 Madrid, Spain
Department of Physical Therapy, OccupationalTherapy, Rehabilitation and Physical Medicine, Universidad Rey Juan Carlos, 28922 Madrid, Spain

Almudena López-López
Department of Psychology, Universidad Rey Juan Carlos Alcorc´on, 28922Madrid, Spain

Davide Blonna, Davide Edoardo Bonasia and Roberto Rossi
AO Ordine Mauriziano Umberto I, Department of Orthopedics and Traumatology, Largo Turati 62, 10128 Turin, Italy

Lorenzo Mattei and Valentina Greco
University of Turin, Via Po 8, 10100 Turin, Italy

Enrico Bellato
San Luigi Gonzaga of Orbassano, Department of Orthopedics and Traumatology, Regione Gonzole 10, 100443 Orbassano, Turin, Italy

Sannie Vester Thorsen and Emil Sundstrup
National Research Centre for the Working Environment, Lersø Parkall´e 105, Copenhagen, Denmark

Kenneth Jay
National Research Centre for the Working Environment, Lersø Parkall´e 105, Copenhagen, Denmark
The Carrick Institute for Graduate studies, Institute of Clinical Neuroscience and Rehabilitation, 8910 Astronaut Blvd, Cape Canaveral, LF 32920, USA

Joaquin Calatayud
National Research Centre for the Working Environment, Lersø Parkall´e 105, Copenhagen, Denmark
Exercise Intervention for Health Research Group (EXINH-RG), Department of Physiotherapy, University of Valencia, Spain

Lars Louis Andersen
National Research Centre for the Working Environment, Lersø Parkall´e 105, Copenhagen, Denmark
Sport Sciences, Department of Health Science and Technology, Aalborg University, Denmark

Ramon Aiguadé
Departamento de Enfermer´ıa y Fisioterapia, Universidad de Lleida, Cataluña, Spain

Jose Casaña
Exercise Intervention for Health Research Group (EXINH-RG), Department of Physiotherapy, University of Valencia, Spain

Sawanya Benchahong, Athita Chanthasenanont, Densak Pongrojpaw and Komsun Suwannarurk
Department of Obstetrics and Gynecology, Faculty of Medicine, Thammasat University, PathumThani, Thailand

Junya Pattaraarchachai
Chulabhorn International College of Medicine, Thammasat University, PathumThani, Thailand

Kornkarn Bhamarapravatana
Department of Preclinical Science, Faculty of Medicine, Thammasat University, PathumThani, Thailand

Juan Antonio García García
Pain Unit, Hospital Infanta Cristina, 28981 Madrid, Spain

Patricia Hernández-Puiggròs
Pain Unit, Hospital Son Ll`atzer, 07198 Palma de Mallorca, Spain

Javier Tesedo Nieto and Alfredo Carrera González
Pain Unit, Hospital Cl´ınico Universitario de Valladolid, 47003 Valladolid, Spain

María Pilar Acín Lázaro and Miguel José Arranz Soler
Pain Unit, Hospital Royo Villanova, 50015 Zaragoza, Spain

Sergio Maldonado Vega
Pain Unit, Hospital Universitario Marqu´es de Valdecilla, 39008 Santander, Spain

Mohammad Rababa
Assistant Professor, Jordan University of Science and Technology, Jordan

Maria Beatrice Passavanti, Vincenzo Pota, Pasquale Sansone, Caterina Aurilio, Lorenzo De Nardis and Maria Caterina Pace
Department of Woman, Child, General and Specialized Surgery, University of Campania L. Vanvitelli, Naples, Italy

Goswami, S. Dasgupta, A. Samanta, G. Talukdar and D. Bhattacharya
ESI Institute of Pain Management, ESI Hospital, Sealdah, 301/3A, A. P. C. Road, Kolkata, West Bengal 700009, India

A. Chanda
Department of Mechanical Engineering, Jadavpur University, 188 Raja S. C. Mallick Road, Kolkata 700032, India

P. Ray Karmakar
Department of Community Medicine, R. G. Kar Medical College and Hospital, 1 Kshudiram Bose Sarani, Kolkata 700004, India

A. Majumdar
The Jute Corporation of India Ltd., 15N Nellie Sengupta Sarani, Kolkata 700087, India

A. Chakrabarti
Regional Occupational Health Centre (Eastern), Indian Council of Medical Research (ICMR), Block DP1, Sector V, Salt Lake, Kolkata 700091, India

Index